Melanoma Development

Anja K. Bosserhoff
Editor

Melanoma Development

Molecular Biology, Genetics and Clinical Application

Second Edition

Springer

Editor
Anja K. Bosserhoff
Institute for Biochemistry
Erlangen
Germany

ISBN 978-3-319-41317-4 ISBN 978-3-319-41319-8 (eBook)
DOI 10.1007/978-3-319-41319-8

Library of Congress Control Number: 2016959044

Printed on acid-free paper

This Springer imprint is published by Springer Nature
The registered company is Springer International Publishing AG
The registered company address is: Gewerbestrasse 11, 6330 Cham, Switzerland

Preface

This book, *Melanoma Development: Molecular Biology, Genetics and Clinical Application*, in its second edition provides a comprehensive insight into the molecular changes of malignant melanoma and implications for therapeutic approaches. In this updated version, all chapters were revised and important new developments and findings of the recent 4 years were added.

The recent clinical success in treating melanoma by inhibitors to mutated BRAF or activated MEK or by stimulating the immune system by checkpoint blockage is very encouraging. After years without strong effects of therapeutical attempts, there is hope that melanoma is curable or at least can be shifted into chronic disease. Of course, more research is strongly needed for a comprehensive understanding of the molecular processes leading to melanoma and of ways to therapy resistance. Nevertheless, the first steps are made with possibilities leading to significantly prolonged survival of the patients with metastasized melanoma. This is a highly inspiring and promising development which should further boost melanoma research.

I am again very grateful to all the authors for their interesting, forward-looking contributions and for their support of this book project. I feel that this book, after the success on the first edition, will further enhance the development in the field of melanoma research. *Melanoma Development: Molecular Biology, Genetics and Clinical Application* aims to contribute to this body of knowledge.

Erlangen, Germany Anja K. Bosserhoff, PhD
June 2016

Contents

Clinicopathologic Overview of Melanoma

1

Anja Bosserhoff and Luigi Strizzi

Human melanoma is the most rapidly increasing malignant skin disease in Caucasians (Siegel et al. 2015). Once considered a rare disease, the lifetime risk for developing melanoma in the US has increased from approximately 1 in 1500 during the 1930s to its present risk of approximately 1 in 60 (Giblin and Thomas 2007). The American Cancer Society's recent cancer report estimates that 76,380 new cases of melanoma will be diagnosed and 10,130 deaths will result from melanoma during 2016 in the United States (American Cancer Society 2016). Important risk factors for developing melanoma include increased number of melanocytic nevi, a family history of melanoma, or a history of previous melanoma (Seykora and Elder 1996; Psaty et al. 2010). Prolonged sun exposure associated with increased outdoor activity has been suggested to play an important role in the epidemiologic increase in the incidence of melanoma (Leiter and Garbe 2008; Moan et al. 2008). Acute exposure of the skin to ultraviolet radiation (UVR) can induce varying degrees of erythema, pigmentation, and impairment of immune function (Matsumura and Ananthaswamy 2004). Increased numbers of melanocytic nevi associated with sunburn and intermittent or "holiday" sun exposure has been suggested as a major risk factor for developing melanoma in different studies (Elwood and Jopson 1997; Newton-Bishop et al. 2010). In fact, the Clark model for melanoma suggests a stepwise progression from hyperplastic and dysplastic nevi to melanoma (Clark et al. 1984).

From a clinical perspective, melanocytic nevi are benign proliferations that appear as flat or slightly raised pigmented growths generally found on sun-exposed skin. Histologically, these are formed by proliferating melanocytes that gradually

A. Bosserhoff (✉)
Institute for Biochemistry, Erlangen, Germany
e-mail: anja.bosserhoff@fau.de

L. Strizzi
Children's Memorial Research Center,
Northwestern University, Feinberg School of Medicine, Chicago, IL, USA

A. Bosserhoff (ed.), *Melanoma Development*,
DOI 10.1007/978-3-319-41319-8_1

assume a more round or oval shape from their normal dendritic-like morphology, forming nests along the basal layer and growing towards the dermis as cords. As the nevus cells grow into the dermis, melanin production significantly decreases as tyrosinase activity is progressively lost in a process known as "maturation." Dysplastic nevi can progress from preexisting benign nevi or form ex novo in a new location. Clinically, they are larger than most benign nevi, have irregular borders, and appear with varying degree of pigmentation. Dysplastic nevi are composed of irregularly shaped cells with hyperchromic nuclei. Discordance in the diagnosis of benign, dysplastic, and melanoma based on morphology alone, however, has continued to plague even experienced pathologists (Ackerman 1996; Lodha et al. 2008; Shoo et al. 2010). Different molecular biomarkers have been proposed to help to differentiate benign nevi from malignant melanomas and are still being validated. Recent studies, for example, have claimed high success rates in discriminating benign lesions from melanoma with the use of multiple tissue marker arrays (Kashani-Sabet et al. 2009) or different fluorescence in situ hybridization (FISH) DNA probes (Gerami et al. 2009). The ideal goal would be to develop high throughput analytical systems that would increase the feasibility of adopting such multimarker approaches at all diagnostic centers.

There remains the fact that some melanomas can also form in areas of the body not exposed to the sun, such as mucous membranes (DeMatos et al. 1998; Das et al. 2010) or arise independently of previous nevi suggesting that other factors, alone or in combination, are also involved in the pathogenesis of melanoma. Recent advances in the understanding of the different cellular signaling events in melanoma have shed some light on the identification of potential underlying molecular mechanisms. To this regard, downstream signaling events caused by mutations in NRAS and BRAF as well as PI3K/Akt, MAPK/ERK, and c-KIT activity have been found to play a role in melanoma signaling (Kyrgidis et al. 2010). Since exposure to UVR can lead to DNA damage, sun exposure may represent an obvious cause of these mutations. However, the identification of some of these genetic mutations in congenital nevi as well seems to argue against the fact that UVR is the sole culprit of these mutations. As mentioned previously, a family history of melanoma is an important predictor of melanoma risk (Psaty et al. 2010), indicating that genetic predisposing factor(s) must also play a role during melanomagenesis, as for instance, with CDKN2A, where up to 40% of members of melanoma-prone families show germ-line mutations in this tumor suppressor gene (Hansson 2010).

As described in the Clark model for melanoma progression, early melanoma is characterized by localized growth referred to as "radial growth phase" or "thin melanoma." During this phase, the melanoma cells tend to grow between the layers of the epidermis and superficial dermis with significantly low risk for metastasis. Surgical excision of these relatively flat lesions is associated with high cure rates. With time, the melanoma assumes a more nodular appearance as the relatively larger and irregular melanoma cells begin to penetrate vertically and invade the dermis ("vertical growth phase"). The depth of invasion of the melanoma related to the anatomical structures of the dermis and subcutaneous tissue or measured directly in millimeters is used to predict clinical outcome with deeper (or thicker) lesions associated with reductions in overall patient survival (Balch et al. 2009). Other factors, such as the presence of tumor ulceration or increased mitotic rates, also negatively affect prognosis (Balch et al. 2009). The metastatic process of melanoma is facilitated once melanoma cells begin to invade vascular and lymphatic structures. At this point chemotherapy is the therapeutic option of choice. Current treatment strategies for advanced stage melanoma employing cytotoxic agents are often accompanied by important side effects and associated with relatively low percentages of objective response rates (Atallah and Flaherty 2005). Similarly, molecular redundancy and cross-talk between multiple signaling pathways appear to have undermined the efficacy hoped to achieve with targeted molecular biotherapy (Shain and Bastian 2016). Generally, anti-cancer drugs appear to have some initial effect usually due to killing of the majority of the cancer cells sensitive to the chemotherapeutic agent. However, increased signaling of cell survival pathways, enhanced DNA repair mechanisms or mutations of molecular targets in melanoma cells often lead to resistance to therapy. Attempts continue at identifying novel diagnostic markers and molecular targets important for melanomagenesis and disease progression. Work is also needed to detect and quantify chemoresistance and to better understand the molecular mechanisms that are involved in inducing drug resistance in melanoma. Results from these efforts could help to identify those patients most likely to present resistance to treatment and that would otherwise benefit from a combinatorial approach.

1.1 Chapters of the Book

In the individual chapters of this book, all aspects of basic biology of melanoma are addressed. Further, general mechanisms and therapeutic approaches based on this knowledge are described.

The second chapter by Zalpha Abdel-Malek, Viki B. Swope, and Arup Indra concentrates on melanocytes, the cellular origin of malignant melanoma. For a general understanding of the molecular processes in melanoma development, epidemiology, as illustrated in Chap. 3 by Marianne Berwick, is of major importance enhancing our knowledge of the tumor inducing stimuli. Basic genetic and genomic changes are summarized in Chap. 4 by Allen Ho, Göran Jönsson, and Hensin Tsao.

The following chapters are focusing on changes in basic molecular regulation. Here, chapters on transcriptional regulation by Satoru Yokoyama and David Fisher; on miRNAs by Maria Mione, Leonel Munoz, Janika Liebig, and Anja Bosserhoff; on cell signaling by Yann Cheli, Eric Lau, and Ze'ev A. Ronai; on proteases by Paola Zigrino and Cornelia Mauch; and on molecules in cell–cell and cell–matrix contacts by Silke Kuphal and Nicolas Haass give insight into molecular details.

The next chapters summarize characteristics of molecular processes in melanoma. The chapter by Jürgen Eberle Lothar F. Fecker describes changes in apoptotic processes in malignant melanoma, and Helen Rizos, Sebastian Haferkamp, and Lyndee L Scurr summarize the knowledge on the role of senescence.

As melanoma is a complex disease understanding is enforced by looking at general biological mechanisms and the analysis of other cell types than melanoma cells existing in a melanoma tumor. Chapters on melanoma stem cell by Markus Frank; on lessons from embryology by Alec Gramann, William Tyler Frantz, and Craig J. Ceol; and on the influence of the tumor microenvironment by Lawrence W. Wu, Meenhard Herlyn, and Gao Zhang are summarizing the available information.

A chapter by Birgit Schittek and Thomas Tüting concentrates on model systems which are available in melanoma research.

The last two chapters comment on the current status of melanoma therapy: Ryan J. Sullivan and Keith T. Flaherty summarize the new approaches targeting cellular signaling whereas the chapter of Alexander M.M. Eggermont, Caroline Robert, and Dirk Schadendorf focuses on the new era of immunotherapy in melanoma.

References

Ackerman AB (1996) Discordance among expert pathologists in diagnosis of melanocytic neoplasms. Hum Pathol 27:1115–1116

American Cancer Society Cancer Facts & Figures 2016 Atlanta: American Cancer Society; 2016

Atallah E, Flaherty L (2005) Treatment of metastatic malignant melanoma. Curr Treat Options Oncol 6:185–193

Balch CM, Gershenwald JE, Soong SJ, Thompson JF, Atkins MB, Byrd DR, Buzaid AC, Cochran AJ, Coit DG, Ding S, Eggermont AM, Flaherty KT, Gimotty PA, Kirkwood JM, McMasters KM, Mihm MC Jr, Morton DL, Ross MI, Sober AJ, Sondak VK (2009) Final version of 2009 AJCC melanoma staging and classification. J Clin Oncol 27:6199–6206

Clark WH Jr, Elder DE, Guerry D, Epstein MN, Greene MH, Van Horn M (1984) A study of tumor progression: the precursor lesions of superficial spreading and nodular melanoma. Hum Pathol 15:1147–1165

Das P, Kumar N, Ahuja A, Jain A, Ray R, Sarkar C, Gupta SD (2010) Primary malignant melanoma at unusual sites: an institutional experience with review of literature. Melanoma Res 20:233–239

DeMatos P, Tyler DS, Seigler HF (1998) Malignant melanoma of the mucous membranes: a review of 119 cases. Ann Surg Oncol 5:733–742

Elwood JM, Jopson J (1997) Melanoma and sun exposure: an overview of published studies. Int J Cancer 73:198–203

Gerami P, Jewell SS, Morrison LE, Blondin B, Schulz J, Ruffalo T, Matushek P 4th, Legator M, Jacobson K, Dalton SR, Charzan S, Kolaitis NA, Guitart J, Lertsbarapa T, Boone S, LeBoit PE, Bastian BC (2009) Fluorescence in situ hybridization (FISH) as an ancillary diagnostic tool in the diagnosis of melanoma. Am J Surg Pathol 33:1146–1156

Giblin AV, Thomas JM (2007) Incidence, mortality and survival in cutaneous melanoma. J Plast Reconstr Aesthet Surg 60:32–40

Hansson J (2010) Familial cutaneous melanoma. Adv Exp Med Biol 685:134–145

Kashani-Sabet M, Rangel J, Torabian S, Nosrati M, Simko J, Jablons DM, Moore DH, Haqq C, Miller JR 3rd, Sagebiel RW (2009) A multi-marker assay to distinguish malignant melanomas from benign nevi. Proc Natl Acad Sci U S A 106:6268–6272

Kyrgidis A, Tzellos TG, Triaridis S (2010) Melanoma: stem cells, sun exposure and hallmarks for carcinogenesis, molecular concepts and future clinical implications. J Carcinog 9:1–15

Leiter U, Garbe C (2008) Epidemiology of melanoma and nonmelanoma skin cancer--the role of sunlight. Adv Exp Med Biol 624:89–103

Lodha S, Saggar S, Celebi JT, Silvers DN (2008) Discordance in the histopathologic diagnosis of difficult melanocytic neoplasms in the clinical setting. J Cutan Pathol 35:349–352

Matsumura Y, Ananthaswamy HN (2004) Toxic effects of ultraviolet radiation on the skin. Toxicol Appl Pharmacol 195:298–308
Moan J, Porojnicu AC, Dahlback A (2008) Ultraviolet radiation and malignant melanoma. Adv Exp Med Biol 624:104–116
Newton-Bishop JA, Chang YM, Iles MM, Taylor JC, Bakker B, Chan M, Leake S, Karpavicius B, Haynes S, Fitzgibbon E, Elliott F, Kanetsky PA, Harland M, Barrett JH, Bishop DT (2010) Melanocytic nevi, nevus genes, and melanoma risk in a large case–control study in the United Kingdom. Cancer Epidemiol Biomarkers Prev 19:2043–2054
Psaty EL, Scope A, Halpern AC, Marghoob AA (2010) Defining the patient at high risk for melanoma. Int J Dermatol 49:362–376
Seykora J, Elder D (1996) Dysplastic nevi and other risk markers for melanoma. Semin Oncol 23:682–687
Shain AH, Bastian BC (2016) From melanocytes to melanomas. Nat Rev Cancer 16(6): 345–358
Shoo BA, Sagebiel RW, Kashani-Sabet M (2010) Discordance in the histopathologic diagnosis of melanoma at a melanoma referral center. J Am Acad Dermatol 62:751–756
Siegel RL, Miller KD, Jemal A (2015) Cancer statistics, 2015. CA Cancer J Clin 65:5–29

Revisiting Epidermal Melanocytes: Regulation of Their Survival, Proliferation, and Function in Human Skin

2

Zalfa A. Abdel-Malek, Viki B. Swope, and Arup Indra

2.1 Introduction

Melanocytes are cells specialized in the synthesis of the pigment melanin, in the form of eumelanin, the brown/black, and pheomelanin, the red/yellow pigment (Ito and Wakamatsu 2003). Melanocytes reside in the cutaneous epidermis, within hair follicles, in the eye, the leptomeninges, the inner ear, and in the heart (Brito and Kos 2008; Goldgeier et al. 1984; Tachibana 1999; Yajima and Larue 2008). Melanin produced by melanocytes provides the skin, hair, and eyes with their distinctive coloration. In this chapter, we focus on epidermal melanocytes, since they have been the most thoroughly investigated due to their importance in photoprotection against sun-induced skin cancers, and for being the precursors for cutaneous melanoma, the deadliest form of skin cancer, and their involvement in pigmentary disorders, such as albinism and vitiligo. We, hereby, provide a brief summary of the properties of melanocytes, review how cutaneous pigmentation is regulated, and discuss the significance of paracrine and autocrine factors and their signaling pathways in modulating the survival, proliferation, and function of melanocytes,

Z.A. Abdel-Malek (✉) • V.B. Swope
Department of Dermatology, University of Cincinnati College of Medicine, Cincinnati, OH, USA
e-mail: abdelmza@uc.edu

A. Indra
Department of Pharmaceutical Sciences, College of Pharmacy, Oregon State University-Oregon Health and Science University, Corvallis, OR, USA

Molecular Cell Biology Program, Oregon State University OSU, Corvallis, OR, USA

Linus Pauling Science Institute, Oregon State University OSU, Corvallis, OR, USA

Department of Dermatology, Oregon Health and Science University OHSU, Portland, OR, USA

Knight Cancer Institute, Oregon Health and Science University OHSU, Portland, OR, USA

A. Bosserhoff (ed.), *Melanoma Development*,
DOI 10.1007/978-3-319-41319-8_2

constitutively, and in response to solar ultraviolet radiation (UV), a major environmental stressor and etiological factor for skin cancers, including melanoma (Gilchrest et al. 1999). We end by briefly describing how the knowledge gained about the regulation of melanocytes can be translated into preventative and therapeutic strategies for melanoma.

2.2 Unique Properties of Melanocytes

In the human epidermis, melanocytes reside on the basement membrane, at the epidermal–dermal junction (Jimbow and Fitzpatrick 1975). Melanocytes differ from keratinocytes, the main structural cells of the epidermis, in many respects. Unlike basal keratinocytes that are highly proliferative and capable of regenerating the epidermal layers, melanocytes have a low proliferation potential. Keratinocytes undergo a well-defined differentiation program that culminates in their death by an apoptosis-like process (reviewed by Eckert et al. 1997). On the other hand, most melanoblasts, the precursors for melanocytes, become fully differentiated upon reaching their final destination, the epidermis, after their migration during embryonic development from the neural crest (Bronner-Fraser 1993). Melanocytes are resistant to apoptosis, as they are endowed with anti-apoptotic mechanisms, exemplified by constitutive expression of the anti-apoptotic protein Bcl2 (Plettenberg et al. 1995). Contrary to keratinocytes, melanocytes have a very long life span and survive for decades in the epidermis (Quevedo et al. 1969). However, the longevity of melanocytes and their resistance to apoptosis is a double-edged sword, since these properties make them vulnerable to mutations that arise over the years, particularly due to repetitive sun exposure, and might culminate in melanoma formation in high-risk individuals. These properties also explain the resistance of melanoma tumors to various chemotherapeutic agents and to radiation therapy. Given the significance of melanocytes in protection of the skin from UV-induced skin cancers, it is critical to maintain genomic stability of these cells to insure their proper function and ability to preserve epidermal homeostasis.

2.3 Factors That Determine Cutaneous Pigmentation

Cutaneous pigmentation is determined by the rate of synthesis of melanins (eumelanin and pheomelanin) by melanocytes, the relative eumelanin and pheomelanin contents, and the rate of transfer of melanosomes, melanin-containing organelles, from melanocytes to keratinocytes (Pathak et al. 1980). These are the main factors that account for individual differences in skin pigmentation. Melanosomes contain enzymes that catalyze melanin synthesis, namely, tyrosinase, the rate-limiting enzyme for melanin synthesis, tyrosinase-related protein (TYRP-1), and dopachrome tautomerase (DCT), also known as tyrosinase-related protein 2 (TRP-2) (reviewed by Hearing 2005). The activity of tyrosinase and the protein levels of these three melanogenic enzymes correlate directly with melanin content of melanocytes (Abdel-Malek et al. 1993; Wakamatsu et al. 2006). Melanosomes also express on their membrane OA1, a G-protein-coupled receptor that is activated by L-DOPA, an intermediate in the melanin synthetic pathway, and a substrate for tyrosinase (Hearing 2005). The number of melanocytes does not significantly differ among individuals with different pigmentary phenotypes (Szabo 1954). The difference in pigmentation lies primarily in the rate of melanin synthesis, which is determined by many genes expressed in melanocytes, and code for regulatory proteins, including melanogenic enzymes, growth factor receptors, and transcription factors, as well as structural proteins that make up the melanosome. The difference in constitutive pigmentation among individuals is primarily dictated by eumelanin, which correlates directly with the extent of pigmentation (Hennessy et al. 2005; Wakamatsu et al. 2006).

Melanocytes interact with keratinocytes by donating fully melanized (mature) melanosomes (Pathak et al. 1980). Melanocytes are dendritic cells, and their dendrites serve as conduits for the transport of melanosomes to surrounding keratinocytes. In turn, keratinocytes participate in regulating the transfer of melanosomes by expressing protease-activated receptor 2 (PAR-2), a G-protein-coupled receptor that is activated upon proteolytic cleavage by trypsin, or by binding of its agonist, Ser-Leu-Ile-Gly-Arg-Leu-NH_2 (SLIGRL), resulting in increased melanosome phagocytosis in a Rho-dependent manner (Scott et al. 2003; Seiberg et al. 2000). Expression of PAR-2 by keratinocytes is up-regulated by UV exposure in vitro and in vivo (Scott et al. 2001). In the epidermis, the ratio of melanocytes to keratinocytes is 1:34, and the interaction of these cells via transfer of melanosomes has been coined the epidermal melanin unit. Melanosome transfer is important for normal and uniform skin pigmentation, is increased upon stimulation of melanogenesis, and is critical for optimal photoprotection.

2.4 Pigmentation: The Main Photoprotective Mechanism in the Skin Against Solar UV

Solar UV is the main environmental factor that affects skin pigmentation and the main etiological factor for skin cancers, including melanoma (Epstein 1983; Gilchrest et al. 1999; Pathak 1991). Melanin synthesized by melanocytes is the main photoprotective mechanism in the skin (Gilchrest et al. 1999; Halder and Bridgeman-Shah 1995; Pathak et al. 1980). Melanosomes transferred to keratinocytes form supranuclear caps that protect the nucleus from impinging UV rays (Kobayashi et al. 1998). Melanin in the epidermis is also photoprotective for dermal fibroblasts, preventing photoaging caused by UV, particularly long wavelength UVA (Gilchrest and Rogers 1993). An interesting paradigm is that increased melanin synthesis is part of the DNA damage response of melanocytes, as treatment of human skin with DNA oligonucleotides that are homologous to the telomere 3′ overhang sequence (T-oligos) enhanced nucleotide excision repair and subsequently increased epidermal melanin content (Arad et al. 2006).

The photoprotective effects of melanin are mainly conferred by eumelanin, since pheomelanin seems to have detrimental rather than beneficial effects. Eumelanin acts as a scavenger of reactive oxygen species produced upon exposure to UV, and thus reduces the oxidative damage to DNA, proteins, and lipids (Bustamante et al. 1993). On the other hand, pheomelanin might be a pro-oxidant, resulting in oxidative DNA damage that causes melanoma formation in melanoma-prone mice expressing the activating mutation in Braf, Braf ^{v600E}, in the absence of UV or any other carcinogen (Mitra et al. 2012). Additionally, pheomelanin seems to exacerbate the formation or the effects of peroxynitrite in UV-irradiated melanocytes, resulting in increased formation of cyclobutane pyrimidine dimers (CPDs), the major form of DNA photoproducts, even after cessation of UV exposure (Premi et al. 2015).

There is overwhelming clinical and epidemiological evidence for the role of melanin in prevention of sun-induced skin cancers (Epstein 1983; Halder and Bridgeman-Shah 1995; Newton Bishop and Bishop 2005). The incidence of these cancers is by far higher in individuals with fair skin and low melanin content, than in individuals with dark skin containing high levels of melanin, mainly eumelanin. Experimental evidence shows that exposure to UV results in less DNA photoproducts in dark-skinned individuals with high melanin (mainly eumelanin) content than in light-skinned individuals with low melanin content (Tadokoro et al. 2003). Similarly, an inverse relationship between eumelanin content and the induction of DNA photoproducts was found in cultured human melanocytes derived from donors with different pigmentary phenotypes, with CPDs being lowest in melanocytes with the highest eumelanin content, and highest in melanocytes that have least eumelanin content (Hauser et al. 2006; Smit et al. 2001).

2.5 Evidence for a Paracrine/Autocrine Network in Human Skin

A symbiotic relationship exists between cutaneous melanocytes, keratinocytes, and fibroblasts. It is well established that a complex and well-regulated paracrine/autocrine network is present in human skin and that this network is modulated in response to stress, such as in response to UV or inflammation. In turn, the paracrine/autocrine factors mediate many of the stress responses of epidermal cells. Many of the cytokines and growth factors synthesized by keratinocytes and fibroblasts play important roles in regulating melanocyte function and survival (summarized in Table 2.1 and Fig. 2.1). The first evidence for keratinocyte-derived paracrine factors that affect melanocytes came from the observation that medium conditioned by cultured human keratinocytes stimulated the proliferation and melanogenesis of cultured normal human melanocytes (Gordon et al. 1989). Additional evidence came from the observation that melanocytes co-cultured with keratinocytes exhibited a dose-dependent increase in melanogenesis following irradiation with very low doses of UVB, while melanocytes in monoculture required irradiation with at least a ten-fold higher dose of UVB in order to stimulate pigmentation (Duval et al. 2001). These latter results implicated keratinocyte-derived factors in the melanogenic response of melanocytes to UVB. Medium conditioned with human fibroblasts also stimulated the proliferation of cultured human melanocytes (Imokawa et al. 1998). Mutations in genes that code for paracrine factors or their receptors,

Table 2.1 Summary of known paracrine/autocrine factors, their cell of origin in the skin, and their effects on melanocytes

Factor	Synthesized by	Role in pigmentation	Melanocyte function
POMC derived: α-MSH, ACTH	KC, MC	↑	MC1R agonist (↑ cAMP)
POMC derived: β-endorphin	KC, MC	↑	Inhibits cAMP, unknown signaling pathway
Agouti signaling protein (ASIP)	Skin, cell of origin Unknown	↓	MC1R antagonist
Human β defensin 3 (HBD3)	KC	↑ In dog and mouse; ? In human	MC1R antagonist
Bone morphogenetic factor (BMP-4)	KC, MC	↓	↓ Tyrosinase activity, ↓ TRP-1, ↓ MC1R
Noggin	Cell of origin in human skin unknown	↑	Antagonist of BMP-4
Interleukin-1 α/β	KC, MC	↓	↓ Tyrosinase activity, ↓ proliferation
Tumor necrosis factor-α (TNF-α)	KC	↓	↓ Tyrosinase activity, ↓ proliferation
Endothelin-1 (ET-1)	KC	↑	↑ Tyrosinase activity, ↑ proliferation, ↑ survival
Stem cell factor (SCF)	KC, FB	↑	↑ Proliferation, ↑ survival, ↑ dendricity
Hepatocyte growth factor (HGF)	KC, FB	↑	↑ Proliferation, ↑migration
Basic fibroblast growth factor (bFGF)	KC, FB	↑	↑ Proliferation
Prostaglandins PGE_2 and $PGF_{2\alpha}$	KC, MC	↑	↑ Dendricity, ↑ tyrosinase activity
Leukotrienes LTC4 and LTD4	KC	↑	↑ Proliferation
Corticotropin releasing hormone	KC, MC	↑	↑ cAMP, ↑ *POMC* gene (↑ACTH)
Nerve growth factor (NGF)	KC	–	↑ Dendricity, ↑ migration, ↑ survival
Neurotrophin 3 (NT-3)	KC, FB	–	↑ Survival
Semaphorin 7a	KC, FB	–	↑ Spreading, ↑ dendricity
Neuregulin-1 (NRG-1)	KC, FB	↑	↑ Pigmentation, ↑ dendricity, ↑ MC size
Nitric oxide	KC, MC	↑	↑ Melanogenesis

such as stem cell factor or its receptor c-kit, or endothelin (ET)-3 and the endothelin-B receptor (ENDBR), result in pigmentary abnormalities (piebaldism or Hirschprung's disease, respectively) due to reduced melanoblast survival and migration during embryonic development (Giebel and Spritz 1991; Puffenberger et al.

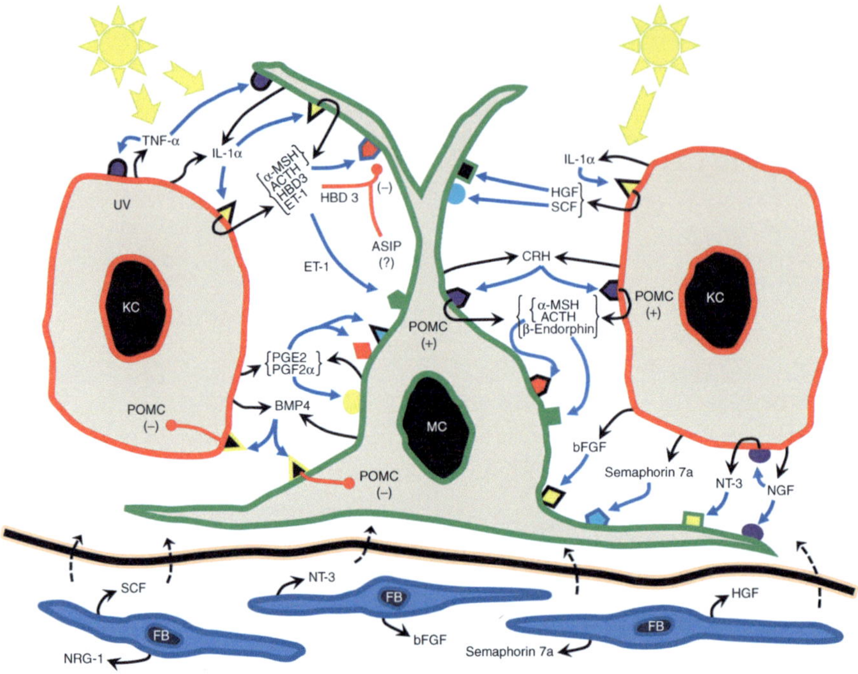

Fig. 2.1 Summary of the major participants in the paracrine/autocrine network that regulates melanocyte function, survival, and proliferation and the regulation of this network by UV. Irradiation of the skin with UV up-regulates the expression of the primary cytokines TNF-α and IL-1α by keratinocytes, both of which directly affect melanocytes. In turn, IL-1α increases the production of α-MSH and ACTH by keratinocytes and melanocytes, as well as HBD3, ET-1, HGF, and SCF by keratinocytes. In response to UV, CRH production is increased by both keratinocytes and melanocytes. CRH affects melanocytes directly and indirectly by increasing the expression of POMC, and hence its derivatives α-MSH, ACTH, and β-endorphin. Melanocytes and keratinocytes synthesize BMP-4, which affects melanocytes directly, and might also inhibit POMC production by keratinocytes and melanocytes. Additionally, both keratinocytes and melanocytes synthesize PGE_2 and $PGF_{2\alpha}$. Keratinocytes synthesize bFGF and semaphorin 7a, and also NGF, which affects melanocytes directly, as well as indirectly by enhancing the production of NT-3 by keratinocytes. Fibroblasts contribute to the paracrine network by synthesizing HGF, SCF, NT-3, semaphorin 7a, and NRG-1

1994). Collectively, these results provide evidence for the existence of a paracrine network in human skin that modulates melanocyte function, proliferation, and survival under constitutive conditions and in response to UV.

2.5.1 The Melanocortin 1 Receptor Physiological Agonists and Antagonists Are Epidermal-Derived Factors That Regulate Eumelanin and Pheomelanin Synthesis

There has been particular interest in understanding the regulation of eumelanin and pheomelanin synthesis by melanocytes, given the significance of eumelanin in photoprotection, and to elucidate the underlying causes for the diversity of human pigmentation. Stimulation of eumelanin synthesis results mainly from activation of the melanocortin 1 receptor (MC1R), a G_s-protein-coupled receptor expressed on melanocytes (Chhajlani and Wikberg 1992; Hunt et al. 1995; Mountjoy et al. 1992; Suzuki et al. 1996). The physiological agonists for the human MC1R are α-melanocyte-stimulating hormone (α-MSH) and adrenocorticotropic hormone (ACTH), which bind the MC1R with the same affinity (Suzuki et al. 1996). Pro-opiomelanocortin, the precursor for ACTH and α-MSH, is synthesized and processed by cultured keratinocytes and melanocytes, and its expression in the skin is increased by UV exposure (Chakraborty et al. 1996; Corre et al. 2006; Suzuki et al. 2002; Wakamatsu et al. 1997). Actually, the presence of MSH peptides in human skin was reported decades ago, long before a physiological role for these peptides in human pigmentation was identified (Thody et al. 1983). Therefore, MC1R agonists are paracrine/autocrine factors that are expected to participate in the UV response of melanocytes (as described later in this review). This is supported by the observation that activation of the cAMP pathway by α-MSH is critical for UV-induced melanogenesis (i.e., tanning response), and enables human melanocytes to overcome the UV-induced growth arrest (Im et al. 1998a).

Agouti signaling protein (ASIP) is the physiological antagonist of the MC1R that acts as an inverse agonist, competing with α-MSH for receptor binding, and abrogating the activation of the cAMP pathway, the main signaling pathway of the activated MC1R (Suzuki et al. 1997). Concomitant treatment of cultured human melanocytes with α-MSH and ASIP blocked the mitogenic and melanogenic effects of α-MSH. In mice, the recessive yellow mutation that causes loss of function of the mc1r results in a yellow coat color (Robbins et al. 1993). Similarly, overexpression of *agouti* results in the same pigmentary phenotype, due to inhibition of eumelanin synthesis, in addition to other pleiotropic effects resulting from interaction of ASIP with other melanocortin receptors, which include obesity, diabetes, and increased susceptibility to develop tumors (Siracusa 1994). Pheomelanin synthesis is considered to be the default pathway, which takes place in the absence of MC1R signaling, unlike eumelanin synthesis that has stringent requirements, including high concentrations of tyrosine, the substrate for tyrosinase, and activation of the MC1R, which leads to stimulation of cAMP formation and increase in activities and protein levels of the melanogenic enzymes tyrosinase, TYRP-1, and TRP-2 (Abdel-Malek et al. 1995; Sakai et al. 1997).

Another factor that affects eumelanin/pheomelanin synthesis is human β-defensin 3 (HBD3), an antimicrobial peptide which was cloned from human keratinocytes and is best known for its role in innate immunity (Candille et al. 2007; Harder et al. 2001). Genetic studies on dogs revealed that mutation in the *HBD3* gene resulted in black coat color, an effect that was postulated to be due to inhibition of ASIP binding to the MC1R (Candille et al. 2007). Receptor binding assays revealed that HBD3 acts as a competitive inhibitor of α-MSH binding to the MC1R. HBD3 acts as an antagonist of the MC1R expressed on human melanocytes, abrogating the effects of α-MSH on cAMP formation (Swope et al. 2012). Brief pretreatment with either HBD3 or ASIP prevented cultured human melanocytes from responding to α-MSH with stimulation of cAMP synthesis. This effect might be due to MC1R desensitization, another mechanism of limiting the response to α-MSH.

2.5.2 Antagonistic Effects of Bone Morphogenetic Protein and Noggin on Pigmentation and Their Potential Regulation of MC1R Agonists and Antagonists

Two interesting modulators of melanogenesis are bone morphogenetic protein-4 (BMP-4) and noggin, which modulate melanogenesis directly, and possibly indirectly, by regulating the expression of the MC1R agonists and ASIP. BMP-4 is a member of the TGF-β superfamily and has been shown to be produced by both human melanocytes and keratinocytes and to inhibit melanogenesis in human melanocytes (Yaar et al. 2006). The inhibitory effect of BMP-4 involved reduction in the levels of the melanogenic enzymes tyrosinase, and TYRP-1, as well as MC1R (Park et al. 2009; Yaar et al. 2006). The BMP-4 receptors-1A, -1B, and -2 are expressed by human melanocytes, confirming the role of BMP-4 as a paracrine/autocrine factor (Yaar et al. 2006). Irradiation of melanocytes with UV down-regulated the expression of BMP-4 receptor-1B, which might be one mechanism by which UV stimulates melanogenesis (i.e., tanning), which requires activation of MC1R and its cAMP signaling pathway (Im et al. 1998b). Studies on mouse coat color showed that noggin acts as an antagonist of BMP-4, and noggin overexpression reduced the expression of ASIP (Sharov et al. 2005). On the other hand, BMP-4 enhanced the expression of ASIP by primary mouse keratinocytes and fibroblasts. Moreover, in the pituitary gland, BMP-4 repressed the expression of *Pro-opiomelanocortin (POMC)* by corticotrophs (Nudi et al. 2005). In addition to increasing ASIP, potential inhibition of POMC production in the skin and reduction of MC1R expression in melanocytes might be a mechanism by which BMP-4 inhibits pigmentation, and reversal of these effects by noggin might be a mechanism to stimulate melanogenesis. The effects of BMP-4 and noggin add another layer of complexity to the regulation of melanogenesis upstream of POMC and ASIP, and the modulation of MC1R expression.

2.5.3 Identification of the Nature of Paracrine Factors for Melanocytes in the Skin

Basic fibroblast growth factor (bFGF), basic fibroblast growth factor (bFGF), the cytokines interleukin (IL)-1α and tumor necrosis factor (TNF)-α, as well as hepatocyte growth factor (HGF) and stem cell factor (SCF) that are induced by these cytokines (Imokawa et al. 1998). It has long been known that production of primary cytokines, namely, IL-1 α and TNF-α, by keratinocytes is up-regulated by UV (Kock et al. 1990; Kupper et al. 1987) and that these cytokines regulate the synthesis of potent mitogenic and melanogenic factors by keratinocytes, such as α-MSH and endothelin-1 (ET-1) (Chakraborty et al. 1996; Imokawa et al. 1992). Human melanocytes were also found to synthesize IL-1α and β and to respond to IL-1α and TNF-α with inhibition of proliferation and melanogenesis, suggesting that these cytokines directly modulate melanocyte function and proliferation (Swope et al. 1991, 1994). Using whole human genome microarray analysis, it was shown that repetitive irradiation of human skin in situ by UVB resulted in altered expression of genes that encode for paracrine factors or their receptors. These genes included those that encode for HGF, bFGF, IL-1 α and β, and GM-CSF, and for the PAR-2 receptor, the SCF receptor c-kit, the endothelin-1 B receptor ENDBR, and MC1R. These in vitro and in vivo findings provide compelling evidence that many factors that regulate melanocytes are synthesized locally in the skin.

The first keratinocyte-derived paracrine factor for melanocytes to be identified was bFGF, an essential mitogen for melanocytes (Halaban et al. 1988). Basic FGF stimulates melanocyte proliferation by binding and activating a specific tyrosine kinase receptor (Pittelkow and Shipley 1989). Another important keratinocyte-derived paracrine factor is ET-1, which induces melanocyte proliferation, melanogenesis, and migration (Horikawa et al. 1995; Tada et al. 1998b; Yada et al. 1991; Yohn et al. 1993). Human melanocytes predominantly express ENDBR, a G_q-coupled receptor, which when bound by either ET-1 or ET-3, activates PKC, intracellular calcium mobilization, and nonreceptor tyrosine kinases (Imokawa et al. 1992; Tada et al. 1998b). Mutations in either the gene for endothelin-3 (which during embryonic development, mimics ET-1 in its effects and mechanism of action) or ENDBR result in Hirschprung's disease Type II, which is characterized by hypopigmentation due to inefficient migration of melanoblasts from the embryonic neural crest and their reduced survival, and by aganglionic megacolon due to absence of neural crest-derived ganglia (Puffenberger et al. 1994). Treatment of cultured human keratinocytes with IL-1α or irradiation of human skin in vivo induced the production of ET-1 (Imokawa et al. 1992). These results suggest a role for ET-1 in the UV response of melanocytes, which is described later in this review.

Two important paracrine factors that are synthesized by both keratinocytes and fibroblasts are SCF and HGF (Imokawa et al. 1998; Matsumoto et al. 1991). Stem cell factor elicits its mitogenic and survival effects on melanocytes by activating a specific tyrosine kinase receptor, c-kit, and mutations in the *Kit* gene result in piebaldism, which is characterized by depigmented skin patches as a consequence of death of melanocytes during their migratory route during embryonic development to populate the epidermis (Giebel and Spritz 1991). In adult skin, SCF is required for melanocyte maintenance, since injection of c-kit antibody resulted in loss of pigmentation due to melanocyte death (Grichnik et al. 1998). Hepatocyte growth factor, which activates the tyrosine kinase receptor c-Met, allows for melanocyte homing to the epidermis during embryonic development and stimulates human melanocyte proliferation (Matsumoto et al. 1991). The observation that HGF transgenic mice have extensive skin melanosis provides genetic evidence for the significance of HGF in directing the migration of melanocytes to the epidermis (Otsuka et al. 1998).

2.5.4 Eicosanoids as Paracrine/Autocrine Factors for Melanocytes

The eicosanoids, prostaglandins (PGs), and leukotrienes (LTs) are lipid-signaling intermediates that are derived from arachidonic acid via the cyclooxygenase and lipooxygenase pathway, respectively. Although the major source of PGs in the skin is the keratinocytes, experimental evidence showed that melanocytes also synthesize the major two forms of PGs, PGE_2 and $PGF_{2\alpha}$, in response to UV irradiation (Scott et al. 2005). Human melanocytes express cyclooxygenase (COX)-1 and −2, the latter of which is the inducible form, and the rate-limiting enzyme for the synthesis of PGs (Nicolaou et al. 2004). Si-RNA mediated knock-down of COX-2 in melanocytes decreased the expression of tyrosinase, TYRP-1, TRP-2, gp100, and MITF and also reduced tyrosinase enzyme activity, suggesting utility of COX2 inhibitors against hyperpigmentary disorder such as melasma, postinflammatory hyperpigmentation, and solar lentigo (Kim et al. 2012). Human melanocytes express FP receptor, the receptor for $PGF_{2\alpha}$ in vitro and in vivo, and expression of this receptor is up-regulated upon UV exposure (Scott et al. 2005; Starner et al. 2010). Melanocytes responded to $PGF_{2\alpha}$ with stimulation of dendricity and melanogenesis that was evidenced by increased activity and protein levels of tyrosinase. Multiple irradiations of cultured melanocytes with moderate noncytotoxic doses of UV induced the synthesis of PGE_2 via activation of cytoplasmic phospholipase A_2 ($cPLA_2$), the rate-limiting enzyme in eicosanoid synthesis (Starner et al. 2010). Epidermal melanocytes were found to produce PGE_2 under basal conditions, which further increased after arachidonic acid stimulation (Gledhill et al. 2010). Human melanocytes express two of the four PGE_2 G-protein-coupled receptors, EP2 and EP4, and treatment with PGE_2 increased cAMP formation and stimulated proliferation and tyrosinase activity (Starner et al. 2010). Recently, PGE_2 has been shown to drive melanosome transfer by promoting filopodia formation in melanocytes (Ma et al. 2014). The leukotrienes (LT)C_4 and D_4 were found to be potent mitogens for cultured human melanocytes (Morelli et al. 1989). These results demonstrate the participation of eicosanoids and their receptors in the autocrine/paracrine network that regulates melanocyte proliferation and functions and the response to UV.

2.5.5 An Equivalent of the Hypothalamic/Pituitary/Adrenal Axis Is Present in Human Skin

Studies from various laboratories provided evidence that the skin is a "neuroendocrine organ," which contains an equivalent of the systemic stress-induced hypothalamic/pituitary/adrenal axis. Skin cells, including melanocytes, express corticotropin-releasing hormone (CRH) mRNA and protein, and also its receptor CRH-R1 (Funasaka et al. 1999; Slominski 1998; Slominski et al. 1995). Treatment of human melanocytes with CRH resulted in increased cAMP levels and up-regulated the expression of *POMC* gene. The latter effect led to increased production of the POMC derivative ACTH, which contains within its structure the entire amino acid sequence of α-MSH. These two bioactive peptides are produced upon processing of POMC by the enzymes pro-convertase 1 and 2, respectively. The significance of POMC in human pigmentation was supported by the observation that mutations in the human *POMC* gene that affected its expression resulted in red hair phenotype, in addition to metabolic abnormalities, such as adrenal insufficiency and obesity (Krude et al. 1998). In melanocytes, ACTH induced the production of cortisol and corticosterone, which feedback negatively to inhibit the production of ACTH and thus terminate the response to stress (Slominski et al. 2005). These series of events recapitulate the functional hierarchy in the hypothalamic/pituitary/adrenal axis and provide further evidence for the participation of the melanocyte in the cutaneous stress response by producing and responding to stress-induced factors.

In addition to α-MSH and ACTH, β-endorphin, a third POMC-derived bioactive peptide, is produced in vitro and in situ by keratinocytes and melanocytes upon the cleavage of β-lipotropic hormone (β-LPH) (Kauser et al. 2003; Slominski 1998). Production of β-endorphin by melanocytes correlated with their differentiation status, as determined by their dendricity and pigmentation, indicating that β-endorphin functions as an autocrine factor (Kauser et al. 2003). Melanocytes and keratinocytes express functional μ-opiate receptors, and treatment of cultured human melanocytes with β-endorphin stimulated proliferation, dendricity, and melanogenesis (Kauser et al. 2003). In melanocytes, both β-endorphin and μ-opiate receptors co-localized in premelanosomes and stage II melanosomes, suggesting that the ligand and receptor internalize into immature melanosomes where they induce melanogenesis. Unlike melanocortins, which elicit their effects by activating the cAMP pathway, β-endorphin inhibited adenylate cyclase, thus reduced cAMP levels. The signaling pathway(s) that mediates the effects of β-endorphin on melanocytes is yet to be determined. The increase in β-endorphin production in response to UV might explain the "addictive" behavior of sun worshippers and the feeling of wellness associated with sun exposure.

2.5.6 Neurotrophins as Members of the Cutaneous Neuroendocrine Paracrine Network

Given that the cutaneous epidermis and the nervous system arise from a common ectodermal origin, it was postulated that growth factors that regulate the survival and function of neurons play a role in the maintenance of epidermal homeostasis. Neutrophins (NTs) are family of neuronal growth factors comprised of nerve growth factor (NGF), brain-derived neurotrophic factor (BDNF), NT-3, and NT-4, two of which, namely, NGF and NT-3, are synthesized in the skin (reviewed by Botchkarev et al. 2006). Human keratinocytes, particularly basal keratinocytes with the highest proliferation capacity, were found to synthesize and release NGF, which in turn enhanced the secretion of NT-3, also synthesized by dermal fibroblasts (Marconi et al. 2003; Yaar et al. 1994). Neurotrophins share about 50 % amino acid sequence homology and interact with tyrosine kinase receptors (Trk) A, B, and C, the high affinity receptors for NGF, BDNF, and NT-3, respectively. All NTs interact with the low-affinity p75 NT receptor, a member of the TNF-α family of receptors. Depending on the intracellular adaptor molecules that interact with p75 receptor, its signaling may be linked to the JNK-p53-Bax pro-apoptotic pathway, or to the NF-kB survival pathway. Human melanocytes responded to NGF with increased migration and dendricity, and additionally, with inhibition of apoptosis after UV irradiation via increasing the levels of the anti-apoptotic Bcl2 (Stefanato et al. 2003; Yaar et al. 1991; Zhai et al. 1996). Both NGF and NT-3 increase the survival of human melanocytes maintained in growth factor-depleted culture medium (Yaar et al. 1994; Zhai et al. 1996). Human melanocytes express p75NT receptor, and this is increased upon UV irradiation (Yaar et al. 1994). Melanocytes also express low levels of TrkC, the receptor for NT-3, and TrkA expression is induced upon stimulation of protein kinase C. Based on these studies, it was concluded that NGF, which is the most prevalent NT that is constitutively produced by keratinocytes, insures the survival of melanocytes by inhibiting UV-induced apoptosis, and NT-3 that is strongly expressed in fibroblasts might also contribute to melanocyte maintenance.

2.5.7 Semaphorin 7a: A Neuronal Factor Synthesized in Human Skin

Sempahorin 7 is a member of the secreted and membrane-bound semaphorin family of proteins that function in neuronal pathfinding and axonal guidance (Yazdani and Terman 2006). It was the first glycosylphosphatidylinositol-linked semaphorin to be identified and shown to bind plexin C1 and β1-integrin receptor (Pasterkamp et al. 2003; Sato and Takahashi 1998; Tamagnone et al. 1999). Semaphorin 7a was found to be expressed in the skin in vivo and in keratinocytes and fibroblasts, as demonstrated in vitro (Scott et al. 2008). In response to UV, fibroblasts exhibited a marked increase in semaphorin 7a expression. The role of semaphorin 7a as a paracrine factor for melanocytes was demonstrated by the finding that co-culturing of melanocytes with cells expressing semaphorin 7a led to increased spreading and dendricity and that melanocytes responded directly to treatment with exogenous semaphorin 7a. These effects were mediated by binding the β1-integrin receptor and were inhibited by plexin C1. These results identify a novel neuronal factor expressed in the skin, which regulates melanocyte spreading and dendricity positively via β1-integrin receptor, or negatively by interacting with Plexin C1. These effects might have significant implications on melanosome transfer, an important determinant of cutaneous pigmentation.

2.5.8 Neuregulin-1: A Neuroendocrine Factor Synthesized by Human Epidermal and Dermal Cells

The neuroendocrine factor Neuregulin-1 (NRG-1) was identified as a fibroblast-derived factor that regulates constitutive human pigmentation (Choi et al. 2010). Neuregulin-1 is a secreted growth factor that is expressed in the central nervous system and is critical for neuronal differentiation, migration, and dendrite formation (Krivosheya et al. 2008). The effects of NRG-1 are mediated by binding to ErbB3 and ErbB4 receptors, tyrosine kinase receptors that belong to the family of epidermal growth factor receptors, which dimer upon ligand binding. NRG1/ErbB3 signaling has been shown to inhibit later stage differentiation of melanoblasts derived from neural tubes of mouse embryos but is dispensable for melanoblast specification and melanocyte maturation and promotes undifferentiated, migratory, and proliferative features (Buac et al. 2009). Neuregulin-1 treatment increased melanocyte proliferation, invasion, and altered morphology together with decreased levels of differentiation genes (Buac et al. 2009). Cultured human fibroblasts derived from skin type VI donors expressed higher levels of NRG-1 than fibroblasts derived from skin type II donors (Choi et al. 2010). In vivo, NRG-1 was highly expressed in the epidermis as well as the dermis of skin type VI donors but was expressed at very low levels only in the dermis of skin type II donors (Choi et al. 2010). Furthermore, treatment with exogenous NRG-1 gave rise to increase in pigmentation, melanocyte size, and dendricity in cultured skin substitutes, and these effects were more pronounced in skin substitutes representative of skin type VI than in their counterparts representative of skin types IV or II. The bioactive motif of NRG1 that is involved in modulating melanin production in human melanocytes has been characterized and was found to increase melanin production without affecting proliferation (Choi et al. 2012). ErbB3 expression was higher in melanocytes derived from dark skin than in melanocytes cultured from light skin, suggesting that activation of this receptor is responsible for the melanogenic effects of NRG-1 (Choi et al. 2012). On the other hand, ErbB4 expression was expressed at higher levels in melanocytes derived from light skin, compared to melanocytes from dark skin. These findings implicate NRG-1 and its receptors in regulating constitutive pigmentation.

2.6 Role of Melanocyte- and Keratinocyte-Derived Nitric Oxide in Regulating Pigmentation

In addition to enhancing the production of a large panel of paracrine and autocrine growth factors, UV stimulates the production of nitric oxide (NO) by both keratinocytes and melanocytes (Romero-Graillet et al. 1996, 1997). In keratinocytes, this effect was mediated by increased constitutive NO synthase (Romero-Graillet et al. 1997) and might involve the activation of Akt (Dimmeler et al. 1999). In lipopolysaccharide (LPS)-treated human melanocytes, the inducible NO synthase (iNOS) gene expression was suppressed by activin, which also inhibited toll-like receptors (TLR) and cytokine expression (Kim et al. 2015). The melanogenic effect of UV was abrogated to a large extent upon treatment with NO scavengers, while treatment of melanocytes with exogenous NO donors stimulated melanogenesis and dendricity, lending direct evidence for the melanogenic effect of NO (Romero-Graillet et al. 1997). This effect of NO was mediated by increasing the levels of cGMP, and treatment of melanocytes with guanylate cyclase inhibitors blocked the UV-induced melanogenesis (Romero-Graillet et al. 1996). It is possible that the melanogenic effect of cGMP is indirect, resulting from inhibition of cAMP phosphodiesterase, which leads to increased cAMP levels, the principle mechanism for stimulation of melanogenesis. In B16 and human melanoma cells, α-MSH increased the UV-induced NO levels, and as in normal human melanocytes, NO stimulated melanogenesis (Tsatmali et al. 2000). This melanogenic effect was abrogated by inhibition of iNOS. The findings that α-MSH modulates the production of NO raises the question whether NO functions as an autocrine factor or as a second messenger that mediates the effects of α-MSH.

Abnormal levels of NO can have detrimental effects on melanocytes. It has been recently shown that variants of *iNOS* gene, −954 G/C and Ex 16+14 C/T, might be genetic susceptibility markers for nonsegmental vitiligo among Egyptians (Zayed et al. 2015). Exposure of human melanocytes to UV induced the formation of superoxide and NO, which combine to form peroxynitrite that excites an electron in fragments of the pigment melanin leading to the formation of CPDs even after cessation of UV exposure (Premi et al. 2015). Peroxynitrite solubilizes melanin into fragments or releases pre-melanin monomers from melanosomes, leading to migration of these fragments or monomers to the nucleus, where they induce CPDS. Not only the initial induction of CPDs but also latent formation of CPDs, coined "dark CPDs," was found to be twice as high in the skin of UVA-irradiated *K14-Kitle/e* mice (homozygous for the loss of function recessive yellow mutation in *Mc1r*) than in the skin of their counterparts with black coat color. These results suggest that pheomelanin sensitizes melanocytes to excessive CPDs, which might be attributed to either increased peroxynitrite formation or sensitivity of pheomelanin to peroxynitrite. Further investigation of the role of NO in the UV response of human melanocytes should shed light on its effects on UV-induced DNA damage in individuals with different pigmentary phenotypes, and on the risk for melanoma.

2.7 Signaling Pathways Responsible for Regulating Melanocyte Proliferation, Survival, and Function

The first melanocyte growth medium was based on the use of phorbol esters that activate protein kinase C, and cAMP inducers, such as cholera toxin (Eisinger and Marko 1982). This underscored the significance of these signaling pathways in sustaining the survival, proliferation, and function of human melanocytes. Later, it was shown that paracrine growth factors for melanocytes that activate tyrosine kinase receptors, such as bFGF, SCF, and HGF, as well as ET-1, can substitute for phorbol esters in the culture medium and stimulate proliferation by activating the MAP kinases ERK1/2 (Bohm et al. 1995; Swope et al. 1995a; Tada et al. 1998b). Activation of ERK1/2 resulted in phosphorylation, hence activation of the transcription factor cyclic AMP response element binding protein (CREB), upstream from the melanocyte master regulator, the transcription factor MITF (Bohm et al. 1995; Tada et al. 2002). Signaling pathways that were involved in ERK1/2 activation included protein kinasec (PKC), tyrosine kinases, and intracellular calcium mobilization. The cAMP pathway has long been known to be essential for stimulating melanogenesis in pigment cells (Hirobe and Takeuchi 1977; Pawelek et al. 1973). The main signaling pathway for α-MSH is the cAMP-dependent pathway, and α-MSH is primarily a melanogenic factor for human melanocytes (Abdel-Malek et al. 1992). In contrast to other growth factors, such as bFGF or ET-1, α-MSH and other cAMP inducers are poor activators of the ERK1/2 pathway, yet α-MSH interacts synergistically with factors that stimulate PKC, tyrosine kinases, or intracellular calcium mobilization to activate these MAP kinases and their downstream targets, leading to increased melanocyte proliferation and melanogenesis (Herraiz et al. 2011; Tada et al. 2002). Based on these findings, a melanocyte growth medium supplemented with bFGF, ET-1, and α-MSH was described and found to support the long-term proliferation of human melanocytes (Swope et al. 1995b).

The transcription factor Mitf is a member of the basic helix–loop–helix leucine zipper transcription factors and is considered the "master regulator" in melanocytes (reviewed by Steingrimsson et al. 2004). Germline mutations in *Mitf* result in Waardenburg Syndrome type 2, characterized by congenital white forelock, sensoneural deafness, and asymmetric iris color. The significance of Mitf lies in its ability to regulate the expression of many target genes that are involved in melanin synthesis, proliferation, and survival of melanocytes (reviewed by Cheli et al. 2009). Direct targets for Mitf are the genes for the melanogenic enzymes *Tyrosinase*, *TYRP1*, *DCT*, and the melanosomal genes PMel 17, OA1, as well as Rab27A that is involved in melanosome transfer. Other Mitf target genes are Bcl2, BIRC7, and DICER that are involved in regulating melanocyte survival, KIT, NGFR, and ENDBR genes that encode for receptors for melanocyte growth and survival factors (SCF, NGF, and ET-1, respectively), and APE/Ref1 that regulates the redox state, as well as HIF1α, which is induced by hypoxia. Additional targets for Mitf include the cell cycle regulatory genes TBX2 and CDK2, as well as CDKN1A (p21) and CDKN2A.

It is well-established that Mitf is regulated by the ERK1/2 pathway. Treatment of melanoma cells with SCF activated ERK, which resulted in the phosphorylation of Mitf on Ser 73 and Ser 409 (Wu et al. 2000). The SCF-induced phosphorylation of Mitf on Ser 73 transiently increased its transcriptional activity, as evidenced by increasing tyrosinase expression, and subsequently targeted Mitf for ubiquitination (Hemesath et al. 1998; Wu et al. 2000). Activation of the cAMP pathway in mouse and human melanoma cells by α-MSH or forskolin also resulted in the phosphorylation of Mitf (Price et al. 1998). Treatment of cultured human melanocytes with α-MSH and/or ET-1 in the presence of bFGF increased total protein levels of Mitf, as well as its phosphorylated form (Kadekaro et al. 2005). Mitf was also regulated transcriptionally, as shown by global gene analysis of melanocytes treated with α-MSH (Kadekaro et al. 2010). Loss of Zinc Finger E-box binding protein 2 (ZEB1) in melanocytes has been shown to induce melanoblast migration defects and melanocyte differentiation defects in vivo, accompanied by down-regulation of MITF (Denecker et al. 2014). Results identified a signaling network in which transcription factor ZEB2 regulates MITF to control melanocyte differentiation. Phosphodiesterase 4D3 has been identified as a direct target of the MSH/cAMP/MITF pathway, which creates a negative feedback loop inducing refractoriness to sustained stimulation of the cAMP pathway in melanocytes (Khaled et al. 2010). Wnt3a has been shown to play an important role in melanocyte homeostasis by up-regulating the expression of MITFA and its downstream targets in vitro (Guo et al. 2012a). In vivo, Wnt3a signaling is activated in mouse follicular melanocytes during anagen stage of the hair cycling and promotes melanin synthesis through induction of MITF (Guo et al. 2012b).

Exposure to UV activated the stress MAP kinases p38 and JNK/SAPK, which regulate the activity of downstream transcription factors that mediate the stress response (Ono and Han 2000; Rosette and Karin 1996). Increase in pigmentation, i.e., tanning, is considered part of the stress response, which is mediated by the paracrine/autocrine network that is activated by UV. The transcription factor Upstream Stimulating Factor-1 (USF-1) was activated by p38 and proved to be an important regulator of *MC1R* and *POMC* expression in melanocytes exposed to UV (Corre et al. 2004). In addition, USF-1 up-regulated the expression of *Tyrosinase*, *TYRP-1*, and *DCT*. Phosphorylation of USF-1 resulted in its activation and enhanced its ability to bind DNA (Galibert et al. 1997). Another transcription factor, ATF2, known to regulate genes involved in DNA repair, such as *XPC* and *ERCC1*, apoptosis, such as *Bcl2*, and the cell cycle, such as *CDK4*, was also activated by p38, as well as by JNK (Fuchs et al. 2000; Hayakawa et al. 2004), and thus is expected to play an important role in the DNA damage response of melanocytes to UV. Global gene analysis of human melanocytes irradiated with UV or treated with α-MSH revealed that ATF2 and its target genes *Bcl2*, *CDK4*, and *ERCC1* were reduced in expression by UV, and up-regulated in expression by α-MSH (Kadekaro et al. 2010). The modulation of ATF2 and Bcl2 expression by UV and α-MSH was confirmed by Western blotting, indicating that ATF2 participates in the UV response of human melanocytes. Recently, it was reported that exposure of human melanocytes to UV induced the phosphorylation of ATF2 on Tyrosine 69 and 71, and pretreatment with ET-1 augmented this effect (von Koschembahr et al. 2015). Interestingly, ET-1 induced ATF2 phosphorylation even without any UV exposure, suggesting that this potent paracrine factor primes melanocytes to respond avidly in order to counteract the genotoxic effects of UV. The impact of phospho-ATF2 on repair of UV-induced DNA damage remains to be determined.

The p53 transcription factor is considered a universal sensor of genotoxic stress (Chouinard et al. 2002; Huang et al. 1999; Liu et al. 1996). It is known to accumulate following UV exposure due to its stabilization and induces growth arrest in order to allow for DNA repair, and this was shown to occur in human melanocytes (Liu et al. 1996; Marrot et al. 2005; Medrano et al. 1995). P53 was regulated by p38, and in turn, it regulated the expression of *Tyrosinase* and *TYRP-1* (Chouinard et al. 2002; Khlgatian et al. 2002; Nylander et al. 2000). In mouse skin, p53 was found to up-regulate the expression of POMC, the precursor for melanocortins, and β-endorphin that stimulate melanogenesis (Cui et al. 2007). Another study found that mutations in the ribosomal protein s (Rps) genes, *Rps6*, *Rps19*, and *Rps20* gave rise to dark skin, due to epidermal melanocytosis (McGowan et al. 2008). The dark skin phenotype was dependent on increased p53 in keratinocytes, which led to increased expression of *SCF* that encodes for a potent mitogen and melanogenic factor for melanocytes. These intriguing results observed in mouse skin implicate p53 in regulating the expression of important paracrine factors known to have significant impact on melanocytes.

Recently, a positive feedback loop between p53, SCF, and ET-1 was described (Murase et al. 2009). Inducing high levels of p53 in cultured human keratinocytes resulted in increased production of SCF and ET-1, and treatment of cultured human melanocytes with either SCF or ET-1 increased phosphorylation of p53 on Ser 15, which led to its stabilization. In contrast, silencing or inhibition of p53 in melanocytes resulted in decreased Kit expression, inhibition of Mitf, as well as reduced tyrosinase levels and melanin content. In cultured skin substitutes, inhibition of p53 suppressed melanogenesis and led to reduced pigmentation, and silencing of p53 in vivo inhibited pigmentation of UV-irradiated mouse ears. These effects of p53 confirm its significance in regulating pigmentation, particularly the tanning response to UV. It was recently shown that p53 directly regulates ET-1 expression in human epidermal keratinocytes, as well as mouse epidermis, and controls UV-induced melanocyte homeostasis in the skin of adult mice (Hyter et al. 2013). These results underscore the significance of p53 in the maintenance of melanocyte homeostasis via regulating expression of paracrine factors that regulate melanocyte proliferation, pigmentation, and survival.

The type II nuclear hormone receptor and transcription factor Retinoid-X-Receptor α (RXRα) has been shown to regulate mouse keratinocyte and melanocyte homeostasis following acute UV irradiation (Wang et al. 2011). Activation of RXRα expressed in keratinocytes regulated in a cell-autonomous manner their proliferation through secretion of heparin-binding EGF-like growth factor, GM-CSF, IL-1α, and cyclooxygenase-2 and activation of mitogen-activated protein kinase pathways. Expression of several keratinocyte-derived paracrine growth factors such as ET-1, hepatocyte growth factor, α-MSH, stem cell factor, and fibroblast growth factor-2 was elevated/altered in skin of mice lacking RXRα in epidermal keratinocytes, which in a non-cell-autonomous manner modulated melanocyte proliferation and activation after UV exposure (Wang et al. 2011).

In comparison, in vivo melanocyte-specific ablation of RXRα and RXRβ in mice led to altered expression of pro- and anti-apoptotic genes following UV exposure and increased survival of these melanocytes, as compared to their wild-type counterpart (Coleman et al. 2014). These results underscore a "cell autonomous" role of melanocytic RXRs in controlling melanocyte survival post-UV exposure.

2.8 The *MC1R*: A Main Determinant of the Diversity of Human Pigmentation and a Melanoma Susceptibility Gene

The *MC1R* is a highly polymorphic gene, with about 200 allelic variants expressed in different human populations (reviewed by Garcia-Borron et al. 2005, 2014). The *MC1R* is considered a main determinant of the diversity of human pigmentation, with the wild-type *MC1R* predominantly expressed in Africa, where high eumelanin content in the skin is critical for optimal photoprotection. A few of the *MC1R* variants, mainly R151C, R160W, and D294H, are strongly associated with red hair phenotype (Box et al. 1997; Smith et al. 1998). Expression of any two of these variants in the homozygous or compound heterozygous state results in loss of function of the receptor, disrupting its ability to signal when bound by its agonists (Kadekaro et al. 2010; Scott et al. 2002). Epidemiological studies from different populations in different geographical locations demonstrated that these allelic variants are also associated with poor tanning ability and increased risk for melanoma and nonmelanoma skin cancers (Box et al. 2001; Kadekaro et al. 2010; Kennedy et al. 2001; Palmer et al. 2000). The *MC1R* gene is considered a low penetrance melanoma susceptibility gene. However, co-expression of one of the *MC1R* red hair-associated variants with a mutation in the highly penetrant *p16* gene significantly increases the risk for melanoma above that caused by the p16 mutation alone (Demenais et al. 2010). Stimulation of eumelanin synthesis by activation of the MC1R confers photoprotection; however, the effect of *MC1R* genotype on melanoma risk is independent of the effect on pigmentation, suggesting that MC1R determines the risk for melanoma by other mechanisms (Kennedy et al. 2001; Landi et al. 2005; Palmer et al. 2000; Stratigos et al. 2006). That the MC1R plays a central role in regulating human pigmentation is further supported by the findings that its expression is up-regulated by its agonist α-MSH and by ET-1 (Kadekaro et al. 2010; Swope et al. 2012; Tada et al. 1998a).

2.9 Role of ET-1 and Melanocortins in the DNA Damage Response of Melanocytes

In 2005, novel roles for melanocortins and ET-1 were discovered. In addition to the well-known effects of these factors on melanogenesis and proliferation, they increased the survival of UV-irradiated human melanocytes, enhanced nucleotide excision repair, and reduced oxidative damage by inhibiting the generation of hydrogen peroxide (Kadekaro et al. 2005). The global effects of ET-1 and α-MSH are shown in Fig. 2.2. Genetic deletion of ET-1 in murine epidermis decreased dermal melanocytes in adult skin without altering melanocyte homeostasis in newborn skin (Hyter et al. 2013). Topical treatment with the EDNRB antagonist BQ788 abrogated UV-induced melanocyte activation and recapitulated the phenotype of ET-1 deletion in mice. Endothelin-1 from epidermal keratinocytes in a non-cell autonomous manner controlled melanocyte proliferation, DNA damage, and apoptosis following UVB irradiation (Hyter et al. 2013). Treatment of cultured human melanocytes with ET-1 reduced the induction and enhanced the repair of CPDs (von Koschembahr et al. 2015). These effects were mediated by increased phosphorylation of p38 and JNK, mainly due to increased intracellular Ca^{2+} mobilization, a signaling pathway activated by ENDBR. Treatment with ET-1 also increased the phosphorylation of ATF-2, known to be involved in DNA repair.

Enhancement of nucleotide excision repair capacity by α-MSH was reported independently by other investigative teams (Bohm et al. 2005; Smith et al. 2008). Treatment of human melanocytes with the potent α-MSH analog NDP-MSH increased the transcription of NR4A subfamily of orphan nuclear receptors, which played a role in the MC1R-mediated repair of DNA photoproducts (Bohm et al. 2005; Smith et al. 2008). Furthermore, treatment of cultured human melanocytes with α-MSH reduced the induction of 8-oxo-guanosine, thus confirming reduction of oxidative DNA damage (Song et al. 2009). The survival effects of α-MSH and

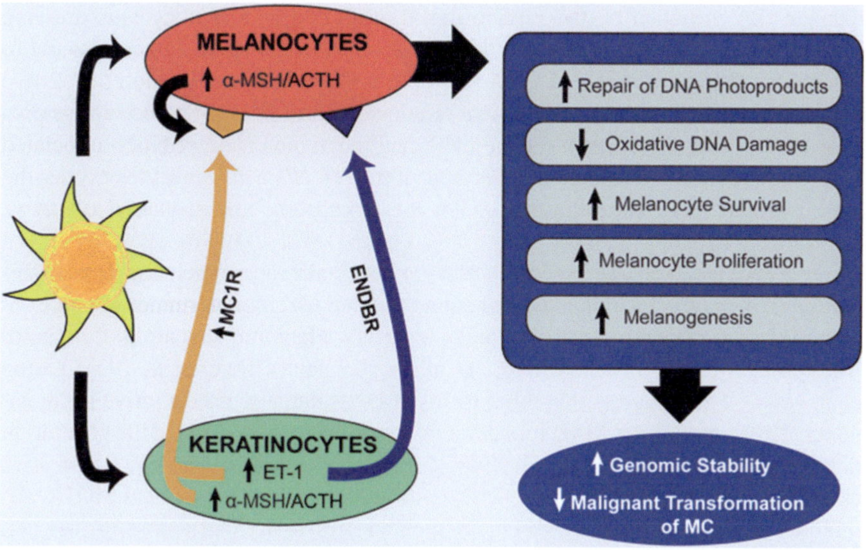

Fig. 2.2 The global effects of α-MSH and ACTH, and ET-1 on melanocytes and their response to UV exposure. Exposure to UV increases the production of ET-1 by keratinocytes, and α-MSH and ACTH by keratinocytes and melanocytes. The melanocortins α-MSH and ACTH, as well as ET-1, up-regulate the expression of the MC1R. Activation of MC1R and ENDBR results in enhanced repair of DNA photoproducts, reduction in generation of reactive oxygen species that lead to oxidative DNA damage, increased melanocyte survival and proliferation, as well as melanogenesis. The effects of these factors on UV-induced DNA damage are expected to maintain genomic stability of melanocytes and reduce the chance for malignant transformation to melanoma

ET-1 on UV-irradiated human melanocytes were mediated by activating the MC1R and ENDBR, respectively, and were independent of increased melanogenesis, since they were observed in tyrosinase-negative albino melanocytes (Kadekaro et al. 2005). These survival effects were mediated by activating Akt and Mitf, and maintaining high levels of Bcl2, a known Mitf target (Kadekaro et al. 2005; McGill et al. 2002). The recent finding that Mitf activation by α-MSH up-regulated the expression of DICER, a RNase II endonuclease that digests premature miRNA to yield mature miRNA, which reduced the expression of the pro-apoptotic BIM (Levy et al. 2010), suggested that decreased BIM expression is involved in the survival effects of α-MSH and ET-1.

The effects of α-MSH on nucleotide excision repair, generation of reactive oxygen species, and oxidative DNA damage received considerable attention, given the high polymorphism of the *MC1R* that results in the differential responses of melanocytes derived from donors with different *MC1R* genotypes to α-MSH and UV (Kadekaro et al. 2010; Scott et al. 2002). These effects required functional MC1R as they were absent in melanocytes that express loss of function receptors. The cAMP pathway mediated the effects of α-MSH on DNA damage, since these effects were also induced by forskolin, a direct activator of adenylate cyclase. Further evidence for the significance of MC1R in reducing the burden of UV-induced DNA damage was provided by the finding that transfection of melanocytes expressing loss-of-function MC1R with the wild-type gene restored the ability to respond to α-MSH by enhanced repair of DNA photoproducts, reduced generation of reactive oxygen species, and increased survival (Kadekaro et al. 2010). These findings provide a molecular mechanism for the increased melanoma susceptibility associated with expression of loss of function variants of the *MC1R*, as melanocytes expressing these variants have compromised DNA repair capacity and sustained oxidative stress.

Oxidative DNA damage seems to play an important role in melanocyte transformation to melanoma. Unlike basal or squamous cell carcinomas that originate from keratinocytes, melanoma tumors rarely have UV signature mutations that result from unrepaired pyrimidine dimers, as in the *p53* gene (Brash et al. 1991; Lubbe et al. 1994). This suggests that other forms of DNA damage are causative for melanoma. Treatment with α-MSH immediately (within minutes) reduced the generation of hydrogen peroxide in UV-irradiated melanocytes (Kadekaro et al. 2005; Kadekaro et al. 2010; Song et al. 2009). This effect absolutely required functional MC1R was inhibited by ASIP and was absent in melanocytes that express loss-of-function receptor. Additionally, α-MSH increased the activity of catalase, a first-line-of-defense antioxidant enzyme, and counteracted the inhibitory effect of UV on catalase activity and protein levels in melanocytes expressing functional MC1R (Song et al. 2009). Recently, it was reported that catalase was transported with melanosomes to keratinocytes (Maresca et al. 2010). This intriguing finding suggests that melanocytes protect keratinocytes not only by transferring melanin contained within melanosomes that reduce the penetration of UV rays to nuclear DNA but also by providing additional catalase, which might further reduce reactive oxygen species, and prevent oxidative damage. Besides increasing the activity and levels of catalase, α-MSH also up-regulated the protein levels of ferritin, an iron sequestrant in melanocytes (Song et al. 2009). Treatment with α-MSH also activated the transcription factor Nrf-2, which regulates the expression of phase II detoxifying enzymes that contain antioxidant response element (ARE) in their promoter (Kokot et al. 2009). Examples of such enzymes are hemeoxygenase-1 (HO-1), γ-glutamylcysteine-synthase, γ-glutathione S-transferase, which were up-regulated by α-MSH in UV-irradiated melanocytes (Kokot et al. 2009).

Microarray analysis of genes altered in expression by α-MSH and/or UV in melanocytes expressing functional versus nonfunctional MC1R revealed that the former responded to α-MSH by altered expression of many genes, particularly those that regulate melanogenesis (e.g., melanogenic enzymes, melanosome biogenesis, transcription factors, growth factor receptors), survival, cell cycle, DNA repair, and oxidative stress, while the latter showed no changes in gene expression, further confirming the refractoriness of these cells to α-MSH (Kadekaro et al. 2010). In general, α-MSH up-regulated, while UV down-regulated transcription. Importantly, α-uMSH reversed the effects of UV on many genes, including some that are involved in the DNA damage response to UV, particularly melanogenesis, DNA repair, cell cycle, oxidative stress, and apoptosis. These effects of α-MSH were only evident in melanocytes expressing functional MC1R and were absent in melanocytes expressing loss-of-function receptor, lending further explanation for why certain *MC1R* genotypes that cause loss of function of MC1R are associated with increased susceptibility to mutagenesis and melanoma formation.

Further evidence for the involvement of the α-MSH/MC1R axis in the DNA damage response of melanocytes was provided by the following findings. Treatment of human melanocytes with α-MSH was shown to phosphorylate the DNA damage sensors ataxia telangiectasia Rad3-related (ATR) and ataxia telangiectasia mutated (ATM) and their downstream kinases Chk1 and Chk2 (Swope et al. 2014). These phosphorylation events led to increased formation of γ-H2AX, the phosphorylated form of histone 2AX (H2AX) known to be critical for recruitment of DNA repair enzymes involved in nucleotide excision repair, the main pathway for repair of DNA photoproducts, to the sites of DNA damage. An increase in the protein levels of XPC, the DNA damage recognition enzyme, was also observed in response to α-MSH treatment. These effects were recapitulated by treatment with forskolin, providing evidence that they are mediated by activating the cAMP pathway, and were absent in melanocytes expressing loss-of-function MC1R. Subsequently, it was reported that activation of the cAMP-dependent protein kinase A (PKA) by α-MSH or forskolin resulted in the phosphorylation of ATR on Ser 435 and the binding of ATR to XPA and their co-localization to DNA photoproducts (Jarrett et al. 2014). As expected, these events that lead to activation of nucleotide excision repair by α-MSH were absent in melanocytes expressing nonfunctional MC1R. The same authors showed that these effects of α-MSH were negated by the MC1R antagonists ASIP and HBD3 (Jarrett et al. 2015), thus providing unequivocal evidence for the significance of the activated MC1R in modulating nucleotide excision repair in melanocytes. The findings that reactive oxygen and nitrogen species can contribute to the formation of CPDs in melanin-containing cells, i.e., melanocytes as well as keratinocytes, following cessation of UV exposure points to the importance of repair of DNA photoproducts for maintenance of genomic stability in these cells, and for prevention of melanoma as well as nonmelanoma skin cancers (Premi et al. 2015).

2.10 Targeting the MC1R by Melanocortin Analogs

Since decades, there has been interest in targeting the MC1R to increase skin pigmentation (tanning). This strategy was initially based on utilizing potent melanocortin analogs for sunless safe tanning that is photoprotective. Injecting human subjects with the potent and best known α-MSH analog NDP-MSH was found to be effective in inducing tanning in the absence of sun exposure (Levine et al. 1991). Later, this analog was found to reduce the induction of DNA photoproducts in sun-exposed human skin (Barnetson et al. 2006). Recently, clinical trials demonstrated the efficacy of NDP-MSH in repigmentation of vitiligo skin (Lim et al. 2015), which may be attributed to the known mitogenic and survival effects of α-MSH (Abdel-Malek et al. 1995; Kadekaro et al. 2005). Given that vitiligo skin is under oxidative stress due to high levels of hydrogen peroxide (Rokos et al. 2002), treatment with

NDP-MSH is expected to have antioxidant effects, thus inhibiting melanocyte death. However, despite the effectiveness of NDP-MSH, it is not specific to the MC1R, as it can bind the other melanocortin receptors, MC3, 4, and 5R, which account for its off-target effects. For the goal of developing small analogs of α-MSH for topical application to prevent skin cancers, including melanoma, tetrapeptide analogs of α-MSH were developed, and shown to surpass α-MSH in their potency to stimulate melanogenesis, and to reduce UV-induced DNA damage and apoptosis (Abdel-Malek et al. 2006). More recently, tripeptide analogs were developed and shown to be capable of activating the MC1R and reducing UV-induced DNA damage (Abdel-Malek et al. 2009). Developing MC1R-selective analogs of α-MSH will reduce the off-target effects, and developing small analogs will facilitate their topical delivery, which should reduce systemic effects. These analogs require functional MC1R and are expected to confer photoprotection for individuals with wild type *MC1R*, or who are heterozygous for *MC1R* variants that reduce receptor function, or mutant for other melanoma susceptibility genes, such as the highly penetrant *p16* or *PTEN* (Demenais et al. 2010; Sosman and Margolin 2009). Others have proposed the use of forskolin, an activator of adenylate cyclase, for melanoma prevention (D'Orazio et al. 2006). Since forskolin activates the cAMP pathway, it has similar photoprotective effects as α-MSH (Kadekaro et al. 2010). However, forskolin is nonspecific, and its target, adenylate cyclase, is ubiquitously expressed in all cell types, which precludes its selective use for photoprotection.

The effects of ET-1 on repair of DNA photoproducts was evident in human melanocytes regardless of their *MC1R* genotype, as these effects were observed in melanocytes expressing loss-of-function MC1R (von Koschembahr et al. 2015). These results suggest that the ET-1/ENDBR axis might be an attractive target for photoprotective strategies. Given that ET-1 and its receptors are ubiquitously expressed, they cannot be targeted directly to activate the DNA damage response of melanocytes. However, the downstream effectors of ENDBR that are involved in the DNA damage response in melanocytes might be targeted, and this would have global benefit against UV-induced genotoxicity and melanomagenesis, independent of *MC1R* genotype.

2.11 What Normal Melanocytes Teach About Melanoma: Revise

Normally, melanocytes in the skin are quiescent, and their homeostasis is maintained via their interaction with keratinocytes and with their microenvironment. During the early stages of melanomagenesis, melanocytes acquire the ability to proliferate and escape from cell cycle regulation by uncoupling from keratinocytes (reviewed by Haass and Herlyn 2005). This is achieved by down-regulating the expression of the adhesion molecules E-cadherin, P-cadherin, and desmoglein in response to binding of the paracrine factor HGF to c-Met and activation of ERK1/2 and IP3 kinase (Li et al. 2001). Similarly, ET-1 can down-regulate E-cadherin (Jamal and Schneider 2002). Further studies showed that overexpression of bFGF in a human xenograft model followed by UVB irradiation gave rise to hyperplastic melanocytic cells with high-grade atypia, reminiscent of lentiginous melanoma (Berking et al. 2001). Overexpression of bFGF concomitantly with ET-3 and SCF, followed by UVB exposure, led to the formation of nests of atypical melanocytes representing melanoma in situ, some of which progressed into invasive melanoma (Berking et al. 2004). These paracrine factors are up-regulated in expression by UV, and sun exposure might lead in vivo to deregulation of their expression, or expression of their receptors, e.g., ENDBR (Demunter et al. 2001). It is not known how the UV-induced levels of these factors compare to their levels when they are overexpressed in xenograft models. Until this is determined, the role of bFGF, ET-3 (or ET-1), and SCF in melanomagenesis remains unclear. As discussed earlier, some paracrine factors for melanocytes are synthesized by fibroblasts. Given the importance of tumor-associated fibroblasts in melanoma progression and invasion, it is critical to understand how these factors might be deregulated and their role in melanomagenesis.

The MAP kinase ERK1/2 and IP3 kinase pathways are important regulators of melanocyte homeostasis. Mutations that disrupt these pathways, such as the activating $BRAF^{V900E}$ mutation, upstream of ERK1/2, and loss of PTEN that causes continuous activation of AKT, thus increased proliferation and survival, are common in melanoma (Davies et al. 2002; Sosman and Margolin 2009). Therefore, understanding the regulation of normal melanocytes provides insight into the pathways that lead to melanoma formation, and the opportunity to target components of these pathways for melanoma therapy, as in the currently used BRAF inhibitors that hold promise for melanoma treatment.

References

Abdel-Malek Z, Swope VB, Pallas J, Krug K, Nordlund JJ (1992) Mitogenic, melanogenic and cAMP responses of cultured neonatal human melanocytes to commonly used mitogens. J Cell Physiol 150:416–425

Abdel-Malek Z, Swope V, Collins C, Boissy R, Zhao H, Nordlund J (1993) Contribution of melanogenic proteins to the heterogeneous pigmentation of human melanocytes. J Cell Sci 106:1323–1331

Abdel-Malek Z, Swope VB, Suzuki I, Akcali C, Harriger MD, Boyce ST, Urabe K, Hearing VJ (1995) Mitogenic and melanogenic stimulation of normal human melanocytes by melanotropic peptides. Proc Natl Acad Sci U S A 92:1789–1793

Abdel-Malek ZA, Kadekaro AL, Kavanagh RJ, Todorovic A, Koikov LN, Mcnulty JC, Jackson PJ, Milhauser GL, Schwemberger S, Babcock G et al (2006) Melanoma prevention strategy based on using tetrapeptide alpha-MSH analogs that protect human melanocytes from UV-induced damage and cytotoxicity. FASEB J 20:1561–1563

Abdel-Malek ZA, Ruwe A, Kavanagh-Starner R, Kadekaro AL, Swope V, Haskell-Luevano C, Koikov L, Knittel JJ (2009) alpha-MSH tripeptide analogs activate the melanocortin 1 receptor and reduce UV-induced DNA damage in human melanocytes. Pigment Cell Melanoma Res 22:635–644

Arad S, Konnikov N, Goukassian DA, Gilchrest BA (2006) T-oligos augment UV-induced protective responses in human skin. FASEB J 20:1895–1897

Barnetson RS, Ooi TK, Zhuang L, Halliday GM, Reid CM, Walker PC, Humphrey SM, Kleinig MJ (2006) [Nle4-D-Phe7]-alpha-melanocyte-stimulating hormone significantly increased pigmentation and decreased UV damage in fair-skinned Caucasian volunteers. J Invest Dermatol 126:1869–1878

Berking C, Takemoto R, Satyamoorthy K, Elenitsas R, Herlyn M (2001) Basic fibroblast growth factor and ultraviolet B transform melanocytes in human skin. Am J Pathol 158:943–953

Berking C, Takemoto R, Satyamoorthy K, Shirakawa T, Eskandarpour M, Hansson J, Vanbelle PA, Elder DE, Herlyn M (2004) Induction of melanoma phenotypes in human skin by growth factors and ultraviolet B. Cancer Res 64:807–811

Bohm M, Moellmann G, Cheng E, Alvarez-Franco M, Wagner S, Sassone-Corsi P, Halaban R (1995) Identification of $p90^{RSK}$ as the probable $CREB\text{-}Ser^{133}$ kinase in human melanocytes. Cell Growth Differ 6:291–302

Bohm M, Wolff I, Scholzen TE, Robinson SJ, Healy E, Luger TA, Schwarz T, Schwarz A (2005) alpha-Melanocyte-stimulating hormone protects from ultraviolet radiation-induced apoptosis and DNA damage. J Biol Chem 280:5795–5802

Botchkarev VA, Yaar M, Peters EM, Raychaudhuri SP, Botchkareva NV, Marconi A, Raychaudhuri SK, Paus R, Pincelli C (2006) Neurotrophins in skin biology and pathology. J Invest Dermatol 126:1719–1727

Box NF, Wyeth JR, O'gorman LE, Martin NG, Sturm RA (1997) Characterization of melanocyte stimulating hormone receptor variant alleles in twins with red hair. Hum Mol Genet 6:1891–1897

Box NF, Duffy DL, Irving RE, Russell A, Chen W, Griffiths LR, Parsons PG, Green AC, Sturm RA (2001) Melanocortin-1 receptor genotype is a risk factor for basal and squamous cell carcinoma. J Invest Dermatol 116:224–229

Brash DE, Rudolph JA, Simon JA, Lin A, Mckenna GJ, Baden HP, Halperin AJ, Pontén JN (1991) A role for sunlight in skin cancer: UV-induced p53 mutations in squamous cell carcinoma. Proc Natl Acad Sci U S A 88:10124–10128

Brito FC, Kos L (2008) Timeline and distribution of melanocyte precursors in the mouse heart. Pigment Cell Melanoma Res 21:464–470

Bronner-Fraser M (1993) Neural development: crest destiny. Curr Biol CB 3:201–203

Buac K, Xu M, Cronin J, Weeraratna AT, Hewitt SM, Pavan WJ (2009) NRG1/ERBB3 signaling in melanocyte development and melanoma: inhibition of differentiation and promotion of proliferation. Pigment Cell Melanoma Res 22:773–784

Bustamante J, Bredeston L, Malanga G, Mordoh J (1993) Role of melanin as a scavenger of active oxygen species. Pigment Cell Res 6:348–353

Candille SI, Kaelin CB, Cattanach BM, Yu B, Thompson DA, Nix MA, Kerns JA, Schmutz SM, Millhauser GL, Barsh GS (2007) A {beta}-defensin mutation causes black coat color in domestic dogs. Science Sciencexpress, www.sciencexpress.org. 18 Oct 2007. 10.1126/science.1147880

Chakraborty AK, Funasaka Y, Slominski A, Ermak G, Hwang J, Pawelek JM, Ichihashi M (1996) Production and release of proopiomelanocortin (POMC) derived peptides by human melanocytes and keratinocytes in culture: regulation by ultraviolet B. Biochim Biophys Acta 1313:130–138

Cheli Y, Ohanna M, Ballotti R, Bertolotto C (2009) Fifteen-year quest for microphthalmia-associated transcription factor target genes. Pigment Cell Melanoma Res 23:27–40

Chhajlani V, Wikberg JES (1992) Molecular cloning and expression of the human melanocyte stimulating hormone receptor cDNA. FEBS Lett 309:417–420

Choi W, Kolbe L, Hearing VJ (2012) Characterization of the bioactive motif of neuregulin-1, a fibroblast-derived paracrine factor that regulates constitutive color and the function of melanocytes in human skin. Pigment Cell Melanoma Res 25:477–481

Choi W, Wolber R, Gerwat W, Mann T, Batzer J, Smuda C, Liu H, Kolbe L, Hearing VJ (2010) The fibroblast-derived paracrine factor neuregulin-1 has a novel role in regulating the constitutive color and melanocyte function in human skin. J Cell Sci 123:3102–3111

Chouinard N, Valerie K, Rouabhia M, Huot J (2002) UVB-mediated activation of p38 mitogen-activated protein kinase enhances resistance of normal human keratinocytes to apoptosis by stabilizing cytoplasmic p53. Biochem J 365:133–145

Coleman DJ, Garcia G, Hyter S, Jang HS, Chagani S, Liang X, Larue L, Ganguli-Indra G, Indra AK (2014) Retinoid-X-receptors (alpha/beta) in melanocytes modulate innate immune responses and differentially regulate cell survival following UV irradiation. PLoS Genet 10:e1004321

Corre S, Primot A, Sviderskaya E, Bennett DC, Vaulont S, Goding CR, Galibert MD (2004) UV-induced expression of key component of the tanning process, the POMC and MC1R genes, is dependent on the p-38-activated upstream stimulating factor-1 (USF-1). J Biol Chem 279:51226–51233

Corre S, Mekideche K, Adamski H, Mosser J, Watier E, Galibert MD (2006) In vivo and ex vivo UV-induced analysis of pigmentation gene expressions. J Invest Dermatol 126:916–918

Cui R, Widlund HR, Feige E, Lin JY, Wilensky DL, Igras VE, D'orazio J, Fung CY, Schanbacher CF, Granter SR et al (2007) Central role of p53 in the suntan response and pathologic hyperpigmentation. Cell 128:853–864

D'orazio JA, Nobuhisa T, Cui R, Arya M, Spry M, Wakamatsu K, Igras V, Kunisada T, Granter SR, Nishimura EK et al (2006) Topical drug rescue strategy and skin protection based on the role of Mc1r in UV-induced tanning. Nature 443:340–344

Davies H, Bignell GR, Cox C, Stephens P, Edkins S, Clegg S, Teague J, Woffendin H, Garnett MJ, Bottomley W et al (2002) Mutations of the *BRAF* gene in human cancer. Nature 417:949–954

Demenais F, Mohamdi H, Chaudru V, Goldstein AM, Newton Bishop JA, Bishop DT, Kanetsky PA, Hayward NK, Gillanders E, Elder DE et al (2010) Association of MC1R variants and host phenotypes with melanoma risk in CDKN2A mutation carriers: a GenoMEL study. J Natl Cancer Inst 102:1568–1583

Demunter A, De Wolf-Peeters C, Degreef H, Stas M, Van Den Oord JJ (2001) Expression of the endothelin-B receptor in pigment cell lesions of the skin. Evidence for its role as tumor progression marker in malignant melanoma. Virchows Arch Int J pathol 438:485–491

Denecker G, Vandamme N, Akay O, Koludrovic D, Taminau J, Lemeire K, Gheldof A, De Craene B, Van Gele M, Brochez L et al (2014) Identification of a ZEB2-MITF-ZEB1 transcriptional network that controls melanogenesis and melanoma progression. Cell Death Differ 21:1250–1261

Dimmeler S, Fleming I, Fisslthaler B, Hermann C, Busse R, Zeiher AM (1999) Activation of nitric oxide synthase in endothelial cells by Akt-dependent phosphorylation. Nature 399:601–605

Duval C, Regnier M, Schmidt R (2001) Distinct melanogenic response of human melanocytes in mono-culture, in co-culture with keratinocytes and in reconstructed epidermis, to UV exposure. Pigment Cell Res 14:348–355

Eckert RL, Crish JF, Robinson NA (1997) The epidermal keratinocyte as a model for the study of gene regulation and cell differentiation. Physiol Rev 77:397–424

Eisinger M, Marko O (1982) Selective proliferation of normal human melanocytes in vitro in the presence of phorbol ester and cholera toxin. Proc Natl Acad Sci U S A 79:2018–2022

Epstein JH (1983) Photocarcinogenesis, skin cancer and aging. J Am Acad Dermatol 9:487–502

Fuchs SY, Tappin I, Ronai Z (2000) Stability of the ATF2 transcription factor is regulated by phosphorylation and dephosphorylation. J Biol Chem 275:12560–12564

Funasaka Y, Sato H, Chakraborty AK, Ohashi A, Chrousos GP, Ichihashi M (1999) Expression of proopiomelanocortin, corticotropin-releasing hormone (CRH), and CRH receptor in melanoma cells, nevus cells, and normal human melanocytes. J Investig Dermatol Symp Proc 4:105–109

Galibert MD, Boucontet L, Goding CR, Meo T (1997) Recognition of the E-C4 element from the C4 complement gene promoter by the upstream stimulatory factor-1 transcription factor. J Immunol 159:6176–6183

Garcia-Borron JC, Sanchez-Laorden BL, Jimenez-Cervantes C (2005) Melanocortin-1 receptor structure and functional regulation. Pigment Cell Res 18:393–410

Garcia-Borron JC, Abdel-Malek Z, Jimenez-Cervantes C (2014) MC1R, the cAMP pathway, and the response to solar UV: extending the horizon beyond pigmentation. Pigment Cell Melanoma Res 27:699–720

Giebel LB, Spritz RA (1991) Mutation of the *KIT* (mast/stem cell growth factor receptor) protooncogene in human piebaldism. Proc Natl Acad Sci U S A 88:8696–8699

Gilchrest BA, Rogers GS (1993) Photoaging. In: Lim HW, Soter NA (eds) Clinical photomedicine. Marcel Dekker, Inc., New York, pp 95–111
Gilchrest BA, Eller MS, Geller AC, Yaar M (1999) The pathogenesis of melanoma induced by ultraviolet radiation. N Engl J Med 340:1341–1348
Gledhill K, Rhodes LE, Brownrigg M, Haylett AK, Masoodi M, Thody AJ, Nicolaou A, Tobin DJ (2010) Prostaglandin-E2 is produced by adult human epidermal melanocytes in response to UVB in a melanogenesis-independent manner. Pigment Cell Melanoma Res 23:394–403
Goldgeier MH, Klein LE, Klein-Angerer S, Moellmann G, Nordlund JJ (1984) The distribution of melanocytes in the leptomeninges of the human brain. J Invest Dermatol 82:235–238
Gordon PR, Mansur CP, Gilchrest BA (1989) Regulation of human melanocyte growth, dendricity, and melanization by keratinocyte derived factors. J Invest Dermatol 92:565–572
Grichnik JM, Burch JA, Burchette J, Shea CR (1998) The SCF/KIT pathway plays a critical role in the control of normal human melanocyte homeostasis. J Invest Dermatol 111:233–238
Guo H, Yang K, Deng F, Xing Y, Li Y, Lian X, Yang T (2012a) Wnt3a inhibits proliferation but promotes melanogenesis of melan-a cells. Int J Mol Med 30:636–642
Guo H, Yang K, Deng F, Ye J, Xing Y, Li Y, Lian X, Yang T (2012b) Wnt3a promotes melanin synthesis of mouse hair follicle melanocytes. Biochem Biophys Res Commun 420:799–804
Haass NK, Herlyn M (2005) Normal human melanocyte homeostasis as a paradigm for understanding melanoma. J Investig Dermatol Symp Proc 10:153–163
Halaban R, Langdon R, Birchall N, Cuono C, Baird A, Scott G, Moellmann G, Mcguire J (1988) Basic fibroblast growth factor from human keratinocytes is a natural mitogen for melanocytes. J Cell Biol 107:1611–1619
Halder RM, Bridgeman-Shah S (1995) Skin cancer in African Americans. Cancer 75:667–673
Harder J, Bartels J, Christophers E, Schroder JM (2001) Isolation and characterization of human beta -defensin-3, a novel human inducible peptide antibiotic. J Biol Chem 276:5707–5713
Hauser JE, Kadekaro AL, Kavanagh RJ, Wakamatsu K, Terzieva S, Schwemberger S, Babcock G, Rao MB, Ito S, Abdel-Malek ZA (2006) Melanin content and MC1R function independently affect UVR-induced DNA damage in cultured human melanocytes. Pigment Cell Res 19:303–314
Hayakawa J, Mittal S, Wang Y, Korkmaz KS, Adamson E, English C, Ohmichi M, Mcclelland M, Mercola D (2004) Identification of promoters bound by c-Jun/ATF2 during rapid large-scale gene activation following genotoxic stress. Mol Cell 16:521–535
Hearing VJ (2005) Biogenesis of pigment granules: a sensitive way to regulate melanocyte function. J Dermatol Sci 37:3–14
Hemesath TJ, Price ER, Takemoto C, Badalian T, Fisher DE (1998) MAP kinase links the transcription factor microphthalmia to c-kit signalling in melanocytes. Nature 391:298–301
Hennessy A, Oh C, Diffey B, Wakamatsu K, Ito S, Rees J (2005) Eumelanin and pheomelanin concentrations in human epidermis before and after UVB irradiation. Pigment Cell Res 18:220–223
Herraiz C, Journe F, Abdel-Malek Z, Ghanem G, Jimenez-Cervantes C, Garcia-Borron JC (2011) Signaling from the human melanocortin 1 receptor to ERK1 and ERK2 mitogen-activated protein kinases involves transactivation of cKIT. Mol Endocrinol 25:138–156
Hirobe T, Takeuchi T (1977) Induction of melanogenesis in the epidermal melanoblasts of newborn mouse by MSH. J Embryol Exp Morphol 37:79–90
Horikawa T, Norris DA, Yohn JJ, Zekman T, Travers JB, Morelli JG (1995) Melanocyte mitogens induce both melanocyte chemokinesis and chemotaxis. J Invest Dermatol 104:256–259
Huang C, Ma W-Y, Maxinert A, Sun Y, Dong Z (1999) p38 Kinase mediates UV-induced phosphorylation of p53 protein at serine 389. J Biol Chem 274:12229–12235
Hunt G, Kyne S, Wakamatsu K, Ito S, Thody AJ (1995) Nle^4DPhe^7 α-melanocyte-stimulating hormone increases the eumelanin:phaeomelanin ratio in cultured human melanocytes. J Invest Dermatol 104:83–85
Hyter S, Coleman DJ, Ganguli-Indra G, Merrill GF, Ma S, Yanagisawa M, Indra AK (2013) Endothelin-1 is a transcriptional target of p53 in epidermal keratinocytes and regulates ultraviolet-induced melanocyte homeostasis. Pigment Cell Melanoma Res 26:247–258

Im S, Moro O, Peng F, Medrano EE, Cornelius J, Babcock G, Nordlund J, Abdel-Malek Z (1998a) Activation of the cyclic AMP pathway by α-melanotropin mediates the response of human melanocytes to ultraviolet B radiation. Cancer Res 58:47–54

Im S, Moro O, Peng F, Medrano EE, Cornelius J, Babcock G, Nordlund JJ, Abdel-Malek ZA (1998b) Activation of the cyclic AMP pathway by alpha-melanotropin mediates the response of human melanocytes to ultraviolet B radiation. Cancer Res 58:47–54

Imokawa G, Yada Y, Miyagishi M (1992) Endothelins secreted from human keratinocytes are intrinsic mitogens for human melanocytes. J Biol Chem 267:24675–24680

Imokawa G, Yada Y, Morisaki N, Kimura M (1998) Biological characterization of human fibroblast-derived mitogenic factors for human melanocytes. Biochem J 330:1235–1239

Ito S, Wakamatsu K (2003) Quantitative analysis of eumelanin and pheomelanin in humans, mice and other animals: a comparative review. Pigment Cell Res 16(5):523–531

Jamal S, Schneider RJ (2002) UV-induction of keratinocyte endothelin-1 downregulates E-cadherin in melanocytes and melanoma cells. J Clin Invest 110:443–452

Jarrett SG, Horrell EM, Christian PA, Vanover JC, Boulanger MC, Zou Y, D'orazio JA (2014) PKA-mediated phosphorylation of ATR promotes recruitment of XPA to UV-induced DNA damage. Mol Cell 54:999–1011

Jarrett SG, Wolf Horrell EM, Boulanger MC, D'orazio JA (2015) Defining the contribution of MC1R physiological ligands to ATR phosphorylation at Ser435, a predictor of DNA repair in melanocytes. J Invest Dermatol 135:3086–3095

Jimbow K, Fitzpatrick TB (1975) Changes in distribution patterns of cytoplasmic filaments in human melanocytes during ultraviolet-mediated melanin pigmentation. J Cell Biol 65:481–488

Kadekaro AL, Kavanagh R, Kanto H, Terzieva S, Hauser J, Kobayashi N, Schwemberger S, Cornelius J, Babcock G, Shertzer HG et al (2005) alpha-Melanocortin and endothelin-1 activate antiapoptotic pathways and reduce DNA damage in human melanocytes. Cancer Res 65:4292–4299

Kadekaro AL, Leachman S, Kavanagh RJ, Swope V, Cassidy P, Supp D, Sartor M, Schwemberger S, Babcock G, Wakamatsu K et al (2010) Melanocortin 1 receptor genotype: an important determinant of the damage response of melanocytes to ultraviolet radiation. FASEB J 24:3850–3860

Kauser S, Schallreuter KU, Thody AJ, Gummer C, Tobin DJ (2003) Regulation of human epidermal melanocyte biology by beta-endorphin. J Invest Dermatol 120:1073–1080

Kennedy C, Ter Huurne J, Berkhout M, Gruis N, Bastiaens M, Bergman W, Willemze R, Bouwes Bavinck JN (2001) Melanocortin 1 receptor (*MC1R*) gene variants are associated with an increased risk for cutaneous melanoma which is largely independent of skin type and hair color. J Invest Dermatol 117:294–300

Khaled M, Levy C, Fisher DE (2010) Control of melanocyte differentiation by a MITF-PDE4D3 homeostatic circuit. Genes Dev 24:2276–2281

Khlgatian MK, Hadshiew IM, Asawanonda P, Yaar M, Eller MS, Fujita M, Norris DA, Gilchrest BA (2002) Tyrosinase gene expression is regulated by p53. J Invest Dermatol 118:126–132

Kim JY, Shin JY, Kim MR, Hann SK, Oh SH (2012) siRNA-mediated knock-down of COX-2 in melanocytes suppresses melanogenesis. Exp Dermatol 21:420–425

Kim YI, Park SW, Shin MK, Lee MH (2015) Activin suppresses LPS-induced toll-like receptor, cytokine and inducible nitric oxide synthase expression in normal melanocytes by inhibiting NFκB and MAPK pathway activation. Int J Mol Med 1165–1172

Kobayashi N, Nakagawa A, Muramatsu T, Yamashina Y, Shirai T, Hashimoto MW, Ishigaki Y, Ohnishi T, Mori T (1998) Supranuclear melanin caps reduce ultraviolet induced DNA photoproducts in human epidermis. J Invest Dermatol 110:806–810

Kock A, Schwarz T, Kirnbauer R, Urbanski A, Perry P, Ansel JC, Luger TA (1990) Human keratinocytes are a source for tumor necrosis factor α: evidence for synthesis and release upon stimulation with endotoxin or ultraviolet light. J Exp Med 172:1609–1614

Kokot A, Metze D, Mouchet N, Galibert MD, Schiller M, Luger TA, Bohm M (2009) Alpha-melanocyte-stimulating hormone counteracts the suppressive effect of UVB on Nrf2 and Nrf-dependent gene expression in human skin. Endocrinology 150:3197–3206

Krivosheya D, Tapia L, Levinson JN, Huang K, Kang Y, Hines R, Ting AK, Craig AM, Mei L, Bamji SX et al (2008) ErbB4-neuregulin signaling modulates synapse development and dendritic arborization through distinct mechanisms. J Biol Chem 283:32944–32956
Krude H, Biebermann H, Luck W, Horn R, Brabant G, Gruters A (1998) Severe early-onset obesity, adrenal insufficiency and red hair pigmentation caused by *POMC* mutations in humans. Nat Genet 19:155–157
Kupper TS, Chua AO, Flood P, Mcguire J, Gubler U (1987) Interleukin 1 gene expression in cultured human keratinocytes is augmented by ultraviolet irradiation. J Clin Invest 80:430–436
Landi MT, Kanetsky PA, Tsang S, Gold B, Munroe D, Rebbeck T, Swoyer J, Ter-Minassian M, Hedayati M, Grossman L et al (2005) MC1R, ASIP, and DNA repair in sporadic and familial melanoma in a Mediterranean population. J Natl Cancer Inst 97:998–1007
Levine N, Sheftel SN, Eytan T, Dorr RT, Hadley ME, Weinrach JC, Ertl GA, Toth K, Hruby VJ (1991) Induction of skin tanning by the subcutaneous administration of a potent synthetic melanotropin. JAMA 266:2730–2736
Levy C, Khaled M, Robinson KC, Veguilla RA, Chen PH, Yokoyama S, Makino E, Lu J, Larue L, Beermann F et al (2010) Lineage-specific transcriptional regulation of DICER by MITF in melanocytes. Cell 141:994–1005
Li G, Satyamoorthy K, Herlyn M (2001) N-cadherin-mediated intercellular interactions promote survival and migration of melanoma cells. Cancer Res 61:3819–3825
Lim HW, Grimes PE, Agbai O, Hamzavi I, Henderson M, Haddican M, Linkner RV, Lebwohl M (2015) Afamelanotide and narrowband UV-B phototherapy for the treatment of vitiligo: a randomized multicenter trial. JAMA Dermatol 151:42–50
Liu Z-G, Baskaran R, Lea-Chou ET, Wood LD, Chen Y, Karin M, Wang JYJ (1996) Three distinct signalling responses by murine fibroblasts to genotoxic stress. Nature 384:273–276
Lubbe J, Reichel M, Burg G, Kleihues P (1994) Absence of p53 gene mutations in cutaneous melanoma. J Invest Dermatol 102:819–821
Ma HJ, Ma HY, Yang Y, Li PC, Zi SX, Jia CY, Chen R (2014) alpha-Melanocyte stimulating hormone (MSH) and prostaglandin E2 (PGE2) drive melanosome transfer by promoting filopodia delivery and shedding spheroid granules: evidences from atomic force microscopy observation. J Dermatol Sci 76:222–230
Marconi A, Terracina M, Fila C, Franchi J, Bonte F, Romagnoli G, Maurelli R, Failla CM, Dumas M, Pincelli C (2003) Expression and function of neurotrophins and their receptors in cultured human keratinocytes. J Invest Dermatol 121:1515–1521
Maresca V, Flori E, Bellei B, Aspite N, Kovacs D, Picardo M (2010) MC1R stimulation by alpha-MSH induces catalase and promotes its re-distribution to the cell periphery and dendrites. Pigment Cell Melanoma Res 23:263–275
Marrot L, Belaidi JP, Jones C, Perez P, Meunier JR (2005) Molecular responses to stress induced in normal human caucasian melanocytes in culture by exposure to simulated solar UV. Photochem Photobiol 81:367–375
Matsumoto K, Tajima H, Nakamura T (1991) Hepatocyte growth factor is a potent stimulator of human melanocyte DNA synthesis and growth. Biochem Biophys Res Commun 176:45–51
Mcgill GG, Horstmann M, Widlund HR, Du J, Motyckova G, Nishimura EK, Lin Y-L, Ramaswamy S, Avery W, Ding H-F et al (2002) Bcl2 regulation by the melanocyte master regulator Mitf modulates lineage survival and melanoma cell viability. Cell 109:707–718
Mcgowan KA, Li JZ, Park CY, Beaudry V, Tabor HK, Sabnis AJ, Zhang W, Fuchs H, De Angelis MH, Myers RM et al (2008) Ribosomal mutations cause p53-mediated dark skin and pleiotropic effects. Nat Genet 40:963–970
Medrano EE, Im S, Yang F, Abdel-Malek Z (1995) UVB light induces G1 arrest in human melanocytes by prolonged inhibition of pRb phosphorylation associated with long term expression of the protein $p21^{Waf-1/SDI/Cip-1}$ protein. Cancer Res 55:4047–4052
Mitra D, Luo X, Morgan A, Wang J, Hoang MP, Lo J, Guerrero CR, Lennerz JK, Mihm MC, Wargo JA et al (2012) An ultraviolet-radiation-independent pathway to melanoma carcinogenesis in the red hair/fair skin background. Nature 491:449–453
Morelli JG, Yohn JJ, Lyons MB, Murphy RC, Norris DA (1989) Leukotrienes C_4 and D_4 as potent mitogens for cultured human melanocytes. J Invest Dermatol 93:719–722

Mountjoy KG, Robbins LS, Mortrud MT, Cone RD (1992) The cloning of a family of genes that encode the melanocortin receptors. Science 257:1248–1251

Murase D, Hachiya A, Amano Y, Ohuchi A, Kitahara T, Takema Y (2009) The essential role of p53 in hyperpigmentation of the skin via regulation of paracrine melanogenic cytokine receptor signaling. J Biol Chem 284:4343–4353

Newton Bishop JA, Bishop DT (2005) The genetics of susceptibility to cutaneous melanoma. Drugs Today (Barc) 41:193–203

Nicolaou A, Estdale SE, Tsatmali M, Herrero DP, Thody AJ (2004) Prostaglandin production by melanocytic cells and the effect of alpha-melanocyte stimulating hormone. FEBS Lett 570:223–226

Nudi M, Ouimette JF, Drouin J (2005) Bone morphogenic protein (Smad)-mediated repression of proopiomelanocortin transcription by interference with Pitx/Tpit activity. Mol Endocrinol 19:1329–1342

Nylander K, Bourdon J-C, Bray SE, Gibbs NK, Kay R, Hart I, Hall PA (2000) Transcriptional activation of tyrosinase and TRP-1 by p53 links UV irradiation to the protective tanning response. J Pathol 190:39–46

Ono K, Han J (2000) The p38 signal transduction pathway. Activation and function. Cell Signal 12:1–13

Otsuka T, Takayama H, Sharp R, Celli G, Larochelle WJ, Bottaro DP, Ellmore N, Vieira W, Owens JW, Anver M et al (1998) c-Met autocrine activation induces development of malignant melanoma and acquisition of the metastatic phenotype. Cancer Res 58:5157–5167

Palmer JS, Duffy DL, Box NF, Aitken JF, O'gorman LE, Green AC, Hayward NK, Martin NG, Sturm RA (2000) Melanocortin-1 receptor polymorphisms and risk of melanoma: is the association explained solely by pigmentation phenotype? Am J Hum Genet 66:176–186

Park HY, Wu C, Yaar M, Stachur CM, Kosmadaki M, Gilchrest BA (2009) Role of BMP-4 and its signaling pathways in cultured human melanocytes. Int J Cell Biol 2009:750482

Pasterkamp RJ, Peschon JJ, Spriggs MK, Kolodkin AL (2003) Semaphorin 7A promotes axon outgrowth through integrins and MAPKs. Nature 424:398–405

Pathak MA (1991) Ultraviolet radiation and the development of non-melanoma and melanoma skin cancer: clinical and experimental evidence. Skin Pharmacol 4(Suppl 1):85–94

Pathak MA, Jimbow K, Fitzpatrick T (1980) Photobiology of pigment cell. In: Seiji M (ed) Phenotypic expression in pigment cells. University of Tokyo Press, Tokyo, pp 655–670

Pawelek J, Wong G, Sansone M, Morowitz J (1973) Molecular biology of pigment cells: molecular controls in mammalian pigmentation. Yale J Biol Med 46:430–443

Pittelkow MR, Shipley GD (1989) Serum-free culture of normal human melanocytes: growth kinetics and growth factor requirements. J Cell Physiol 140:565–576

Plettenberg A, Ballaun C, Pammer J, Mildner M, Strunk D, Weninger W, Tschachler E (1995) Human melanocytes and melanoma cells constitutively express the bcl-2 proto-oncogene in situ and in cell culture. Am J Pathol 146:651–659

Premi S, Wallisch S, Mano CM, Weiner AB, Bacchiocchi A, Wakamatsu K, Bechara EJ, Halaban R, Douki T, Brash DE (2015) Photochemistry. Chemiexcitation of melanin derivatives induces DNA photoproducts long after UV exposure. Science 347:842–847

Price ER, Horstmann MA, Wells AG, Weilbaecher KN, Takemoto CM, Landis MW, Fisher DE (1998) α-Melanocyte-stimulating hormone signaling regulates expression of *microphthalmia*, a gene deficient in Waardenburg syndrome. J Biol Chem 273:33042–33047

Puffenberger EG, Hosoda K, Washington SS, Nakao K, Dewit D, Yanagisawa M, Chakravarti A (1994) A missense mutation of the endothelin-B receptor gene in multigenic Hirschsprung's disease. Cell 79:1257–1266

Quevedo WC Jr, Szabo G, Virks J (1969) Influence of age and UV on the population of DOPA-positive melanocytes in human skin. J Invest Dermatol 52:287–290

Robbins LS, Nadeau JH, Johnson KR, Kelly MA, Roselli-Rehfuss L, Baack E, Mountjoy KG, Cone RD (1993) Pigmentation phenotypes of variant extension locus alleles result from point mutations that alter MSH receptor function. Cell 72:827–834

Rokos H, Beazley WD, Schallreuter KU (2002) Oxidative stress in vitiligo: photo-oxidation of pterins produces H(2)O(2) and pterin-6-carboxylic acid. Biochem Biophys Res Commun 292:805–811

Romero-Graillet C, Aberdam E, Biagoli N, Massabni W, Ortonne JP, Ballotti R (1996) Ultraviolet B radiation acts through the nitric oxide and cGMP signal transduction pathway to stimulate melanogenesis in human melanocytes. J Biol Chem 271:28052–28056
Romero-Graillet C, Aberdam E, Clement M, Ortonne JP, Ballotti R (1997) Nitric oxide produced by ultraviolet-irradiated keratinocytes stimulates melanogenesis. J Clin Invest 99:635–642
Rosette C, Karin M (1996) Ultraviolet light and osmotic stress: activation of the JNK cascade through multiple growth factor and cytokine receptors. Science 274:1194–1197
Sakai C, Ollmann M, Kobayashi T, Abdel-Malek Z, Muller J, Vieira WD, Imokawa G, Barsh GS, Hearing VJ (1997) Modulation of murine melanocyte function *in vitro* by agouti signal protein. EMBO J 16:3544–3552
Sato Y, Takahashi H (1998) Molecular cloning and expression of murine homologue of semaphorin K1 gene. Biochim Biophys Acta 1443:419–422
Scott G, Deng A, Rodriguez-Burford C, Seiberg M, Han R, Babiarz L, Grizzle W, Bell W, Pentland A (2001) Protease-activated receptor 2, a receptor involved in melanosome transfer, is upregulated in human skin by ultraviolet irradiation. J Invest Dermatol 117:1412–1420
Scott MC, Wakamatsu K, Ito S, Kadekaro AL, Kobayashi N, Groden J, Kavanagh R, Takakuwa T, Virador V, Hearing VJ et al (2002) Human *melanocortin 1 receptor* variants, receptor function and melanocyte response to UV radiation. J Cell Sci 115:2349–2355
Scott G, Leopardi S, Parker L, Babiarz L, Seiberg M, Han R (2003) The proteinase-activated receptor-2 mediates phagocytosis in a Rho-dependent manner in human keratinocytes. J Invest Dermatol 121:529–541
Scott G, Jacobs S, Leopardi S, Anthony FA, Learn D, Malaviya R, Pentland A (2005) Effects of PGF2alpha on human melanocytes and regulation of the FP receptor by ultraviolet radiation. Exp Cell Res 304:407–416
Scott GA, Mcclelland LA, Fricke AF (2008) Semaphorin 7a promotes spreading and dendricity in human melanocytes through beta1-integrins. J Invest Dermatol 128:151–161
Seiberg M, Paine C, Sharlow E, Costanzo M, Andrade-Gordon P, Eisinger M, Shapiro SS (2000) The protease-activated receptor-2 regulates pigmentation via keratinocyte-melanocyte interactions. Exp Cell Res 254:25–32
Sharov AA, Fessing M, Atoyan R, Sharova TY, Haskell-Luevano C, Weiner L, Funa K, Brissette JL, Gilchrest BA, Botchkarev VA (2005) Bone morphogenetic protein (BMP) signaling controls hair pigmentation by means of cross-talk with the melanocortin receptor-1 pathway. Proc Natl Acad Sci U S A 102:93–98
Siracusa LD (1994) The *agouti* gene: turned on to yellow. Trends Genet 10:423–428
Slominski A (1998) Identification of beta-endorphin, alpha-MSH and ACTH peptides in cultured human melanocytes, melanoma and squamous cell carcinoma cells by RP-HPLC. Exp Dermatol 7:213–216
Slominski A, Ermak G, Hwang J, Chakraborty A, Mazurkiewicz JE, Mihm M (1995) Proopiomelanocortin, corticotropin releasing hormone and corticotropin releasing hormone receptor genes are expressed in human skin. FEBS Lett 374:113–116
Slominski A, Zbytek B, Szczesniewski A, Semak I, Kaminski J, Sweatman T, Wortsman J (2005) CRH stimulation of corticosteroids production in melanocytes is mediated by ACTH. Am J Physiol Endocrinol Metab 288:E701–E706
Smit NPM, Vink AA, Kolb RM, Steenwinkel M-JST, Van Den Berg PTM, Van Nieuwpoort F, Roza L, Pavel S (2001) Melanin offers protection against induction of cyclobutane pyrimidine dimers and 6–4 photoproducts by UVB in cultured human melanocytes. Photochem Photobiol 74:424–430
Smith R, Healy E, Siddiqui S, Flanagan N, Steijlen PM, Rosdahl I, Jacques JP, Rogers S, Turner R, Jackson IJ et al (1998) Melanocortin 1 receptor variants in Irish population. J Invest Dermatol 111:119–122
Smith AG, Luk N, Newton RA, Roberts DW, Sturm RA, Muscat GE (2008) Melanocortin-1 receptor signaling markedly induces the expression of the NR4A nuclear receptor subgroup in melanocytic cells. J Biol Chem 283:12564–12570

Song X, Mosby N, Yang J, Xu A, Abdel-Malek Z, Kadekaro AL (2009) alpha-MSH activates immediate defense responses to UV-induced oxidative stress in human melanocytes. Pigment Cell Melanoma Res 22:809–818

Sosman JA, Margolin KA (2009) Inside life of melanoma cell signaling, molecular insights, and therapeutic targets. Curr Oncol Rep 11:405–411

Starner RJ, Mcclelland L, Abdel-Malek Z, Fricke A, Scott G (2010) PGE(2) is a UVR-inducible autocrine factor for human melanocytes that stimulates tyrosinase activation. Exp Dermatol 19:682–684

Stefanato CM, Yaar M, Bhawan J, Phillips TJ, Kosmadaki MG, Botchkarev V, Gilchrest BA (2003) Modulations of nerve growth factor and Bcl-2 in ultraviolet-irradiated human epidermis. J Cutan Pathol 30:351–357

Steingrimsson E, Copeland NG, Jenkins NA (2004) Melanocytes and the microphthalmia transcription factor network. Annu Rev Genet 38:365–411

Stratigos AJ, Dimisianos G, Nikolaou V, Poulou M, Sypsa V, Stefanaki I, Papadopoulos O, Polydorou D, Plaka M, Christofidou E et al (2006) Melanocortin receptor-1 gene polymorphisms and the risk of cutaneous melanoma in a low-risk southern European population. J Invest Dermatol 126:1842–1849

Suzuki I, Cone R, Im S, Nordlund J, Abdel-Malek Z (1996) Binding of melanotropic hormones to the melanocortin receptor MC1R on human melanocytes stimulates proliferation and melanogenesis. Endocrinology 137:1627–1633

Suzuki I, Tada A, Ollmann MM, Barsh GS, Im S, Lamoreux ML, Hearing VJ, Nordlund J, Abdel-Malek ZA (1997) Agouti signaling protein inhibits melanogenesis and the response of human melanocytes to α-melanotropin. J Invest Dermatol 108:838–842

Suzuki I, Kato T, Motokawa T, Tomita Y, Nakamura E, Katagiri T (2002) Increase of pro-opiomelanocortin mRNA prior to tyrosinase, tyrosinase-related protein 1, dopachrome tautomerase, Pmel-17/gp100, and P-protein mRNA in human skin after ultraviolet B irradiation. J Invest Dermatol 118:73–78

Swope V, Alexander C, Starner R, Schwemberger S, Babcock G, Abdel-Malek ZA (2014) Significance of the melanocortin 1 receptor in the DNA damage response of human melanocytes to ultraviolet radiation. Pigment Cell Melanoma Res 27:601–610

Swope VB, Abdel-Malek ZA, Kassem L, Nordlund JJ (1991) Interleukins 1α and 6 and tumor necrosis factor-α are paracrine inhibitors of human melanocyte proliferation and melanogenesis. J Invest Dermatol 96:180–185

Swope VB, Sauder DN, Mckenzie RC, Sramkoski RM, Krug KA, Babcock GF, Nordlund JJ, Abdel-Malek ZA (1994) Synthesis of interleukin-1α and β by normal human melanocytes. J Invest Dermatol 102:749–753

Swope VB, Medrano EE, Smalara D, Abdel-Malek Z (1995a) Long-term proliferation of human melanocytes is supported by the physiologic mitogens α-melanotropin, endothelin-1, and basic fibroblast growth factor. Exp Cell Res 217:453–459

Swope VB, Medrano EE, Smalara D, Abdel-Malek ZA (1995b) Long-term proliferation of human melanocytes is supported by the physiologic mitogens alpha-melanotropin, endothelin-1, and basic fibroblast growth factor. Exp Cell Res 217:453–459

Swope VB, Jameson JA, Mcfarland KL, Supp DM, Miller WE, Mcgraw DW, Patel MA, Nix MA, Millhauser GL, Babcock GF et al (2012) Defining MC1R regulation in human melanocytes by its agonist alpha-melanocortin and antagonists agouti signaling protein and beta-defensin 3. J Invest Dermatol 132(9):2255–2262

Szabo G (1954) The number of melanocytes in human epidermis. Br Med J 1:1016–1017

Tachibana M (1999) Sound needs sound melanocytes to be heard. Pigment Cell Res 12:344–354

Tada A, Suzuki I, Im S, Davis MB, Cornelius J, Babcock G, Nordlund JJ, Abdel-Malek ZA (1998a) Endothelin-1 is a paracrine growth factor that modulates melanogenesis of human melanocytes and participates in their responses to ultraviolet radiation. Cell Growth Differ Mol Biol J Am Assoc Cancer Res 9:575–584

Tada A, Suzuki I, Im S, Davis MB, Cornelius J, Babcock G, Nordlund JJ, Abdel-Malek ZA (1998b) Endothelin-1 is a paracrine growth factor that modulates melanogenesis of human melanocytes and participates in their responses to ultraviolet radiation. Cell Growth Differ 9:575–584

Tada A, Pereira E, Beitner Johnson D, Kavanagh R, Abdel-Malek ZA (2002) Mitogen and ultraviolet-B-induced signaling pathways in normal human melanocytes. J Invest Dermatol 118:316–322

Tadokoro T, Kobayashi N, Zmudzka BZ, Ito S, Wakamatsu K, Yamaguchi Y, Korossy KS, Miller SA, Beer JZ, Hearing VJ (2003) UV-induced DNA damage and melanin content in human skin differing in racial/ethnic origin. FASEB J 17:1177–1179

Tamagnone L, Artigiani S, Chen H, He Z, Ming GI, Song H, Chedotal A, Winberg ML, Goodman CS, Poo M et al (1999) Plexins are a large family of receptors for transmembrane, secreted, and GPI-anchored semaphorins in vertebrates. Cell 99:71–80

Thody AJ, Ridley K, Penny RJ, Chalmers R, Fisher C, Shuster S (1983) MSH peptides are present in mammalian skin. Peptides 4:813–816

Tsatmali M, Graham A, Szatkowski D, Ancans J, Manning P, Mcneil CJ, Graham AM, Thody AJ (2000) α-Melanocyte-stimulating hormone modulates nitric oxide production in melanocytes. J Invest Dermatol 114:520–526

Von Koschembahr AM, Swope VB, Starner RJ, Abdel-Malek ZA (2015) Endothelin-1 protects human melanocytes from UV-induced DNA damage by activating JNK and p38 signaling pathways. Exp Dermatol 24:269–274

Wakamatsu K, Graham A, Cook D, Thody AJ (1997) Characterization of ACTH peptides in human skin and their activation of the melanocortin-1 receptor. Pigment Cell Res 10:288–297

Wakamatsu K, Kavanagh R, Kadekaro AL, Terzieva S, Strum RA, Leachman S, Abdel-Malek ZA, Ito S (2006) Diversity of pigmentation in cultured human melanocytes is due to differences in the type as well as quantity of melanin. Pigment Cell Res 19:154–162

Wang Z, Coleman DJ, Bajaj G, Liang X, Ganguli-Indra G, Indra AK (2011) RXRalpha ablation in epidermal keratinocytes enhances UVR-induced DNA damage, apoptosis, and proliferation of keratinocytes and melanocytes. J Invest Dermatol 131(1):177–187

Wu M, Hemesath T, Takemoto CM, Horstmann MA, Wells AG, Price ER, Fisher DZ, Fisher DE (2000) c-Kit triggers dual phosphorylations, which couple activation and degradation of the essential melanocyte factor Mi. Genes Dev 14:301–312

Yaar M, Grossman K, Eller M, Gilchrest BA (1991) Evidence for nerve growth factor-mediated paracrine effects in human epidermis. J Cell Biol 115:821–828

Yaar M, Eller MS, Dibenedetto P, Reenstra WR, Zhai S, Mcquiad T, Archambault M, Gilchrest BA (1994) The trk family of receptors mediates nerve growth factor and neurotrophin-3 effects in melanocytes. J Clin Invest 94:1550–1562

Yaar M, Wu C, Park HY, Panova I, Schutz G, Gilchrest BA (2006) Bone morphogenetic protein-4, a novel modulator of melanogenesis. J Biol Chem 281:25307–25314

Yada Y, Higuchi K, Imokawa G (1991) Effects of endothelins on signal transduction and proliferation in human melanocytes. J Biol Chem 266:18352–18357

Yajima I, Larue L (2008) The location of heart melanocytes is specified and the level of pigmentation in the heart may correlate with coat color. Pigment Cell Melanoma Res 21:471–476

Yazdani U, Terman JR (2006) The semaphorins. Genome Biol 7:211

Yohn JJ, Morelli JG, Walchak SJ, Rundell KB, Norris DA, Zamora MR (1993) Cultured human keratinocytes synthesize and secrete endothelin-1. J Invest Dermatol 100:23–26

Zayed AA, Khorshied MM, Hussein MF (2015) Inducible nitric oxide synthase promoter polymorphism: a molecular susceptibility marker for vitiligo in Egyptians. Int J Dermatol 54:675–679

Zhai S, Yaar M, Doyle S, Gilchrest B (1996) Nerve growth factor rescues pigment cells from ultaviolet-induced apoptosis by upregulating BCL-2 levels. Exp Cell Res 224:335–343

Melanoma Epidemiology

3

Marianne Berwick

3.1 Introduction

The incidence of cutaneous melanoma is steadily increasing, mainly in populations of European origin and is thus an important public health issue throughout the world. The pattern of mortality varies by country, age, and sex. In general, older males continue to have an increase in mortality, while younger males and females have a downward trend. This chapter reviews these trends and suggests a perspective. The chapter covers worldwide incidence and mortality patterns, the relationship of host characteristics to incidence and mortality, and the relationship of environmental factors to risk.

3.2 Rates and Trends

Incidence rates for melanoma have continued to increase since 1960 through 2016 and are highest among the developed countries with some potential increases among developing countries (Table 3.1), pointing to either a change in behavior, a change in screening, or a combination of both. Among non-Caucasian populations, incidence rates are relatively low and quite variable (see Fig. 3.1). World rates vary between a low of 0.2 per 100,000 among females in India to 55.8 per 100,000 among males in Queensland, Australia. Note that rates in this chapter are standardized to the world population, which is generally younger than the populations in developed countries, and so when evaluating rates, it is important to understand the population used for standardization. Thus, for the same time period, the Queensland Cancer Council cites melanoma rates in Queensland among males as 76.4, but this is standardized to the Australian population.

M. Berwick
Department of Internal Medicine, University of New Mexico,
MSC10-5550, Albuquerque, NM 87131-0001, USA
e-mail: mberwick@salud.unm.edu

A. Bosserhoff (ed.), *Melanoma Development*,
DOI 10.1007/978-3-319-41319-8_3

Table 3.1 Rates for age-standardized[a] melanoma incidence (per 100,000; IARC, 2012, Cancer Incidence in Five Continents, Volume X), both sexes, by level of development

Population	Number	Age-standardized rate
World population	232,130	3.0
More developed regions	191,066	9.6
Less developed regions	41,064	0.8

[a]Standardized to the anticipated world population, 2012

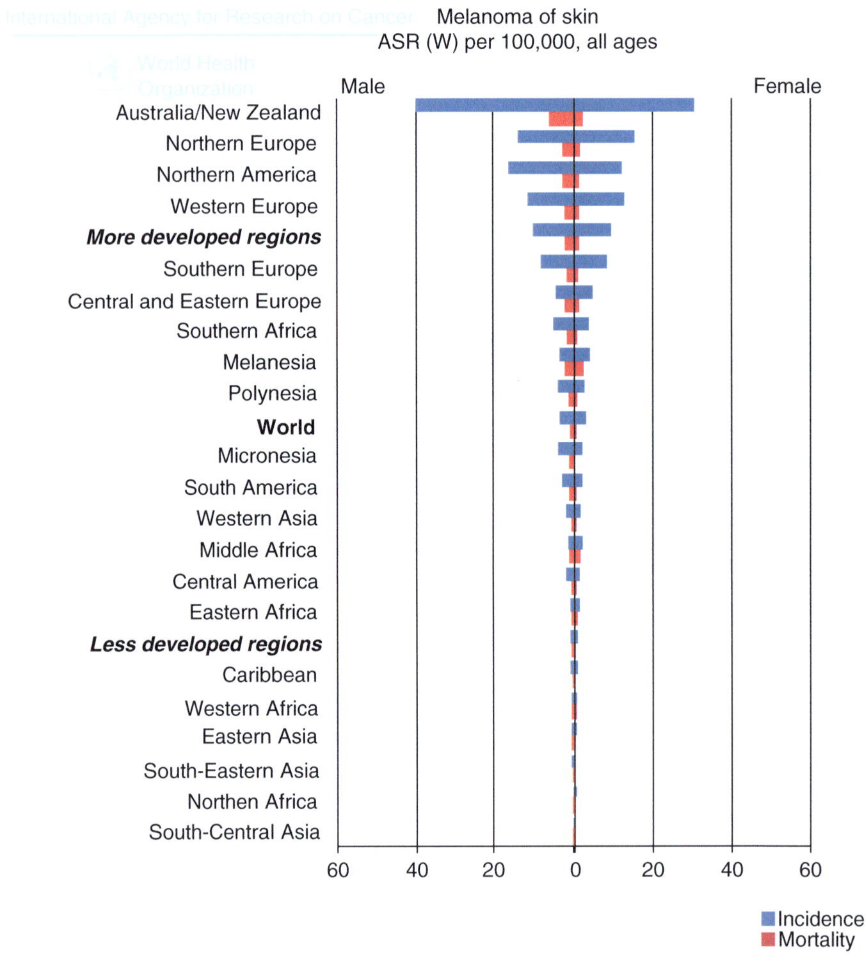

Fig. 3.1 Age standardized incidence and mortality rates of melanoma throughout the world (standardized to the world population)

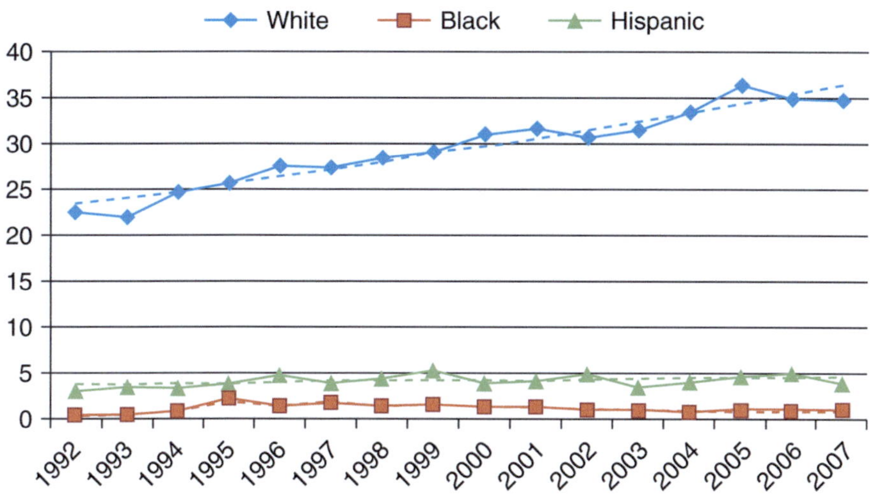

Fig. 3.2 Incidence rates for melanoma among males in the US SEER sites

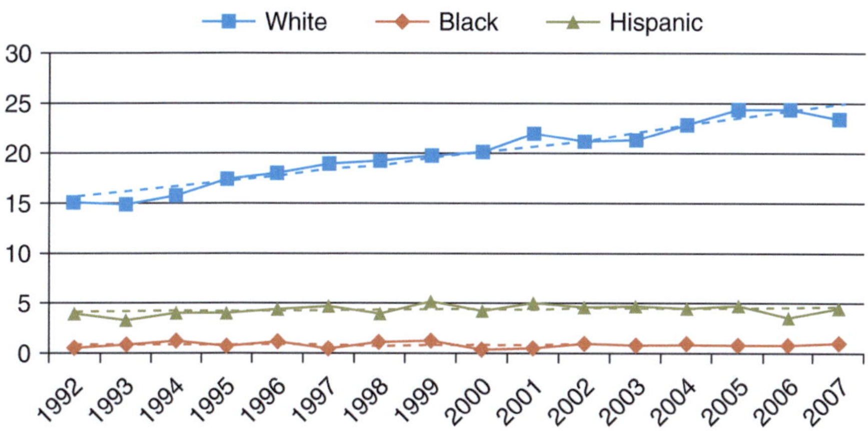

Fig. 3.3 Incidence rates for melanoma among females in the US SEER sites

Melanoma is notable for higher rates among non-Hispanic whites and this is noted in the USA Surveillance, Epidemiology, and End Results (SEER) registries, where the rates for white males are 28/100,000 and white females 17.8/100,000 compared to rates for Hispanic white males of 4.4/100,000 and 4.2/100,000 for Hispanic white females (Guy et al. 2015) (see Figs. 3.2 and 3.3).

Several recent analyses have reported on increasing incidence rates among Hispanics in California and Florida (Cockburn et al. 2006; Rouhani et al. 2010; Clairwood et al. 2014). However, although both groups represent a large proportion of the NCI SEER (Surveillance, Epidemiology, and End Results) analytic group, the overall the age-adjusted melanoma incidence rates do not reflect an increase overall among those who are identified as Hispanic, in either males or females.

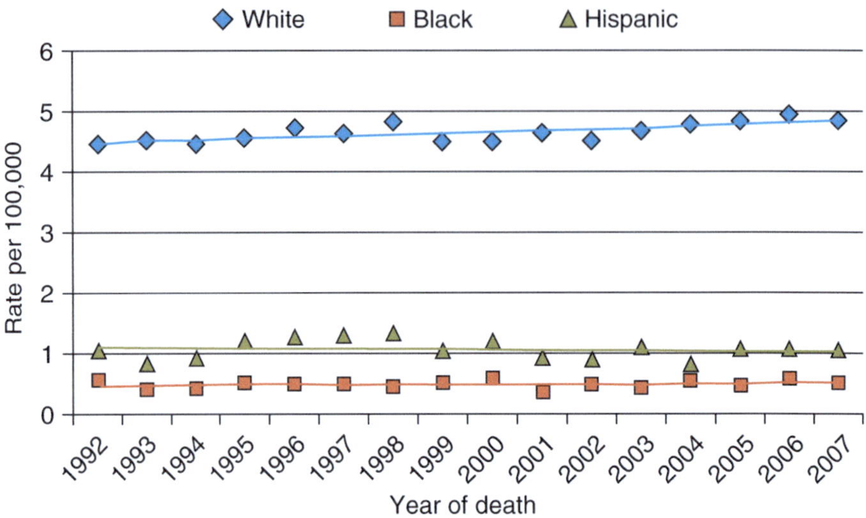

Fig. 3.4 Mortality rates for melanoma among males in the US SEER sites

When melanoma is identified among racial/ethnic groups other than whites, it is often at a deeper Breslow thickness and more advanced stage. This may be due to a lack of awareness of melanoma risk among these groups. Unfortunately, but logically, most risk models (Olsen et al. 2015) and melanoma awareness campaigns have been developed for white subjects, those at highest risk.

Mortality due to melanoma has continued to increase among white males worldwide; however, this may be focused on males over the age of 65. Over three decades (1969–1999), mortality rates from melanoma increased 157 % in men aged 65 and older (Geller et al. 2002) (Fig. 3.4). There has been a trend toward a plateau among females as noted in both the Australian data and the US data (Fig. 3.5). Unfortunately, this trend is not evident worldwide. In the UK, for example, the increase in mortality among women is continuing at a slower rate.

A thoughtful analysis by Erickson and Driscoll (2010) suggests that the discrepancy between a rapid increase in incidence and slower increase in mortality in combination with the increase in thick minimally invasive melanomas relative to thicker melanomas may be the result of intensive surveillance and a concomitantly increased biopsy rate, or "over-diagnosis" (suggested by Welch and Black 2010). Over-diagnosis can be noted when the curve for incidence is relatively steep and that for mortality is flat or relatively so. This situation exists in Australia and the United States, although mortality is not actually flat among the older age groups but is continuing to increase. Such an analysis is supported by Cho et al. (2014) but not by Shaikh et al. (2016) or Criscione and Weinstock (2010). The difference appears to lie in an emphasis by Shaikh et al. on tumor thickness, whereas Cho et al. focus on the pattern of increased 5-year survival (as with kidney and thyroid cancer) accompanied by increased incidence, but no change in mortality. Other projections suggest that incidence and mortality is declining from

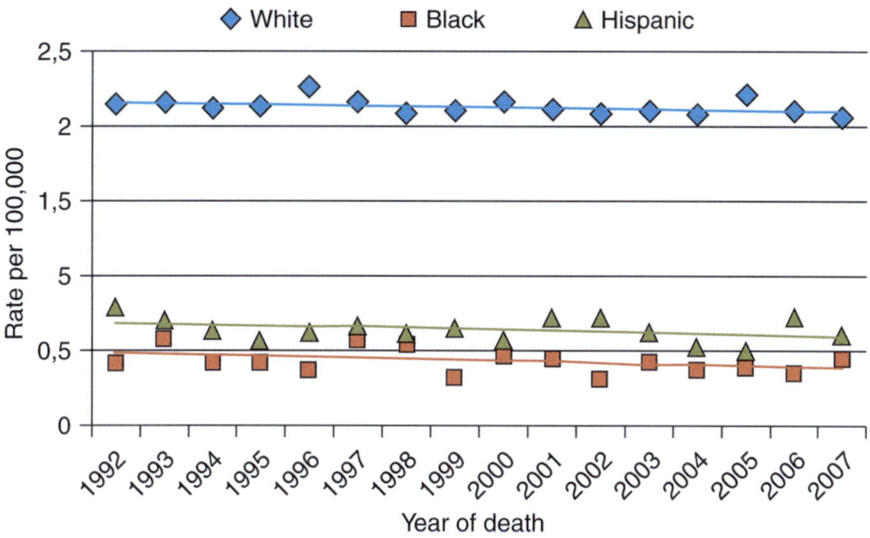

Fig. 3.5 Mortality rates for melanoma among females in the US SEER sites

melanoma (Guy et al. 2015 [mortality]; Autier et al. 2015; and among children and adolescents, Campbell et al. 2015).

In addition, there has been an approximately doubling of in situ tumors between 1988 and 2006. Until we are able to distinguish the faster growing, more aggressive tumors that are likely to lead to death from the more slowly growing tumor that may never cause problems, we will not be able to address this issue in a way to improve public health. Several investigators (Liu et al. 2006; Grob et al. 2002) have made attempts at evaluating these aggressive tumors from more slowly growing tumors; however, these methods are not yet standard and are unlikely to be applied globally.

Years of life lost (YLL) is a particularly salient method for estimating the burden of melanoma on a population. Thiam et al. (2015) estimated the highest YLL in Australia (19.9 years for males, 22.7 years for females) while Brazil appeared to have the lowest estimate (17.2 YLL for males and 19.0 for females).

3.3 Host Factors

3.3.1 Age and Sex

Lachiewicz and colleagues (2008) describe melanoma as a heterogeneous cancer with tumors with different biological mechanisms having different survival patterns. In an analysis of age-specific incidence rates, it is clear that there are two peaks of incidence in melanoma, one at 54 years and one at 74 years, with truncal melanoma peaking earlier and melanoma of the face and ears peaking later. The

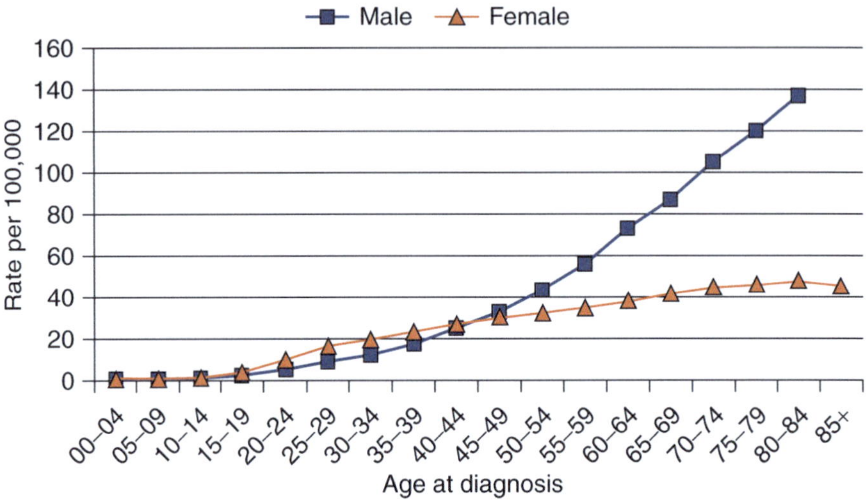

Fig. 3.6 Age at diagnosis for males (*blue squares*) and females (*red triangles*) in the US

median age of melanoma diagnosis overall ranges between 57 and 62 years. Unfortunately, melanoma among young women has been recently increasing in the US and is currently the cancer with the highest incidence among young women aged 15–24 (Purdue et al. 2008), and the site with the highest incidence is the trunk (Bradford et al. 2010). In the US, the age-specific incidence of melanoma among young women has generally been higher than that of males under the age of 40.

This pattern of the age-specific melanoma incidence is quite distinct for males and females, with a higher incidence among females up to the age of 45–50 when the age-specific rate for males climbs steeply while that for females continues to increase at a far slower rate. A "Clemmensen's hook" has been described for melanoma incidence, a similar pattern as seen in breast cancer, where there is a change in the slope of incidence near menopause, indicating a potential role for female hormones in the etiology of the disease (Fig. 3.6). It should be pointed out that while Australia's melanoma incidence rates are approximately three times those in the US, they are approximately nine times those in Ireland (Table 3.1). This statistic is rather startling and underlines the critical importance of the mixture of phenotype and intense solar exposure in Australia where much of the population migrated from Ireland and the UK. Given the great difference in incidence rates, the similarity of the age-specific rates between the US and Australia is all the more striking.

While sex differences in incidence are obvious, there are also differences in survival which are less clear (Crocetti et al. 2015) with women having a 34 % reduced risk of dying from melanoma compared to men. Biological, environmental, and behavioral factors underlie the differences (Roh et al. 2015), but more specifically, there is little understood as to precisely how Roh et al. summarize selected studies of the gender difference and find that the adjusted risk estimate for females compared to males ranges from 0.53 (deVries et al. 2008) to 0.84 (Balch et al. 2001).

Overall, female survival is generally better than males at all stages (Khosrotehrani et al 2015) even when controlling for risk factors such as age, thickness, nodal metastasis, distant metastasis, and ulceration.

3.3.2 Melanoma and Pregnancy

Given the survival advantage of females and the presence of a Clemmensen's hook in the incidence rates as well as the consistent pattern of age-specific incidence rates between an area of high incidence (Australia) and moderate incidence (the US), much speculation has focused on the hormonal aspects of melanoma. The role of pregnancy and melanoma incidence and survival has received the most attention. The bulk of evidence amassed over the past half century, however, suggests that pregnancy does not significantly affect the risk of developing malignant melanoma (Kjems and Krag 1993). Further, pregnancy does not appear to adversely influence overall survival from the disease. Results from some studies suggested that pregnant women with melanoma were more likely than their nonpregnant counterparts to exhibit adverse prognostic indicators, specifically, thicker lesions and shorter time to recurrence. Nonetheless, most studies found no difference in overall survival between pregnant and nonpregnant women with melanoma (Byrom et al. 2015). Recent reports from large-scale, population-based studies support these conclusions. Newly discovered estrogen receptors have led to new hypotheses about the role of estrogen in melanoma and these are under intense investigation (de Giorgi et al. 2009).

3.3.3 Body Site

In addition to the distinctly different pattern of incidence between males and females, the anatomic site for the development of melanoma varies distinctively among males and females. Many observers feel that this is due to specific patterns of sun exposure, but a minority think that there may be a sex-linked genetic factor that influences the distribution of melanomas by anatomic site. This conjecture is yet to be proven. In almost every registry in the world, women have a preponderance of melanomas on the leg while males have a majority of melanomas on the trunk. This difference has been modifying over time as women develop more melanomas on the trunk. Lachiewicz et al. (2008) demonstrated, as others have previously, that males and females have different incidences of melanoma on the trunk and head and neck, with the male excess on the trunk occurring at approximately age 54, while the head and neck incidence among males peaks at age 77.

These data are consistent with Whiteman's "divergent pathway" model (Whiteman et al. 2003) where those with an inherently low propensity for melanocyte proliferation require chronic sun exposure to habitually exposed sites, such as the face, to develop melanoma, whereas those with a high propensity for melanocyte proliferation develop melanomas on sites with unstable melanocytes – or aberrant melanogenesis, such as the trunk – with intermittent solar damage.

3.3.4 Pigmentation

As can be noted in Table 3.1, melanoma occurs most often among light-skinned individuals. Melanin type and content of both melanocytes and keratinocytes are critical for determining skin phenotype. Individual photoprotection of the skin is based primarily on the level of constitutive, or genetically determined, pigmentation afforded by the types and amounts of melanin synthesized and distributed in the skin. Constitutive pigmentation of the skin with higher melanin content protects the epidermis from DNA damage (Yamaguchi et al. 2006). The melanocortin 1 receptor (*MC1R*) seems to regulate the activity of melanocytes and thus is a critical genetic factor in melanin synthesis and is discussed in Chap. 2. Other genes, such as *OCA2*, for example, are clearly involved as well (Barón et al. 2014).

Those with light hair, light eyes, and skin that burns easily are at most risk for developing melanoma from ultraviolet (UV) exposure whether it is from the sun or from artificial tanning devices.

Genetics plays a role in risk to any UV and all the factors involved have not yet been determined. Recent publications show that those exposed to solar UV have a wide variety of responses to UV (see Tran et al. 2008) in terms of cellular response to DNA damage, DNA repair capacity (Wei et al. 2003), and vitamin D synthesis due to vitamin D receptor polymorphisms (Orlow et al. 2012), among others.

It is critical to note that individuals with similar levels of constitutive pigmentation may have different responses to UV (Bykov et al. 2000; Wagner et al. 2002). These differences may be due to variation in pigmentation genes. Data from the University of Pennsylvania (Kanetsky et al. 2010) and Australia (Palmer et al. 2000) demonstrate that pigmentary phenotype alone is not an adequate indicator of melanoma risk. Individuals who display darker phenotype characteristics (dark hair, brown eyes, and ability to tan) and who carry any variant *MC1R* alleles show an increased risk for melanoma (Pasquali et al. 2015).

3.3.5 Nevi

An important pigmentary-related factor is nevus density; individuals with many nevi are at consistently higher risk for developing melanoma. In fact, a large number of nevi have been shown to be the strongest known risk factor for developing melanoma among Caucasians (Armstrong and Kricker 2001). Even in the absence of clinically atypical nevi, a very high number of nevi (e.g., more than 100) have been shown to significantly increase risk for melanoma (Huynh et al. 2003). Patients with great many nevi may be missing a genetic checkpoint, the absence of which may permit the development of a higher number of nevi and increase melanoma risk. Nevus density is a simple characteristic that is likely to be useful in determining risk for melanoma among all persons and measuring genetic factors underlying nevus density should improve risk estimation.

There is an apparent interaction between sun exposure and nevus density with regard to the site of the melanoma (Karlsson et al. 2015). For example, in Australia, sex differences in nevus density on the back and lower extremities are similar to sex differences for melanoma – men having higher rates on the back, women having higher rates on the legs – areas that are not chronically exposed to the sun (Green 1992). A similar distribution of nevi and melanoma has been noted (Juhl et al. 2009). Whiteman et al. (2003) have proposed a model for cutaneous melanoma in which two pathways – chronic exposure to the sun and melanocyte instability – represent divergent pathways for developing melanoma. Under this model, people with an inherently low propensity for melanocyte proliferation require chronic sun exposure to drive clonal expansion of transformed epidermal melanocytes. Melanomas arising in this group of people would occur on habitually sun-exposed body sites, such as the face. In contrast, the model would predict that in individuals with an inherently high propensity for melanocyte proliferation (e.g., high nevus counts), exposure to sunlight early in life would be required to start the process of carcinogenesis. These individuals would be expected to develop tumors on body sites with unstable melanocyte populations such as the trunk.

3.3.6 Family History

First-degree relatives of melanoma patients have a higher risk of the disease than individuals without positive family history (Greene and Fraumeni 1979), suggesting that a distinct hereditary component exists. Familial melanoma accounts for an estimated 5–10 % of all cases of melanoma, and characteristics that distinguish the familial from the nonfamilial form of the disease include younger age at first diagnosis, better survival, thinner lesions, multiple primary lesions, and increased occurrence of non-melanoma cancers (Begg et al. 2004; Aguilera et al. 2014). Ford pooled data from eight case–control studies and found that an individual's risk of melanoma increases by about twofold if he has an affected first-degree relative (Ford et al. 1995), and this effect was independent of host factors such as age, nevus count, hair and eye color, and freckling. Familial relative risk remained similar in all of the studies, even though melanoma incidence varied by about ten-fold in the study areas.

3.3.7 Immunologic Factors

A major enigma is that the host immune system is clearly associated with the development and progression of melanoma, but the mechanism by which it does so is not established. In some studies, melanoma incidence increased in frequency and aggressiveness after organ transplantation and immunosuppressive therapy (Vajdic et al. 2009; Dinh and Chong 2007). There is also evidence that immune reactions are altered after UV exposure in the skin (locally) and perhaps throughout the body (systemically) (Murphy et al. 1993; Hersey et al. 1983; Norval 2006). Thus, melanoma represents a unique model for studying the human immune system and the role of vitamin D in coordinating important changes in cancer development. Clearly, the new more effective therapies that target the immune system underscore the importance of the immune system in the development and progression of melanoma (Naidoo et al. 2014).

Some data are available as to how the human immune system may alter during or as a result of UVB radiation exposure (Bechetoille et al. 2007; Muller et al. 2008; Seité et al. 2003; Berthier-Vergnes et al. 2001). However, very little is known about how and why the immune surveillance mechanism actually fails to destroy melanoma precursor lesions. Melanomas are extremely antigenic because melanoma cells produce high amounts of melanoma-specific proteins (Gould Rothberg and Rimm 2010). Even though certain T cell clones can recognize those proteins, they remain in a suppressed status; therefore, they cannot actively eradicate cancerous melanocyte growths. Lymphocytic infiltrates, mostly CD8+ or CD4+ CD25+ Fox3+ T regulator cells, have been detected in and around tumor sites in several cancers (Nedergaard et al. 2007). It is generally thought that UV exposure can induce direct immunosuppression; however, there are no strong data relating systemic and local immune reactions to UV with the etiology of melanoma. Finally, tumor-infiltrating lymphocyte status of the tumor is strongly associated with survival, indicating that immunological factors are critical for the development and prognosis of melanoma (Thomas et al. 2014).

3.4 Environmental Factors

3.4.1 Sun Exposure

Sun exposure is generally equated with ultraviolet radiation exposure, although the evidence does not rule out other unmeasured exposures associated with the sun. In the public mind, a major correlation exists between increased outdoor activity and increased skin cancer rates. In fact, there are no data available to substantiate such a relationship; that is, although there has been a dramatic increase in melanoma incidence over the last 50 years, no data show that there has been an increase in outdoor activity during the past 50 or so years although the trend toward wearing less clothing is self-evident (Chang et al. 2014).

The data to support an association between sun exposure and the development of melanoma are indirect. There has been a latitude gradient for the incidence of melanoma among Caucasians, such that the highest rates are nearest the equator. In Europe, this gradient has been confounded by the fact that those with darker pigmentary phenotype live in the Southern areas of Europe and those with lighter phenotype in the Northern, so that the gradient in Italy, for example, was actually reversed. However, this does not explain the higher melanoma rates in Norway than in Sweden. Furthermore, new data suggest that trends for incidence and mortality are "evening out" in terms of latitude. Armstrong and Kricker (1993) estimate that between 68 % and 90 % of all melanomas are caused by sun exposure. Most would not dispute this estimate; however, the major point here is that it is likely intermittent sun exposure among susceptible individuals that leads to melanoma as noted among the UK migrants to Australia. Noticing that personal annual UV doses are low and melanoma is increasing rapidly, Merrill et al. (2015) suggest that low vitamin D and possibly viral infections may play a role in this paradox.

3.4.1.1 Patterns of Sun Exposure: Intermittent, Chronic, and Cumulative Sun Exposure

Although there is no standard measure of sun exposure in research, sun exposure can be generally classified as "Intermittent" or "Chronic," and the effects may be considered as acute or cumulative. *Intermittent sun exposure* is that obtained sporadically, during recreational activities usually, and particularly by indoor workers who have only weekends or vacations to be outdoors and have not adapted to the sun. *Chronic sun exposure* is incurred by consistent sun exposure, usually by outdoor work, but also among those people who are outdoors a great deal. *Cumulative sun exposure* is the additive amount of sun exposure that one receives over a lifetime. Cumulative sun exposure may reflect the additive effects of intermittent sun exposure or chronic sun exposure or both. Thomas et al. (2010) recently demonstrated that solar elastosis, a breakdown of collagen and elastin in the epidermis, when located near the site of a melanoma is directly linked to high levels of ultraviolet radiation at the site. Surprisingly, Berwick et al. (2005) demonstrated that solar elastosis is associated with better survival from melanoma, independent of age or histologic subtype of the tumor.

Indeed, different patterns of sun exposure appear to lead to different types of skin cancer among susceptible individuals. In Europe, Rosso et al. (1996) quantified suggestions by Kricker et al. (1995) that basal cell carcinoma and squamous cell carcinoma have different patterns such that squamous cell carcinoma appears to have a threshold at approximately 70,000 h of exposure to sun after which incidence increases sharply, regardless of whether it is chronic sun exposure or intermittent sun exposure. This is highly consistent with the molecular genetic evidence (Kraemer et al. 1994) where combined analysis of skin cancer mutations from several laboratories found the p53 tumor suppressor gene mutated in 90 % of human squamous cell carcinomas and approximately 50 % of basal cell carcinoma. Approximately 70 % of tumors exhibited the characteristic UVB footprint, a C to T or a CC to TT mutation at specific codons.

It is a surprise to many that analytic epidemiologic studies have shown only modest risks at best for the role of sun exposure in the development of melanoma incidence, and three systematic reviews have demonstrated extremely similar estimates of effect for the role of intermittent sun exposure, an odds ratio of 1.6 (Gandini et al. 2005; Nelemans et al. 1995; Elwood and Jopson 1997). It is important to note that chronic sun exposure, as in those occupationally exposed to sunlight, is protective for the development of melanoma, with an odds ratio of 0.7–0.9, equivocal for the development of basal cell carcinoma, and a risk factor for squamous cell carcinoma. As Elwood and Jopson point out, the measurement of sun exposure is complex and any discrepancies among studies could be sorted out by conducting new studies using compatible protocols in different populations with different levels of sun exposure.

A clearer explanation for the rise in melanoma incidence that takes into account the different effects of chronic and intermittent sun exposure, proposed by Gallagher et al. (1989), is that as people have replaced outdoor occupations with indoor, they have engaged in more intermittent sun exposure. Gallagher showed that the decrease in outdoor occupations, or chronic exposure which is not a risk factor for melanoma, could explain the increase in melanoma incidence in Canada.

The evidence for cumulative exposure comes from two sources to date: migrant studies and studies of lifetime exposure, controlling for intermittent and occupational exposure. Data from Australia and Italy show that individuals who migrate at a young age (less than 10 years) from areas of low exposure, such as the UK, to areas of high exposure, such as Australia or Israel, have a lifetime risk of developing melanoma that is similar to that of the new country. On the other hand, individuals who migrate later in life, adolescence or older, from areas of low solar exposure to areas of high solar exposure, have a risk that is quite reduced (Whiteman et al. 2001; see Table 3.1). These data have often been cited to indicate that childhood sun exposure is more important than adult sun exposure in the development of melanoma. However, they can also be interpreted to indicate that the length of exposure is critical rather than the time of exposure; that is, those who migrate early in life have a longer period for intense exposure compared to those who migrate later in life.

3.4.1.2 Effect Varies by Skin Type

The pattern of sun exposure that appears to induce melanoma development is complex and is clearly different by skin type (i.e., propensity to burn, ability to tan). Armstrong et al. (1997) have proposed a model consistent with data from other epidemiologic studies (White et al. 1994, among others) where risk for melanoma increases with increasing sun exposure among those who tan easily, but only with a small amount after which risk decreases with increasing exposure. Among subjects who are intermediate in their ability to tan, risk continues to increase slowly and then at some point declines with increasing exposure. On the other hand, those subjects who have great difficulty tanning have an almost linear increase in risk with increasing sun exposure. This model recognizes that individuals are differentially susceptible to sun exposure and have different levels of risk based on skin type. Moreover, it suggests that different types or patterns of sun exposure are associated with different levels of risk for melanoma.

It is worthwhile looking at the estimates of effect of sun exposure on the development of melanoma in tandem with the other major risk factors for the development of melanoma – nevi number and pigmentary phenotype. Work is ongoing to determine the interrelationship of genetic susceptibility and these phenotypic characteristics (Begg and Berwick 1997). In unpublished data from a population-based case control study in Connecticut (Berwick et al. 1996), the investigators estimated the risk for developing melanoma for nevus number, pigmentary phenotype, and sun exposure in early life as well as sun exposure 10 years prior to the diagnosis of melanoma, adjusting for age and sex. The risk for melanoma with numerous nevi in this study is six times that of someone with few nevi. The risk for melanoma with the most sensitive pigmentary phenotype is almost six times that of someone with the least sensitive phenotype. However, the risk for melanoma with increasing early life sun exposure or increasing later life sun exposure is only two times that of someone with the least sun exposure. Clearly, genetically determined characteristics such as nevi and pigmentary phenotype are more powerful determinants of melanoma risk than is sun exposure.

3.4.1.3 Sunburn

The role of sunburns in the development of melanoma is a critical issue. This aspect of sun exposure is the one most often cited as key to determining melanoma risk. In fact, it can be forcefully argued that sunburn itself is not on the pathway to the development of melanoma, but that it is an important marker for the combination of genetically susceptible phenotype and excessive sun exposure. Numerous articles in the lay media as well as dermatology journals stress the importance of a specific number of sunburns in increasing risk for melanoma. However, a critical look at these studies will show that the relative risk for developing melanoma, when adjusted for host characteristics, is often not statistically significant and is not always impressive. Data from Europe (Autier and Dore 1998) support the concept that childhood sun exposure is not fully represented by sunburning episodes.

While sunburn is the most visible and immediate effect of overexposure to UV, it is also the one that the public is most likely to associate with the development of melanoma. The emerging consensus, however, is that it is unlikely that sunburn is causally associated with melanoma; it is more likely that sunburn is a clear indicator of the interaction between too much sun exposure and a susceptible phenotype, that is severe solar exposure to skin unaccustomed to it.

3.4.1.4 Suberythemic Exposure

Indeed, a great deal of research is currently being focused on suberythemic exposures, that is, those doses of ultraviolet radiation that do not cause an actual burn but that may have biologic significance. Certainly, exposures to the UVA portion of the UV spectrum may lead to the development of melanoma (Moan et al. 1999; Vogel et al. 2014).

Measurement error is a more serious problem in evaluating sunburn history than other sun-associated variables (English et al. 1998; Westerdahl et al. 1996; Berwick and Chen 1995). At least three studies have conducted test–retest reliability studies and concluded that sunburn history is poorly recalled with only a little over half the subjects giving the same answer at two points in time to the question: “Have you ever been sunburned severely enough to cause pain or blisters for 2 days or more?” Other sun-associated variables, such as time spent outdoors during recreation, for example, appear to be more reliably remembered (English et al. 1998; Petersen et al. 2013).

3.4.1.5 Timing of Sun Exposure

Much has been made of the critical time of sun exposure in the development of melanoma. This concept has not yet been proven. In fact, it is likely that all times in life are important in the development of melanoma. Data from a case–control study of melanoma conducted in Connecticut show that intermittent exposure in the 10 years prior to the diagnosis of melanoma is just as important as intermittent exposure in early life. The argument that 70 % of one's sun exposure is likely obtained before the age of 20 may be true; however, this often-quoted statistic is merely an estimate (Stern 2005). With the changes in lifestyle of the 1990s and the early twenty-first century, it is quite possible that individuals in the latter half of life receive a very substantial amount of sun exposure as a result of early retirement and flexible work schedules. At the same time, there are numerous forces at work to diminish the outdoor experiences of young people: the tremendous increase in video games and computers as well as the increasing atomization of neighborhoods, so that "pick up" games of kick the can are no longer as easy to organize.

The preponderance of data shows that excessive intermittent sun exposure at any age increases risk for melanoma. Although the public and many researchers feel that sun exposure during early childhood is the critical period for melanoma induction, there are no empirical data to support this view, attractive though it is.

Autier and Dore (1998) attempted to address the issue as to whether early life or later life sun exposure was the critical factor in determining melanoma risk. They found that both time periods were important. An interesting comparison shows the joint effects of sun exposure during childhood and adulthood. They find, as one might expect, that the highest risk among adults is for those who had high intermittent sun exposure as children. Conversely, those who had low sun exposure during childhood and high sun exposure in adulthood had a similar risk to those who had high exposure during childhood and low exposure during adulthood.

Other data support the idea that intermittent sun exposure leads to increased risk at any age. Holly et al. (1995) showed that more than seven painful sunburns during elementary school increased risk twofold ($OR = 2.0$, 95 % $CI = 1.4, 2.9$) and that more than seven sunburns after the age of 30 (the age of women in this study ranged from 18 to 59) increased risk twofold ($OR = 2.0$, 95 % $CI = 1.1, 3.8$). In sum, data from very different setting seem to suggest that intermittent sun exposure is critical to the risk for developing melanoma. In the published studies that looked at both early life and adult sun exposure, there is very little difference between the effects of sun exposure at either stage, but that lifelong intermittent sun exposure is indeed cumulative.

3.4.1.6 Occupational or Chronic Sun Exposure

The reasons for the differing trends in melanoma risk between occupational and intermittent sun exposure are not well understood. Analyses of melanoma time trends from Canada (Bulliard and Cox 1999), New Zealand (Bulliard and Cox 2000), Germany (Garbe et al. 1994), Australia (Garbe et al. 2000; Marrett et al. 2001), and Denmark indicate that changes in lifestyle factors, such as sun exposure behaviors and fashion, correlate (Osterlind et al. 1988) strongly with increases in melanoma on skin areas exposed intermittently to the sun (trunk, upper arms, and upper legs). With regard to chronic occupational sun exposure, it is also possible that additional phenotypic differences among workforce members may be influencing the direction and intensity of melanoma risk. In a study of occupational melanoma from Spain (Espinosa Arranz et al. 1999), higher melanoma risk was observed among construction workers than among farmers. The melanoma risk in construction workers became more significant when adjusted for skin type, age, freckle count (odds ratio (OR) 4.3; 95 % confidence interval (CI) 1.8, 9.9), and number of nevi (OR 2.8; 95 % CI 1.4, 5.8), while the risk in farmers remained protective even with these adjustments.

3.4.2 Tanning Beds

Tanning beds have been increasing in number and popularity throughout the world, particularly but not exclusively in more northern latitude. Great concern has been expressed by the International Agency on Cancer (IARC) that this increase will lead to increases in melanoma risk. IARC convened an expert panel of epidemiologists (IARC 2007) who performed a meta-analysis of 19 studies that have evaluated the association between sunbed exposure and melanoma and other skin cancers to that time. This analysis showed a significant summary, or overall, relative risk for melanoma of 1.8 (95 % CI 1.4, 2.3) for "first exposure under the age of 35"; a relative risk of 1.2 that was statistically significant (95 % CI 1.0, 1.3) for "ever use." Controversy has, however, continued over the carcinogenic properties of tanning beds. The tanning industry "sells" tanning beds as a safe alternative to UV exposure for both tanning as well as vitamin D biosynthesis. As most tanning beds are not regulated (Nilsen et al. 2016), the amount of UV exposure from using tanning beds is far higher than the same amount of time spent in the sun. Usage of tanning beds have been subject to regulations, with Brazil in 2009 and Australia in 2015 banning all tanning beds and the EU and many states in the US banning them for use by minors (Sinclair et al. 2014; Bulger et al 2015).

A recent study conducted in Minnesota has published high and significant risks for developing melanoma among tanning bed users. Among 1,167 cases and 1,101 controls, 62.9 % of cases and 51.1 % of controls had tanned indoors (adjusted OR 1.7; 95 % CI 1.4, 2.1). Melanoma risk was pronounced among users of both UVB-enhanced (adjusted OR 2.9; 95 % CI 2.0, 4.0) and primarily UVA-emitting devices (adjusted OR 4.4; 95 % CI 2.5, 8.0). Risk increased with use: years ($P<0.006$), hours ($P<0.0001$), or sessions ($P=0.0002$). ORs were elevated within each initiation age category; among indoor tanners, years used was more relevant for melanoma development (Lazovich et al. 2010). Thus, epidemiologic data suggest that tanning beds are not safer than solar ultraviolet radiation and that they may have independent effects from solar exposure that increase risk for melanoma.

A major problem in evaluating the risk from tanning beds and sunlamps is that they have changed over time in terms of their usage and their spectral output. In addition, the dosage of UV is extremely difficult to obtain as most tanning parlors do not calibrate their equipment or measure their output. When comparing dosage of tanning lamps to solar radiation, it is important to estimate the proportion of the body irradiated. From 15 % to 50 % of the total body is uncovered during outdoor activities, but up to 95–100 % of the total body is uncovered during indoor tanning. Therefore, the dosage is likely to be far greater than from a similar amount of outdoor solar exposure.

Females tend to use sunbeds more than males, particularly young women. Recent data from the United States National Cancer Institute show that the incidence of melanoma is growing among young females (Purdue et al. 2008). In addition, sunbed usage in the US is most prevalent among young women (Lazovich and Forster 2005). These statistics point up the fact that sunbed usage is an area for serious concern. In fact, Veierød et al.'s (2003) evaluation of use of sunbeds found that those who used sunbeds at ages 20–29 years once or more per month had a statistically significant relative risk of developing melanoma of 2.6 (95 % CI 1.5, 4.5). This fact will be crucial to guide prevention in the future.

Most studies have shown an increased risk for melanoma associated with sunbed use, but there are multiple qualifications that need to be taken into account. In the first place, it is difficult to disentangle the use of artificial UV from natural UV exposure. Many authors, for example, Wester et al. (1999), have found frequent tanning in sunlight correlated with sunbed use.

Gallagher et al. (2005) asks the critical question: "If there is a causal relationship, how important is the risk?" This is a difficult question to respond to at this point in time for a number of reasons: (1) Assessment of sunbed use needs improvement as well as assessment of spectral output. Although we see good agreement for individual's recall of sunbed usage, it is likely that the timing and the exposure are not all the same for all individuals. (2) It is unclear whether one can compare sunbed use and sunbathing; is there the same biological mechanism? (3) Most studies have taken place in higher latitudes in North America and Europe where the background ambient ultraviolet radiation is low; it would be useful to have more data from lower latitudes with higher levels of ambient UV, such as Australia and Southern US. (4) Ecological studies are inconsistent – even at similar latitudes with very good data. In Denmark Faurschou and Wulf (2007) concluded that sunbed risk for BCC is important but not CMM. However, in the UK, Diffey (2007) estimated that sunbed risk for CMM in women is dramatic and may have caused as many as 182 cases of CMM in women and 49 in males in the last 8 years.

3.4.3 Other Environmental Factors

Other environmental factors are receiving new attention.

3.4.3.1 Pesticides and Herbicides

Dennis' group evaluated data from the Agricultural Health Workers' Study and found significant associations between cutaneous melanoma and maneb/mancozeb (trend $P=0.006$), parathion (trend $P=0.003$), and carbaryl (trend $P=0.013$). Other associations with benomyl and ever use of arsenical pesticides were also suggested (Dennis et al. 2010). Seggato et al. (2015) found that indoor domestic use of pesticides may be an independent environmental risk factor for melanoma. Lerro et al. (2015) reported borderline associations for the use of acetochlor and melanoma incidence among acetochlor users in the Agricultural Health Workers' Study.

3.4.3.2 Arsenic

Arsenic has been suspected of involvement, since it is a known cocarcinogen with UV in exacerbating development of non-melanoma skin cancer (Rossman et al. 2004). However, most elevated levels of As are found in areas with populations who are highly resistant to UV-induced melanoma (Taiwan, Bangladesh) and so even a significant increase in malignant melanoma skin cancer rate would not be detected in epidemiology studies in those populations. A significant positive association has been shown between body arsenic levels (toenail arsenic) and melanoma risk in a (predominantly) Caucasian Iowa population, demonstrating that interactions between sunlight and arsenic may contribute to melanoma in these populations (Beane Freeman et al. 2004). Yager et al. (2016) found an interaction between DNA damage and UV among cases with melanoma, suggesting genetic predisposition

3.4.3.3 Polychlorinated Biphenyls (PCBs)

Some epidemiologic studies have suggested that exposure to organochlorine compounds might increase the risk of melanoma, but these studies have lacked biological measures of exposure and have not been able to control for the major environmental risk factor for melanoma – sun exposure. Gallagher and co-workers (2011) were able to conduct a pilot study with the ability to adjust for sun sensitivity and sun exposure. Plasma was collected from 80 cases and 310 controls in British Columbia. Assays for 14 PCB congeners and 11 organochlorine pesticide residues were conducted: risk of melanoma and plasma levels of non-dioxin-like PCBs (adjusted OR 7.0, 95 % CI 2.3, 21.4 among those in the highest quartile) as well as several PCB congeners, organochlorine pesticides, or metabolites. This study suggests that other environmental factors in addition to UV radiation may play an important role in the etiology of melanoma.

3.4.3.4 Diet

Although dietary behaviors have not previously been shown to be associated with the development of melanoma, there is current interest in the role of coffee consumption. A meta-analysis and systematic review (Yew et al. 2016) of coffee consumption shows that the pooled relative risk for coffee drinkers for melanoma was 0.75 (95 % CI 0.63–0.89, $P=0.001$), although there is some suggestion of publication bias. This conclusion was supported by another meta-analysis by Wang et al. (2016) which reached similar conclusions. A study evaluating the quality of the diet and risk of melanoma in an Italian population (Malagoli et al. 2015) found that the DASH diet (Dietary Approaches to Stop Hypertension) was significantly inversely associated with melanoma in women. Data on alcohol's relationship to melanoma have been mixed. A thorough pooled analysis by Miura et al. (2015) finds no strong support for such an hypothesis.

3.5 Summary

Melanoma is clearly a complex disease for which we do not have simple answers. This chapter has attempted to delineate some of the challenges in understanding the trends for melanoma incidence and mortality. Although we do not yet understand fully the etiology of melanoma, there seems to be a relatively clear message for the public: "Be cautious all your life. Enjoy the sun in moderation. Stay away from large bursts of sun exposure, particularly on untanned skin."

Acknowledgments I acknowledge assistance with the SEER and IARC data from Angela Meisner and Dr. Charles Wiggins. This work was supported by NCI R01 CA 112425 and by the University of New Mexico Cancer Center and the University of New Mexico Department of Internal Medicine.

References

Aguilera P, Malvehy J, Carrera C, Palou J, Puig-Buille JA, Alos L, Badenas C, Puig S (2014) Clinical and histopathological characteristics between familial and sporadic melanoma in Barcelona, Spain. J Clin Exp Dermatol Res 5:231

Armstrong BK, Kricker A (1993) How much melanoma is caused by sun exposure? Melanoma Res 3:395–401

Armstrong BK, Kricker A (2001) The epidemiology of UV induced skin cancer. J Photochem Photobiol B 63:8–18

Armstrong BK, Kricker A, English DR (1997) Sun exposure and skin cancer. Australas J Dermatol 38(Suppl 1):S1–S6

Autier P, Dore JF (1998) Influence of sun exposures during childhood and during adulthood on melanoma risk. EPIMEL and EORTC Melanoma Cooperative Group. European Organisation for Research and Treatment of Cancer. Int J Cancer 77:533–537

Autier P, Koechlin A, Boniol M (2015) The forthcoming inexorable decline of cutaneous melanoma mortality in light-skinned populations. Eur J Cancer 51:869–878

Balch CM, Soong SJ, Gershenwald JE, Thompson JF, Reintgen DS, Cascinelli N, Urist M, McMasters KM, Ross MI, Kirkwood JM, Atkins MB, Thompson JA, Coit DG, Byrd D, Desmond R, Zhang Y, Liu PY, Lyman GH, Morabito A (2001) Prognostic factors analysis of 17,600 melanoma patients: validation of the American Joint Committee on Cancer melanoma staging system. J Clin Oncol 19:3622–3634

Barón AE, Asdigian NL, Gonzalez V, Aalborg J, Terzian T, Stiegmann RA, Torchia EC, Berwick M, Dellavalle RP, Morelli JG, Modrohisky ST, Crane LA, Box NF (2014) Interactions between ultraviolet light and MC1R and OCA2 variants are determinants of childhood nevus and freckle phenotypes. Cancer Epidemiol Biomarkers Prev 23:2829–2839

Beane Freeman LE, Dennis LK, Lynch CF, Thorne PS, Just CL (2004) Toenail arsenic content and cutaneous melanoma in Iowa. Am J Epidemiol 160:679–687

Bechetoille N, Dezutter-Dambuyant C, Damour O, Andre V, Orly I, Perrier E (2007) Effects of solar ultraviolet radiation on engineered human skin equivalent containing both Langerhans cells and dermal dendritic cells. Tissue Eng 13:2667–2679

Begg C, Berwick M (1997) A note on the estimation of relative risks of rare genetic susceptibility markers. Cancer Epidemiol Biomarkers Prev 6:99–103

Begg CB, Hummer A, Mujumdar U, Armstrong BK, Kricker A, Marrett LD, Millikan RC, Gruber SB, Anton-Culver H, Klotz JB, Zanetti R, Gallagher RP, Dwyer T, Rebbeck TR, Berwick M, GEM Study Group (2004) Familial aggregation of melanoma risks in a large population-based sample of melanoma cases. Cancer Causes Control 15:957–965

Berthier-Vergnes O, Gaucherand M, Péguet-Navarro J, Plouet J, Pageaux JF, Schmitt D, Staquet MJ (2001) Human melanoma cells inhibit the earliest differentiation steps of human Langerhans cell precursors but failed to affect the functional maturation of epidermal Langerhans cells. Br J Cancer 85:1944–1951

Berwick M, Begg C, Fine JA, Roush GC, Barnhill RL. Screening for malignant melanoma by skin self-examination. J Natl Cancer Inst 1996:88:17–23. PMID 8847720

Berwick M, Chen YT (1995) Reliability of reported sunburn history in a case–control study of cutaneous malignant melanoma. Am J Epidemiol 141:1033–1037

Berwick M, Armstrong BK, Ben-Porat L, Fine J, Kricker A, Eberle C, Barnhill R (2005) Sun exposure and mortality from melanoma. J Natl Cancer Inst 97:195–199
Bradford PT, Anderson WF, Purdue MP, Goldstein AM, Tucker MA (2010) Rising melanoma incidence rates of the trunk among younger women in the United States. Cancer Epidemiol Biomarkers Prev 19:2401–2406
Bulliard J, Cox B (1999) Trends by anatomical site in Incidence of cutaneous malignant melanoma in Canada: 1963–1993. Cancer Causes Control 10:407–416
Bulger AL, Mayer JE, Gershenwald JE, Guild SR, Gottlieb MA, Geller AC (2015) Enforcement provisions of indoor tanning bans for minors: an analysis of the first 6 US states. Am J Public Health 105:310–312
Bulliard J, Cox B (2000) Incidence of cutaneous malignant melanoma in New Zealand by anatomical site: 1963–1993. Int J Epidemiol 29:416–423
Bykov VJ, Marcusson JA, Hemminki K (2000) Effect of constitutional pigmentation on ultraviolet B-induced DNA damage in fair-skinned people. J Invest Dermatol 114:40–43
Byrom L, Olsen CM, Knight L, Khosrotehrani K, Green AC (2015) Does pregnancy after a diagnosis of melanoma affect prognosis? Systematic review and meta-analysis. Dermatol Surg 41:875–882
Campbell LB, Kreicher BA, Gittleman HR, Strodtbeck K, Barnholtz-Sloan J, Bordeaux JS (2015) Melanoma incidence in children and adolescents: decreasing trends in the United States. J Pediatr 166:1505–1513
Chang C, Murzaku EC, Penn L, Abbasi NR, Davis PD, Berwick M, Polsky D (2014) More skin, more sun, more tan, more melanoma. Am J Public Health 104:e92–e99
Cho H, Mariotto AB, Schwartz LM, Luo J, Woloshin S (2014) When do changes in cnacer survival mean progress? the insight from population incidence and mortality. J Natl Cancer Inst Monogr 49:187–197
Clairwood M, Ricketts J, Grant-Kels J, Gonsalves L (2014) Melanoma in skin of color in Connecticut: an analysis of melanoma incidence and stage at diagnosis in non-Hispanic blacks, non-Hispanic whites, and Hispanics. Int J Dermatol 53:425–433
Cockburn MG, Zadnick J, Deapen D (2006) Developing epidemic of melanoma in the Hispanic population of California. Cancer 106:1162–1168
Criscione VD, Weinstock MA (2010) Melanoma thickness trends in the United States, 1988–2006. J Invest Dermatol 130:793–797
Crocetti E, Fancelli L, Manneschi G, Caldarella A, Pimpinelli N, Chiarugi A, Nardini P, Buzzoni C (2016) Melanoma survival: sex does matter, but we do not know how. Eur J Cancer Prev 25(5):404–409
de Giorgi V, Mavilla C, Massi D, Gozzini A, Aragona P, Tanini A, Sestini S, Paglieranti M, Boddi V, Brandi ML, Lottti T (2009) Estrogen receptor expression in cutaneous melanoma. Arch Dermatol 145:30–36
Dennis LK, Lynch CF, Sandler DP, Alavanja MC (2010) Pesticide use and cutaneous melanoma in pesticide applicators in the agricultural heath study. Environ Health Perspect 118:812–817
deVries E, Nijsten TE, Visser O, Bastiaannet E, van Hattem S, Janssen-Heijnen ML, Coebergh JW (2008) Superior survival of females among 19,538 Dutch melanoma patients is independent of Breslow thickness, histologic type and tumor site. Ann Oncol 19:583–589
Diffey BL (2007) Sunbeds, beauty and melanoma. Br J Dermatol 157:215–216
Dinh QQ, Chong AH (2007) Melanoma in organ transplant recipients: the old enemy finds a new battleground. Australas J Dermatol 48:199–207
Elwood JM, Jopson J (1997) Melanoma and sun exposure: an overview of published studies. Int J Cancer 73:198–203
English DR, Armstrong BK, Kricker A (1998) Reproducibility of reported measurements of sun exposure in a case–control study. Cancer Epidemiol Biomarkers Prev 7:857–863
Erickson C, Driscoll MS (2010) Melanoma epidemic: facts and controversies. Clin Dermatol 28:281–286
Espinosa Arranz J, Sanchez Hernandez JJ, Bravo Fernandez P, Gonzalez-Baron M, Zamora Auñon P, Espinosa Arranz E, Jalon Lopez JI, Ordoñez GA (1999) Cutaneous malignant melanoma and sun exposure in Spain. Melanoma Res 2:199–205
Faurschou A, Wulf HC (2007) Ecological analysis of the relation between sunbeds and skin cancer. Photodermatol Photoimmunol Photomed 23:120–125

Ford D, Bliss JM, Swerdlow AJ, Armstrong BK, Franceschi S, Green A, Holly EA, Mack T, Mackie RM, Østerlind A, Walter SD, Peto J, Easton DF (1995) Risk of cutaneous melanoma associated with a family history of the disease. Int J Cancer 62:377–381

Gallagher RP, Elwood JM, Yang CP (1989) Is chronic sunlight exposure important in accounting for increases in melanoma incidence? Int J Cancer 44:813–815

Gallagher RP, Spinelli JJ, Lee TK (2005) Tanning beds, sunlamps and risk of cutaneous malignant melanoma. Cancer Epidemiol Biomarkers Prev 4:562–566

Gallagher RP, MacArthur AC, Lee TK, Weber J-P, Leblanc A, Elwood JM, Borugian M, Zbanto Z, Spinelli JJ (2011) Plasma levels of polychlorinated biphenyls and risk of cutaneous malignant melanoma: a preliminary study. Int J Cancer 128(8):1872–1880

Gandini S, Sera F, Cattaruzza MS, Pasquini P, Picconi O, Boyle P, Melchi CF (2005) Meta-analysis of risk factors for cutaneous melanoma: II. Sun exposure. Eur J Cancer 41:45–60

Garbe C, Buettner PG, Weiss J, Soyer HP, Stocker U, Krüger S, Roser M, Weckbecker J, Panizzon R, Bahmer F et al (1994) Risk factors for developing cutaneous melanoma and criteria for identifying persons at risk: multicenter case–control study of central malignant melanoma registry of the German dermatological society. J Invest Dermatol 102:695–699

Garbe C, McLeod GR, Buettner PG (2000) Time trends in cutaneous melanoma in Queensland, Australia and Central Europe. Cancer 89:1269–1278

Geller AC, Miller DR, Annas GD, Demierre MF, Gilchrest BA, Koh HK (2002) Melanoma incidence and mortality among US whites, 1969–1999. JAMA 288:1719–1720

Gould Rothberg BE, Rimm DL (2010) Biomarkers: the useful and the not so useful–an assessment of molecular prognostic markers for cutaneous melanoma. J Invest Dermatol 130:1971–1987

Green A (1992) A theory of the site distribution of melanomas: Queensland, Australia. Cancer Causes Control 3:513–516

Greene MH, Fraumeni JJ (1979) The hereditary variant of malignant melanoma. In: Clark WH, Goldman LI, Mastrangelo MJ (eds) Human malignant melanoma. Grune & Stratton, New York

Grob JJ, Richard MA, Gouvernet J, Avril MF, Delaunay M, Wolkenstein P, Souteyrand P, Bonerandi JJ, Machet L, Guillaume JC, Chevrant-Breton J, Vilmer C, Aubin F, Guillot B, Beylot-Barry M, Lok C, Raison-Peyron N, Chemaly P (2002) The kinetics of the visible growth of a primary melanoma reflects the tumor aggressiveness and is an independent prognostic marker: a prospective study. Int J Cancer 102:34–38

Guy GP Jr, Thomas CC, Thompson T, Watson M, Massetti GM, Richardson LC (2015) Vital signs: Melanoma incidence and mortality trends and projections – United States, 1982–2030. MMWR Morb Mortal Wkly Rep 64(21):591–596

Hersey P, Bradley DE, Hasic E, Haran G, Edwards A, McCarthy WH (1983) Immunological effects of solarium exposure. Lancet 1:545–548

Holly EA, Aston DA, Cress RD, Ahn DK, Kristiansen JJ (1995) Cutaneous melanoma in women. I. Exposure to sunlight, ability to tan, and other risk factors related to ultraviolet light. Am J Epidemiol 141:923–933

Huynh PM, Glusac EJ, Alvarez-Franco M, Berwick M, Bolognia J (2003) Numerous small darkly pigmented melanocytic nevi: the cheetah phenotype. J Am Acad Dermatol 48:707–713

International Agency for Research on Cancer (WHO) and International Association of Cancer Registries; Curado MP, Edwards B, Shin HR, Storm H, Ferlay J, Heanue M, Boyle P (eds) (2007) Cancer incidence in five continents, vol 9. IARC Scientific Publication No. 160. International Agency for Research on Cancer, Lyon

International Agency for Research on Cancer Working Group on artificial ultraviolet (UV) light and skin cancer (2007) The association of use of sunbeds with cutaneous malignant melanoma and other skin cancers: a systematic review. Int J Cancer 120:1116–1122

Juhl AL, Byers TE, Robison WA, Morelli JG, Crane LA (2009) The anatomic distribution of melanoma and relationships with childhood nevus distribution in Colorado. Melanoma Res 19:252–259

Kanetsky PA, Panossian S, Elder DE et al (2010) Does MC1R genotype convey information about melanoma risk beyond risk phenotypes? Cancer 116:2416–2428

Karlsson MA, Rodvall Y, Wahlgren CF, Wiklund K, Lindelof B (2015) Similar anatomical distributions of childhood naevi and cutaneous melanoma in young adults residing in northern and southern Sweden. Eur J Cancer 51:2067–2075
Khosrotehrani K, Dasgupta P, Byrom L, Youlden DR, Baade PD, Green AC (2015) Melanoma survival is superior in females across all tumour stages but is influenced by age. Arch Dermatol Res 307:731–740
Kjems E, Krag C (1993) Melanoma and pregnancy. A review. Acta Oncol 32:371–378
Kraemer KH, Lee MM, Andrews AD, Lambert WC (1994) The role of sunlight and DNA repair in melanoma and nonmelanoma skin cancer. The xeroderma pigmentosum paradigm. Arch Dermatol 130:1018–1021
Kricker A, Armstrong BK, English DR, Heenan PJ (1995) A dose–response curve for sun exposure and basal cell carcinoma. Int J Cancer 60:482–488
Lachiewicz A, Berwick M, Wiggins CL, Thomas NE (2008) Epidemiologic support for melanoma heterogeneity using the surveillance, epidemiology, and end results program. J Invest Dermatol 128:1340–1342
Lazovich D, Forster J (2005) Indoor tanning by adolescents: prevalence, practices and policies. Eur J Cancer 41:20–27
Lazovich D, Vogel RI, Berwick M, Weinstock MA, Anderson KE, Warshaw EM (2010) Indoor tanning and risk of melanoma: a case–control study in a highly exposed population. Cancer Epidemiol Biomarkers Prev 19:1557–1568
Lerro CC, Coutros S, Adreotti G, Hines CJ, Blair A, Lubin J, Ma X, LE Zhang B-F (2015) Use of acetochlor and cancer incidence in the Agricultural Health Study. Int J Cancer 137:1167–1175
Liu W, Dowling JP, Murray WK, McArthur GA, Thompson JF, Wolfe R, Kelly JW (2006) Rate of growth in melanomas: characteristics and associations of rapidly growing melanomas. Arch Dermatol 142:1551–1558
Malagoli C, Malavolti M, Agnoli C, Crespi CM, Fiorentini CFarnetani F, Longo C, Ricci C, Albertini G, Lanzoni A, Venziano L, An V, Pagliarello C, Santini M, Fanti PA, Em D, Sieri S, Krogh V, Pellacani G, Vinceti M (2015) Diet quality and risk of melanoma in an Italian population. J Nutr 145:1800–1807
Marrett LD, Nguyen HL, Armstrong BK (2001) Trends in the incidence of cutaneous malignant melanoma in New South Wales, 1983–1996. Int J Cancer 92:457–462
Merrill SJ, Ashrafi S, Subramanian M, Godar DE (2015) Exponentially increasing incidences of cutaneous malignant melanoma in Europe correlate with low personal annual UV doses and suggests 2 major risk factors. Dermato Endocrinol 7(1): e1004018. Open access.
Miura K, Zens MS, Peart T, Holly EA, Berwick M, Gallagher RP, Mack TM, Elwood JM, Karagas MR, Green AC (2015) Alcohol consumption and risk of melanoma among women: pooled analysis of eight case–control studies. Arch Dermatol Res 307:819–828
Moan J, Dahlback A, Setlow RB (1999) Epidemiological support for an hypothesis for melanoma induction indicating a role for UVA radiation. Photochem Photobiol 70:243–247
Muller HK, Malley RC, McGee HM, Scott DK, Wozniak T, Woods GM (2008) Effect of UV radiation on the neonatal skin immune system – implications for melanoma. Photochem Photobiol 84:47–54
Murphy GM, Norris PG, Young AR, Corbett MF, Hawk JL (1993) Low-dose ultraviolet-B irradiation depletes human epidermal Langerhans cells. Br J Dermatol 129:674–677
Naidoo J, Page DB, Wolchok JD (2014) Immune modulation for cancer therapy. Br J Cancer 111:2214–2219
Nedergaard BS, Ladekarl M, Thomsen HF, Nyengaard JR, Nielsen K (2007) Low density of CD3+, CD4+ and CD8+ cells is associated with increased risk of relapse in squamous cell cervical cancer. Br J Cancer 97:1135–1138
Nelemans PJ, Rampen FHJ, Ruiter DJ, Verbeek ALM (1995) An addition to the controversy on sunlight exposure and melanoma risk: a meta-analytical approach. J Clin Epidemol 58:1331–1342

Nilsen LTN, Hannevik M, Veierod MB (2016) UV exposure from indoor tanning devices: a systematic review. Br J Dermatol 174(4):730–740
Norval M (2006) The mechanisms and consequences of ultraviolet-induced immunosuppression. Prog Biophys Mol Biol 92:108–118
Olsen CM, Neale RE, Green AC, Webb PM, QSkin Study, Epigene Study, Whiteman DC (2015) Independent validation of six melanoma risk prediction models. J Invest Dermatol 135:1377–1384
Orlow I, Roy P, Reiner AS, Yoo S, Patel H, Paine S, Armstrong BK, Kricker A, Marrett LD, Millikan RC, Thomas NE, Gruber SB, Anton-Culver H, Rosso S, Gallgaher RP, Dwyer T, Kanetsky PA, Busam K, From L, Begg CB, Berwick M, GEM Study Group (2012) Vitamin D receptor polymorphisms in patients with cutaneous melanoma. Int J Cancer 130:405–418
Osterlind A, Engholm G, Jensen OM (1988) Trends in cutaneous malignant melanoma in Denmark 1943–1982 by anatomical site. APMIS 96:953–963
Palmer JS, Duffy DL, Box NF et al (2000) Melanocortin-1 receptor polymorphisms and risk of melanoma: is the association explained solely by pigmentation phenotype? Am J Hum Genet 66:176–186
Pasquali E, Garcia-Borrón JC, Fargnoli MC, Gandini S, Maisonneuve P, Bagnardi V, Specchia C, Liu F, Kayser M, Nijsten T, Nagore E, Kumar R, Hansson J, Kanetsky PA, Ghiorzo P, Debniak T, Branicki W, Gruis NA, Han J, Dwyer T, Blizzard L, Landi MT, Palmieri G, Ribas G, Stratigos A, Council ML, Autier P, Little J, Newton-Bishop J, Sera F, Raimondi S, M-SKIP Study Group (2015) MC1R variants increase the risk of sporadic cutaneous melanoma in darker-pigmentd Caucasians: a pooled-analysis from the M-SKIP project. Int J Cancer 136:618–631
Petersen B, Thieden E, Lerche CM, Wulf HC (2013) Validation of self-reported erythema: comparison of self-reports, researcher assessment and objective measurements in sun worshippers and skiers. J Eur Acad Dermatol Venereol 27:214–219
Purdue MP, Freeman LE, Anderson WF, Tucker MA (2008) Recent trends in incidence of cutaneous melanoma among US Caucasian young adults. J Invest Dermatol 128:2905–2908
Roh MR, Eliades P, Gupta SM, Grant-Kels JM, Tsao H (2015) Cutaneous melanoma in women. Int J Womens Dermatol 1:21–25
Rossman TG, Uddin AN, Burns FJ (2004) Evidence that arsenite acts as a cocarcinogen in skin cancer. Toxicol Appl Pharmacol 198:394–404
Rosso S, Zanetti R, Martinez C, Tormo MJ, Schraub S, Sancho-Garnier H, Franceschi S, Gafa L, Perea E, Navarro C, Laurent R, Schrameck C, Talamini R, Tumino R, Wechsler J (1996) The multicentre south European study "Helios" II: different sun exposure patterns in the aetiology of basal cell and squamous cell carcinomas of the skin. Br J Cancer 73:1447–1454
Rouhani P, Pinheiro PS, Sherman R, Arheart K, Fleming LE, Mackinnon J, Kirsner RS (2010) Increasing rates of melanoma among nonwhites in Florida compared with the United States. Arch Dermatol 146:741–746
Seggato MM, Bananigo RR, Hohman CB, Müller KR, Bakos L, Matrroeni S, Fortes C (2015) Residential and occupational exposure to pesticides may increase risk for cutaneous melanoma: a case–control study conducted in the south of Brazil. Int J Dermatol 54:e527–e538
Seité S, Zucchi H, Moyal D, Tison S, Compan D, Christiaens F, Gueniche A, Fourtanier A (2003) Alterations in human epidermal Langerhans cells by ultraviolet radiation: quantitative and morphological study. Br J Dermatol 148:291–299
Shaikh WR, Dusza SW, Weinstock MA, Oliveria SA, Geller AC, Halpern AC (2016) Melanoma thickness and survival trends in the United States, 1989 to 2009. J Natl Cancer Inst 108:1–7
Sinclair CA, Makin JK, Tang A, Brozek I, Rock V (2014) The role of public health advocacy in achieving an outright ban on commercial tanning beds in Australia. Am J Public Health 104:e7–e9
Stern RS (2005) Proportion of lifetime UV dose received by age 18, what Stern et al actually said in 1986. J Invest Dermatol 124:1079–1080
Surveillance Epidemiology and End Results (SEER) Program (2009) Cancer statistics review. National Cancer Institute, Bethesda

Thiam A, Zhao Z, Quinn C, Barber B (2015) Years of life lost due to metastatic melanoma in 12 countries. J Med Econ 25:1–6
Thomas NE, Kricker A, From L, Busam KJ, Millikan RC, Ritchey ME, Armstrong BK, Lee-Taylor J, Marrett L, Anton-Culver H, Zanetti R, Rosso S, Gallagher RP, Dwyer T, Goumas C, Kanetsky PA, Begg CB, Orlow I, Wilcox H, Paine S, Berwick M (2010) Associations of cumulative sun exposure and phenotypic characteristics with histologic solar elastosis. Cancer Epidemiol Biomarkers Prev 19:2932–2941
Thomas NE, Busam KJ, From L, Kricker A, Armstrong BK, Anton-Culver H, Gruber SB, Gallagher RP, Zanetti R, Rosso S, Dwyer T, Venn A, Kanetsky PA, Groben PA, Hao H, Orlow I, Reiner AS, Luo L, Paine S, Ollila DW, Wilcox H, Begg CB, Berwick M (2014) Tumor-infiltrating lymphocyte grade in primary melanomas is independently associated with melanoma-specific survival in the population-based genes, environment and melanoma study. J Clin Oncol 31:4252–4259
Tran TT, Schulman J, Fisher DE (2008) UV and pigmentation: molecular mechanisms and social controversies. Pigment Cell Melanoma Res 21:509–516
Vajdic CM, van Leeuwen MT, Webster AC, McCredie MRE, Stewart JH, Chapman JR, Amin J, McDonald SP, Grulich AE (2009) Cutaneous melanoma is related to immune suppression in kidney transplant recipients. Cancer Epidemiol Biomarkers Prev 18:2297–2303
Veierød MB, Weiderpass E, Thörn M, Hansson J, Lund E, Armstrong B, Adami HO (2003) A prospective study of pigmentation, sun exposure, and risk of cutaneous malignant melanoma in women. J Natl Cancer Inst 95:1530–1538
Vogel RI, Ahmed RL, Nelson HH, Berwick M, Weinstock MA, Lazovich D (2014) Exposure to indoor tanning without burning and melanoma risk by sunburn history. J Natl Cancer Inst 106:dju112
Wagner JK, Parra EJ, Norton HL, Jovel C, Shriver MD (2002) Skin responses to ultraviolet radiation: effects of constitutive pigmentation, sex, and ancestry. Pigment Cell Res 15:385–390
Wang J, Li X, Zhang D (2016) Coffee consumption and the risk of cutaneous melanoma: a meta-analysis. Eur J Nutr 55(4):1317–1329
Wei Q, Lee JE, Gershenwald JE, Ross MI, Mansfield PF, Strom SS, Wang LE, Guo Z, Qiao Y, Amos CI, Spitz MR, Duvic M (2003) Repair of UV light-induced DNA damage and risk of cutaneous malignant melanoma. J Natl Cancer Inst 95:308–315
Welch HG, Black WC (2010) Overdiagnosis in cancer. J Natl Cancer Inst 102:605–613
Wester U, Boldemann C, Jansson B, Ullén H (1999) Population UV-dose and skin area – do sunbeds rival the sun? Health Phys 77:436–440
Westerdahl J, Anderson H, Olsson H, Ingvar C (1996) Reproducibility of a self-administered questionnaire for assessment of melanoma risk. Int J Epidemiol 25:245–251
White E, Kirkpatrick CS, Lee JA (1994) Case–control study of malignant melanoma in Washington State. I. Constitutional factors and sun exposure. Am J Epidemiol 139:857–868
Whiteman DC, Watt P, Purdie DM, Hughes MC, Hayward NK, Green AC (2003) Melanocytic nevi, solar keratoses and divergent pathways to cutaneous melanoma. J Natl Cancer Inst 95:806–812
Whiteman DC, Whiteman CA, Green AC (2001) Childhood sun exposure as a risk factor for melanoma: a systematic review of epidemiologic studies. Cancer Causes Control 12:69–82
Yager JW, Erdei E, Myers O, Siegel M, Berwick M (2016) Arsenic and ultraviolet radiation exposure: melanoma in a New Mexico no-Hispanic white population. Environ Geochem Health 38(3):897–910
Yamaguchi Y, Takahashi K, Zmudzka BZ, Kornhauser A, Miller SA, Tadokoro T, Berens W, Beer JZ, Hearing VJ (2006) Human skin responses to UV radiation: pigment in the upper epidermis protects against DNA damage in the lower epidermis and facilitates apoptosis. FASEB J 20(9):1486–1488
Yew YW, Lai YC, Schwartz RA (2016) Coffee consumption and melanoma: a systematic review and meta-analysis of observational studies. Am J Clin Dermatol 17(2):113–123

Melanoma Genetics and Genomics

4

Allen Ho, Göran Jönsson, and Hensin Tsao

4.1 MAPK and PI3K Pathways and Melanoma

There is substantial evidence that two of the major pathways central for melanoma development are the mitogen-activated protein kinase (MAPK) and phosphatidylinositol 3-kinase (PI3K) pathways. Indeed, nearly 25 % of melanomas have activating mutations of *NRAS*, an additional 15 % have loss of Nf1 function, and a small fraction of melanomas have either *KIT* activating changes or translocations/fusions of *ALK* or *ROS* with other genes, which result in increased MAPK signaling (Bastian 2014). Moreover, the clinical success of targeting the MAPK pathway in the treatment of metastatic melanoma underscores the central role this pathway plays in melanoma pathogenesis. The first oncogene to be identified in melanoma was *NRAS* (Padua et al. 1984), which is known to be mutated not only in melanoma but also in other cancers. It would take an additional 20 years before the next established melanoma oncogene was discovered. In a comprehensive mutation screen of protein kinases in human cancer conducted by the Wellcome Trust Sanger Institute, *BRAF*, the immediate downstream effector of *NRAS*, was found to be somatically mutated

A. Ho
Institute for Biochemistry, Erlangen, Germany

Harvard Combined Dermatology Residency Program,
Harvard Medical School, Boston, MA, USA

G. Jönsson
Institute for Biochemistry, Erlangen, Germany

Melanoma Genetics Unit, Division of Oncology and Pathology,
Lund University, Lund, Sweden

H. Tsao (✉)
Wellman Center for Photomedicine, Department of Dermatology,
Melanoma and Pigmented Lesion Center, Massachusetts General Hospital and Harvard
Medical School, Boston, MA, USA
e-mail: htsao@mgh.harvard.edu

A. Bosserhoff (ed.), *Melanoma Development*,
DOI 10.1007/978-3-319-41319-8_4

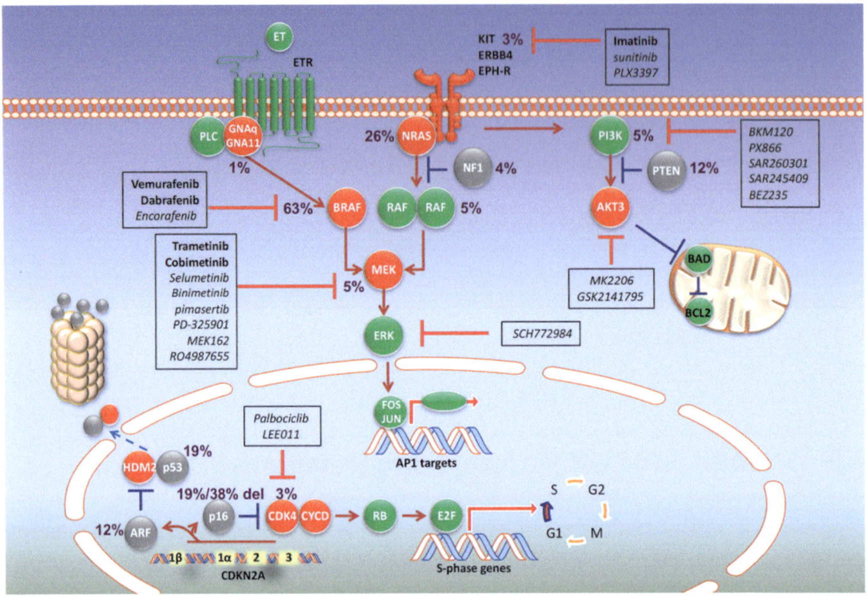

Fig. 4.1 Molecular lesions in melanoma signaling genes. Many components of the melanoma growth signaling cascade are mutated and activated. *Red* activated, *gray* inactivated, *green* normal function. Drugs (*shown in boxes*) that have been approved (*bold*), or in trial (*non-bold, italics*), are indicated

in >60 % of metastatic melanomas (Davies et al. 2002). The dual role of Nras in activating both the MAPK and PI3K pathways and Braf in activating the MAPK pathway underscores the importance and therapeutic opportunities the defects in these pathways presents. Here, we summarize the genetic alterations found in these pathways and their consequences.

4.1.1 MAPK Pathway

Braf is a serine threonine kinase and a member of the "classical" MAPK pathway, which regulates cell growth, survival, and differentiation. Braf is highly expressed in melanocytes and neuronal tissue, both of which are of neural crest origin. MAPK pathway activation is mediated by receptor tyrosine kinases and G-protein-coupled receptors, which subsequently activates the Ras family members and then the Raf kinase family (Araf, Braf, and Craf). The Raf kinases activate Mek1/2, which in turn stimulates Erk1/2, thereby triggering the eventual expression of genes involved in proliferation or differentiation (Fig. 4.1). It was demonstrated early on that mutations in *BRAF* was a common genetic event in nevi, suggesting that it is an early event in melanoma progression (Pollock et al. 2003). This led several groups to investigate whether *BRAF* germline mutations were present in melanoma kindreds not accounted for by *CDKN2A* mutation; however, no germline mutations were identified thereby excluding the role of *BRAF* as a melanoma susceptibility gene

(Casula et al. 2004; Jackson et al. 2005; Laud et al. 2003). The single most common mutation found in *BRAF* is the T1799A point mutation leading to an amino acid substitution of glutamic acid to valine at position 600 located in the kinase domain of the *BRAF* gene and in total >80 % of all *BRAF* mutations occur at this locus (Hocker and Tsao 2007). Other putative oncogenic mutations occur at other codons in exon 15 or in exon 11, both of which correspond to the kinase domain as well (Hocker and Tsao 2007). The frequency of mutations in melanoma varies from 30 to 70 % depending on the study; in the largest study on primary cutaneous melanomas, a *BRAF* mutation rate of 48.9 % was reported (Ellerhorst et al. 2011). Studies have demonstrated that *BRAF/RAS* mutant melanomas are driven, at least in part, by MAPK signaling (Hodis et al. 2012; Krauthammer et al. 2012). Noteworthy, *BRAF* mutation frequency differs in melanoma depending on certain clinical and pathological subsets. In melanomas arising from chronically sun-exposed body sites as well as in melanomas not related to sun exposure (mucosal and acral melanomas), the rate of *BRAF* mutagenesis is quite low, whereas the opposite is observed for melanomas arising on intermittently sun-exposed areas (such as trunk and back) (Curtin et al. 2005; Maldonado et al. 2003). Whether the difference is actually based on body site or histological subtype is difficult to tease apart since melanomas arising on chronically sun-exposed sites often are lentigo maligna melanomas (LMM) and melanomas on intermittently sun-exposed sites often are superficial spreading (SSM) or nodular melanomas (NMM) (Curtin et al. 2005). *NRAS*, the second most commonly mutated oncogene in cutaneous melanoma (~15–25 %), is known to activate both the MAPK and the PI3K pathways (Ellerhorst et al. 2011; Bastian 2014). Although some associate *NRAS* mutations with chronic actinic damage and nodular melanomas, *NRAS* mutations were not found to be specific for a melanoma subtype and were noted among melanomas from non-sun-damaged skin (Curtin et al. 2005). Most importantly, *BRAF* and *NRAS* mutations occur in a mutually exclusive manner and in all about 75 % of all melanomas harbor mutations in either of the genes (Hocker and Tsao 2007; Curtin et al. 2005). Additional *RAS* genes seem to have only a minor impact in melanoma. In recent studies, a few somatic mutations were detected in *KRAS* (Brose et al. 2002; Reifenberger et al. 2004). Likewise, *HRAS* mutations are rare in melanomas; however, 12 % of Spitz nevi harbor a genomic gain of the *HRAS* locus and simultaneously 67 % of nevi harboring a gain concomitantly carry a mutation in the *HRAS* gene (Bastian et al. 2000). In some rarer forms of melanoma, such as uveal melanoma, *BRAF*, *KIT*, and *NRAS* mutations are extremely rare. Instead, mutations in the heterotrimeric *GNAQ* gene were identified in 46 % of uveal melanomas. Mutations occurred at a single locus ($\text{Gnaq}^{\text{Q209L}}$) located in the Ras-like domain, and in vitro studies verified that the Q209L mutation activated the MAPK pathway suggesting an alternative route for *BRAF* and *NRAS* mutation (Onken et al. 2008; Van Raamsdonk et al. 2010). Indeed, pre-clinical studies examining inhibition of Mek and Akt pathways in uveal melanoma cells demonstrate decreased cell viability in a synergistic manner (Ambrosini et al. 2013). *GNAQ* mutations are also frequently detected in blue nevi, suggesting that it is an early genetic event similar to the findings of *BRAF* mutations in nevi (Van Raamsdonk et al. 2009). Additionally, in vivo analysis indicates that mutation of *GNAQ* is not sufficient for full progression to melanoma. This is also true for *BRAF* and *NRAS* mutations suggesting overlapping functional properties of these three proteins. The discovery of somatic mutations of *GNAQ* in uveal melanoma led research groups to investigate mutation patterns of heterotrimeric G proteins in melanoma. The group of Yardena Samuels examined the mutation spectrum of 35 genes in melanoma samples. Somatic changes were detected in 17 % of all samples with *GNG10* and *GNAZ* having highest frequency of mutations (Cardenas-Navia et al. 2010). Mutations in *GNA11* were found in 32 % of uveal melanomas in a mutually exclusive pattern with *GNAQ* mutations (Van Raamsdonk et al. 2010).

Patients with high-risk ocular melanomas in the context of COMMON (*c*utaneous/*o*cular *m*elanoma, atypical *m*elanocytic proliferations and *o*ther *n*eoplasms) syndrome have somatic-inactivating mutations of *BAP1* (Njauw et al. 2012). Furthermore, a germline mutation of *BAP1* has been associated with uveal melanoma, suggesting a tumor suppression function (Höiom et al. 2013). However, the role of Bap1 in cutaneous melanoma may be more nuanced as Bap1 has been shown to have a growth-sustaining role in cutaneous melanoma cells (Kumar et al. 2015).

Genome-wide screens to discern whether molecular patterns associated to *BRAF* mutation exist have been performed. Pavey et al. used microarray expression profiling to distinguish *BRAF* and *NRAS* mutant and wild-type cell lines. A set of 83 genes was identified to clearly discriminate *BRAF* mutant and *BRAF* wild-type cells (Pavey et al. 2004), and the approach was later verified in additional data sets (Johansson et al. 2007). It has also been demonstrated that distinct genomic changes in *BRAF*-mutated cells where chromosomes 7 (harboring *BRAF*), 10q (harboring *PTEN*), 11q, 14q, and 20q were identified are discriminatory (Jonsson et al. 2007). The observation of concomitant *BRAFV600* mutation and *PTEN* loss is further enforced by a significant association between *BRAFV600* mutation and *PTEN* somatic mutation (Jonsson et al. 2007; Tsao et al. 2004). These genetic data are corroborated by a recent study where a mouse model with conditional melanocyte-specific expression of *BRAFV600E* developed melanocytic hyperplasias. Moreover, when *PTEN* was abrogated, mice developed melanomas with 100 % penetrance and subsequently induced metastases in the lymph nodes and lungs (Dankort et al. 2009). These data emphasize the cooperativity between the PI3K and the MAPK pathways for melanoma tumorigenesis, and thus activating mutations of *BRAF* as well as inactivating changes in *PTEN* represent one molecular partnership to attain the desired effect. Taken together, these results suggest that *BRAF* mutant melanomas develop via a distinct genetic pathway.

The success of therapeutic targeting of Braf in metastatic melanoma underscores the importance of understanding the genetics underlying melanoma pathogenesis (see Chap. 16). The first drug tested that targets Braf was Sorafenib, which was later found to be ineffective in the clinical setting (Eisen et al. 2006). Vemurafenib, a potent Braf inhibitor, is approved for patients with $Braf^{V600E}$-mutated melanomas that are unresectable or metastatic (Chapman et al. 2011). The phase III trial, BRIM-3, comparing vemurafenib versus dacarbazine as a first-line therapy for $Braf^{V600E}$-mutated metastatic melanoma demonstrated improved median progression-free survival (PFS; 5.3 versus 1.6 months) and better overall survival (OS; 84 % versus 64 %) at 6 months in the vemurafenib versus dacarbazine groups, respectively. The early positive results of BRIM-3 led to unblinding, allowing patients on the dacarbazine arm to cross over to vemurafenib. Dabrafenib is another selective Braf inhibitor recently approved for the treatment of $Braf^{V600E}$ mutation positive, unresectable, or metastatic melanoma. The phase III trial, BREAK-3, comparing dabrafenib versus dacarbazine demonstrated improved median PFS when compared to those in the dacarbazine arm, 5.1 versus 2.7 months, respectively, with a hazard ratio (HR) for progression of 0.30 (95 % CI 0.18–0.51; $p<0.0001$) (Hauschild et al. 2012). The true difference in overall survival cannot be assessed due to the predefined crossover of progressing dacarbazine patients into the dabrafenib arm.

The discovery of *BRAF* mutations suggested that other members of the MAPK pathway may prove to be attractive therapeutic targets. Mek 1/2 are effector proteins downstream of Braf. Moreover, exome sequencing of metastatic melanoma specimens identified somatic mutations in *MEK1* and *MEK2* as potential clinically significant aberrations, characterizing *MEK1* and *MEK2* mutations in 8 % of melanomas (Nikolaev et al. 2011). Trametinib is a selective Mek 1/2 inhibitor recently approved for the treatment of patients with $Braf^{V600E/K}$—mutant metastatic melanoma. The phase III trial, METRIC, comparing trametinib to chemotherapy (dacarbazine or paclitaxel) in the treatment of patients with $Braf^{V600E/K}$ mutant-positive metastatic melanoma demonstrated significant improvement in median PFS (1.5 versus 4.8 months; HR = 0.45; 95 % CI 0.33–0.63; $p<0.001$) and 6-month OS (67 % versus 81 %; HR = 0.54; 95 % CI 0.32–0.92; $p=0.01$), despite being permitted to crossover to trametinib (Flaherty et al. 2012a).

Notwithstanding these promising results with single agent selective Braf inhibitor use, clinical responses are typically short-lived with a PFS of approximately 7 months (Chapman et al. 2011; Hauschild et al. 2012). This led to several approaches to improve the durability of response, including using combination strategies and intermittent dosing schedules to delay selection of resistant tumor cells (Das Thakur et al. 2013; Flaherty et al. 2012b; Long et al. 2014; Robert et al. 2015). A phase III trial, COMBI-v, comparing first-line trametinib plus dabrafenib to dabrafenib alone in patients with $Braf^{V600E/K}$ mutant metastatic melanoma demonstrated improvements in the median PFS (9.3 months versus 8.8 months; HR = 0.75; 95 % CI 0.57–0.99; $p=0.03$) in the combination group (Long et al. 2014). Furthermore, an open-label phase III trial comparing first line dabrafenib plus trametinib to vemurafenib alone in patients with $Braf^{V600E/K}$ mutant metastatic melanoma showed a significant improvement in OS with combination therapy versus vemurafenib (HR = 0.69; 95 % CI 0.53–0.89; $p=0.005$); median PFS was 11.4 versus 7.3 months, respectively (HR = 0.56; 95 % CI 0.46–0.69; $p<0.001$) (Robert et al. 2015). A phase III study demonstrated the combination of vemurafenib and the MEK inhibitor cobimetinib improved PFS (9.9 versus 6.2 months; HR = 0.51; 95 % CI 0.39–0.68; $p<0.001$) and OR (68 % versus 45 %; $p<0.001$) when compared to vemurafenib alone (Larkin et al 2014). Taken together, these results suggest that combination therapy can attenuate resistance to Braf inhibition and has replaced single agent targeted therapy.

Genetic studies into the molecular mechanisms underlying resistance to Braf-targeted therapy can provide future avenues to prolong responses to therapy. Potential mechanisms of resistance include intrinsic and acquired modes of resistance. There are a number of proposed intrinsic mechanisms of resistance related to cell cycle regulation. The amplification of cyclin D1, observed in 15–20 % of Braf mutant melanomas, has been associated with high rates of resistance to Braf inhibitors by allowing for cell cycle entry when MAPK signaling is abrogated (Smalley et al. 2008). Additionally, one study methodically screened kinase-coding genes for any that conferred resistance to a Braf inhibitor and identified Cot overexpression as a mediator of Braf inhibitor resistance. COT activation, which functions upstream of Mek, results in Raf-independent MEK and Erk activation (Johannessen et al. 2010). Loss or inactivation of Pten has also been associated with resistance to Braf inhibitors (Paraiso et al. 2011). However, Pten expression has been correlated with shorter PFS in patients treated with dabrafenib (Nathanson et al. 2013). Moreover, the deletion of the retinoblastoma protein (Rb) attenuates Raf dependence in $Braf^{V600E}$-mutated melanoma cells (Xing et al. 2012).

Acquired Braf inhibitor resistance in melanoma cells is mediated through a number of different proposed mechanisms. The reactivation of the MAPK pathway by bypassing mutant Braf is the most frequently described mechanism of acquired resistance to mutant Braf inhibition. Nras activating mutations promote enhanced Raf dimerization. Upon binding of the Braf inhibitor to one member of the dimer, allosteric transactivation of the drug-free Raf protein results in the downstream signaling (Nazarian et al. 2010). Furthermore, constitutive signaling by receptor tyrosine kinases results in signal transduction either through Craf or through the PI3K pathway (Nazarian et al. 2010; Sun et al. 2014). A number of different resistance mechanisms within the PI3K pathway that results in MAPK reactivation have been described including mutations in *AKT* and regulatory members of the PI3K pathway (Rizos et al. 2014). Alternative splicing of mutant Braf and copy number amplification of mutant Braf have also been described (Poulikakos et al. 2011; Shi et al. 2012). These results suggest that understanding the genetic alterations in melanoma cells pre- and post-exposure to targeted therapies can shed light onto the development of more effective therapeutic strategies.

4.1.2 PI3K Pathway

As in the MAPK pathway, Nras is also an essential part of the PI3K pathway. Here, Ras induces membrane translocation and activates PI3K, which in turn leads to phosphorylation and activation of one of the major targets of the PI3K pathway, AKT. Mutations in members of the PI3K pathway have been extensively studied in several cancers. Although *PIK3CA* (p110α subunit of PI3K) is a common oncogene in breast (~30 %) and colon (~15 %) cancers (Ogino et al. 2009; Saal et al. 2005), it is rarely altered in melanoma (Omholt et al. 2006). It appears that melanomas preferentially activate the PI3K pathway through inactivation of *PTEN*—another key component of the PI3K pathway. *PTEN*, located on chromosome 10, is deleted in 30–50 % of melanomas and is a major tumor suppressor gene commonly abrogated in human tumors. Somatic mutations of *PTEN* are rare in primary melanomas (Reifenberger et al. 2004; Tsao et al. 2004), whereas the frequency increases in metastases and melanoma cell line cultures (Guldberg et al. 1997; Pollock et al. 2002; Tsao et al. 2004); this may indicate a selective advantage for cells with a

PTEN deficiency. There are three isoforms of Akt—Akt1, 2, and 3; however, there are several lines of evidence suggesting that Akt3 is the main player in melanoma. It has been shown that Akt3 is the predominant active form in melanoma cells and the *AKT3* gene is located on chromosome 1q a region commonly gained in primary melanoma. At least one metastatic tumor has been described to harbor the focal amplification of the *AKT3* locus (Jonsson et al. 2007). Moreover, a rare point mutation (E17K) in the pleckstrin homology domain, which results in constitutive activation, was identified in melanoma cells (Davies et al. 2008).

Regulators of the PI3K pathway also impact melanoma pathogenesis. Prex2 is a PTEN-regulating protein that was demonstrated to accelerate tumor formation of in vivo immortalized human melanocytes (Berger et al. 2012). *PREX2* alterations were initially identified on sequencing of genomes of 25 metastatic melanomas and matched germline DNA. It was then confirmed in 14 % of an independent extension cohort of 107 human melanomas. Other attractive targets in the PI3K pathway have been identified including *MTOR*, *IRS4*, *PIK3R4*, *PIK3R5*, and *NFKB1* (Shull et al. 2012).

Therapeutic targeting of the PI3K pathway in melanoma has shown early promise in pre-clinical studies. The dual inhibition of Braf and the PI3K pathway demonstrated induction of melanoma cell apoptosis via a mechanism independent of Mek signaling (Sánchez-Hernández et al. 2012). Furthermore, combinations of Braf, Mek, and PI3K inhibitors overcame acquired resistance to the Braf inhibitor dabrafenib (Greger et al. 2012). However, phase II trials examining the combinations of everolimus with temozolomide and temsirolimus or tipifarnib with sorafenib failed to demonstrate promising clinical activity for metastatic melanoma (Margolin et al. 2012; Dronca et al. 2014). The reason for this appears to be interruption of negative feedback loops mediated by mTorc1, causing activation of PI3K, Akt, and Erk (Carracedo et al. 2008).

As mentioned above, the activation of the PI3K pathway is one proposed mechanism of resistance to Braf and MEK inhibitors. Furthermore, vemurafenib and selumetinib, a selective MEK inhibitor, co-resistant Braf mutant melanoma cell lines have been shown to be dependent on AKT induction for survival (Atefi et al. 2011). Therefore, efforts to target the PI3K pathway for inhibition as a means of combating Braf and MEK inhibitor resistance are underway (Greger et al. 2012). AKT inhibition overcame acquired resistance to both Braf and MEK inhibition with the exception of vemurafenib-resistant melanoma cells that acquired a *NRAS* mutation (Atefi et al. 2011). $BRAF^{V600E}$ mutant melanoma cells harboring *MEK* or *NRAS* mutations demonstrated resistance to dabrafenib and trametinib monotherapy. However, the addition of a PI3K inhibitor to dabrafenib resulted in improved growth inhibition (Greger et al. 2012). These studies suggest that combination therapy that includes concomitant inhibition of the PI3K pathway may prolong clinical responses in Braf mutant melanoma.

4.1.3 The CDKN2A Network

The chromosome 9p21 locus is commonly targeted by loss-of-heterozygosity (LOH) or deletions in melanoma. The importance of this locus is underscored by the identification of somatic as well as germline mutations in *CDKN2A*

(Hayward 2003; Jonsson et al. 2007). Patients with *CDKN2A* mutations carry an increased risk of melanoma of 70 % over their lifetimes (Hayward 2003). *CDKN2A* is unique in the way that it encodes for two different proteins, $p16^{INK4A}$ and $p14^{ARF}$, each transcribed in a separate reading frame. The two genes share one exon but have two distinct first exons (exon 1α and exon 1β). The *CDKN2A* locus was discovered through linkage analysis of melanoma kindreds and molecular assays showing limited homozygous deletions in some melanoma cell lines (Kamb et al. 1994; Weaver-Feldhaus et al. 1994). It was subsequently shown that germline mutations in *CDKN2A* could explain a substantial fraction of melanoma kindreds (Hayward 2003; Lin et al. 2008). Mutations in *CDKN2A* are also detected in sporadic multiple primary melanoma patients with a frequency around 9 % (Puig et al. 2005). In cultured melanoma cells, *CDKN2A* is frequently inactivated by homozygous deletions whereas small deletions or mutations are more common as germline changes. For both germline and somatic mutations, many of the reported changes reside in exon 2, which impinges on both $p16^{INK4A}$ and $p14^{ARF}$ while mutations only affecting the $p14^{ARF}$ transcript are rare. Within the retinoblastoma (RB) pathway, both the Rb protein and the $p16^{INK4A}$ act as tumor suppressors by regulating the cell cycle. Whereas Rb has been shown to have a limited role in melanoma development, $p16^{INK4A}$ appears to be the major tumor suppressor in this pathway for melanoma. The key function of $p16^{INK4A}$ is as an inhibitor at the G1-to-S cell cycle restriction point where it binds to Cdk4 and thus unable Cdk4 to bind to cyclinD1, which subsequently would lead to phosphorylation and inactivation of Rb. This ultimately releases the E2f transcription factors thereby transcriptionally upregulating S-phase-related genes. The $p16^{INK4A}$ also plays an important role in cellular senescence, a mechanism that restricts the emergence of immortalized cells; however, the explanation for this is elegantly reviewed elsewhere (Bennett 2003). By contrast, $p14^{ARF}$ suppresses oncogenic transformation by binding and inhibiting Hdm2 whose function is to abrogate p53 function by targeting it for degradation via the ubiquitin pathway (Momand et al. 1992). The amplification of both *CDK4* and *MDM2* has been observed in a subset of melanomas and has also been associated with preserved expression of $p16^{INK4A}$ and $p14^{ARF}$ (Muthusamy et al. 2006). Additionally, melanomas with wild-type *BRAF* and *NRAS* frequently display increased gene copy number of *CDK4* and *CCND1*, which are direct downstream targets of the MAPK pathway (Curtin et al. 2005). These melanomas frequently represent chronically sun-damaged, acral- or mucosal-type lesions. The relevance of the *TP53* gene is uncertain since 22 % of melanoma cell lines are mutated at this locus while only 12 % of primary cutaneous melanomas are mutated (Hocker and Tsao 2007). In one study, a mutation frequency of 30 % of mucosal melanomas was found (Ragnarsson-Olding et al. 2002), suggesting subtype-specific mutation patterns. The low prevalence of p53 mutations in melanoma as compared to other cancers might be explained by the high frequency of *CDKN2A* inactivation. Evidence on the functional association between $p14^{ARF}$ and p53 became clear when the interaction between Hdm2 and $p14^{ARF}$ was elucidated (Zhang et al. 1998).

4.2 Somatic Changes in the Pigmentation Pathway of Melanoma

It was early demonstrated that the biology of pigmentation is an essential part of melanoma development. Several epidemiological studies demonstrate that dark skinned individuals have a decreased risk of developing melanoma and red-haired and light skinned people are at an increased risk of melanoma (Cho et al. 2005; Swerdlow et al. 1986). One of the key regulators of pigmentation is *MC1R* located on chromosome 16q and acts by inducing production of dark eumelanin over the red pheomelanin (Rouzaud et al. 2005). The dark eumelanin is thought to be more protective against UV radiation than the red pheomelanin. Genetic variants of the *MC1R* gene are, not unexpectedly, associated with an increased risk of melanoma as reviewed elsewhere (Nelson and Tsao 2009). Also, genetic variants in other genes or loci (*TYR*, *ASIP*, *OCA2*, *TYRP1*, *SLC24A4*, *TPCN2*, and 9p21) connected to the pigmentation pathway have been shown to confer melanoma risk through a recent set of with genome-wide association (GWAS) studies (Bishop et al. 2009; Brown et al. 2008; Gudbjartsson et al. 2008). Although these GWAS results clearly link *MC1R* to risk, no *MC1R* somatic mutations were identified in a cohort of 103 primary melanomas suggesting that *MC1R* is not a frequent target of somatic alteration (Kim et al. 2008). Furthermore, there are studies that demonstrate that the presence of *MC1R* variants increase the melanoma penetrance in *CDKN2A* carriers (Fargnoli et al. 2010). The r variant p.R163Q is associated with increased risk of melanoma in high sun exposed geographies (Córdoba-Lanús et al. 2014). In 2005, Garraway et al. used the NCI 60 panel of cell lines and an integrative genomics approach to map novel oncogenes. High-resolution genomic maps indicated lineage restricted copy number changes and integrated with gene expression profiling data-supervised methods identified *MITF* as amplified and highly expressed in a subset of melanomas (Garraway et al. 2005). It was at that time known that Mitf was a master regulator of the melanocyte lineage. When investigating *MITF* gene copy number status in a set of primary melanomas, an inverse relationship was observed between gene copy number and survival. Intriguingly, all *MITF*-amplified cell lines harbored *BRAF* mutation as well as inactivated p16^{INK4A}, suggesting a cooperative effect of these genetic defects. Consequently, the overexpression of *MITF* in combination with oncogenic *BRAF* in immortalized melanocytes transformed these thereby confirming the oncogenic potential of *MITF* in melanoma. Furthermore, two independent studies identified the rare functional variant in *MITFE318K* that increases melanoma risk and also predisposes to renal cell carcinoma. *MITFE318K* occurs at a conserved SUMOylation position, decreasing the number of SUMO-modified Mitf isoforms. This leads to increased Mitf transcriptional activity (Yokoyama et al. 2011; Bertolotto et al. 2011). Several major pathways such as normal pigment cell physiology, melanocyte survival, cell cycle regulation, and growth are known to be downstream activities of Mitf. An elegant study by McGill et al. showed that *BCL2* is a transcriptional target of Mitf confirming the growth regulatory function of Mitf since Bcl2 is an antiapoptotic factor (McGill et al. 2002). Moreover, additional targets of Mitf include Tbx2, Met, and Cdk2 representing mechanisms that provide growth advantage (Carreira et al. 2000; Du et al. 2004; McGill et al. 2006). The regulation of Mitf has been investigated and regulatory pathways include Notch, Mc1r, Wnt, endothelin receptor, KIT, and MAPK pathways. These pathways are known to genetically interact with *MITF*, such as *PAX3* and *SOX10*, and are involved in neural crest development (Potterf et al. 2000; Verastegui et al. 2000) (see Chaps. 2 and 4). The critical function of Mitf in melanoma as well as the finding of *MITF*-amplified melanomas led to the discovery of somatic mutations of *MITF* in a subset of melanomas. In the study by Cronin et al., eight cases of 50 metastatic melanoma lines were either amplified or mutated for *MITF*. In line with these results, an additional three cases harbored mutation of the *SOX10* gene, an upstream regulator of *MITF*, in a mutually exclusive fashion with *MITF* alterations (Cronin et al. 2009). Correlation between mutations in the Mitf pathway and *BRAF*/*NRAS* mutation status supported the observation made by Garraway et al. that these alterations are cooperative genetic events (Garraway et al. 2005). Overall, this study observed that approximately 20 % of metastatic melanoma harbors genetic alterations of the Mitf pathway. Chromosome 7p gains/amplifications is commonly found in melanoma and with this in mind, Jane-Valbuena et al. set out to search for a potential novel oncogene in melanoma. Using high-density SNP arrays, *ETV1* was pinpointed as an attractive target (Jane-Valbuena et al. 2010). Functional analysis revealed that the oncogenic potential of *ETV1* was dependent on concomitant activation of the MAPK pathway and upregulated mRNA levels of *MITF*. Additional studies of other members of the Mitf pathway will most likely unravel additional gene alterations.

As an initiator of several melanocytic signaling pathways, *KIT* has a central role in the development of melanoma. It has been demonstrated that *KIT* mutations in melanoma are mutually exclusive with *BRAF* and *NRAS* mutations. c-Kit is a receptor tyrosine kinase and has been proven to be able to activate both the MAPK and PI3K pathways (Fig. 4.1). Particular high frequency of mutations was identified in melanomas arising on palms, soles, and subungual sites (acral melanomas) as well as on mucosal membranes (mucosal melanomas) (Curtin et al. 2006). Additionally, the gain or amplification of the *KIT* locus (chromosome 4q12) was observed preferentially in mucosal, acral, or chronically sun-damaged melanomas and a substantial number of mutated tumors also harbored amplification suggesting an additive effect of amplification and mutation. In melanomas that harbor c-kit mutations, mutations leading to substitutions at L576P and K642E have been shown to account for 55 % of c-Kit mutated melanomas (Beadling et al. 2008). These findings set the stage for clinical targeting of c-Kit in melanoma patients. Initial trials with imatinib, an ATP-competitive inhibitor of several tyrosine kinases including c-Kit, did not demonstrate statistically significant results, likely because these early trials did not select for patients with known c-Kit mutated tumors (Ugurel et al. 2005). More recent trials have selected for patients with known c-kit mutated metastatic melanoma. In one phase II, single-group, open-label trial exploring the effect of c-Kit inhibition with imatinib mesylate in patients with *KIT*-altered melanoma, clinically significant results were found. In this study, 23.4 % of the patients had *KIT* mutations and/or amplifications, with a median PFS of 12.0 weeks and an OS of 46.3 weeks. The K642E or L576P substitutions within c-Kit were present in all responses observed

(Carvajal et al. 2011). Further molecular studies are required to characterize specific genetic alterations in c-kit to allow for more effective therapeutic targeting.

Like *KIT*, β-catenin is also involved in melanocyte lineage development. Wnt ligand binding results in nuclear translocation of β-catenin, resulting in gene transduction. The overexpression of β-catenin in neural crest cells results in pigment cell formation, while conditional inactivation of β-catenin led to loss of melanoblasts (Dorsky et al. 1998; Hari et al. 2002). Many studies have shown that β-catenin is critical for the transformation of melanocytes. Increased level of nuclear β-catenin is a consequence of a cascade initially started by canonical Wnt signaling and has been found in 50 % of melanomas (Kielhorn et al. 2003). In mice, functional analysis has revealed that β-catenin cooperates with *NRAS* oncogenesis by repressing *p16INK4A* (Delmas et al. 2007). However, somatic mutations of β-catenin are detected in only a small fraction of melanomas suggesting that there are other unknown mechanisms responsible for the localization of β-catenin in the nucleus. Recent work has suggested that Wnt signaling in melanoma cells regulates their interaction with the tumor microenvironment. One study demonstrated that Wnt1 is anti-lymphangiogenic by suppressing melanoma derived VEGF-C expression (Niederleithner et al. 2012). Intriguingly, recent evidence has demonstrated that melanoma intrinsic β-catenin signaling results in the lack of T cell infiltration in melanoma animal models and patient-derived biopsies (Spranger et al. 2015). Further work will be required to define strategies to effectively target β-catenin signaling in melanoma cells as this has implications for not only targeted therapies in melanoma but also checkpoint blockade regimens.

4.3 Novel Pathways in Melanoma

To identify novel key regulators of melanoma oncogenesis and metastasis several approaches have been taken where an integrative approach combining gene expression profiling and SNP arrays identified *MITF* as lineage-specific oncogene in melanoma as discussed previously. An alternative approach employed by Kim et al. includes comparative oncogenomics using a Ras inducible nonmetastatic mouse model to identify clones that had accumulated genetic changes conferring metastatic capacity (Kim et al. 2006). With this approach, a focal amplification on mouse chromosome 13 containing eight genes was identified using high-resolution comparative genomic hybridization. When analyzing mRNA transcript levels, *NEDD9* was pinpointed as the target gene. To confirm the results found in the mouse model, a number of primary and metastatic melanomas were genome-wide screened for copy number changes. In all, 36 % of metastatic and 8 % of primary melanomas harbored the amplification of 6p25-p24 (syntenic to mouse chromosome 13) as well as increased gene and protein expression of *NEDD9*. Furthermore, the knockdown of *NEDD9* inhibited proliferation and invasion corroborating the metastatic capacity of Nedd9-activated melanoma cells.

There has also been a systematic genetic screen of the matrix metalloproteinase (MMP) superfamily of genes (Palavalli et al. 2009) in melanomas. Matrix metalloproteinases (MMPs) are proteolytic enzymes that degrade the basement membrane and the extracellular matrix. This suggests an involvement of MMPs in cancer metastasis; however, clinical trials using MMP inhibitors are largely unsuccessful in clinical trials.

MMP8-deficient mice, however, exhibit an increased skin cancer risk suggesting a tumor suppressor role of *MMP8* in skin cancers including melanoma (Lopez-Otin et al. 2009). Notably, *MMP8* and *MMP27* were mutated in 6–8 %, respectively, of the melanoma cases investigated. Furthermore, mutations of *MMP8* were frequently accompanied by LOH, suggesting that *MMP8* acts as a tumor suppressor gene in melanoma. Functional analysis of *MMP8* mutant cells displayed decreased proliferation as compared to *MMP8* wild-type cells. By contrast, when investigating migratory capacity of *MMP8* mutant cells these displayed decreased migration ability. Taken together, MMPs seem to play some role in melanoma development.

Recent work has identified alterations in genes that play a role in telomere maintenance as promoting susceptibility to melanoma. Telomeres consist of tandem nucleotide repeats located at chromosomal ends and maintain genomic stability and chromosomal stability by protecting chromosome ends from degradation, end-to-end fusion, and atypical recombination. The enzyme telomerase replenishes telomeres as the telomere ends become shorter with each cell division. In one recent study, Horn et al. used multipoint linkage analyses and target-enriched high-throughput sequencing to identify a germline mutation in the promoter of telomerase reverse transcriptase (*TERT*) in a melanoma-prone family. Tert is part of a ribonucleoprotein complex that maintains telomere length. They also found recurrent ultraviolet signature somatic mutations within the *TERT* promoter in 74 % of human cell lines derived from metastatic melanomas that they examined (Horn et al. 2013). In another recent report, germline mutations in *ACD* and *TERF2IP*, two members of the shelterin complex that protects telomeres, were found in melanoma-prone families using next-generation sequencing. The study included 510 melanoma-prone families without mutations in known melanoma-susceptibility genes (Aoude et al. 2015). Furthermore, two independent studies identified germline variants in protection of telomere 1 (*POT1*) in *CDKN2A* wild-type melanoma-prone families. Pot1 plays a role in protecting telomere ends by preventing inappropriate processing of the exposed chromosome ends and regulating telomerase function (Robles-Espinoza et al. 2014; Shi et al. 2014). These findings suggest that telomere maintenance plays a role in melanoma susceptibility.

4.4 Genome-Wide Screening Approaches in Melanoma

Recent technical developments have allowed researchers to investigate gene copy number changes on a global basis. In melanoma, the availability of frozen tissue is a major drawback when it comes to genome-wide analyses; hence, many studies in melanoma have been performed with melanoma cell lines or short-term cultures. Several research groups have investigated the detailed landscape of gene copy number changes in melanoma lines (Gast et al. 2010; Jonsson et al. 2007; Stark and Hayward 2007). Interestingly, a fairly homogenous pattern of DNA copy number changes was observed with several chromosomes altered in more than 50 % of the cases. Frequent losses were observed on chromosomes 4, 6, 8, 9, 10, and 11, whereas frequent gains were found on chromosomes 1, 7, 8, 17, and 20. These regions are corroborated by high-density SNP array analysis with frequent LOH at these regions (Stark and Hayward 2007). Additionally, 11q13, 3p14, and 1p12 were recurrently amplified including candidate oncogenes such as *CCND1*, *MITF*, and *NOTCH2*. Homozygous deletions are frequently identified in melanoma lines with the *CDKN2A* locus being affected in 40–60 % and *PTEN* in 10–15 %. Moreover, less frequent deletions include genes such as *PTPRD*, *HDAC4*, and *PARD3* suggesting novel tumor suppressor genes in melanoma.

In 2005, a vanguard study described genome-wide assessment of DNA copy number changes in 126 primary melanomas (Curtin et al. 2005). Tumors were divided into four groups based on sun-induced damage and on whether the tumor was classified as acral or mucosal melanoma. Specifically, acral and mucosal melanomas were found to harbor an increased frequency of genomic alterations as well as higher frequency of gene amplifications. Furthermore, chromosome 10q deletions were more common in melanomas without chronic sun-damaged skin, whereas focal gains of the *CCND1* locus were more frequent in the group with chronic sun-damaged skin. This elegant analysis of genetic alterations displayed that subgroups can be identified in melanoma and a strong relationship between sun exposure and genome-wide DNA copy number patterns exist.

Primary and metastatic melanomas have been subjected to transcriptomic analysis. Using supervised and integrative methods a number of genes with a significant expression deregulation between primary and metastatic melanoma were identified. The proinvasive ability of these genes was subsequently validated with functional assays (Kabbarah et al. 2010).

New genome-wide sequencing approaches have been used to identify epigenetic targets in melanoma pathogenesis. More specifically, regulators of chromatin remodeling such as members of the SWI/SNF complex, a nucleosome remodeling complex, have recently been implicated. Inactivating mutations in SWI/SNF family member genes (*ARID1A*, *ARID1B*, *ARID2*, and *SMARCA4*) and in members of another chromatin remodeling complex, the poly comb complex, (*EZH2*, *BMI1*, and *JARID1B/KDM5B*) were altered in melanoma (Hodis et al. 2012; Kuźbicki et al. 2013; Chang et al. 2015; Tiffen et al. 2015). While the exact mechanism of how alterations in chromatin remodeling drive melanoma disease progression is unclear, cellular de-differentiation is one proposed mechanism (Sarris et al. 2014). Preliminary studies have demonstrated that EZH2, a member of the poly comb complex, is overexpressed in melanoma cells and suppresses tumor suppressor proteins (Tiffen et al. 2015). Other epigenetic alterations that have been suggested as mediating melanoma disease progression are noncoding RNAs. These molecules have been known to be aberrantly expressed in melanoma; however, the specific role in melanoma pathogenesis is yet unknown (Greenberg et al. 2014). As new technologies emerge to identify genetic alterations in melanoma, functional studies will be required to characterize the mechanism by which these alterations contribute to disease progression.

In summary, during the past few years there have been an explosion of genomic analyses in melanoma. The heterogeneous nature of melanoma is clearly reflected in genome-wide DNA copy number changes and the numerous genetic alterations found.

4.5 Progression of Melanoma: The Genomic Approach

The classical histopathological pathway of progression described by Clark is initiated in the benign nevus where proliferation of normal melanocytes begins. The next step includes the formation of dysplastic nevi and this may occur in pre-existing nevi or at a new location. The formation of radial growth phase melanomas occurs when melanocytes acquire the ability to proliferate intraepidermally. One of the most critical steps in the development of melanoma includes the progression from radially growing melanomas (i.e., radial growth phase, RGP) to vertically advancing melanomas (i.e., vertical growth phase, VGP) where cells have the ability to invade the dermis. This deep invasion allows melanoma cells to spread to distant organs, form metastases, and potentially create a lethal event. Dissemination can occur by either lymphatic or hematogenous routes. Since access to these vascular structures is a prerequisite for metastatic spread, it is not surprising that a simple measure of vertical invasion, i.e., Breslow thickness, has survived the test of time.

The genetic factors related to this histopathological progression are starting to emerge. The presence of somatic *BRAF* mutations in nevi (Pollock et al. 2003) suggests that this is an early event and that *BRAF* activation alone is not sufficient for melanocytes to transform into a malignant state. Moreover, there is no significant difference in the frequency *BRAF or NRAS* mutations within control nevi or melanoma-associated nevi (Tschandl et al. 2013). Subsequent genetic events are more uncertain, though $p16^{INK4A}$ loss is considered to be an important early step since germline mutations in *CDKN2A* have been found in a significant fraction of melanoma kindreds and homozygous deletions and deleterious mutations of *CDKN2A* occur in a large fraction of melanoma cell lines. Also, it is evident that mice with *Cdkn2a* loss cooperate with activating MAPK lesions to drive melanoma formation (Chin et al. 1997). In addition to *CDKN2A*, loss of *PTEN* should also be considered to be a critical event. This is supported by human studies where deleterious *PTEN* alterations have been described (Tsao et al. 2000, 2004) and also by mice studies where *Pten* loss has been shown to induce metastatic melanoma in combination with activating *Braf* alleles (Dankort et al. 2009). Moreover, *PTEN* depletion and subsequent PI3K pathway activation abrogates $Braf^{V600E}$-induced senescence in melanocytes (Vredeveld et al. 2012). Furthermore, simultaneous *CDKN2A* and *LKB1* inactivation in $Braf^{V600E}$ melanocytes results in activation of both mTorc1 and Akt, resulting in rapid melanoma formation in mice (Damsky et al. 2015).

Beyond discrete genetic events, markers that define the switch from RGP to VGP have also been examined. One of the hallmarks in the switch between RGP and VGP include the loss of E-cadherin expression and simultaneously increased expression of N-cadherin affecting cell adhesion mechanisms. In addition, these expression differences stimulate β-catenin and thereby increase the survival of melanoma cells. In a more comprehensive screen, Haqq et al. investigated gene expression difference between RGP and VGP (Haqq et al. 2005). Interestingly, loss of expression for a set of genes was observed in the vertical growth phase of the melanoma; these include *CDH3* and *MMP10* among other genes. Furthermore, the same gene set effectively partitions metastatic melanomas into two groups, which might indicate that metastases could develop from either the radial growth or the vertical growth phase of melanoma. The authors also identified gene sets that differed between normal skin, nevi, primary melanoma, and two types of metastatic melanoma suggesting that molecular patterns of progression do exist. Likewise, Sabatino et al. characterized melanoma cell lines derived from metachronous metastases from a single melanoma patient (Sabatino et al. 2008). Genome-wide copy number analysis supported a cancer stem cell model where a suggestive progenitor cell harbors a core set of genomic aberrations and that metastatic progression is not a sequential event. In a similar study by Harbst et al. metastases obtained from five patients were investigated for genomic imbalances, gene expression profiles, and methylation profiles (Harbst et al. 2010). Here, evidence for two models of metastatic progression was provided. The first model was supported by genomic aberration patterns of a case with three metachronous metastases. Homozygous deletions at chromosomes 3p26 and 6q23 were found in two consecutive metastases originating from the same primary tumor in a mutually exclusive manner corroborating the findings of Sabatino et al. (2008). Investigation of the E-cadherin and N-cadherin mRNA levels indicates variability as to when the actual switch in expression occurs. For one case the switch had obviously occurred prior to the metastases investigated, whereas in two of the cases the switch became apparent at the development of the second metastasis (Fig. 4.2). Interestingly, methylation analysis provided additional evidence for *PTEN*'s role in melanoma progression. Silencing of the *PTEN* gene was evident in the last of three consecutive metastases originating from a single primary melanoma. An alternative model of sequential progression was also found. In another case, the primary tumor as well as two consecutive metastases displayed almost indistinguishable genomic profiles. Furthermore, gene expression and methylation profiles support a common origin for metastases originating from the same primary tumor. In all, this indicates that at least two types of mechanisms can contribute to melanoma metastases.

To further detail the genetic landscape of melanoma progression, high-throughput DNA sequencing has begun to provide a framework of melanoma evolution. One recent study investigated the succession of genetic events contributing to the malignant transformation of melanocytes. In 37 melanocytic neoplasms specifically chosen for melanomas with histologically distinct precursors, benign lesions had *BRAFV600* mutations exclusively. Intermediate lesions harbored *NRAS* and additional driver mutations. Of the lesions examined, 77 % of intermediate lesions and melanomas in situ harbored *TERT* promoter mutations, suggesting that these mutations a selected for early in the malignant transformation. *CDKN2A* inactivation was found exclusively in invasive melanomas. *PTEN* and *TP53* mutations were found only in advanced primary melanomas. Moreover, the mutational burden characteristic of ultraviolet radiation

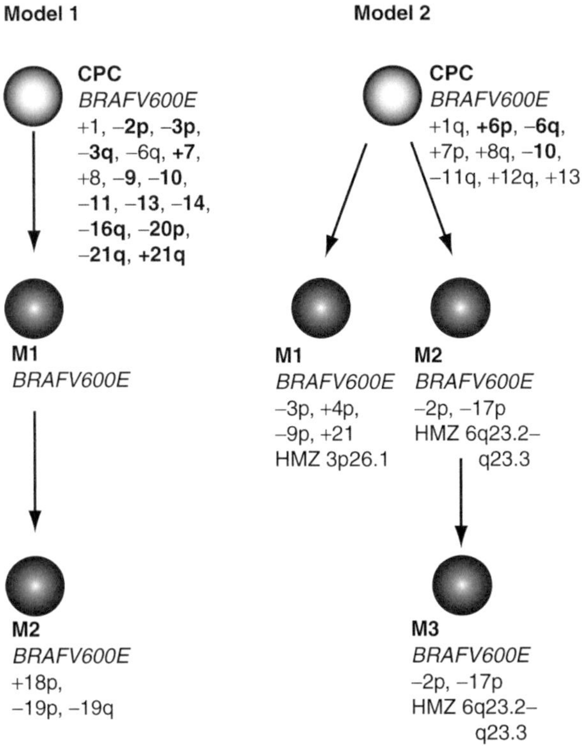

Fig. 4.2 Two models of tumor progression as suggested by Harbst et al. (2010). *Model 1*: The indistinguishable genomic profiles, as well as inheritance of the *BRAF* mutation, suggest sequential tumor progression. *Model 2*: Metastasis-specific gene copy number aberrations exclude the possibility of a sequential process and indicate to the evolvement of at least two distinct subclones with metastatic potential. However, both a core set of genomic aberrations and presence of the *BRAF* mutation in all lesions confirm common origin of the tumors. Major chromosomal changes are indicated. CPC indicates a common metastatic precursor cell/clone that harbors indicated chromosomal aberrations inherited by all the metastases from that tumor. In *bold*, copy number aberrations observed in the primary tumor. *HMZ* homozygous deletion

increased from benign through intermediate lesions to melanoma (Hunter Shain et al. 2015). In seeming contradiction to the traditional models of sequential genetic alterations and subsequent clonal selection leading the melanoma pathogenesis, recent studies have demonstrated that normal skin already contains a high burden of driver mutations. There are six genes (*Notch 1*, *2*, *3*, *P53*, *FAT1*, and *RBM10*) that were demonstrated to have an excess of nonsilent mutations, suggesting there is a selection pressure for these mutations, and as such, represent drivers. One-quarter of middle-aged skin contains a mutation in one of these genes (Martincorena et al. 2015). However, the sizes of clones containing these mutations are relatively limited and similar across individuals, indicating that the growth of clones slows early in their expansion. How this occurs is unknown at this time and warrants further investigation as it likely represents a checkpoint preventing malignant transformation.

These recent studies where a genomic approach was taken indicates the extensive complexity in progression of malignant melanoma and more in-depth genetic studies are eagerly awaited.

4.6 Molecular Classification of Melanoma

Several groups have used molecular parameters in an attempt to recover a subclassification of melanoma. Viros et al. used a combination of histomorphologic and genetic features to classify a comprehensive set of melanomas (Viros et al. 2008). Interestingly, *BRAF*-mutated melanomas displayed characteristic features such as nest formation of intraepidermal melanocytes and larger, rounder, and more pigmented tumor cells. By contrast, *NRAS*-mutated melanomas did not show any specific morphologic characteristics. A survival benefit was also identified in patients predicted to be *BRAF* mutated, most likely due to a different route of metastasis. As mentioned previously, Curtin et al. described a classification based on genetic alterations and primary tumor location and sun-damaged tumor surrounding skin (Curtin et al. 2005). A more recent study also used genome-wide DNA copy number changes as a way of subclassifying melanoma metastases. Here, three classes were found and showed different event-free survival (Kabbarah et al. 2010). An alternative way of molecularly classifying cancer is by using genome-wide assessment of mRNA transcript levels though the lack of frozen tissue from primary melanomas has led to only one study with sufficient clinical annotation (Kabbarah et al. 2010). In that study, 83 primary melanomas in the vertical growth phase with a Breslow thickness of at least 1 mm were subjected to global gene expression profiling. Applying supervised methods on melanomas from patients with or without 4-year distant metastasis-free survival a prognostic set of 254 genes was identified. The investigation of clinical parameters in the two prognostic groups revealed differences with regard to Breslow thickness, AJCC stage, melanoma type, ulceration, and mitotic rate—features all known to be strong prognostic factors in melanoma. Indeed, a comparison of the prognostic gene set and a gene set derived based on Breslow thickness revealed a considerable overlap. Genes related to DNA repair and cell cycle increased with thickness as well as with poor prognosis. A more careful analysis of the prognostic gene set showed that DNA replication and DNA repair are the most significant pathways (Kauffmann et al. 2008). These results have also been corroborated by a recent study applying an alternative microarray platform (Jewell et al. 2010).

Technical developments have enabled researchers to start exploring global gene expression profiles from formalin-fixed paraffin-embedded (FFPE) tissue (April et al. 2009). In melanoma, the first studies used a microarray platform consisting of a restricted set of cancer-related genes ($n = 502$) (Conway et al. 2009; Jewell et al. 2010; Mitra et al. 2010). However, these have been directed toward identifying single molecular biomarkers and not in classifying melanomas. Through such approaches, the expression level of osteopontin was identified as the gene with strongest association with reduced relapse-free survival (Conway et al. 2009).

Subsequent studies with sentinel lymph node status confirmed the prognostic significance of osteopontin and DNA repair genes (Jewell et al. 2010; Mitra et al. 2010). Studies using whole-genome approaches of gene expression analysis of archival FFPE RNA open up a wide range of opportunities for investigating the genomic landscape of primary malignant melanoma.

Global gene expression patterns have to a larger extent been applied to advanced stage or metastatic melanomas where availability of frozen tissue is not the main limitation. As alluded to earlier, one study used a gene set derived from a discriminatory analysis between radial growth and vertical growth phase of a single primary melanoma (Haqq et al. 2005). In this study, the investigators also detected two subtypes of metastatic melanoma. Type I metastases displayed increased expression of genes presumably downregulated in the vertical growth phase of primary melanoma, whereas type II metastases were characterized by increased expression of genes related to pigmentation such as *MITF*, *MLANA*, and *TYR*. More recently, Jönsson et al. set out to discern a biological subclassification with clinical impact in stage IV melanoma (Jonsson et al. 2010). Gene expression profiles were obtained for 57 lymph node or subcutaneous metastases. Unsupervised hierarchical clustering algorithms identified four molecular classes. These were subsequently characterized and named according to the gene expression pattern of the class. The first group, high-immune response, expressed high levels of immune response-related genes such as *LCK*, *CXCL12*, and *HLA* class I and II antigen. The second class, proliferative, expressed decreased levels of immune response-related genes as well as a trend toward higher Ki67 staining. High levels of genes such as *MITF*, *TYR*, *DCT*, and *MLANA* characterized the third class (pigmentation class). This is in line with the findings of Haqq et al. who identified a subclass in metastatic melanoma that had high expression of genes that characterize the radial growth phase of a single primary melanoma as well as high expression of pigmentation-related genes (Haqq et al. 2005). Finally, the normal-like subclass was characterized by melanomas expressing genes such as *TRIM29*, *KRT17*, and *KRT10*. Most importantly, this biological subclassification scheme displayed a significant association to clinical outcome with the proliferative subtype as a poor prognostic group, which was validated in an independent cohort of stage III melanomas (Fig. 4.3). In a study by Bugonvic et al., a prognostic gene expression signature supports the finding of improved survival in patients with tumors having increased expression of immune response-related genes (Bogunovic et al. 2009). Additionally, all patients included in the Jönsson et al. study were enrolled in a prospective trial of DTIC treatment. This allowed the investigators to correlate treatment response with molecular subclass. Indeed, a significant association between the pigmentation subclass and a stable disease at 3 months of treatment was identified suggesting that pigmentation might be a predictive target of DTIC response. Further molecular characterization of subclasses implied different frequencies of genomic imbalances and targeted gene deletions, e.g., *CDKN2A* homozygous deletion was significantly associated with the proliferative class. In all, this study indicates that a molecular classification is tenable and could be clinically meaningful. These results have

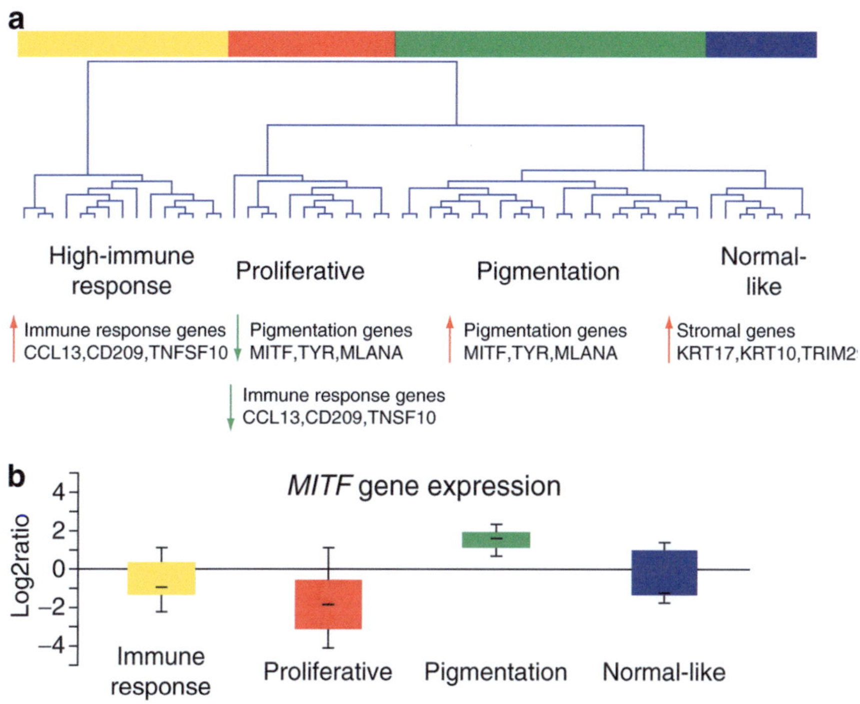

Fig. 4.3 Molecular classification of malignant melanoma. (**a**) Subclassification of stage IV melanomas based on gene expression patterns as suggested by Jönsson et al. (2010). Four classes were identified each broadly characterized by expression of set of genes involved in immune response and pigmentation. (**b**) Box plot of *MITF* gene expression levels in each class displaying an increased expression in the Pigmentation class

subsequently been validated in primary and metastatic melanomas (Harbst et al. 2012 and Cirenajwis et al. 2015). Finally, it has been demonstrated that tumors from CDKN2A germline mutation carriers are indistinguishable from sporadic melanomas and found in all four molecular subclasses (Staaf et al. 2014).

In one recent hallmark study, an integrative analysis of cutaneous melanomas establishes a genetic framework for molecular classification into four subtypes: mutant *BRAF*, mutant *RAS*, mutant *NF1*, and triple wild-type. Enrichment of *KIT* mutations, focal amplifications, and structural rearrangements were features of the triple-wild-type subgroup. There was no significant difference in clinical outcome between subtypes. However, a subset of each molecular subtype with a significant immune signature was associated with improved survival, which has significant implications for immunotherapy (Cancer Genome Atlas Network 2015).

In summary, the classification of melanoma based on molecular patterns will most likely be an important parameter in future medical oncology since the advent of targeted and immunotherapy showing promising results in melanoma will require molecular stratification prior to treatment.

4.7 Next-Generation Sequencing: Approaches in Melanoma

The availability of novel high-throughput sequencing methods such as human genome sequencing has revolutionized cancer research during the past few years. In a pioneering study from the Wellcome Trust Sanger Institute, a single melanoma cancer genome was sequenced with a tremendous gain in biologic insight (Pleasance et al. 2010). One of the main findings of the study was the observation that the melanoma genome was littered with C>T mutations 3′ to a pyrimidine site, a hallmark of mutations attributed by UV-induced DNA damage. This single finding puts to rest the controversy that melanomas are in fact not subject to UV mutagenesis (Hocker and Tsao 2007) (see also Chap. 3). It is also possible to sequence RNA transcripts using next-generation sequencing. An elegant study by Berger et al. used this approach to analyze short-term melanoma cultures (Berger et al. 2010). In the analysis, 11 novel melanoma gene fusions produced by underlying genomic rearrangements were found. However, none of these changes were recurrent suggesting that the gene fusions could be "passenger" events. Interestingly, in a screen for novel prostate cancer fusion genes, *BRAF* was identified and because of the high mutation rate of somatic mutations of *BRAF* in melanoma the screen was extended to include melanomas; however, only one case out of 131 harbored a rearranged *BRAF* gene corroborating the low prevalence of recurrent gene fusions in melanoma (Palanisamy et al. 2010).

A very important study demonstrating the significance and enormous potential of next-generation sequencing was published in 2009 (Emery et al. 2009). Here, a somatic *MEK* mutation was observed in a metastatic lesion showing resistance to treatment of an MEK inhibitor. In vitro analysis displaying further evidence of *MEK*-mutated clones demonstrated resistance to both a MEK inhibitor as well as to a Raf inhibitor. However, when combining Mek and Raf inhibitors resistance to targeted therapies of the MAPK pathway is circumvented.

As has been described above, next-generation sequencing has been leveraged to identify mechanisms of resistance to targeted therapy in metastatic melanoma. As an example, Van Allen et al. performed whole-exome sequencing on formalin-fixed, paraffin-embedded tumors and demonstrated that common pathways of selective Braf inhibitor resistance in melanoma cells include *BRAF* mutant amplification, STAT3 upregulation, or mutations in other members of the MAPK pathway (Van Allen et al. 2014). Mutations in downstream MAPK members results in constitutive activation of Mek, independent of the upstream Braf kinase and insensitive to Mek inhibitors.

With the recent success of immunotherapy in the treatment of metastatic melanoma (see Chap. 17), novel high-throughput technologies have been used to predict those patients that will likely benefit from immunotherapy targeting CTLA-4 or PD1/PD-L1. Whole exome sequencing was performed on tumor and blood samples from melanoma patients treated with the CTLA-4 inhibitors ipilimumab or tremelimumab. This revealed a neoantigen peptide landscape specifically present in tumors with a strong response to CTLA-4 blockade. More specifically, there was an association between high mutational load and clinical benefit with CTLA-4 immune checkpoint blockade (Snyder et al. 2014). In another recent study, whole exomes from CTLA-4 blockade pretreatment melanoma tumor biopsies and matched germline tissue samples were examined. Clinical benefit was associated with overall mutational load, neoantigen load, and expression of cytolytic markers in the immune microenvironment (Van Allen et al. 2015). Similar findings have been demonstrated with respect to PD-1 immune checkpoint inhibitors. Tumors that have a high somatic mutational frequency, above 10 somatic mutations per megabase of coding DNA, such as melanomas, were shown to respond best to PD-1 inhibitors (Lawrence et al. 2013).

4.8 Summary

In summary, the genetic and genomic landscape of melanoma has radically changed over the past decade. Advances in our understanding of cancer genetics and the advent of powerful technologies will undoubtedly transform our vision of the molecular underpinnings of melanoma within the next few years. In this chapter, we have been able to survey only some of the principles and technologies that underlie the ongoing genomic revolution. It is clear that only the tip of the iceberg has come into view.

References

Ambrosini G, Musi E, Ho AL, de Stanchina E, Schwartz GK (2013) Inhibition of mutant GNAQ signaling in uveal melanoma induces AMPK-dependent autophagic cell death. Mol Cancer Ther 12(5):768–776

Aoude LG, Pritchard AL, Robles-Espinoza CD, Wadt K, Harland M, Choi J, Gartside M, Quesada V, Johansson P, Palmer JM, Ramsay AJ, Zhang X, Jones K, Symmons J, Holland EA, Schmid H, Bonazzi V, Woods S, Dutton-Regester K, Stark MS, Snowden H, van Doorn R, Montgomery GW, Martin NG, Keane TM, López-Otín C, Gerdes AM, Olsson H, Ingvar C, Borg A, Gruis NA, Trent JM, Jönsson G, Bishop DT, Mann GJ, Newton-Bishop JA, Brown KM, Adams DJ, Hayward NK (2015) Nonsense mutations in the shelterin complex genes ACD and TERF2IP in familial melanoma. J Natl Cancer Inst 107(2). pii: dju408

April C, Klotzle B, Royce T, Wickham-Garcia E, Boyaniwsky T, Izzo J, Cox D, Jones W, Rubio R, Holton K, Matulonis U, Quackenbush J, Fan JB (2009) Whole-genome gene expression profiling of formalin-fixed, paraffin-embedded tissue samples. PLoS One 4:e8162

Atefi M, von Euw E, Attar N, Ng C, Chu C, Guo D, Nazarian R, Chmielowski B, Glaspy JA, Comin-Anduix B, Mischel PS, Lo RS, Ribas A (2011) Reversing melanoma cross-resistance to BRAF and MEK inhibitors by co-targeting the AKT/mTOR pathway. PLoS One 6(12):e28973

Bastian BC (2014) The molecular pathology of melanoma: an integrated taxonomy of melanocytic neoplasia. Annu Rev Pathol 9:239–271

Bastian BC, LeBoit PE, Pinkel D (2000) Mutations and copy number increase of HRAS in Spitz nevi with distinctive histopathological features. Am J Pathol 157:967–972

Beadling C, Jacobson-Dunlop E, Hodi FS, Le C, Warrick A, Patterson J, Town A, Harlow A, Cruz F 3rd, Azar S, Rubin BP, Muller S, West R, Heinrich MC, Corless CL (2008) KIT gene mutations and copy number in melanoma subtypes. Clin Cancer Res 14(21):6821–6828

Bennett DC (2003) Human melanocyte senescence and melanoma susceptibility genes. Oncogene 22:3063–3069

Berger MF, Levin JZ, Vijayendran K, Sivachenko A, Adiconis X, Maguire J, Johnson LA, Robinson J, Verhaak RG, Sougnez C, Onofrio RC, Ziaugra L, Cibulskis K, Laine E, Barretina J, Winckler W, Fisher DE, Getz G, Meyerson M, Jaffe DB, Gabriel SB, Lander ES, Dummer R, Gnirke A, Nusbaum C, Garraway LA (2010) Integrative analysis of the melanoma transcriptome. Genome Res 20:413–427

Berger MF, Hodis E, Heffernan TP, Deribe YL, Lawrence MS, Protopopov A, Ivanova E, Watson IR, Nickerson E, Ghosh P, Zhang H, Zeid R, Ren X, Cibulskis K, Sivachenko AY, Wagle N, Sucker A, Sougnez C, Onofrio R, Ambrogio L, Auclair D, Fennell T, Carter SL, Drier Y, Stojanov P, Singer MA, Voet D, Jing R, Saksena G, Barretina J, Ramos AH, Pugh TJ, Stransky N, Parkin M, Winckler W, Mahan S, Ardlie K, Baldwin J, Wargo J, Schadendorf D, Meyerson M, Gabriel SB, Golub TR, Wagner SN, Lander ES, Getz G, Chin L, Garraway LA (2012) Melanoma genome sequencing reveals frequent PREX2 mutations. Nature 485(7399): 502–506

Bertolotto C, Lesueur F, Giuliano S, Strub T, de Lichy M, Bille K, Dessen P, d'Hayer B, Mohamdi H, Remenieras A, Maubec E, de la Fouchardière A, Molinié V, Vabres P, Dalle S, Poulalhon N, Martin-Denavit T, Thomas L, Andry-Benzaquen P, Dupin N, Boitier F, Rossi A, Perrot JL, Labeille B, Robert C, Escudier B, Caron O, Brugières L, Saule S, Gardie B, Gad S, Richard S, Couturier J, Teh BT, Ghiorzo P, Pastorino L, Puig S, Badenas C, Olsson H, Ingvar C, Rouleau E, Lidereau R, Bahadoran P, Vielh P, Corda E, Blanché H, Zelenika D, Galan P, Group FFMS, Aubin F, Bachollet B, Becuwe C, Berthet P, Bignon YJ, Bonadona V, Bonafe JL, Bonnet-Dupeyron MN, Cambazard F, Chevrant-Breton J, Coupier I, Dalac S, Demange L, d'Incan M, Dugast C, Faivre L, Vincent-Fétita L, Gauthier-Villars M, Gilbert B, Grange F, Grob JJ, Humbert P, Janin N, Joly P, Kerob D, Lasset C, Leroux D, Levang J, Limacher JM, Livideanu C, Longy M, Lortholary A, Stoppa-Lyonnet D, Mansard S, Mansuy L, Marrou K, Matéus C, Maugard C, Meyer N, Nogues C, Souteyrand P, Venat-Bouvet L, Zattara H, Chaudru V, Lenoir GM, Lathrop M, Davidson I, Avril MF, Demenais F, Ballotti R, Bressac-de Paillerets B (2011) A SUMOylation-defective MITF germline mutation predisposes to melanoma and renal carcinoma. Nature 480(7375):94–98

Bishop DT, Demenais F, Iles MM, Harland M, Taylor JC, Corda E, Randerson-Moor J, Aitken JF, Avril MF, Azizi E, Bakker B, Bianchi-Scarra G, Bressac-de Paillerets B, Calista D, Cannon-Albright LA, Chin AWT, Debniak T, Galore-Haskel G, Ghiorzo P, Gut I, Hansson J, Hocevar M, Hoiom V, Hopper JL, Ingvar C, Kanetsky PA, Kefford RF, Landi MT, Lang J, Lubinski J, Mackie R, Malvehy J, Mann GJ, Martin NG, Montgomery GW, van Nieuwpoort FA, Novakovic S, Olsson H, Puig S, Weiss M, van Workum W, Zelenika D, Brown KM, Goldstein AM, Gillanders EM, Boland A, Galan P, Elder DE, Gruis NA, Hayward NK, Lathrop GM, Barrett JH, Bishop JA (2009) Genome-wide association study identifies three loci associated with melanoma risk. Nat Genet 41:920–925

Bogunovic D, O'Neill DW, Belitskaya-Levy I, Vacic V, Yu YL, Adams S, Darvishian F, Berman R, Shapiro R, Pavlick AC, Lonardi S, Zavadil J, Osman I, Bhardwaj N (2009) Immune profile and mitotic index of metastatic melanoma lesions enhance clinical staging in predicting patient survival. Proc Natl Acad Sci U S A 106:20429–20434

Brose MS, Volpe P, Feldman M, Kumar M, Rishi I, Gerrero R, Einhorn E, Herlyn M, Minna J, Nicholson A, Roth JA, Albelda SM, Davies H, Cox C, Brignell G, Stephens P, Futreal PA, Wooster R, Stratton MR, Weber BL (2002) BRAF and RAS mutations in human lung cancer and melanoma. Cancer Res 62:6997–7000

Brown KM, Macgregor S, Montgomery GW, Craig DW, Zhao ZZ, Iyadurai K, Henders AK, Homer N, Campbell MJ, Stark M, Thomas S, Schmid H, Holland EA, Gillanders EM, Duffy DL, Maskiell JA, Jetann J, Ferguson M, Stephan DA, Cust AE, Whiteman D, Green A, Olsson H, Puig S, Ghiorzo P, Hansson J, Demenais F, Goldstein AM, Gruis NA, Elder DE, Bishop JN, Kefford RF, Giles GG, Armstrong BK, Aitken JF, Hopper JL, Martin NG, Trent JM, Mann GJ, Hayward NK (2008) Common sequence variants on 20q11.22 confer melanoma susceptibility. Nat Genet 40:838–840

Cancer Genome Atlas Network (2015) Genomic classification of cutaneous melanoma. Cell 161(7):1681–1696

Cardenas-Navia LI, Cruz P, Lin JC, Rosenberg SA, Samuels Y (2010) Novel somatic mutations in heterotrimeric G proteins in melanoma. Cancer Biol Ther 10:33–37

Carracedo A, Ma L, Teruya-Feldstein J, Rojo F, Salmena L, Alimonti A, Egia A, Sasaki AT, Thomas G, Kozma SC, Papa A, Nardella C, Cantley LC, Baselga J, Pandolfi PP (2008) Inhibition of mTORC1 leads to MAPK pathway activation through a PI3K-dependent feedback loop in human cancer. J Clin Invest 118(9):3065–3074

Carreira S, Liu B, Goding CR (2000) The gene encoding the T-box factor Tbx2 is a target for the microphthalmia-associated transcription factor in melanocytes. J Biol Chem 275:21920–21927

Carvajal RD, Antonescu CR, Wolchok JD, Chapman PB, Roman RA, Teitcher J, Panageas KS, Busam KJ, Chmielowski B, Lutzky J, Pavlick AC, Fusco A, Cane L, Takebe N, Vemula S, Bouvier N, Bastian BC, Schwartz GK (2011) KIT as a therapeutic target in metastatic melanoma. JAMA 305(22):2327–2334

Casula M, Colombino M, Satta MP, Cossu A, Ascierto PA, Bianchi-Scarra G, Castiglia D, Budroni M, Rozzo C, Manca A, Lissia A, Carboni A, Petretto E, Satriano SM, Botti G, Mantelli M, Ghiorzo P, Stratton MR, Tanda F, Palmieri G (2004) BRAF gene is somatically mutated but does not make a major contribution to malignant melanoma susceptibility: the Italian Melanoma Intergroup Study. J Clin Oncol 22:286–292

Chang X, Sun Y, Han S, Zhu W, Zhang H, Lian S (2015) MiR-203 inhibits melanoma invasive and proliferative abilities by targeting the polycomb group gene BMI1. Biochem Biophys Res Commun 456(1):361–366

Chapman PB, Hauschild A, Robert C, Haanen JB, Ascierto P, Larkin J, Dummer R, Garbe C, Testori A, Maio M, Hogg D, Lorigan P, Lebbe C, Jouary T, Schadendorf D, Ribas A, O'Day SJ, Sosman JA, Kirkwood JM, Eggermont AM, Dreno B, Nolop K, Li J, Nelson B, Hou J, Lee RJ, Flaherty KT, McArthur GA, BRIM-3 Study Group (2011) Improved survival with vemurafenib in melanoma with BRAF V600E mutation. N Engl J Med 364(26):2507–2516

Chin L, Pomerantz J, Polsky D, Jacobson M, Cohen C, Cordon-Cardo C, Horner JW 2nd, DePinho RA (1997) Cooperative effects of INK4a and ras in melanoma susceptibility in vivo. Genes Dev 11:2822–2834

Cho E, Rosner BA, Colditz GA (2005) Risk factors for melanoma by body site. Cancer Epidemiol Biomarkers Prev 14:1241–1244

Cirenajwis H, Ekedahl H, Lauss M, Harbst K, Carneiro A, Enoksson J, Rosengren F, Werner-Hartman L, Törngren T, Kvist A, Fredlund E, Bendahl PO, Jirström K, Lundgren L, Howlin J, Borg Å, Gruvberger-Saal SK, Saal LH, Nielsen K, Ringnér M, Tsao H, Olsson H, Ingvar C, Staaf J, Jönsson G (2015) Molecular stratification of metastatic melanoma using gene expression profiling: prediction of survival outcome and benefit from molecular targeted therapy. Oncotarget 6(14):12297–12309

Conway C, Mitra A, Jewell R, Randerson-Moor J, Lobo S, Nsengimana J, Edward S, Sanders DS, Cook M, Powell B, Boon A, Elliott F, de Kort F, Knowles MA, Bishop DT, Newton-Bishop J (2009) Gene expression profiling of paraffin-embedded primary melanoma using the DASL assay identifies increased osteopontin expression as predictive of reduced relapse-free survival. Clin Cancer Res 15:6939–6946

Córdoba-Lanús E, Hernández-Jiménez JG, Medina-Coello C, Espinoza-Jiménez A, González A, Rodríguez-Pérez MD, Carretero-Hernández G, Almeida P, Suárez-Hernández J, Perera-Molinero A, Fernández-de-Misa R (2014) MC1R gene variants and sporadic malignant melanoma susceptibility in the Canary Islands population. Arch Dermatol Res 306(1):51–58

Cronin JC, Wunderlich J, Loftus SK, Prickett TD, Wei X, Ridd K, Vemula S, Burrell AS, Agrawal NS, Lin JC, Banister CE, Buckhaults P, Rosenberg SA, Bastian BC, Pavan WJ, Samuels Y (2009) Frequent mutations in the MITF pathway in melanoma. Pigment Cell Melanoma Res 22:435–444

Curtin JA, Fridlyand J, Kageshita T, Patel HN, Busam KJ, Kutzner H, Cho KH, Aiba S, Brocker EB, LeBoit PE, Pinkel D, Bastian BC (2005) Distinct sets of genetic alterations in melanoma. N Engl J Med 353:2135–2147

Curtin JA, Busam K, Pinkel D, Bastian BC (2006) Somatic activation of KIT in distinct subtypes of melanoma. J Clin Oncol 24:4340–4346

Damsky W, Micevic G, Meeth K, Muthusamy V, Curley DP, Santhanakrishnan M, Erdelyi I, Platt JT, Huang L, Theodosakis N, Zaidi MR, Tighe S, Davies MA, Dankort D, McMahon M, Merlino G, Bardeesy N, Bosenberg M (2015) mTORC1 activation blocks BrafV600E-induced growth arrest but is insufficient for melanoma formation. Cancer Cell 27(1):41–56

Dankort D, Curley DP, Cartlidge RA, Nelson B, Karnezis AN, Damsky WE Jr, You MJ, DePinho RA, McMahon M, Bosenberg M (2009) Braf(V600E) cooperates with Pten loss to induce metastatic melanoma. Nat Genet 41:544–552

Das Thakur M, Salangsang F, Landman AS, Sellers WR, Pryer NK, Levesque MP, Dummer R, McMahon M, Stuart DD (2013) Modelling vemurafenib resistance in melanoma reveals a strategy to forestall drug resistance. Nature 494(7436):251–255

Davies H, Bignell GR, Cox C, Stephens P, Edkins S, Clegg S, Teague J, Woffendin H, Garnett MJ, Bottomley W, Davis N, Dicks E, Ewing R, Floyd Y, Gray K, Hall S, Hawes R, Hughes J, Kosmidou V, Menzies A, Mould C, Parker A, Stevens C, Watt S, Hooper S, Wilson R, Jayatilake H, Gusterson BA, Cooper C, Shipley J, Hargrave D, Pritchard-Jones K, Maitland N, Chenevix-Trench G, Riggins GJ, Bigner DD, Palmieri G, Cossu A, Flanagan A, Nicholson A, Ho JW, Leung SY, Yuen ST, Weber BL, Seigler HF, Darrow TL, Paterson H, Marais R, Marshall CJ, Wooster R, Stratton MR, Futreal PA (2002) Mutations of the BRAF gene in human cancer. Nature 417:949–954

Davies MA, Stemke-Hale K, Tellez C, Calderone TL, Deng W, Prieto VG, Lazar AJ, Gershenwald JE, Mills GB (2008) A novel AKT3 mutation in melanoma tumours and cell lines. Br J Cancer 99:1265–1268

Delmas V, Beermann F, Martinozzi S, Carreira S, Ackermann J, Kumasaka M, Denat L, Goodall J, Luciani F, Viros A, Demirkan N, Bastian BC, Goding CR, Larue L (2007) Beta-catenin induces immortalization of melanocytes by suppressing p16INK4a expression and cooperates with N-Ras in melanoma development. Genes Dev 21:2923–2935

Dorsky RI, Moon RT, Raible DW (1998) Control of neural crest cell fate by the Wnt signalling pathway. Nature 396(6709):370–373

Dronca RS, Allred JB, Perez DG, Nevala WK, Lieser EA, Thompson M, Maples WJ, Creagan ET, Pockaj BA, Kaur JS, Moore TD, Marchello BT, Markovic SN (2014) Phase II study of temozolomide (TMZ) and everolimus (RAD001) therapy for metastatic melanoma: a North Central Cancer Treatment Group study, N0675. Am J Clin Oncol 37(4):369–376

Du J, Widlund HR, Horstmann MA, Ramaswamy S, Ross K, Huber WE, Nishimura EK, Golub TR, Fisher DE (2004) Critical role of CDK2 for melanoma growth linked to its melanocyte-specific transcriptional regulation by MITF. Cancer Cell 6:565–576

Eisen T, Ahmad T, Flaherty KT, Gore M, Kaye S, Marais R, Gibbens I, Hackett S, James M, Schuchter LM, Nathanson KL, Xia C, Simantov R, Schwartz B, Poulin-Costello M, O'Dwyer PJ, Ratain MJ (2006) Sorafenib in advanced melanoma: a phase II randomised discontinuation trial analysis. Br J Cancer 95:581–586

Ellerhorst JA, Greene VR, Ekmekcioglu S, Warneke CL, Johnson MM, Cooke CP, Wang LE, Prieto VG, Gershenwald JE, Wei Q, Grimm EA (2011) Clinical correlates of NRAS and BRAF mutations in primary human melanoma. Clin Cancer Res 17:229–235

Emery CM, Vijayendran KG, Zipser MC, Sawyer AM, Niu L, Kim JJ, Hatton C, Chopra R, Oberholzer PA, Karpova MB, MacConaill LE, Zhang J, Gray NS, Sellers WR, Dummer R, Garraway LA (2009) MEK1 mutations confer resistance to MEK and B-RAF inhibition. Proc Natl Acad Sci U S A 106:20411–20416

Fargnoli MC, Gandini S, Peris K, Maisonneuve P, Raimondi S (2010) MC1R variants increase melanoma risk in families with CDKN2A mutations: a meta-analysis. Eur J Cancer 46(8):1413–1420

Flaherty KT, Robert C, Hersey P, Nathan P, Garbe C, Milhem M, Demidov LV, Hassel JC, Rutkowski P, Mohr P, Dummer R, Trefzer U, Larkin JM, Utikal J, Dreno B, Nyakas M, Middleton MR, Becker JC, Casey M, Sherman LJ, Wu FS, Ouellet D, Martin AM, Patel K, Schadendorf D, METRIC Study Group (2012a) Improved survival with MEK inhibition in BRAF-mutated melanoma. N Engl J Med 367(2):107–114

Flaherty KT, Infante JR, Daud A, Gonzalez R, Kefford RF, Sosman J, Hamid O, Schuchter L, Cebon J, Ibrahim N, Kudchadkar R, Burris HA 3rd, Falchook G, Algazi A, Lewis K, Long GV, Puzanov I, Lebowitz P, Singh A, Little S, Sun P, Allred A, Ouellet D, Kim KB, Patel K, Weber J (2012b) Combined BRAF and MEK inhibition in melanoma with BRAF V600 mutations. N Engl J Med 367(18):1694–1703

Garraway LA, Widlund HR, Rubin MA, Getz G, Berger AJ, Ramaswamy S, Beroukhim R, Milner DA, Granter SR, Du J, Lee C, Wagner SN, Li C, Golub TR, Rimm DL, Meyerson ML, Fisher DE, Sellers WR (2005) Integrative genomic analyses identify MITF as a lineage survival oncogene amplified in malignant melanoma. Nature 436:117–122

Gast A, Scherer D, Chen B, Bloethner S, Melchert S, Sucker A, Hemminki K, Schadendorf D, Kumar R (2010) Somatic alterations in the melanoma genome: a high-resolution array-based comparative genomic hybridization study. Genes Chromosomes Cancer 49:733–745

Greenberg ES, Chong KK, Huynh KT, Tanaka R, Hoon DS (2014) Epigenetic biomarkers in skin cancer. Cancer Lett 342(2):170–177

Greger JG, Eastman SD, Zhang V, Bleam MR, Hughes AM, Smitheman KN, Dickerson SH, Laquerre SG, Liu L, Gilmer TM (2012) Combinations of BRAF, MEK, and PI3K/mTOR inhibitors overcome acquired resistance to the BRAF inhibitor GSK2118436 dabrafenib, mediated by NRAS or MEK mutations. Mol Cancer Ther 11(4):909–920

Gudbjartsson DF, Sulem P, Stacey SN, Goldstein AM, Rafnar T, Sigurgeirsson B, Benediktsdottir KR, Thorisdottir K, Ragnarsson R, Sveinsdottir SG, Magnusson V, Lindblom A, Kostulas K, Botella-Estrada R, Soriano V, Juberias P, Grasa M, Saez B, Andres R, Scherer D, Rudnai P, Gurzau E, Koppova K, Kiemeney LA, Jakobsdottir M, Steinberg S, Helgason A, Gretarsdottir S, Tucker MA, Mayordomo JI, Nagore E, Kumar R, Hansson J, Olafsson JH, Gulcher J, Kong A, Thorsteinsdottir U, Stefansson K (2008) ASIP and TYR pigmentation variants associate with cutaneous melanoma and basal cell carcinoma. Nat Genet 40:886–891

Guldberg P, thor Straten P, Birck A, Ahrenkiel V, Kirkin AF, Zeuthen J (1997) Disruption of the MMAC1/PTEN gene by deletion or mutation is a frequent event in malignant melanoma. Cancer Res 57:3660–3663

Haqq C, Nosrati M, Sudilovsky D, Crothers J, Khodabakhsh D, Pulliam BL, Federman S, Miller JR 3rd, Allen RE, Singer MI, Leong SP, Ljung BM, Sagebiel RW, Kashani-Sabet M (2005) The gene expression signatures of melanoma progression. Proc Natl Acad Sci U S A 102:6092–6097

Harbst K, Staaf J, Masback A, Olsson H, Ingvar C, Vallon-Christersson J, Ringner M, Borg A, Jonsson G (2010) Multiple metastases from cutaneous malignant melanoma patients may display heterogeneous genomic and epigenomic patterns. Melanoma Res 20:381–391

Harbst K, Staaf J, Lauss M, Karlsson A, Måsbäck A, Johansson I, Bendahl PO, Vallon-Christersson J, Törngren T, Ekedahl H, Geisler J, Höglund M, Ringnér M, Lundgren L, Jirström K, Olsson H, Ingvar C, Borg Å, Tsao H, Jönsson G (2012) Molecular profiling reveals low- and high-grade forms of primary melanoma. Clin Cancer Res 18(15):4026–4036

Hari L, Brault V, Kléber M, Lee HY, Ille F, Leimeroth R, Paratore C, Suter U, Kemler R, Sommer L (2002) Lineage-specific requirements of beta-catenin in neural crest development. J Cell Biol 159(5):867–880

Hauschild A, Grob JJ, Demidov LV, Jouary T, Gutzmer R, Millward M, Rutkowski P, Blank CU, Miller WH Jr, Kaempgen E, Martín-Algarra S, Karaszewska B, Mauch C, Chiarion-Sileni V, Martin AM, Swann S, Haney P, Mirakhur B, Guckert ME, Goodman V, Chapman PB (2012) Dabrafenib in BRAF-mutated metastatic melanoma: a multicentre, open-label, phase 3 randomised controlled trial. Lancet 380(9839):358–365

Hayward NK (2003) Genetics of melanoma predisposition. Oncogene 22:3053–3062

Hocker T, Tsao H (2007) Ultraviolet radiation and melanoma: a systematic review and analysis of reported sequence variants. Hum Mutat 28:578–588

Hodis E, Watson IR, Kryukov GV, Arold ST, Imielinski M, Theurillat JP, Nickerson E, Auclair D, Li L, Place C, Dicara D, Ramos AH, Lawrence MS, Cibulskis K, Sivachenko A, Voet D, Saksena G, Stransky N, Onofrio RC, Winckler W, Ardlie K, Wagle N, Wargo J, Chong K, Morton DL, Stemke-Hale K, Chen G, Noble M, Meyerson M, Ladbury JE, Davies MA,

Gershenwald JE, Wagner SN, Hoon DS, Schadendorf D, Lander ES, Gabriel SB, Getz G, Garraway LA, Chin L (2012) A landscape of driver mutations in melanoma. Cell 150(2):251–263
Höiom V, Edsgärd D, Helgadottir H, Eriksson H, All-Ericsson C, Tuominen R, Ivanova I, Lundeberg J, Emanuelsson O, Hansson J (2013) Hereditary uveal melanoma: a report of a germline mutation in BAP1. Genes Chromosomes Cancer 52(4):378–384
Horn S, Figl A, Rachakonda PS, Fischer C, Sucker A, Gast A, Kadel S, Moll I, Nagore E, Hemminki K, Schadendorf D, Kumar R (2013) TERT promoter mutations in familial and sporadic melanoma. Science 339(6122):959–961
Hunter Shain A, Ye I, Kovalyshyn I, Sriharan A, Talevich E, Gagnon A, Dummer R, North J, Pincus L, Ruben B, Rickaby W, D'Arrigo C, Robson A, Bastian B (2015) The genetic evolution of melanoma from precursor lesions. N Engl J Med 373:1926–1936
Jackson S, Harland M, Turner F, Taylor C, Chambers PA, Dos Randerson-Moor J, Swerdlow AJ, Santos Silva I, Beswick S, Bishop DT, Newton Bishop JA (2005) No evidence for BRAF as a melanoma/nevus susceptibility gene. Cancer Epidemiol Biomarkers Prev 14:913–918
Jane-Valbuena J, Widlund HR, Perner S, Johnson LA, Dibner AC, Lin WM, Baker AC, Nazarian RM, Vijayendran KG, Sellers WR, Hahn WC, Duncan LM, Rubin MA, Fisher DE, Garraway LA (2010) An oncogenic role for ETV1 in melanoma. Cancer Res 70:2075–2084
Jewell R, Conway C, Mitra A, Randerson-Moor J, Lobo S, Nsengimana J, Harland M, Marples M, Edward S, Cook M, Powell B, Boon A, de Kort F, Parker KA, Cree IA, Barrett JH, Knowles MA, Bishop DT, Newton-Bishop J (2010) Patterns of expression of DNA repair genes and relapse from melanoma. Clin Cancer Res 16:5211–5221
Johannessen CM, Boehm JS, Kim SY, Thomas SR, Wardwell L, Johnson LA, Emery CM, Stransky N, Cogdill AP, Barretina J, Caponigro G, Hieronymus H, Murray RR, Salehi-Ashtiani K, Hill DE, Vidal M, Zhao JJ, Yang X, Alkan O, Kim S, Harris JL, Wilson CJ, Myer VE, Finan PM, Root DE, Roberts TM, Golub T, Flaherty KT, Dummer R, Weber BL, Sellers WR, Schlegel R, Wargo JA, Hahn WC, Garraway LA (2010) COT drives resistance to RAF inhibition through MAP kinase pathway reactivation. Nature 468(7326):968–972
Johansson P, Pavey S, Hayward N (2007) Confirmation of a BRAF mutation-associated gene expression signature in melanoma. Pigment Cell Res 20:216–221
Jonsson G, Dahl C, Staaf J, Sandberg T, Bendahl PO, Ringner M, Guldberg P, Borg A (2007) Genomic profiling of malignant melanoma using tiling-resolution arrayCGH. Oncogene 26:4738–4748
Jonsson G, Busch C, Knappskog S, Geisler J, Miletic H, Ringner M, Lillehaug JR, Borg A, Lonning PE (2010) Gene expression profiling-based identification of molecular subtypes in stage IV melanomas with different clinical outcome. Clin Cancer Res 16:3356–3367
Kabbarah O, Nogueira C, Feng B, Nazarian RM, Bosenberg M, Wu M, Scott KL, Kwong LN, Xiao Y, Cordon-Cardo C, Granter SR, Ramaswamy S, Golub T, Duncan LM, Wagner SN, Brennan C, Chin L (2010) Integrative genome comparison of primary and metastatic melanomas. PLoS One 5:e10770
Kamb A, Shattuck-Eidens D, Eeles R, Liu Q, Gruis NA, Ding W, Hussey C, Tran T, Miki Y, Weaver-Feldhaus J et al (1994) Analysis of the p16 gene (CDKN2) as a candidate for the chromosome 9p melanoma susceptibility locus. Nat Genet 8:23–26
Kauffmann A, Rosselli F, Lazar V, Winnepenninckx V, Mansuet-Lupo A, Dessen P, van den Oord JJ, Spatz A, Sarasin A (2008) High expression of DNA repair pathways is associated with metastasis in melanoma patients. Oncogene 27:565–573
Kielhorn E, Provost E, Olsen D, D'Aquila TG, Smith BL, Camp RL, Rimm DL (2003) Tissue microarray-based analysis shows phospho-beta-catenin expression in malignant melanoma is associated with poor outcome. Int J Cancer 103:652–656
Kim M, Gans JD, Nogueira C, Wang A, Paik JH, Feng B, Brennan C, Hahn WC, Cordon-Cardo C, Wagner SN, Flotte TJ, Duncan LM, Granter SR, Chin L (2006) Comparative oncogenomics identifies NEDD9 as a melanoma metastasis gene. Cell 125:1269–1281
Kim RD, Curtin JA, Bastian BC (2008) Lack of somatic alterations of MC1R in primary melanoma. Pigment Cell Melanoma Res 21:579–582

Krauthammer M, Kong Y, Ha BH, Evans P, Bacchiocchi A, McCusker JP, Cheng E, Davis MJ, Goh G, Choi M, Ariyan S, Narayan D, Dutton-Regester K, Capatana A, Holman EC, Bosenberg M, Sznol M, Kluger HM, Brash DE, Stern DF, Materin MA, Lo RS, Mane S, Ma S, Kidd KK, Hayward NK, Lifton RP, Schlessinger J, Boggon TJ, Halaban R (2012) Exome sequencing identifies recurrent somatic RAC1 mutations in melanoma. Nat Genet 44(9):1006–1014

Kumar R, Taylor M, Miao B, Ji Z, Njauw JC, Jönsson G, Frederick DT, Tsao H (2015) BAP1 has a survival role in cutaneous melanoma. J Invest Dermatol 135(4):1089–1097

Kuźbicki L, Lange D, Strączyńska-Niemiec A, Chwirot BW (2013) JARID1B expression in human melanoma and benign melanocytic skin lesions. Melanoma Res 23(1):8–12

Larkin J, Ascierto PA, Dréno B, Atkinson V, Liszkay G, Maio M, Mandalà M, Demidov L, Stroyakovskiy D, Thomas L, de la Cruz-Merino L, Dutriaux C, Garbe C, Sovak MA, Chang I, Choong N, Hack SP, McArthur GA, Ribas A (2014) Combined vemurafenib and cobimetinib in BRAF-mutated melanoma. N Engl J Med 371(20):1867–1876

Laud K, Kannengiesser C, Avril MF, Chompret A, Stoppa-Lyonnet D, Desjardins L, Eychene A, Demenais F, Lenoir GM, Bressac-de Paillerets B (2003) BRAF as a melanoma susceptibility candidate gene? Cancer Res 63:3061–3065

Lawrence MS, Stojanov P, Polak P, Kryukov GV, Cibulskis K, Sivachenko A, Carter SL, Stewart C, Mermel CH, Roberts SA, Kiezun A, Hammerman PS, McKenna A, Drier Y, Zou L, Ramos AH, Pugh TJ, Stransky N, Helman E, Kim J, Sougnez C, Ambrogio L, Nickerson E, Shefler E, Cortés ML, Auclair D, Saksena G, Voct D, Noble M, DiCara D, Lin P, Lichtenstein L, Heiman DI, Fennell T, Imielinski M, Hernandez B, Hodis E, Baca S, Dulak AM, Lohr J, Landau DA, Wu CJ, Melendez-Zajgla J, Hidalgo-Miranda A, Koren A, McCarroll SA, Mora J, Lee RS, Crompton B, Onofrio R, Parkin M, Winckler W, Ardlie K, Gabriel SB, Roberts CW, Biegel JA, Stegmaier K, Bass AJ, Garraway LA, Meyerson M, Golub TR, Gordenin DA, Sunyaev S, Lander ES, Getz G (2013) Mutational heterogeneity in cancer and the search for new cancer-associated genes. Nature 499(7457):214–218

Lin J, Hocker TL, Singh M, Tsao H (2008) Genetics of melanoma predisposition. Br J Dermatol 159:286–291

Long GV, Stroyakovskiy D, Gogas H, Levchenko E, de Braud F, Larkin J, Garbe C, Jouary T, Hauschild A, Grob JJ, Chiarion Sileni V, Lebbe C, Mandalà M, Millward M, Arance A, Bondarenko I, Haanen JB, Hansson J, Utikal J, Ferraresi V, Kovalenko N, Mohr P, Probachai V, Schadendorf D, Nathan P, Robert C, Ribas A, DeMarini DJ, Irani JG, Casey M, Ouellet D, Martin AM, Le N, Patel K, Flaherty K (2014) Combined BRAF and MEK inhibition versus BRAF inhibition alone in melanoma. N Engl J Med 371(20):1877–1888

Lopez-Otin C, Palavalli LH, Samuels Y (2009) Protective roles of matrix metalloproteinases: from mouse models to human cancer. Cell Cycle 8:3657–3662

Maldonado JL, Fridlyand J, Patel H, Jain AN, Busam K, Kageshita T, Ono T, Albertson DG, Pinkel D, Bastian BC (2003) Determinants of BRAF mutations in primary melanomas. J Natl Cancer Inst 95:1878–1890

Margolin KA, Moon J, Flaherty LE, Lao CD, Akerley WL 3rd, Othus M, Sosman JA, Kirkwood JM, Sondak VK (2012) Randomized phase II trial of sorafenib with temsirolimus or tipifarnib in untreated metastatic melanoma (S0438). Clin Cancer Res 18(4):1129–1137

Martincorena I, Roshan A, Gerstung M, Ellis P, Van Loo P, McLaren S, Wedge DC, Fullam A, Alexandrov LB, Tubio JM, Stebbings L, Menzies A, Widaa S, Stratton MR, Jones PH, Campbell PJ (2015) Tumor evolution. High burden and pervasive positive selection of somatic mutations in normal human skin. Science 348(6237):880–886

McGill GG, Horstmann M, Widlund HR, Du J, Motyckova G, Nishimura EK, Lin YL, Ramaswamy S, Avery W, Ding HF, Jordan SA, Jackson IJ, Korsmeyer SJ, Golub TR, Fisher DE (2002) Bcl2 regulation by the melanocyte master regulator Mitf modulates lineage survival and melanoma cell viability. Cell 109:707–718

McGill GG, Haq R, Nishimura EK, Fisher DE (2006) c-Met expression is regulated by Mitf in the melanocyte lineage. J Biol Chem 281:10365–10373

Mitra A, Conway C, Walker C, Cook M, Powell B, Lobo S, Chan M, Kissin M, Layer G, Smallwood J, Ottensmeier C, Stanley P, Peach H, Chong H, Elliott F, Iles MM, Nsengimana J, Barrett JH,

Bishop DT, Newton-Bishop JA (2010) Melanoma sentinel node biopsy and prediction models for relapse and overall survival. Br J Cancer 103:1229–1236

Momand J, Zambetti GP, Olson DC, George D, Levine AJ (1992) The mdm-2 oncogene product forms a complex with the p53 protein and inhibits p53-mediated transactivation. Cell 69:1237–1245

Muthusamy V, Hobbs C, Nogueira C, Cordon-Cardo C, McKee PH, Chin L, Bosenberg MW (2006) Amplification of CDK4 and MDM2 in malignant melanoma. Genes Chromosomes Cancer 45:447–454

Nathanson KL, Martin AM, Wubbenhorst B, Greshock J, Letrero R, D'Andrea K, O'Day S, Infante JR, Falchook GS, Arkenau HT, Millward M, Brown MP, Pavlick A, Davies MA, Ma B, Gagnon R, Curtis M, Lebowitz PF, Kefford R, Long GV (2013) Tumor genetic analyses of patients with metastatic melanoma treated with the BRAF inhibitor dabrafenib (GSK2118436). Clin Cancer Res 19(17):4868–4878

Nazarian R, Shi H, Wang Q, Kong X, Koya RC, Lee H, Chen Z, Lee MK, Attar N, Sazegar H, Chodon T, Nelson SF, McArthur G, Sosman JA, Ribas A, Lo RS (2010) Melanomas acquire resistance to B-RAF(V600E) inhibition by RTK or N-RAS upregulation. Nature 468(7326):973–977

Nelson AA, Tsao H (2009) Melanoma and genetics. Clin Dermatol 27:46–52

Niederleithner H, Heinz M, Tauber S, Bilban M, Pehamberger H, Sonderegger S, Knöfler M, Bracher A, Berger W, Loewe R, Petzelbauer P (2012) Wnt1 is anti-lymphangiogenic in a melanoma mouse model. J Invest Dermatol 132(9):2235–2244

Nikolaev SI, Rimoldi D, Iseli C, Valsesia A, Robyr D, Gehrig C, Harshman K, Guipponi M, Bukach O, Zoete V, Michielin O, Muehlethaler K, Speiser D, Beckmann JS, Xenarios I, Halazonetis TD, Jongeneel CV, Stevenson BJ, Antonarakis SE (2011) Exome sequencing identifies recurrent somatic MAP2K1 and MAP2K2 mutations in melanoma. Nat Genet 44(2):133–139

Njauw CN, Kim I, Piris A, Gabree M, Taylor M, Lane AM, DeAngelis MM, Gragoudas E, Duncan LM, Tsao H (2012) Germline BAP1 inactivation is preferentially associated with metastatic ocular melanoma and cutaneous-ocular melanoma families. PLoS One 7(4):e35295

Ogino S, Nosho K, Kirkner GJ, Shima K, Irahara N, Kure S, Chan AT, Engelman JA, Kraft P, Cantley LC, Giovannucci EL, Fuchs CS (2009) PIK3CA mutation is associated with poor prognosis among patients with curatively resected colon cancer. J Clin Oncol 27:1477–1484

Omholt K, Krockel D, Ringborg U, Hansson J (2006) Mutations of PIK3CA are rare in cutaneous melanoma. Melanoma Res 16:197–200

Onken MD, Worley LA, Long MD, Duan S, Council ML, Bowcock AM, Harbour JW (2008) Oncogenic mutations in GNAQ occur early in uveal melanoma. Invest Ophthalmol Vis Sci 49:5230–5234

Padua RA, Barrass N, Currie GA (1984) A novel transforming gene in a human malignant melanoma cell line. Nature 311:671–673

Palanisamy N, Ateeq B, Kalyana-Sundaram S, Pflueger D, Ramnarayanan K, Shankar S, Han B, Cao Q, Cao X, Suleman K, Kumar-Sinha C, Dhanasekaran SM, Chen YB, Esgueva R, Banerjee S, LaFargue CJ, Siddiqui J, Demichelis F, Moeller P, Bismar TA, Kuefer R, Fullen DR, Johnson TM, Greenson JK, Giordano TJ, Tan P, Tomlins SA, Varambally S, Rubin MA, Maher CA, Chinnaiyan AM (2010) Rearrangements of the RAF kinase pathway in prostate cancer, gastric cancer and melanoma. Nat Med 16:793–798

Palavalli LH, Prickett TD, Wunderlich JR, Wei X, Burrell AS, Porter-Gill P, Davis S, Wang C, Cronin JC, Agrawal NS, Lin JC, Westbroek W, Hoogstraten-Miller S, Molinolo AA, Fetsch P, Filie AC, O'Connell MP, Banister CE, Howard JD, Buckhaults P, Weeraratna AT, Brody LC, Rosenberg SA, Samuels Y (2009) Analysis of the matrix metalloproteinase family reveals that MMP8 is often mutated in melanoma. Nat Genet 41:518–520

Paraiso KH, Xiang Y, Rebecca VW, Abel EV, Chen YA, Munko AC, Wood E, Fedorenko IV, Sondak VK, Anderson AR, Ribas A, Palma MD, Nathanson KL, Koomen JM, Messina JL, Smalley KS (2011) PTEN loss confers BRAF inhibitor resistance to melanoma cells through the suppression of BIM expression. Cancer Res 71(7):2750–2760

Pavey S, Johansson P, Packer L, Taylor J, Stark M, Pollock PM, Walker GJ, Boyle GM, Harper U, Cozzi SJ, Hansen K, Yudt L, Schmidt C, Hersey P, Ellem KA, O'Rourke MG, Parsons PG, Meltzer P, Ringner M, Hayward NK (2004) Microarray expression profiling in melanoma reveals a BRAF mutation signature. Oncogene 23:4060–4067

Pleasance ED, Cheetham RK, Stephens PJ, McBride DJ, Humphray SJ, Greenman CD, Varela I, Lin ML, Ordonez GR, Bignell GR, Ye K, Alipaz J, Bauer MJ, Beare D, Butler A, Carter RJ, Chen L, Cox AJ, Edkins S, Kokko-Gonzales PI, Gormley NA, Grocock RJ, Haudenschild CD, Hims MM, James T, Jia M, Kingsbury Z, Leroy C, Marshall J, Menzies A, Mudie LJ, Ning Z, Royce T, Schulz-Trieglaff OB, Spiridou A, Stebbings LA, Szajkowski L, Teague J, Williamson D, Chin L, Ross MT, Campbell PJ, Bentley DR, Futreal PA, Stratton MR (2010) A comprehensive catalogue of somatic mutations from a human cancer genome. Nature 463:191–196

Pollock PM, Walker GJ, Glendening JM, Que Noy T, Bloch NC, Fountain JW, Hayward NK (2002) PTEN inactivation is rare in melanoma tumours but occurs frequently in melanoma cell lines. Melanoma Res 12:565–575

Pollock PM, Harper UL, Hansen KS, Yudt LM, Stark M, Robbins CM, Moses TY, Hostetter G, Wagner U, Kakareka J, Salem G, Pohida T, Heenan P, Duray P, Kallioniemi O, Hayward NK, Trent JM, Meltzer PS (2003) High frequency of BRAF mutations in nevi. Nat Genet 33:19–20

Potterf SB, Furumura M, Dunn KJ, Arnheiter H, Pavan WJ (2000) Transcription factor hierarchy in Waardenburg syndrome: regulation of MITF expression by SOX10 and PAX3. Hum Genet 107:1–6

Poulikakos PI, Persaud Y, Janakiraman M, Kong X, Ng C, Moriceau G, Shi H, Atefi M, Titz B, Gabay MT, Salton M, Dahlman KB, Tadi M, Wargo JA, Flaherty KT, Kelley MC, Misteli T, Chapman PB, Sosman JA, Graeber TG, Ribas A, Lo RS, Rosen N, Solit DB (2011) RAF inhibitor resistance is mediated by dimerization of aberrantly spliced BRAF(V600E). Nature 480(7377):387–390

Puig S, Malvehy J, Badenas C, Ruiz A, Jimenez D, Cuellar F, Azon A, Gonzàlez U, Castel T, Campoy A, Herrero J, Martí R, Brunet-Vidal J, Milà M (2005) Role of the CDKN2A locus in patients with multiple primary melanomas. J Clin Oncol 23(13):3043–3051

Ragnarsson-Olding BK, Karsberg S, Platz A, Ringborg UK (2002) Mutations in the TP53 gene in human malignant melanomas derived from sun-exposed skin and unexposed mucosal membranes. Melanoma Res 12:453–463

Reifenberger J, Knobbe CB, Sterzinger AA, Blaschke B, Schulte KW, Ruzicka T, Reifenberger G (2004) Frequent alterations of Ras signaling pathway genes in sporadic malignant melanomas. Int J Cancer 109:377–384

Rizos H, Menzies AM, Pupo GM, Carlino MS, Fung C, Hyman J, Haydu LE, Mijatov B, Becker TM, Boyd SC, Howle J, Saw R, Thompson JF, Kefford RF, Scolyer RA, Long GV (2014) BRAF inhibitor resistance mechanisms in metastatic melanoma: spectrum and clinical impact. Clin Cancer Res 20(7):1965–1977

Robert C, Karaszewska B, Schachter J, Rutkowski P, Mackiewicz A, Stroiakovski D, Lichinitser M, Dummer R, Grange F, Mortier L, Chiarion-Sileni V, Drucis K, Krajsova I, Hauschild A, Lorigan P, Wolter P, Long GV, Flaherty K, Nathan P, Ribas A, Martin AM, Sun P, Crist W, Legos J, Rubin SD, Little SM, Schadendorf D (2015) Improved overall survival in melanoma with combined dabrafenib and trametinib. N Engl J Med 372(1):30–39

Robles-Espinoza CD, Harland M, Ramsay AJ, Aoude LG, Quesada V, Ding Z, Pooley KA, Pritchard AL, Tiffen JC, Petljak M, Palmer JM, Symmons J, Johansson P, Stark MS, Gartside MG, Snowden H, Montgomery GW, Martin NG, Liu JZ, Choi J, Makowski M, Brown KM, Dunning AM, Keane TM, López-Otín C, Gruis NA, Hayward NK, Bishop DT, Newton-Bishop JA, Adams DJ (2014) POT1 loss-of-function variants predispose to familial melanoma. Nat Genet 46(5):478–481

Rouzaud F, Kadekaro AL, Abdel-Malek ZA, Hearing VJ (2005) MC1R and the response of melanocytes to ultraviolet radiation. Mutat Res 571:133–152

Saal LH, Holm K, Maurer M, Memeo L, Su T, Wang X, Yu JS, Malmstrom PO, Mansukhani M, Enoksson J, Hibshoosh H, Borg A, Parsons R (2005) PIK3CA mutations correlate with hormone receptors, node metastasis, and ERBB2, and are mutually exclusive with PTEN loss in human breast carcinoma. Cancer Res 65:2554–2559

Sabatino M, Zhao Y, Voiculescu S, Monaco A, Robbins P, Karai L, Nickoloff BJ, Maio M, Selleri S, Marincola FM, Wang E (2008) Conservation of genetic alterations in recurrent melanoma supports the melanoma stem cell hypothesis. Cancer Res 68:122–131

Sánchez-Hernández I, Baquero P, Calleros L, Chiloeches A (2012) Dual inhibition of (V600E) BRAF and the PI3K/AKT/mTOR pathway cooperates to induce apoptosis in melanoma cells through a MEK-independent mechanism. Cancer Lett 314(2):244–255

Sarris M, Nikolaou K, Talianidis I (2014) Context-specific regulation of cancer epigenomes by histone and transcription factor methylation. Oncogene 33(10):1207–1217

Shi H, Moriceau G, Kong X, Lee MK, Lee H, Koya RC, Ng C, Chodon T, Scolyer RA, Dahlman KB, Sosman JA, Kefford RF, Long GV, Nelson SF, Ribas A, Lo RS (2012) Melanoma whole-exome sequencing identifies (V600E)B-RAF amplification-mediated acquired B-RAF inhibitor resistance. Nat Commun 3:724

Shi J, Yang XR, Ballew B, Rotunno M, Calista D, Fargnoli MC, Ghiorzo P, Bressac-de Paillerets B, Nagore E, Avril MF, Caporaso NE, McMaster ML, Cullen M, Wang Z, Zhang X, NCI DCEG Cancer Sequencing Working Group, NCI DCEG Cancer Genomics Research Laboratory, French Familial Melanoma Study Group, Bruno W, Pastorino L, Queirolo P, Banuls-Roca J, Garcia-Casado Z, Vaysse A, Mohamdi H, Riazalhosseini Y, Foglio M, Jouenne F, Hua X, Hyland PL, Yin J, Vallabhaneni H, Chai W, Minghetti P, Pellegrini C, Ravichandran S, Eggermont A, Lathrop M, Peris K, Scarra GB, Landi G, Savage SA, Sampson JN, He J, Yeager M, Goldin LR, Demenais F, Chanock SJ, Tucker MA, Goldstein AM, Liu Y, Landi MT (2014) Rare missense variants in POT1 predispose to familial cutaneous malignant melanoma. Nat Genet 46(5):482–486

Shull AY, Latham-Schwark A, Ramasamy P, Leskoske K, Oroian D, Birtwistle MR, Buckhaults PJ (2012) Novel somatic mutations to PI3K pathway genes in metastatic melanoma. PLoS One 7(8):e43369

Smalley KS, Lioni M, Dalla Palma M, Xiao M, Desai B, Egyhazi S, Hansson J, Wu H, King AJ, Van Belle P, Elder DE, Flaherty KT, Herlyn M, Nathanson KL (2008) Increased cyclin D1 expression can mediate BRAF inhibitor resistance in BRAF V600E-mutated melanomas. Mol Cancer Ther 7(9):2876–2883

Snyder A, Makarov V, Merghoub T, Yuan J, Zaretsky JM, Desrichard A, Walsh LA, Postow MA, Wong P, Ho TS, Hollmann TJ, Bruggeman C, Kannan K, Li Y, Elipenahli C, Liu C, Harbison CT, Wang L, Ribas A, Wolchok JD, Chan TA (2014) Genetic basis for clinical response to CTLA-4 blockade in melanoma. N Engl J Med 371(23):2189–2199

Spranger S, Bao R, Gajewski TF (2015) Melanoma-intrinsic β-catenin signalling prevents anti-tumour immunity. Nature 523(7559):231–235

Staaf J, Harbst K, Lauss M, Ringnér M, Måsbäck A, Howlin J, Jirström K, Harland M, Zebary A, Palmer JM, Ingvar C, Olsson H, Newton-Bishop J, Hansson J, Hayward N, Gruis N, Jönsson G, Melanoma Genetics Consortium (2014) Primary melanoma tumors from CDKN2A mutation carriers do not belong to a distinct molecular subclass. J Invest Dermatol 134(12):3000–3003

Stark M, Hayward N (2007) Genome-wide loss of heterozygosity and copy number analysis in melanoma using high-density single-nucleotide polymorphism arrays. Cancer Res 67:2632–2642

Sun C, Wang L, Huang S, Heynen GJ, Prahallad A, Robert C, Haanen J, Blank C, Wesseling J, Willems SM, Zecchin D, Hobor S, Bajpe PK, Lieftink C, Mateus C, Vagner S, Grernrum W, Hofland I, Schlicker A, Wessels LF, Beijersbergen RL, Bardelli A, Di Nicolantonio F, Eggermont AM, Bernards R (2014) Reversible and adaptive resistance to BRAF(V600E) inhibition in melanoma. Nature 508(7494):118–122

Swerdlow AJ, English J, MacKie RM, O'Doherty CJ, Hunter JA, Clark J, Hole DJ (1986) Benign melanocytic naevi as a risk factor for malignant melanoma. Br Med J (Clin Res Ed) 292:1555–1559

Tiffen J, Gallagher SJ, Hersey P (2015) EZH2: an emerging role in melanoma biology and strategies for targeted therapy. Pigment Cell Melanoma Res 28(1):21–30

Tsao H, Zhang X, Fowlkes K, Haluska FG (2000) Relative reciprocity of NRAS and PTEN/MMAC1 alterations in cutaneous melanoma cell lines. Cancer Res 60:1800–1804

Tsao H, Goel V, Wu H, Yang G, Haluska FG (2004) Genetic interaction between NRAS and BRAF mutations and PTEN/MMAC1 inactivation in melanoma. J Invest Dermatol 122:337–341

Tschandl P, Berghoff AS, Preusser M, Burgstaller-Muehlbacher S, Pehamberger H, Okamoto I, Kittler H (2013) NRAS and BRAF mutations in melanoma-associated nevi and uninvolved nevi. PLoS One 8(7):e69639

Ugurel S, Hildenbrand R, Zimpfer A, La Rosée P, Paschka P, Sucker A, Keikavoussi P, Becker JC, Rittgen W, Hochhaus A, Schadendorf D (2005) Lack of clinical efficacy of imatinib in metastatic melanoma. Br J Cancer 92(8):1398–1405

Van Allen EM, Wagle N, Sucker A, Treacy DJ, Johannessen CM, Goetz EM, Place CS, Taylor-Weiner A, Whittaker S, Kryukov GV, Hodis E, Rosenberg M, McKenna A, Cibulskis K, Farlow D, Zimmer L, Hillen U, Gutzmer R, Goldinger SM, Ugurel S, Gogas HJ, Egberts F, Berking C, Trefzer U, Loquai C, Weide B, Hassel JC, Gabriel SB, Carter SL, Getz G, Garraway LA, Schadendorf D, Dermatologic Cooperative Oncology Group of Germany (DeCOG) (2014) The genetic landscape of clinical resistance to RAF inhibition in metastatic melanoma. Cancer Discov 4(1):94–109

Van Allen EM, Miao D, Schilling B, Shukla SA, Blank C, Zimmer L, Sucker A, Hillen U, Foppen MH, Goldinger SM, Utikal J, Hassel JC, Weide B, Kaehler KC, Loquai C, Mohr P, Gutzmer R, Dummer R, Gabriel S, Wu CJ, Schadendorf D, Garraway LA (2015) Genomic correlates of response to CTLA-4 blockade in metastatic melanoma. Science 350(6257):207–211

Van Raamsdonk CD, Bezrookove V, Green G, Bauer J, Gaugler L, O'Brien JM, Simpson EM, Barsh GS, Bastian BC (2009) Frequent somatic mutations of GNAQ in uveal melanoma and blue naevi. Nature 457:599–602

Van Raamsdonk CD, Griewank KG, Crosby MB, Garrido MC, Vemula S, Wiesner T, Obenauf AC, Wackernagel W, Green G, Bouvier N, Sozen MM, Baimukanova G, Roy R, Heguy A, Dolgalev I, Khanin R, Busam K, Speicher MR, O'Brien J, Bastian BC (2010) Mutations in GNA11 in uveal melanoma. N Engl J Med 363(23):2191–2199

Verastegui C, Bille K, Ortonne JP, Ballotti R (2000) Regulation of the microphthalmia-associated transcription factor gene by the Waardenburg syndrome type 4 gene, SOX10. J Biol Chem 275:30757–30760

Viros A, Fridlyand J, Bauer J, Lasithiotakis K, Garbe C, Pinkel D, Bastian BC (2008) Improving melanoma classification by integrating genetic and morphologic features. PLoS Med 5:e120

Vredeveld LC, Possik PA, Smit MA, Meissl K, Michaloglou C, Horlings HM, Ajouaou A, Kortman PC, Dankort D, McMahon M, Mooi WJ, Peeper DS (2012) Abrogation of BRAFV600E-induced senescence by PI3K pathway activation contributes to melanomagenesis. Genes Dev 26(10):1055–1069

Weaver-Feldhaus J, Gruis NA, Neuhausen S, Le Paslier D, Stockert E, Skolnick MH, Kamb A (1994) Localization of a putative tumor suppressor gene by using homozygous deletions in melanomas. Proc Natl Acad Sci U S A 91:7563–7567

Xing F, Persaud Y, Pratilas CA, Taylor BS, Janakiraman M, She QB, Gallardo H, Liu C, Merghoub T, Hefter B, Dolgalev I, Viale A, Heguy A, De Stanchina E, Cobrinik D, Bollag G, Wolchok J, Houghton A, Solit DB (2012) Concurrent loss of the PTEN and RB1 tumor suppressors attenuates RAF dependence in melanomas harboring (V600E)BRAF. Oncogene 31(4):446–457

Yokoyama S, Woods SL, Boyle GM, Aoude LG, MacGregor S, Zismann V, Gartside M, Cust AE, Haq R, Harland M, Taylor JC, Duffy DL, Holohan K, Dutton-Regester K, Palmer JM, Bonazzi V, Stark MS, Symmons J, Law MH, Schmidt C, Lanagan C, O'Connor L, Holland EA, Schmid H, Maskiell JA, Jetann J, Ferguson M, Jenkins MA, Kefford RF, Giles GG, Armstrong BK, Aitken JF, Hopper JL, Whiteman DC, Pharoah PD, Easton DF, Dunning AM, Newton-Bishop JA, Montgomery GW, Martin NG, Mann GJ, Bishop DT, Tsao H, Trent JM, Fisher DE, Hayward NK, Brown KM (2011) A novel recurrent mutation in MITF predisposes to familial and sporadic melanoma. Nature 480(7375):99–103

Zhang Y, Xiong Y, Yarbrough WG (1998) ARF promotes MDM2 degradation and stabilizes p53: ARF-INK4a locus deletion impairs both the Rb and p53 tumor suppression pathways. Cell 92:725–734

Transcriptional Regulation in Melanoma

5

Satoru Yokoyama and David E. Fisher

5.1 MITF (Microphthalmia-Associated Transcription Factor)

MITF is a basic helix–loop–helix leucine zipper protein, which binds to E-box sequences (5′-CA(C/T)GTG-3′) as a homo- or heterodimer with other MiT family members (itself, TFE3, TFEB, or TFEC) (Hemesath et al. 1994; Yasumoto et al. 1994). MITF has many isoforms, which are transcribed from different initial exons and exhibit tissue-specific expression patterns depending upon promoter usage (Hershey and Fisher 2005). Among isoforms, MITF-M, with its exon1M, is highly expressed in melanocyte-lineage cells (Fuse et al. 1996).

MITF has been shown to be required for melanocyte development, differentiation, and survival (see also Chap. 2). Mutations of MITF in humans cause Waardenburg syndrome (WS) 2A, which is an autosomal dominant auditory–pigmentary syndrome characterized by pigmentary abnormalities of the hair, skin, and eyes and congenital sensorineural hearing loss (Tassabehji et al. 1994). Appropriate regulation of MITF is required for cell growth/survival in melanocytes and MITF amplification has been reported in 10–20 % of human melanomas (Garraway et al. 2005). In addition, human clear cell sarcoma is a frequently pigmented soft tissue sarcoma, which harbors a chromosomal translocation producing the EWS-ATF1 fusion protein (Davis et al. 2006). This chimeric oncoprotein is thought to mimic the normally cAMP-regulated ability of ATF1 to activate M-MITF expression, instead of constitutively activating the *M-MITF* promoter. The result is dysregulated M-MITF expression in clear cell sarcoma which likely accounts for the tumor's

S. Yokoyama, Ph.D.
Division of Pathogenic Biochemistry, Institute of Natural Medicine, University of Toyama, 2630 Sugitani, Toyama 930-0194, Japan
e-mail: yokoyama@inm.u-toyama.ac.jp

D.E. Fisher (✉)
Department of Dermatology, Massachusetts General Hospital, 55 Fruit Street, Boston, MA 02114, USA
e-mail: dfisher3@partners.org

A. Bosserhoff (ed.), *Melanoma Development*,
DOI 10.1007/978-3-319-41319-8_5

melanin production as well as oncogenic behavior (Davis et al. 2006). In addition, ~20 % of metastatic melanomas were found to harbor somatic coding mutations, which may represent an additional oncogenic mechanism (Cronin et al. 2009) and recently a novel MITF mutation (E318K), which affects sumoylation of MITF, has been identified in familial and sporadic melanoma (Yokoyama et al. 2011).

MITF transactivates multiple genes related to cell cycle (CDK2, p16, p21, and Tbx2), pigmentation/differentiation (TYR, TYRP1, DCT, MART1, AIM-1, TRPM1, and PMEL17), apoptosis (HIF1A, BCL2, BCL2A1), and motility (c-MET, mir-211) (Fig. 5.1).

MITF transcription is regulated by other transcription factors, including PAX3, SOX10, CREB, FOXD3, LEF-1, and ONECUT-2. CREB/ATF1-mediated regulation of MITF is important for physiological expression in melanocytes, under the control of cAMP or other signals. MITF is also posttranslationally regulated by phosphorylation (via MAPK, GSK-3b, and RSK) (Mansky et al. 2002; Takeda et al. 2000; Weilbaecher et al. 2001; Wu et al. 2000), sumoylation (Miller et al. 2005; Murakami and Arnheiter 2005), caspase-dependent cleavage (Larribere et al. 2005), and ubiquitination. The MAPK-phosphorylated MITF is ubiquitinated and degraded via the proteosome pathway. MITF activity can be suppressed by the overexpression of PIAS3, which directly binds to MITF and inhibits DNA binding (Levy et al. 2002).

Recent work has indicated that nonspecific histone deacetylase inhibitors (HDACi) could potently repress MITF expression in melanoma cells. Suppressed MITF expression and cell growth were produced in melanoma cell lines and in mouse xenografts in response to treatment with a variety of HDACi (Yokoyama et al. 2008).

5.2 cAMP-Responsive Element (CRE)-Binding Protein/ Activating Transcription Factor-1 (CREB/ATF-1)

CREB/ATF-1 is one of the most important transcription factors in G-protein-coupled receptor (GPCR) signaling. In normal melanocytes, CREB/ATF-1 is required for pigmentation signaling from melanocortin receptor type 1 (MC1R) to MITF, which plays a central role in pigmentation as mentioned above (Price et al. 1998). α-Melanocyte-stimulating hormone (α-MSH) is produced after UV exposure in human skin (Lin and Fisher 2007; Yamaguchi and Hearing 2009) then bound to MC1R, which is a GPCR, in melanocytes. MC1R activates protein kinase A via cAMP production. Activated PKA phosphorylates CREB at Ser133, which induces transcription activity via a highly conserved CREB-binding site (cAMP-responsive element; CRE) (5′-TGANNTCA-3′) in the *M-MITF* promoter.

EWS-ATF1 fusion protein plays an oncogenic role in human clear cell sarcoma via MITF (Davis et al. 2006). It is reported that the transition of melanoma cells from radial to vertical growth phase is associated with the overexpression of CREB/ATF-1. Dominant-negative CREB (KCREB) can decrease melanoma tumorigenicity (possibly via MITF) and metastatic potential (via MMP-2 and MCAM/MUC18) in nude mice (Xie et al. 1997). Taken together, CREB/ATF1 contributes importantly to melanoma behavior.

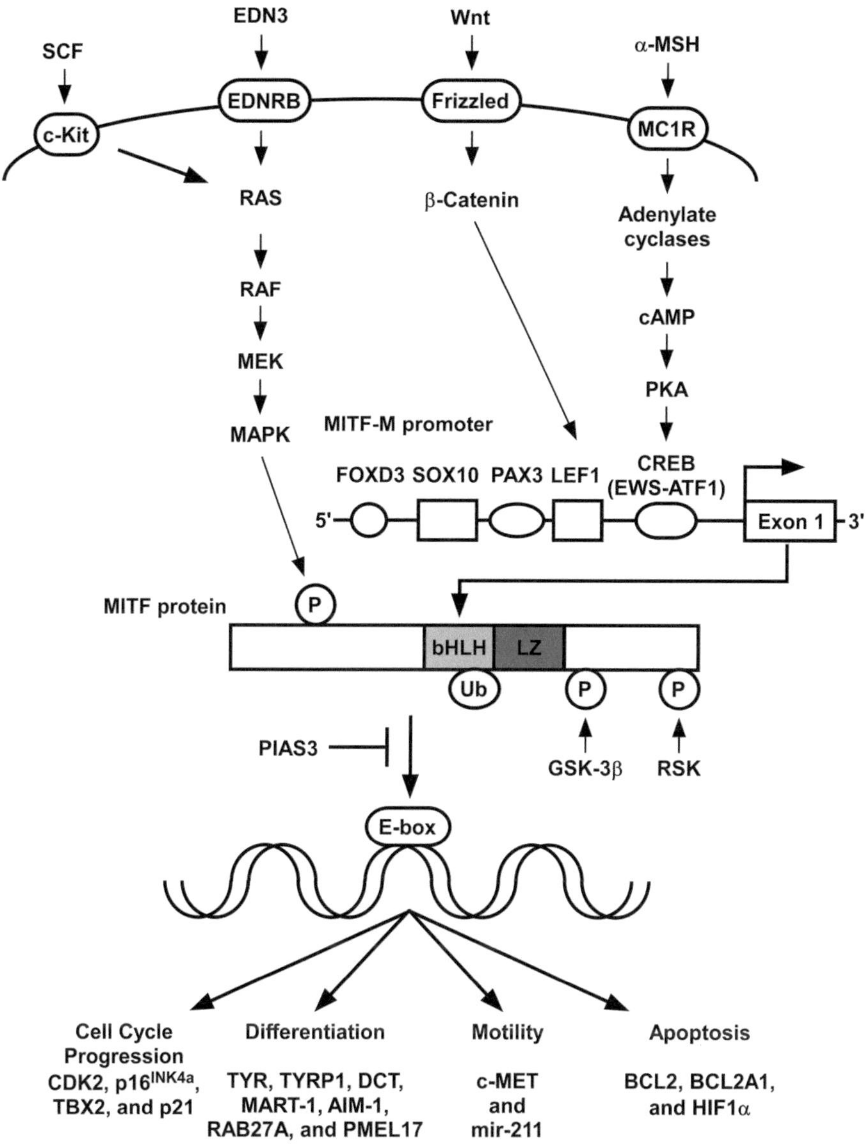

Fig. 5.1 MITF is involved in the induction of melanoma, melanocyte differentiation, cell-cycle progression, and survival. *Black lines* represent some of the signaling pathways connected to MITF, such as steel factor (*SCF*) and endothelin-3 (*EDN3*), and α-melanocyte-stimulating hormone (*α-MSH*). *White circles and squares* represent transcription factor-binding sites on the MITF-M promoter. MITF protein is posttranslationally regulated by phosphorylation via MAPK, GSK-3β, and RSK. PIAS3 suppresses the DNA-binding of MITF. MITF protein binds to consensus sequences, a subset of E-boxes, present in promoter or enhancer elements containing the consensus CATGTG or CACGTG. MITF regulates multiple targets in melanocytes and melanoma cells involved in various cellular processes such as cell-cycle control, survival, motility, invasion, differentiation, and/or pigmentation

5.3 SOX (Sry-Box) Family (SOX9 and SOX10)

The SOX family is comprised of approximately 20 transcription factors named after the original member, Sry (sex-determining region Y), because they all share a similar high-mobility group (HMG) domain (Soullier et al. 1999), which recognizes the consensus sequence (5′-(A/T)(A/T)CAA(A/T)G-3′). SOX proteins bind DNA as a monomer or a dimer and then regulate the transcription of target genes (Jiao et al. 2004; Ludwig et al. 2004; Peirano and Wegner 2000).

Among SOX family members, SOX10 is one of the major players in melanocyte development, and some recent data have suggested a significant role for SOX9 as well. In humans, SOX10 mutation causes WS type 4, which is characterized by sensorineural deafness/hypopigmentation associated with WS and enteric aganglionosis associated with Hirschprung's disease (Herbarth et al. 1998; Southard-Smith et al. 1998). SOX8 and SOX9 play roles in neural crest development, which is the origin of melanocytes (Cheung and Briscoe 2003; Maka et al. 2005).

UV exposure induces SOX9 via a cAMP/PKC-dependent pathway (Passeron et al. 2007) and SOX9 increases MITF and DCT expression in an SOX10-independent manner. In the case of SOX10, there is little information about its own transcriptional regulation. The tyrosine kinase TYRO3 can control SOX10 nuclear localization, resulting in subsequent SOX10-dependent increases in MITF, together with melanoma cell proliferation and survival (Zhu et al. 2009).

SOX10 regulates MITF, EDNRB, and c-ret, which are also related to WS and Hirschprung's disease. The function of SOX10 in melanomagenesis is still unknown, though SOX10 somatic mutations were reported in ~7 % of metastatic melanomas (Cronin et al. 2009) and SOX10 knockdown induced vemurafenib-resistance through activation of TGF-β signaling (Sun et al. 2014). These suggest that SOX10 could have a tumor-suppressive function in melanoma.

5.4 PAX3 (Paired Box 3)

PAX proteins represent a highly conserved family of transcription factors required for the development of multiple tissue types. Pax3 is a particularly interesting member of the Pax family, which coordinates the development of certain neural crest-derived lineages including skeletal muscle and melanocytes (Tassabehji et al. 1993). In humans, specific PAX3 mutations may cause either WS type 1 or type 3 characterized by abnormalities of the central nervous system, face, eye, nose, cochlea, and hair pigmentation.

PAX3 has two DNA binding domains: a paired domain and a homeodomain (Goulding et al. 1991). The paired domain binds the consensus sequence (5′-GT (T/C)(C/A)(C/T)(G/C)(G/C)-3′), whereas the homeodomain recognizes DNA containing a core sequence (5′-TAAT-3′). Pax3 can serve as a transcriptional activator or repressor by binding different partner proteins, such as SOX10 and TAZ (as activators) and TLE4 (Grg4 in mice), KAP1, and HP1γ (as repressors) (Bondurand et al. 2000; Hsieh et al. 2006; Lang et al. 2005; Murakami et al. 2006).

As predicted from WS types1/3, PAX3 regulates MITF, c-Ret, WNT1, and TGF-β2, which are required for the development of neural crest derivatives. PAX3 also regulates pigmentation genes (DCT and TRP1), which are related to melanocyte differentiation.

PAX3 overexpression is observed in many primary melanomas, melanoma cell lines, and melanoma sections (Barr et al. 1999; Medic and Ziman 2010; Plummer et al. 2008; Scholl et al. 2001). Even though Pax3's precise function in melanoma is not known, anti-apoptotic genes (PTEN, BCL-XL), differentiation-related genes (FGFR4, C-MET, MYF-5, MyoD, MSX2, HES1, and NGN2), and metastasis-related genes (CXCR4 and MET) (Kubic et al. 2015a, b) has been identified as PAX3 target genes, suggesting PAX3 could play an important role in melanoma.

5.5 Snail Superfamily (Snail and Slug)

Snail family members encode transcription factors of the zinc-finger type (Boulay et al. 1987). They share a similar organization, being composed of a highly conserved carboxy-terminal region, which contains 4–6 zinc fingers, and a more divergent amino-terminal region. The consensus binding site for Snail-related genes contains a core of six bases, 5′-CAGGTG-3′ (Mauhin et al. 1993), which also corresponds to a subset of the E-box motif (5′-CANNTG-3′). On binding to their E-boxes, Snail family members act as transcriptional repressors (Batlle et al. 2000; Cano et al. 2000). In humans, the mutation of SLUG causes WS type 2D, which is characterized by an auditory–pigmentary syndrome characterized by pigmentary abnormalities of the hair, skin, and eyes and congenital sensorineural hearing loss (Sanchez-Martin et al. 2002). SLUG was also identified as an MITF target gene.

SNAIL/SLUG is related to the epithelial-to-mesenchymal transition (EMT), which is thought to be a key step in development and cancer metastasis (Polyak and Weinberg 2009). The activation of Snail expression plays an important role in downregulation of E-cadherin, contributing to tumorigenesis of malignant melanomas (Poser et al. 2001) (see also Chap. 9). In vitro and in vivo experiments suggest that Slug is required for the metastasis of the transformed melanoma cells (Gupta et al. 2005) and for the survival through PUMA suppression.

5.6 FOXD3 (Forkhead Box D3)

FOX transcription factors represent a closely related family of proteins that mediate cell-cycle progression, survival, and differentiation (Myatt and Lam 2007). The FOX transcription factors contain a conserved FOX or winged helix domain, which is required for binding to a consensus DNA sequence and for activating target gene transcription.

Foxd3 acts as transcriptional repressor via a consensus binding site (5′-A(A/T) T(A/G) TTTGTTT-3′) and is expressed in migratory neural crest (NC) cells that give rise to multiple lineages. The downregulation of FOXD3 results in an increase in the number of differentiating melanocytes in quail NC cultures, and in premature dorsolateral migration of chick NC cells (Kos et al. 2001). Conversely, the misexpression of FOXD3 in melanoblasts results in a failure of NC cells to enter the dorsolateral pathway. The ectopic expression of FOXD3 represses MITF in cultured NC cells and in B16-F10 melanoma cells via inhibition of PAX3 binding to MITF promoter (Thomas and Erickson 2009).

In melanoma, it was reported that B-RAF^{V600E}, which is one of the major mutations, suppresses FOXD3 levels in human melanoma cells and FOXD3 expression represses melanoma growth by inhibiting the G1-S transition (Abel and Aplin 2010). Recently, some of FOXD3 targets were identified such as ERBB3 and TWIST1, both of which are related to melanoma malignant phenotypes (Abel et al. 2013; Weiss et al. 2014).

5.7 ETS Family Members

ETS transcription factors have a conserved DNA-binding domain (the ETS domain) of about 85 amino acids. The ETS domain, which bears a winged helix–turn–helix protein fold, mediates binding to a core DNA sequence (5′-GGA(A/T)-3′), with adjacent sequences influencing binding affinities (Sharrocks 2001). ETS transcription factors are important in many biological settings such as cell growth, differentiation, and survival and in processes that include hematopoiesis, angiogenesis, wound healing, cancer, and inflammation. At least 27 ETS family members have been described in mammalian cells and nearly two-thirds are ubiquitously expressed in adult tissues.

Multiple members of the ETS family undergo oncogenic dysregulation in cancer, often through chromosomal translocation. In Ewing's sarcoma (EWS), EWS-ETV1 translocations result in highly transforming chimeric ETS fusion proteins (Bailly et al. 1994; Ouchida et al. 1995). Chromosomal translocations involving ETV1 and other ETS genes were found in more than 40 % of prostate cancers (Tomlins et al. 2005). Most commonly, these translocations interpose the promoter and 5′ coding exons of the TMPRSS2 gene upstream of an ETS factor gene (ERG, ETV1, ETV4, or ETV5), resulting in androgen-dependent regulation and elevated the expression of these genes.

In melanoma, translocations involving Ets family members have not yet been described. However, the amplification of the ETV1 locus (>40 %) and dependency on ETV1 expression for melanoma proliferation were reported (Jane-Valbuena et al. 2010). The oncogenic activity of ETV1 is thought to be mediated by another oncogene, MITF.

5.8 BRN2 (POU3F2/N-Oct-3)

POU domain transcription factors are present in many cell lineages where they perform varying functions, either as ubiquitous regulators of "house-keeping" genes or as developmental- and lineage-specific coordinators of cell fate decisions. The POU domain is a highly conserved DNA binding structure, which was first found to recognize the canonical octameric sequence (5′-ATGCAAAT-3′) (Pruijn et al. 1986, 1987). Later, two subdomains, POUs and POUh, were identified to bind to DNA sequences 5′-ATGC and 3′-AAAT, respectively (Sturm and Herr 1988). POU proteins are capable of homodimerization on DNA target binding sites and interaction with a variety of other proteins, such as SOX family members (Wegner 2005). A major interaction between the POU family and SOX family involves OCT4 (POU5F1) and SOX2 in embryonic stem cells (Yuan et al. 1995). BRN2, SOX10, SOX9, and PAX3 are expressed in melanocytes and physical interactions among SOX10, PAX3, and BRN2 have been reported (Smit et al. 2000). BRN2 acts as a repressor of MITF expression in melanoma cells via direct binding to a region adjacent to the TATA box, resulting in suppressing the differentiated melanocytic phenotype and enhancing tumor metastasis (Goodall et al. 2008). BRN2 also regulates melanoma invasion and metastasis through suppressing PDE5A expression (Arozarena et al. 2011).

5.9 AP-1 (Activator Protein 1)/ATF2 (Activating Transcription Factor 2)

The AP-1 transcription factor is a dimeric complex that comprises members of the JUN, FOS, ATF (activating transcription factor), and MAF (musculoaponeurotic fibrosarcoma) protein families (Vogt 2002). AP-1 proteins are known as basic leucine-zipper (bZIP) proteins because they dimerize through a leucine-zipper motif and contain a basic domain for interaction with DNA. The AP-1 complex can form various different combinations of heterodimers or homodimers, and these combinations determine the genes that are regulated by AP-1. AP-1 upregulates transcription of genes containing the TPA response element (TRE; 5′-TGA(G/C)TCA-3′).

ATF2 is well characterized and thought to play a key role in melanoma (Bhoumik et al. 2007). ATF2 activity is regulated by phosphorylation on threonine (Thr) residues 69 and 71 via stress-activated kinases JNK, RalGDS-Src-P38 pathway, ATM, and Ras-MEK-ERK (Bhoumik et al. 2005; Gupta et al. 1995; Ouwens et al. 2002). Stimuli that activate these kinases, including exposure to proinflammatory cytokines, UV irradiation, DNA damage, or changes in ROS, are among the inducers of ATF2 transcriptional activity. Following phosphorylation, ATF2 activates transcription through heterodimerization with other transcription factors, among which c-Jun has been best characterized. ATF2/c-Jun heterodimers preferentially bind to the consensus sequence (5′-T(G/T)ACNTCA-3′). In addition to phosphorylation, ATF2 is also regulated by ubiquitin-dependent degradation by the proteasome, which is dependent on the association with JNK (Fuchs et al. 2000). ATF2 also functions in the DNA damage response by associating with the TIP60 HAT complex (Bhoumik et al. 2008). The TIP60 complex is required for ATM self-phosphorylation via acetylation. ATF2 regulates ATM activation by control of TIP60 stability and activity.

Through its dimerization with specific partners, ATF2 regulates the expression of its transcriptional targets. These are stress/DNA damage response genes (c-Jun, c-fos, ATM, XPA, RAD23B, etc.), growth/tumorigenesis genes (cyclin A. cyclin D1, MMP2, TNF-α, etc.), and physiological homeostasis genes (tyrosine hydroxyrase, collagen, VCAM-1, PGC-1α, etc.).

There are several lines of striking evidence regarding ATF2 function in melanoma (Bhoumik et al. 2007). Nuclear ATF2 expression is a strong predictor of poor survival in melanoma patients (Berger et al. 2003) and interfering with ATF2 transcriptional activity can inhibit proliferation of melanoma cells in culture and formation of tumors and metastasis in mouse models. On the other hand, ATF2 located at mitochondria increases mitochondrial permeability and promotes apoptosis, suggesting that cytosolic ATF2 works as a tumor suppressor (Lau et al. 2012). Recent studies shows that AP-1 might be one of the key regulators of the invasive state in melanoma (Kappelmann et al. 2013; Verfaillie et al. 2015).

5.10 AP-2

The AP-2 family of transcription factors consists in humans and mice of five members, AP-2a, AP-2b, AP-2c, AP-2d, and AP-2e (Hilger-Eversheim et al. 2000). All AP-2 proteins share a highly conserved helix–span–helix dimerization motif at the carboxyl terminus, followed by a central basic region and a less conserved domain rich in proline and glutamine at the amino terminus. The proteins are able to form hetero- as well as homodimers. The helix–span–helix motif together with the basic region mediates DNA binding, and the proline- and glutamine-rich region is responsible for transactivation. AP-2 has been shown to bind to the palindromic consensus sequence (5′-GCCNNNGGC-3′) found in various cellular and viral enhancers. AP-2 activity is regulated through a number of signal transduction pathways. Phorbol esters and signals that enhance cAMP levels induce AP-2 activity independent of protein synthesis, whereas retinoic acid treatment of teratocarcinoma cell lines results in transient induction of AP-2 mRNA levels at a transcription level (Buettner et al. 1993; Luscher et al. 1989).

Many experiments have demonstrated the functions of AP-2 in melanoma (Bar-Eli 2001). For example, loss of AP-2 expression increases tumor growth and metastasis in melanoma cells (Jean et al. 1998) and dominant-negative AP-2 (AP-2B) augments melanoma tumor growth in vivo (Gershenwald et al. 2001). AP-2 function is mediated via its regulated expression of target genes, which appear to be involved in proliferation, cell-cycle regulation (HER-2, p21/WAF-1), apoptosis (c-KIT, Bcl-2, FAS/APO-1), adhesion (MCAM/MUC18, E-cadherin), and invasion:angiogenesis (MMP-2, plasminogen activator inhibitor type I, VEGF, and PAR-1).

5.11 LEF/TCF/β-Catenin (Canonical Wnt Signaling)

LEF1/β-catenins are downstream mediators of canonical Wnt signaling and are involved in a variety of processes in development and tumorigenesis. The Wnt family consists of over 19 members, all of which are hydrophobic cysteine-rich secreted molecules that share a high level of homology. The ligand subtype determines which Wnt signaling pathway will be activated. For example, Wnt1, 3a, and 7 activate the canonical pathway, whereas Wnt5a, 5b, and 11 activate the noncanonical pathway (Weeraratna 2005). Receptors of Wnt ligands include the Frizzled (FZD) family of receptors (Zilberberg et al. 2004). The detailed WNT signaling are described in altered signal transdution pathway in melanoma (Chap. 7).

The transcription factors of the LEF/TCF (lymphoid enhancer factor/T-cell-specific factor) family are the most downstream components of the Wnt signaling cascade. Today, four family members are known in mammals: LEF-1, TCF-1, TCF-3, and TCF-4. All share a homologous "HMG box" DNA-binding domain and recognize the conserved consensus sequence (5′-AGATCAAAGGG-3′) in their target gene promoters, including cyclin D1, MITF, c-myc, MMP-7, and others.

Wnt1 and Wnt3A are the predominant family members involved in melanocyte development and both activate β-catenin. β-Catenin mutations were found in 6 out of 26 melanoma cell lines but appeared to be rare among primary melanoma tumor specimens. Truncating mutations of the adenomatous polyposis coli (APC) gene that regulates β-catenin levels are also rare in melanoma. β-Catenin is still required for melanoma survival even though mutations in Wnt signaling are rare (Takeda et al. 2000; Widlund et al. 2002). Recently, active b-catenin signaling in melanoma cells suppresses T-cell infiltration into tumor tissues, resulting in anti-PD-L1/anti-CTLA-4 monoclonal antibody therapy (Spranger et al. 2015).

5.12 Notch Signaling

The Notch signaling pathway is a key developmental cell–cell interaction mechanism, which regulates processes such as cell proliferation, cell fate, differentiation, or stem cell maintenance. All receptors and ligands are single-pass transmembrane proteins with large extracellular domains that consist primarily of epidermal growth factor (EGF)-like repeats. In mammals, four Notch receptors (Notch1-4) and five ligands (Jagged-1 and 2, and Delta-like [Dll] 1, 3, and 4) have been described (Greenwald 1998).

The detailed Notch signaling are described in "Altered Signal Transduction Pathway in Melanoma" (Chap. 7). After proteolytic cleavage of intracellular domain of Notch (NIC), it translocates to the nucleus where it binds to CSL transcription factors (CBF1 in humans) and thereby activates transcription of Notch target genes via consensus Notch-binding site (5′- TGGGAA -3′). In the absence of Notch signaling, CSL functions as a transcriptional repressor via interactions with several corepressors.

The Notch signaling pathway is involved in tumorigenesis, as aberrant Notch signaling is frequently observed in certain cancers. Depending on the cell type and context, Notch can promote cell proliferation and cancer growth, or act as a tumor suppressor (Radtke and Raj 2003; Wilson and Radtke 2006). There is increasing evidence that Notch acts as an oncogene in the development of melanomas, with several receptors (Notch1 and Notch2), ligands (Jagged-1, Jagged-2, and Dll1), as well as target genes (HES1, HEY1, and MCAM) upregulated at early stages of melanocytes transformation and tumor progression (Hoek et al. 2004). Notch1 is thought to play an important role stage-specifically to promote the progression of primary melanoma (Balint et al. 2005). Recently, melanoma–keratinocytes contact could induce Notch signaling activation in melanoma, resulting in the induction of metastatic microRNA, mir-222/221, and finally melanoma metastasis (Golan et al. 2015).

5.13 NF-kB (Nuclear Factor Kappa-Light-Chain-Enhancer of Activated B Cells)

NF-kB proteins were initially identified as pivotal transcription factors in chronic inflammatory diseases (Sen and Baltimore 1986). Accumulating evidence indicates that NF-kB is activated by a wide variety of stimuli such as cytokines and chemokines via AKT-signaling, MAPK-signaling, or NIK (NF-kB interacting kinase) (Perkins 2012). NF-kB is a homo- or heterodimeric complex consisting of proteins of the Rel-family. Rel-proteins can be divided into 2 groups depending on their mode of synthesis and transactivation properties. One class combines p65 (also known as REL A), REL B, and c-REL, which are all directly synthesized in their mature forms. The second class consists of p105 (also known as NFkB1) and p100 (also known as NFkB2), which are synthesized as large precursors and matured via phosphorylation and proteolysis into p52 and p50, respectively. The most commonly detected dimers are p65/p50, p65/p65, and p50/p50. NF-kB recognizes the DNA consensus (5′-GGG(A/G) NN(C/T)(C/T)CC-3′) (Amiri and Richmond 2005).

In the absence of stimuli such as cytokines or chemokines, NF-kB binds with IkBα protein and localizes in the cytoplasm. In the presence of stimuli, IkB kinase (IKK) complex is activated via kinases including AKT, ERK, or NIK and then IkBα is phosphorylated, ubiquitinated, and degraded. IkBα degradation induces translocation of NF-kB from the cytoplasm to the nucleus, and target genes are transcriptionally activated.

Many NF-kB-regulated genes have been reported, which are related to carcinogenesis, including apoptosis (TRAF1, TRAF2, c-IAP1/2, ML-IAP, and survivin), proliferation (cyclin D1 and CDK2), metastasis (COX2, ICAM-1, VCAM-1, ELAM-1, and MMPs), and angiogenesis (CXCL-1/8, IL-1, and TNF).

Constitutive activation of NF-*k*B is an emerging feature in melanoma and various target genes, CXCL1 and CXCL8, are highly expressed in most melanoma cell lines (Yang and Richmond 2001). Recently, RIP1, which is one of the upstream genes of NF-kB, has shown to be upregulated in melanoma, resulting in NF-kB activation and melanoma proliferation (Liu et al. 2015). Furthermore, knockdown of IKKbeta reduces the growth of the melanoma lesions in mouse studies, and conditional deletion of Ikkbeta in melanocytes blocks HRAS-induced melanomagenesis. Taken together, NF-kB-signaling may play an important role in melanoma growth/survival and melanomagenesis (Yang et al. 2010).

5.14 SMAD/SKI

The transforming growth factor-β (TGF-β) family of growth factors comprises more than 40 members, including TGF-β, activins, bone morphogenetic proteins (BMP), and nodal. They are ubiquitous multifunctional cytokines that regulate cellular activities, such as proliferation, differentiation, migration, survival, embryonic development, angiogenesis, or immune surveillance (Massague 2000). Binding of the TGF family to their receptors causes the assembly of a receptor complex that phosphorylates Smad2/3, which in turn bind to Smad4 and accumulate in the nucleus where they act as transcription factors, usually via Smad-binding sites (5′-AGAC-3′) (Nakao et al. 1997).

In normal tissues and cells, including melanocytes, transforming growth factor β (TGF-β) contributes to homeostasis by blocking cell-cycle progression via upregulation of the cyclin-dependent kinase inhibitors p15 and p21Waf-1, and downregulation of c-MYC (Reynisdottir et al. 1995; Warner et al. 1999). There are other targets regulated by TGF-β-smad signaling, including VEGF, BMPR-II, ets2, and PAI-1. Epithelial-to mesenchymal transition is also induced by TGF-β, which is related to tissue development and cancer metastasis.

The ski oncogene was discovered in its viral form, v-ski, as the transforming gene of the defective Sloan–Kettering virus (Stavnezer et al. 1981). SKI has been shown to interact with Smad2/3/4 and to recruit a transcriptional repressor of the N-CoR family and histone deacetylases (HDACs), resulting in repression of Smad-driven transcription (Khan et al. 2001). As the inactivation of the TGF-β pathway has been observed in a variety of human cancers, including melanomas, primary invasive melanomas in vivo exhibit nuclear, and cytoplasmic localization of SKI, whereas in melanoma metastasis, SKI is mostly localized in the cytoplasm and expressed at very high levels (Reed et al. 2001). SKI might inhibit smad-driven transcription of p21 in melanoma, resulting in escaping TGF-β-induced anti-proliferative activity. SKI is also a potent stimulator of Wnt/β-catenin signaling in human melanoma cells by binding to FHL2, which in turn activates MITF and Nr-CAM promoters in a β-catenin-dependent manner (Chen et al. 2003). SKI may participate as a regulator of melanoma progression by activating β-catenin signaling and repressing the TGF-β pathway. Consistent with SKI oncogenic function, TGF-β plays a tumor suppressive role through MITF suppression in melanoma (Pierrat et al. 2012).

5.15 STAT3 (Signal Transducer and Activator of Transcription 3)

STAT proteins were originally discovered as mediators of cytokine receptor signaling and are both cytoplasmic signaling molecules and nuclear transcription factors that activate diverse genes (Schindler et al. 1992; Shuai et al. 1992). There are seven STAT proteins (STAT1–4, 5A, 5B, and 6) in mammals (Li 2008). In the canonical mode of JAK–STAT signaling, the activation of the pathway is initiated by binding of a peptide ligand (e.g., a cytokine) to transmembrane receptors. This leads to receptor dimerization and cross-activation of receptor-associated JAK kinases (JAK1-3 or tyrosine kinase 2 (TYK2)), which in turn phosphorylate tyrosine residues in the cytoplasmic tail of the receptor. These phosphotyrosine residues function as docking sites for latent cytoplasmic STAT proteins, which are then phosphorylated by JAK on a crucial C-terminal tyrosine residue near the 700 amino acid position. Phosphorylated STAT proteins dimerize via Src-homology 2 (SH2)–domain–phosphotyrosine interactions and translocate to the nucleus, where they function as transcriptional activators, inducing the expression of target genes via their consensus binding site (5′-TTC(N)nGAA-3′).

STAT3 regulates genes related to survival/apoptosis (survivin, BCL2-XL, and MCL-1), proliferation (MYC and cyclin D1), metastasis (HIF-1, VEGF, and MMP-2), and immune checkpoint molecule (PD-L1) though some of its targets are not yet known to be directly regulated by STAT3 (i.e., may be indirectly regulated downstream of STAT3).

Protein inhibitor of activated STAT3 (PIAS3) has been identified as an inhibitor of STAT3 and MITF and may also regulate melanocyte growth. The overexpression of PIAS3 in melanoma cell lines inhibits the transcriptional activity of both MITF and STAT3 and induces apoptosis (Levy et al. 2002).

The overexpression of activated Stat3 containing two cysteine residue mutations can mediate cellular transformation (Bromberg et al. 1999). Among the human cancers that display constitutively activated STAT3 are a variety of hematologic malignancies, including myeloma, leukemias, and lymphomas, as well as solid tumors, including breast, lung, prostate, ovarian cancers, and melanoma (Buettner et al. 2002). In melanoma, several receptor tyrosine kinases including c-Met, EGFR, ERRB2, and ERRB4, which are known to activate src kinases, are overexpressed or activated. STAT3 inhibition in melanoma cell lines or melanoma tumor models has been shown to induce cell death/tumor regression (Niu et al. 1999; Niu et al. 2001), inhibit angiogenesis (Xu et al. 2005), prevent metastasis (Xie et al. 2004), and activate antitumor immune responses (Wang et al. 2004).

5.16 HIF1A (Hypoxia-Inducible Factor 1α)

HIF-1 is the key transcriptional regulator of the cellular response to a hypoxic environment. HIF1 plays a key role in many cellular processes that participate in responses to reduced oxygen and energy supply. HIF1 consists of a heterodimer with HIF1α and HIF1β and binds to the hypoxia responsive element (HRE, 5′-RCGTG-3′). Under normoxic conditions, HIF-1α is hydroxylated on proline residue 402 (Pro-402) and/or Pro-564 by prolyl hydroxylase domain protein 2 (PHD2). Prolyl-hydroxylated HIF-1α is bound by the von Hippel–Lindau tumor suppressor protein (VHL), which recruits an E3-ubiquitin ligase that targets HIF-1α for proteasomal degradation (Maxwell et al. 1999). Under hypoxic conditions, the prolyl and asparaginyl hydroxylation reactions are inhibited by substrate (O_2) deprivation and/or the mitochondrial generation of reactive oxygen species (ROS), which may oxidize Fe(II) present in the catalytic center of the hydroxylases.

HIF1 target genes have been identified in tumors, and are related to angiogenesis (VEGF), motility (CXCR4), proliferation (BNIP3), and the reprogramming of cancer metabolism (SLC2A1, SLC2A3, LDHA, MCT4, and PDK1).

HIF1α expression is regulated at the transcriptional and translational levels by the PI3K/AKT and MAPK/ERK pathways. Interestingly, PTEN loss or $BRAF^{V600E}$, which overactivate the PI3K/AKT or MAPK/ERK pathways, respectively, increase HIF1α expression and melanoma survival under hypoxic condition through HIF-1α (Kumar et al. 2007). HIF1α has been reported to be an MITF target gene (Busca et al. 2005) and also an regulator of MITF though DEC1 (Feige et al. 2011).

5.17 Tbx-2/3 (T-Box Binding Protein 2/3)

Members of the T-box family of transcription factors play important roles in the regulation of cell-fate decisions and morphogenesis during development. This family binds the 20 nucleotide partially palindromic sequence T[G/C] ACACCTAGGTGTGAAATT. Brachyury can bind as a monomer or a dimmer whereas Tbx-2 binds as a monomer to brachyury single half-sites, recognizing the consensus sequences GTGTGA, GGGTGA, or GTGTTA (Carreira et al. 2000). Several T-box genes are involved in the progression of cancer. The amplification of Tbx2/3 is reported in breast cancer (Fan et al. 2004; Sinclair et al. 2002). Both are also expressed in normal melanocytes and have been found to be strongly upregulated in a subset of melanoma cell lines (Carreira et al. 1998; Hoek et al. 2004; Vance et al. 2005).

Tbx2 and Tbx3 function as transcriptional repressors. Tbx2 represses TYRP-1, which is one of the pigmentation enzymes, p21, and p19. Through its targeting of p21 and p19, Tbx2 may be required to maintain proliferation and suppress senescence in melanomas (Vance et al. 2005). E-cadherin is also known to be a target gene of Tbx3 and potentially Tbx2. Tbx3 may be related to the transition from radial growth phase (RGP) to vertical growth phase (VGP) and could contribute to metastatic potential via suppression of E-cadherin expression.

TBX2 is regulated transcriptionally and posttranslationally by the p38 stress signaling pathway in response to UVC irradiation (Abrahams et al. 2008). TBX2 is also reported to be an MITF and PAX3 target gene (Carreira et al. 2000; Liu et al. 2013).

5.18 C-MYC

c-Myc is a basic helix–loop–helix leucine zipper protein, which binds to a subset of E-box (5′-CANNTG-3′) consensus sequences. This gene was discovered as a translocated oncogene in Burkitt's lymphoma, resulting in c-MYC overexpression under the control of the immunoglobulin enhancer or promoter (Taub et al. 1982). Dysregulated expression and/or amplification of C-MYC have been known to be an important event for many tumors. The c-myc locus (8q24) is amplified in 30–50 % melanoma (Kraehn et al. 2001). Moreover, the $BRAF^{V600E}$ and $NRAS^{Q61R}$-specific senescence program is suppressed by c-myc overexpression in melanoma (Zhuang et al. 2008). c-MYC also regulates a melanoma oncogene, RAB7 (Alonso-Curbelo et al. 2014).

c-MYC-dependent transactivation requires heterodimerization with a partner protein Max. This dimerization with Max is also essential for Myc proliferative and oncogenic function (Amati et al. 1993; Ferre-D'Amare et al. 1993). The inhibition of the dimerization with Max might be a potential therapeutic target. Thus far, the most "drug-able" transcription factors are ligand-dependent ones (particularly nuclear hormone receptors), although efforts to successfully target other transcription factors will hopefully bear fruit in the future.

5.19 p53

p53 is one of the most important human tumor suppressors (Lozano 2007; Riley et al. 2008). It plays important roles in controlling the DNA damage response, cell-cycle progression (p21, p16, p14, etc.), and apoptosis (APAF-1, PUMA, etc.) by regulating its targets transcriptionally. Deletion or loss-of-function mutations are found in diverse human cancers (see also Chap. 4).

UV causes DNA damage in human skin and correlates with melanoma incidence. Pigmentation may prevent epidermal cells from UV-induced DNA damage. p53 plays a role in the pigmentation response via transcriptional activation of the POMC promoter in keratinocytes, which encodes α-melanocyte-stimulating hormone (Cui et al. 2007).

A number of groups have reported mutational analysis of the *p53* gene in melanoma. Low-frequency (0–10 %) *p53* mutation or loss of heterozygosity in melanoma has been observed (Volkenandt et al. 1991), suggesting that there are additional mechanisms to suppress the function of p53. One mechanism involves the MDM2 gene, which encodes an E3 ubiquitin ligase that binds directly to p53 and ubiquitinates it, targeting p53 for proteosomal degradation. In melanoma progression, MDM2 has been shown to be highly expressed in 6 % of dysplastic nevi, 27 % of melanoma in situ, and 56 % of invasive primary and metastatic melanomas (Polsky et al. 2001).

Conclusions

The importance of transcription factors in melanocyte development and melanomagenesis has been summarized in this chapter (Table 5.1). Multiple transcription factors have been shown to be activators or suppressors of melanoma proliferation, survival, metastasis, and apoptosis. The complexity of their activities remains to be fully elucidated and will undoubtedly employ newer technologies including analyses of epigenetic marks, chromatin remodeling, and identification of coactivator or corepressor multiprotein complexes. For most transcription factors, we do not currently have effective therapeutic strategies available to permit their pharmacologic modulation. Exceptions include nuclear hormone receptors, which require small molecule ligand-dependent activation or certain drug-able strategies affecting pathways that indirectly control

Table 5.1 Overview of relevant transcription factors for melanoma

Gene	Binding sequences	Cancer-related biological function	Cancer-related target genes
MITF	CA[C/T]GTG	Cell-cycle progression, survival	CDK2, p16, p21, TBX2, TRPM1, HIF1A, BCL2, c-MET
CREB	TGANNTCA	Tumorigenicity	CCND1, MITF (by EWS-ATF1)
SOX10	[A/T][A/T]CAA[A/T]G	Unknown	MITF
PAX3	GT[T/C] [C/A] [C/T] [G/C] [G/C], TAAT	Motility (by PAX3-FOXO1)	MITF, PTEN, BCL-XL, c-MET
Snail superfamily	CAGGTG	Epithelial–mesenchymal transition	E-cadherin (CDH1), claudin, occludin
FOXD3	A[A/T]T[A/G]TTTGTTT	Suppressor of growth	MITF
ETS family	GGA[A/T]	Tumorigenicity	MITF (not direct target)
BRN2	ATGC, AAAT	Metastasis	MITF
AP-1	TGA[G/C]TCA	Proliferation, metastasis	ATM, XPA, cyclin A, CCND1, MMP2, TNF-α
AP-2	GCCNNNGGC	Melanoma progression	p21, c-KIT, BCL2, MMP2, CDH1
LEF/TCF/β-catenin	AGATCAAAGGG	Survival	CCND1, MITF, c-MYC, MMP7
Notch (NIC)	TGGGAA	Melanoma progression	HES, HEY1, MCAM
NFkB	GGG[A/G]NN[C/T][C/T]CC	Growth, survival	c-IAP1/2, survivin, CCND1, CDK2, CXCL-1/8
SMAD/SKI	AGAC	Melanoma progression	p21, VEGF, ETS2, PAI-1
STAT3	TTCNnGAA	Melanoma survival, angiogenesis	Survivin, BCL-XL, MCL-1, HIF1A, c-MYC, CCND1, MMP2, VEGF
HIF1A	[A/G]CGTG	Angiogenesis, metastasis, proliferation	VEGF, CXCR4, BNIP
TBX2/3	G[G/T]GTTA, GTGTTA	Metastasis	p21, p19, CDH1
c-MYC	CANNTG	Suppress the senescence	BCL2
p53	[A/G] [A/G] [A/G]C[A/T] [T/A]-G[C/T] [C/T] [C/T]	Cell-cycle progression, DNA damage response	p21, p16, p14, PUMA

transcription factors. Hopefully increasing accumulation of information about transcription factor biochemistry and the pathways which modulate their activities will provide new clues to novel therapeutic targeting strategies aimed at transcription factors in melanoma.

References

Abel EV, Aplin AE (2010) FOXD3 is a mutant B-RAF-regulated inhibitor of G(1)-S progression in melanoma cells. Cancer Res 70:2891–2900

Abel EV, Basile KJ, Kugel CH 3rd, Witkiewicz AK, Le K, Amaravadi RK, Karakousis GC, Xu X, Xu W, Schuchter LM, Lee JB, Ertel A, Fortina P, Aplin AE (2013) Melanoma adapts to RAF/MEK inhibitors through FOXD3-mediated upregulation of ERBB3. J Clin Invest 123:2155–2168

Abrahams A, Mowla S, Parker MI, Goding CR, Prince S (2008) UV-mediated regulation of the anti-senescence factor Tbx2. J Biol Chem 283:2223–2230

Alonso-Curbelo D, Riveiro-Falkenbach E, Perez-Guijarro E, Cifdaloz M, Karras P, Osterloh L, Megias D, Canon E, Calvo TG, Olmeda D, Gomez-Lopez G, Grana O, Sanchez-Arevalo Lobo VJ, Pisano DG, Wang HW, Ortiz-Romero P, Tormo D, Hoek K, Rodriguez-Peralto JL, Joyce JA, Soengas MS (2014) RAB7 controls melanoma progression by exploiting a lineage-specific wiring of the endolysosomal pathway. Cancer Cell 26:61–76

Amati B, Littlewood TD, Evan GI, Land H (1993) The c-Myc protein induces cell cycle progression and apoptosis through dimerization with Max. EMBO J 12:5083–5087

Amiri KI, Richmond A (2005) Role of nuclear factor-kappa B in melanoma. Cancer Metastasis Rev 24:301–313

Arozarena I, Sanchez-Laorden B, Packer L, Hidalgo-Carcedo C, Hayward R, Viros A, Sahai E, Marais R (2011) Oncogenic BRAF induces melanoma cell invasion by downregulating the cGMP-specific phosphodiesterase PDE5A. Cancer Cell 19:45–57

Bailly RA, Bosselut R, Zucman J, Cormier F, Delattre O, Roussel M, Thomas G, Ghysdael J (1994) DNA-binding and transcriptional activation properties of the EWS-FLI-1 fusion protein resulting from the t(11;22) translocation in Ewing sarcoma. Mol Cell Biol 14:3230–3241

Balint K, Xiao M, Pinnix CC, Soma A, Veres I, Juhasz I, Brown EJ, Capobianco AJ, Herlyn M, Liu ZJ (2005) Activation of Notch1 signaling is required for beta-catenin-mediated human primary melanoma progression. J Clin Invest 115:3166–3176

Bar-Eli M (2001) Gene regulation in melanoma progression by the AP-2 transcription factor. Pigment Cell Res 14:78–85

Barr FG, Fitzgerald JC, Ginsberg JP, Vanella ML, Davis RJ, Bennicelli JL (1999) Predominant expression of alternative PAX3 and PAX7 forms in myogenic and neural tumor cell lines. Cancer Res 59:5443–5448

Batlle E, Sancho E, Franci C, Dominguez D, Monfar M, Baulida J, Garcia De Herreros A (2000) The transcription factor snail is a repressor of E-cadherin gene expression in epithelial tumour cells. Nat Cell Biol 2:84–89

Berger AJ, Kluger HM, Li N, Kielhorn E, Halaban R, Ronai Z, Rimm DL (2003) Subcellular localization of activating transcription factor 2 in melanoma specimens predicts patient survival. Cancer Res 63:8103–8107

Bhoumik A, Lopez-Bergami P, Ronai Z (2007) ATF2 on the double - activating transcription factor and DNA damage response protein. Pigment Cell Res 20:498–506

Bhoumik A, Singha N, O'Connell MJ, Ronai ZA (2008) Regulation of TIP60 by ATF2 modulates ATM activation. J Biol Chem 283:17605–17614

Bhoumik A, Takahashi S, Breitweiser W, Shiloh Y, Jones N, Ronai Z (2005) ATM-dependent phosphorylation of ATF2 is required for the DNA damage response. Mol Cell 18:577–587

Bondurand N, Pingault V, Goerich DE, Lemort N, Sock E, Le Caignec C, Wegner M, Goossens M (2000) Interaction among SOX10, PAX3 and MITF, three genes altered in Waardenburg syndrome. Hum Mol Genet 9:1907–1917

Boulay JL, Dennefeld C, Alberga A (1987) The Drosophila developmental gene snail encodes a protein with nucleic acid binding fingers. Nature 330:395–398

Bromberg JF, Wrzeszczynska MH, Devgan G, Zhao Y, Pestell RG, Albanese C, Darnell JE Jr (1999) Stat3 as an oncogene. Cell 98:295–303

Buettner R, Kannan P, Imhof A, Bauer R, Yim SO, Glockshuber R, Van Dyke MW, Tainsky MA (1993) An alternatively spliced mRNA from the AP-2 gene encodes a negative regulator of transcriptional activation by AP-2. Mol Cell Biol 13:4174–4185

Buettner R, Mora LB, Jove R (2002) Activated STAT signaling in human tumors provides novel molecular targets for therapeutic intervention. Clin Cancer Res 8:945–954

Busca R, Berra E, Gaggioli C, Khaled M, Bille K, Marchetti B, Thyss R, Fitsialos G, Larribere L, Bertolotto C, Virolle T, Barbry P, Pouyssegur J, Ponzio G, Ballotti R (2005) Hypoxia-inducible factor 1{alpha} is a new target of microphthalmia-associated transcription factor (MITF) in melanoma cells. J Cell Biol 170:49–59

Cano A, Perez-Moreno MA, Rodrigo I, Locascio A, Blanco MJ, del Barrio MG, Portillo F, Nieto MA (2000) The transcription factor snail controls epithelial-mesenchymal transitions by repressing E-cadherin expression. Nat Cell Biol 2:76–83

Carreira S, Dexter TJ, Yavuzer U, Easty DJ, Goding CR (1998) Brachyury-related transcription factor Tbx2 and repression of the melanocyte-specific TRP-1 promoter. Mol Cell Biol 18:5099–5108

Carreira S, Liu B, Goding CR (2000) The gene encoding the T-box factor Tbx2 is a target for the microphthalmia-associated transcription factor in melanocytes. J Biol Chem 275:21920–21927

Chen D, Xu W, Bales E, Colmenares C, Conacci-Sorrell M, Ishii S, Stavnezer E, Campisi J, Fisher DE, Ben-Ze'ev A, Medrano EE (2003) SKI activates Wnt/beta-catenin signaling in human melanoma. Cancer Res 63:6626–6634

Cheung M, Briscoe J (2003) Neural crest development is regulated by the transcription factor Sox9. Development 130:5681–5693

Cronin JC, Wunderlich J, Loftus SK, Prickett TD, Wei X, Ridd K, Vemula S, Burrell AS, Agrawal NS, Lin JC, Banister CE, Buckhaults P, Rosenberg SA, Bastian BC, Pavan WJ, Samuels Y (2009) Frequent mutations in the MITF pathway in melanoma. Pigment Cell Melanoma Res 22:435–444

Cui R, Widlund HR, Feige E, Lin JY, Wilensky DL, Igras VE, D'Orazio J, Fung CY, Schanbacher CF, Granter SR, Fisher DE (2007) Central role of p53 in the suntan response and pathologic hyperpigmentation. Cell 128:853–864

Davis IJ, Kim JJ, Ozsolak F, Widlund HR, Rozenblatt-Rosen O, Granter SR, Du J, Fletcher JA, Denny CT, Lessnick SL, Linehan WM, Kung AL, Fisher DE (2006) Oncogenic MITF dysregulation in clear cell sarcoma: defining the MiT family of human cancers. Cancer Cell 9:473–484

Fan W, Huang X, Chen C, Gray J, Huang T (2004) TBX3 and its isoform TBX3+2a are functionally distinctive in inhibition of senescence and are overexpressed in a subset of breast cancer cell lines. Cancer Res 64:5132–5139

Feige E, Yokoyama S, Levy C, Khaled M, Igras V, Lin RJ, Lee S, Widlund HR, Granter SR, Kung AL, Fisher DE (2011) Hypoxia-induced transcriptional repression of the melanoma-associated oncogene MITF. Proc Natl Acad Sci U S A 108:E924–E933

Ferre-D'Amare AR, Prendergast GC, Ziff EB, Burley SK (1993) Recognition by Max of its cognate DNA through a dimeric b/HLH/Z domain. Nature 363:38–45

Fuchs SY, Tappin I, Ronai Z (2000) Stability of the ATF2 transcription factor is regulated by phosphorylation and dephosphorylation. J Biol Chem 275:12560–12564

Fuse N, Yasumoto K, Suzuki H, Takahashi K, Shibahara S (1996) Identification of a melanocyte-type promoter of the microphthalmia-associated transcription factor gene. Biochem Biophys Res Commun 219:702–707

Garraway LA, Weir BA, Zhao X, Widlund H, Beroukhim R, Berger A, Rimm D, Rubin MA, Fisher DE, Meyerson ML, Sellers WR (2005) "Lineage addiction" in human cancer: lessons from integrated genomics. Cold Spring Harb Symp Quant Biol 70:25–34

Gershenwald JE, Sumner W, Calderone T, Wang Z, Huang S, Bar-Eli M (2001) Dominant-negative transcription factor AP-2 augments SB-2 melanoma tumor growth in vivo. Oncogene 20:3363–3375

Golan T, Messer AR, Amitai-Lange A, Melamed Z, Ohana R, Bell RE, Kapitansky O, Lerman G, Greenberger S, Khaled M, Amar N, Albrengues J, Gaggioli C, Gonen P, Tabach Y, Sprinzak D, Shalom-Feuerstein R, Levy C (2015) Interactions of melanoma cells with distal keratinocytes trigger metastasis via notch signaling inhibition of MITF. Mol Cell 59:664–676

Goodall J, Carreira S, Denat L, Kobi D, Davidson I, Nuciforo P, Sturm RA, Larue L, Goding CR (2008) Brn-2 represses microphthalmia-associated transcription factor expression and marks a distinct subpopulation of microphthalmia-associated transcription factor-negative melanoma cells. Cancer Res 68:7788–7794

Goulding MD, Chalepakis G, Deutsch U, Erselius JR, Gruss P (1991) Pax-3, a novel murine DNA binding protein expressed during early neurogenesis. EMBO J 10:1135–1147

Greenwald I (1998) LIN-12/Notch signaling: lessons from worms and flies. Genes Dev 12:1751–1762

Gupta PB, Kuperwasser C, Brunet JP, Ramaswamy S, Kuo WL, Gray JW, Naber SP, Weinberg RA (2005) The melanocyte differentiation program predisposes to metastasis after neoplastic transformation. Nat Genet 37:1047–1054

Gupta S, Campbell D, Derijard B, Davis RJ (1995) Transcription factor ATF2 regulation by the JNK signal transduction pathway. Science 267:389–393

Hemesath TJ, Steingrimsson E, McGill G, Hansen MJ, Vaught J, Hodgkinson CA, Arnheiter H, Copeland NG, Jenkins NA, Fisher DE (1994) microphthalmia, a critical factor in melanocyte development, defines a discrete transcription factor family. Genes Dev 8:2770–2780

Herbarth B, Pingault V, Bondurand N, Kuhlbrodt K, Hermans-Borgmeyer I, Puliti A, Lemort N, Goossens M, Wegner M (1998) Mutation of the Sry-related Sox10 gene in Dominant megacolon, a mouse model for human Hirschsprung disease. Proc Natl Acad Sci U S A 95:5161–5165

Hershey CL, Fisher DE (2005) Genomic analysis of the Microphthalmia locus and identification of the MITF-J/Mitf-J isoform. Gene 347:73–82

Hilger-Eversheim K, Moser M, Schorle H, Buettner R (2000) Regulatory roles of AP-2 transcription factors in vertebrate development, apoptosis and cell-cycle control. Gene 260:1–12

Hoek K, Rimm DL, Williams KR, Zhao H, Ariyan S, Lin A, Kluger HM, Berger AJ, Cheng E, Trombetta ES, Wu T, Niinobe M, Yoshikawa K, Hannigan GE, Halaban R (2004) Expression profiling reveals novel pathways in the transformation of melanocytes to melanomas. Cancer Res 64:5270–5282

Hsieh MJ, Yao YL, Lai IL, Yang WM (2006) Transcriptional repression activity of PAX3 is modulated by competition between corepressor KAP1 and heterochromatin protein 1. Biochem Biophys Res Commun 349:573–581

Jane-Valbuena J, Widlund HR, Perner S, Johnson LA, Dibner AC, Lin WM, Baker AC, Nazarian RM, Vijayendran KG, Sellers WR, Hahn WC, Duncan LM, Rubin MA, Fisher DE, Garraway LA (2010) An oncogenic role for ETV1 in melanoma. Cancer Res 70:2075–2084

Jean D, Gershenwald JE, Huang S, Luca M, Hudson MJ, Tainsky MA, Bar-Eli M (1998) Loss of AP-2 results in up-regulation of MCAM/MUC18 and an increase in tumor growth and metastasis of human melanoma cells. J Biol Chem 273:16501–16508

Jiao Z, Mollaaghababa R, Pavan WJ, Antonellis A, Green ED, Hornyak TJ (2004) Direct interaction of Sox10 with the promoter of murine Dopachrome Tautomerase (Dct) and synergistic activation of Dct expression with Mitf. Pigment Cell Res 17:352–362

Kappelmann M, Kuphal S, Meister G, Vardimon L, Bosserhoff AK (2013) MicroRNA miR-125b controls melanoma progression by direct regulation of c-Jun protein expression. Oncogene 32:2984–2991

Khan MM, Nomura T, Kim H, Kaul SC, Wadhwa R, Shinagawa T, Ichikawa-Iwata E, Zhong S, Pandolfi PP, Ishii S (2001) Role of PML and PML-RARalpha in Mad-mediated transcriptional repression. Mol Cell 7:1233–1243

Kraehn GM, Utikal J, Udart M, Greulich KM, Bezold G, Kaskel P, Leiter U, Peter RU (2001) Extra c-myc oncogene copies in high risk cutaneous malignant melanoma and melanoma metastases. Br J Cancer 84(1):72–9.

Kos R, Reedy MV, Johnson RL, Erickson CA (2001) The winged-helix transcription factor FoxD3 is important for establishing the neural crest lineage and repressing melanogenesis in avian embryos. Development 128:1467–1479
Kubic JD, Little EC, Lui JW, Iizuka T, Lang D (2015a) PAX3 and ETS1 synergistically activate MET expression in melanoma cells. Oncogene 34:4964–4974
Kubic JD, Lui JW, Little EC, Ludvik AE, Konda S, Salgia R, Aplin AE, Lang D (2015b) PAX3 and FOXD3 promote CXCR4 expression in melanoma. J Biol Chem 290:21901–21914
Kumar SM, Yu H, Edwards R, Chen L, Kazianis S, Brafford P, Acs G, Herlyn M, Xu X (2007) Mutant V600E BRAF increases hypoxia inducible factor-1alpha expression in melanoma. Cancer Res 67:3177–3184
Lang D, Lu MM, Huang L, Engleka KA, Zhang M, Chu EY, Lipner S, Skoultchi A, Millar SE, Epstein JA (2005) Pax3 functions at a nodal point in melanocyte stem cell differentiation. Nature 433:884–887
Larribere L, Hilmi C, Khaled M, Gaggioli C, Bille K, Auberger P, Ortonne JP, Ballotti R, Bertolotto C (2005) The cleavage of microphthalmia-associated transcription factor, MITF, by caspases plays an essential role in melanocyte and melanoma cell apoptosis. Genes Dev 19:1980–1985
Lau E, Kluger H, Varsano T, Lee K, Scheffler I, Rimm DL, Ideker T, Ronai ZA (2012) PKCepsilon promotes oncogenic functions of ATF2 in the nucleus while blocking its apoptotic function at mitochondria. Cell 148:543–555
Levy C, Nechushtan H, Razin E (2002) A new role for the STAT3 inhibitor, PIAS3: a repressor of microphthalmia transcription factor. J Biol Chem 277:1962–1966
Li WX (2008) Canonical and non-canonical JAK-STAT signaling. Trends Cell Biol 18:545–551
Lin JY, Fisher DE (2007) Melanocyte biology and skin pigmentation. Nature 445:843–850
Liu F, Cao J, Lv J, Dong L, Pier E, Xu GX, Wang RA, Xu Z, Goding C, Cui R (2013) TBX2 expression is regulated by PAX3 in the melanocyte lineage. Pigment Cell Melanoma Res 26:67–77
Liu XY, Lai F, Yan XG, Jiang CC, Guo ST, Wang CY, Croft A, Tseng HY, Wilmott JS, Scolyer RA, Jin L, Zhang XD (2015) RIP1 kinase is an oncogenic driver in melanoma. Cancer Res 75:1736–1748
Lozano G (2007) The oncogenic roles of p53 mutants in mouse models. Curr Opin Genet Dev 17:66–70
Ludwig A, Rehberg S, Wegner M (2004) Melanocyte-specific expression of dopachrome tautomerase is dependent on synergistic gene activation by the Sox10 and Mitf transcription factors. FEBS Lett 556:236–244
Luscher B, Mitchell PJ, Williams T, Tjian R (1989) Regulation of transcription factor AP-2 by the morphogen retinoic acid and by second messengers. Genes Dev 3:1507–1517
Maka M, Stolt CC, Wegner M (2005) Identification of Sox8 as a modifier gene in a mouse model of Hirschsprung disease reveals underlying molecular defect. Dev Biol 277:155–169
Mansky KC, Sankar U, Han J, Ostrowski MC (2002) Microphthalmia transcription factor is a target of the p38 MAPK pathway in response to receptor activator of NF-kappa B ligand signaling. J Biol Chem 277:11077–11083
Massague J (2000) How cells read TGF-beta signals. Nat Rev Mol Cell Biol 1:169–178
Mauhin V, Lutz Y, Dennefeld C, Alberga A (1993) Definition of the DNA-binding site repertoire for the Drosophila transcription factor SNAIL. Nucleic Acids Res 21:3951–3957
Maxwell PH, Wiesener MS, Chang GW, Clifford SC, Vaux EC, Cockman ME, Wykoff CC, Pugh CW, Maher ER, Ratcliffe PJ (1999) The tumour suppressor protein VHL targets hypoxia-inducible factors for oxygen-dependent proteolysis. Nature 399:271–275
Medic S, Ziman M (2010) PAX3 expression in normal skin melanocytes and melanocytic lesions (naevi and melanomas). PLoS One 5:e9977
Miller AJ, Levy C, Davis IJ, Razin E, Fisher DE (2005) Sumoylation of MITF and its related family members TFE3 and TFEB. J Biol Chem 280:146–155
Murakami H, Arnheiter H (2005) Sumoylation modulates transcriptional activity of MITF in a promoter-specific manner. Pigment Cell Res 18:265–277

Murakami M, Tominaga J, Makita R, Uchijima Y, Kurihara Y, Nakagawa O, Asano T, Kurihara H (2006) Transcriptional activity of Pax3 is co-activated by TAZ. Biochem Biophys Res Commun 339:533–539

Myatt SS, Lam EW (2007) The emerging roles of forkhead box (Fox) proteins in cancer. Nat Rev Cancer 7:847–859

Nakao A, Imamura T, Souchelnytskyi S, Kawabata M, Ishisaki A, Oeda E, Tamaki K, Hanai J, Heldin CH, Miyazono K, ten Dijke P (1997) TGF-beta receptor-mediated signalling through Smad2, Smad3 and Smad4. EMBO J 16:5353–5362

Niu G, Heller R, Catlett-Falcone R, Coppola D, Jaroszeski M, Dalton W, Jove R, Yu H (1999) Gene therapy with dominant-negative Stat3 suppresses growth of the murine melanoma B16 tumor in vivo. Cancer Res 59:5059–5063

Niu G, Shain KH, Huang M, Ravi R, Bedi A, Dalton WS, Jove R, Yu H (2001) Overexpression of a dominant-negative signal transducer and activator of transcription 3 variant in tumor cells leads to production of soluble factors that induce apoptosis and cell cycle arrest. Cancer Res 61:3276–3280

Ouchida M, Ohno T, Fujimura Y, Rao VN, Reddy ES (1995) Loss of tumorigenicity of Ewing's sarcoma cells expressing antisense RNA to EWS-fusion transcripts. Oncogene 11:1049–1054

Ouwens DM, de Ruiter ND, van der Zon GC, Carter AP, Schouten J, van der Burgt C, Kooistra K, Bos JL, Maassen JA, van Dam H (2002) Growth factors can activate ATF2 via a two-step mechanism: phosphorylation of Thr71 through the Ras-MEK-ERK pathway and of Thr69 through RalGDS-Src-p38. EMBO J 21:3782–3793

Passeron T, Valencia JC, Bertolotto C, Hoashi T, Le Pape E, Takahashi K, Ballotti R, Hearing VJ (2007) SOX9 is a key player in ultraviolet B-induced melanocyte differentiation and pigmentation. Proc Natl Acad Sci U S A 104:13984–13989

Peirano RI, Wegner M (2000) The glial transcription factor Sox10 binds to DNA both as monomer and dimer with different functional consequences. Nucleic Acids Res 28:3047–3055

Perkins ND (2012) The diverse and complex roles of NF-kappaB subunits in cancer. Nat Rev Cancer 12:121–132

Pierrat MJ, Marsaud V, Mauviel A, Javelaud D (2012) Expression of microphthalmia-associated transcription factor (MITF), which is critical for melanoma progression, is inhibited by both transcription factor GLI2 and transforming growth factor-beta. J Biol Chem 287: 17996–18004

Plummer RS, Shea CR, Nelson M, Powell SK, Freeman DM, Dan CP, Lang D (2008) PAX3 expression in primary melanomas and nevi. Mod Pathol 21:525–530

Polsky D, Bastian BC, Hazan C, Melzer K, Pack J, Houghton A, Busam K, Cordon-Cardo C, Osman I (2001) HDM2 protein overexpression, but not gene amplification, is related to tumorigenesis of cutaneous melanoma. Cancer Res 61:7642–7646

Polyak K, Weinberg RA (2009) Transitions between epithelial and mesenchymal states: acquisition of malignant and stem cell traits. Nat Rev Cancer 9:265–273

Poser I, Dominguez D, de Herreros AG, Varnai A, Buettner R, Bosserhoff AK (2001) Loss of E-cadherin expression in melanoma cells involves up-regulation of the transcriptional repressor Snail. J Biol Chem 276:24661–24666

Price ER, Horstmann MA, Wells AG, Weilbaecher KN, Takemoto CM, Landis MW, Fisher DE (1998) alpha-Melanocyte-stimulating hormone signaling regulates expression of microphthalmia, a gene deficient in Waardenburg syndrome. J Biol Chem 273:33042–33047

Pruijn GJ, van Driel W, van der Vliet PC (1986) Nuclear factor III, a novel sequence-specific DNA-binding protein from HeLa cells stimulating adenovirus DNA replication. Nature 322:656–659

Pruijn GJ, van Driel W, van Miltenburg RT, van der Vliet PC (1987) Promoter and enhancer elements containing a conserved sequence motif are recognized by nuclear factor III, a protein stimulating adenovirus DNA replication. EMBO J 6:3771–3778

Radtke F, Raj K (2003) The role of Notch in tumorigenesis: oncogene or tumour suppressor? Nat Rev Cancer 3:756–767

Reed JA, Bales E, Xu W, Okan NA, Bandyopadhyay D, Medrano EE (2001) Cytoplasmic localization of the oncogenic protein Ski in human cutaneous melanomas in vivo: functional implications for transforming growth factor beta signaling. Cancer Res 61:8074–8078

Reynisdottir I, Polyak K, Iavarone A, Massague J (1995) Kip/Cip and Ink4 Cdk inhibitors cooperate to induce cell cycle arrest in response to TGF-beta. Genes Dev 9:1831–1845

Riley T, Sontag E, Chen P, Levine A (2008) Transcriptional control of human p53-regulated genes. Nat Rev Mol Cell Biol 9:402–412

Sanchez-Martin M, Rodriguez-Garcia A, Perez-Losada J, Sagrera A, Read AP, Sanchez-Garcia I (2002) SLUG (SNAI2) deletions in patients with Waardenburg disease. Hum Mol Genet 11:3231–3236

Schindler C, Shuai K, Prezioso VR, Darnell JE Jr (1992) Interferon-dependent tyrosine phosphorylation of a latent cytoplasmic transcription factor. Science 257:809–813

Scholl FA, Kamarashev J, Murmann OV, Geertsen R, Dummer R, Schafer BW (2001) PAX3 is expressed in human melanomas and contributes to tumor cell survival. Cancer Res 61:823–826

Sen R, Baltimore D (1986) Inducibility of kappa immunoglobulin enhancer-binding protein Nf-kappa B by a posttranslational mechanism. Cell 47:921–928

Sharrocks AD (2001) The ETS-domain transcription factor family. Nat Rev Mol Cell Biol 2:827–837

Shuai K, Schindler C, Prezioso VR, Darnell JE Jr (1992) Activation of transcription by IFN-gamma: tyrosine phosphorylation of a 91-kD DNA binding protein. Science 258:1808–1812

Sinclair CS, Adem C, Naderi A, Soderberg CL, Johnson M, Wu K, Wadum L, Couch VL, Sellers TA, Schaid D, Slezak J, Fredericksen Z, Ingle JN, Hartmann L, Jenkins RB, Couch FJ (2002) TBX2 is preferentially amplified in BRCA1- and BRCA2-related breast tumors. Cancer Res 62:3587–3591

Smit DJ, Smith AG, Parsons PG, Muscat GE, Sturm RA (2000) Domains of Brn-2 that mediate homodimerization and interaction with general and melanocytic transcription factors. Eur J Biochem 267:6413–6422

Soullier S, Jay P, Poulat F, Vanacker JM, Berta P, Laudet V (1999) Diversification pattern of the HMG and SOX family members during evolution. J Mol Evol 48:517–527

Southard-Smith EM, Kos L, Pavan WJ (1998) Sox10 mutation disrupts neural crest development in Dom Hirschsprung mouse model. Nat Genet 18:60–64

Spranger S, Bao R, Gajewski TF (2015) Melanoma-intrinsic beta-catenin signalling prevents anti-tumour immunity. Nature 523:231–235

Stavnezer E, Gerhard DS, Binari RC, Balazs I (1981) Generation of transforming viruses in cultures of chicken fibroblasts infected with an avian leukosis virus. J Virol 39:920–934

Sturm RA, Herr W (1988) The POU domain is a bipartite DNA-binding structure. Nature 336:601–604

Sun C, Wang L, Huang S, Heynen GJ, Prahallad A, Robert C, Haanen J, Blank C, Wesseling J, Willems SM, Zecchin D, Hobor S, Bajpe PK, Lieftink C, Mateus C, Vagner S, Grernrum W, Hofland I, Schlicker A, Wessels LF, Beijersbergen RL, Bardelli A, Di Nicolantonio F, Eggermont AM, Bernards R (2014) Reversible and adaptive resistance to BRAF(V600E) inhibition in melanoma. Nature 508:118–122

Takeda K, Yasumoto K, Takada R, Takada S, Watanabe K, Udono T, Saito H, Takahashi K, Shibahara S (2000) Induction of melanocyte-specific microphthalmia-associated transcription factor by Wnt-3a. J Biol Chem 275:14013–14016

Tassabehji M, Newton VE, Read AP (1994) Waardenburg syndrome type 2 caused by mutations in the human microphthalmia (MITF) gene. Nat Genet 8:251–255

Tassabehji M, Read AP, Newton VE, Patton M, Gruss P, Harris R, Strachan T (1993) Mutations in the PAX3 gene causing Waardenburg syndrome type 1 and type 2. Nat Genet 3:26–30

Taub R, Kirsch I, Morton C, Lenoir G, Swan D, Tronick S, Aaronson S, Leder P (1982) Translocation of the c-myc gene into the immunoglobulin heavy chain locus in human Burkitt lymphoma and murine plasmacytoma cells. Proc Natl Acad Sci U S A 79:7837–7841

Thomas AJ, Erickson CA (2009) FOXD3 regulates the lineage switch between neural crest-derived glial cells and pigment cells by repressing MITF through a non-canonical mechanism. Development 136:1849–1858

Tomlins SA, Rhodes DR, Perner S, Dhanasekaran SM, Mehra R, Sun XW, Varambally S, Cao X, Tchinda J, Kuefer R, Lee C, Montie JE, Shah RB, Pienta KJ, Rubin MA, Chinnaiyan AM (2005) Recurrent fusion of TMPRSS2 and ETS transcription factor genes in prostate cancer. Science 310:644–648

Vance KW, Carreira S, Brosch G, Goding CR (2005) Tbx2 is overexpressed and plays an important role in maintaining proliferation and suppression of senescence in melanomas. Cancer Res 65:2260–2268

Verfaillie A, Imrichova H, Atak ZK, Dewaele M, Rambow F, Hulselmans G, Christiaens V, Svetlichnyy D, Luciani F, Van den Mooter L, Claerhout S, Fiers M, Journe F, Ghanem GE, Herrmann C, Halder G, Marine JC, Aerts S (2015) Decoding the regulatory landscape of melanoma reveals TEADS as regulators of the invasive cell state. Nat Commun 6:6683

Vogt PK (2002) Fortuitous convergences: the beginnings of JUN. Nat Rev Cancer 2:465–469

Volkenandt M, Schlegel U, Nanus DM, Albino AP (1991) Mutational analysis of the human p53 gene in malignant melanoma. Pigment Cell Res 4:35–40

Wang T, Niu G, Kortylewski M, Burdelya L, Shain K, Zhang S, Bhattacharya R, Gabrilovich D, Heller R, Coppola D, Dalton W, Jove R, Pardoll D, Yu H (2004) Regulation of the innate and adaptive immune responses by Stat-3 signaling in tumor cells. Nat Med 10:48–54

Warner BJ, Blain SW, Seoane J, Massague J (1999) Myc downregulation by transforming growth factor beta required for activation of the p15(Ink4b) G(1) arrest pathway. Mol Cell Biol 19:5913–5922

Weeraratna AT (2005) A Wnt-er wonderland – the complexity of Wnt signaling in melanoma. Cancer Metastasis Rev 24:237–250

Wegner M (2005) Secrets to a healthy Sox life: lessons for melanocytes. Pigment Cell Res 18:74–85

Weilbaecher KN, Motyckova G, Huber WE, Takemoto CM, Hemesath TJ, Xu Y, Hershey CL, Dowland NR, Wells AG, Fisher DE (2001) Linkage of M-CSF signaling to Mitf, TFE3, and the osteoclast defect in Mitf(mi/mi) mice. Mol Cell 8:749–758

Weiss MB, Abel EV, Dadpey N, Aplin AE (2014) FOXD3 modulates migration through direct transcriptional repression of TWIST1 in melanoma. Mol Cancer Res 12:1314–1323

Widlund HR, Horstmann MA, Price ER, Cui J, Lessnick SL, Wu M, He X, Fisher DE (2002) Beta-catenin-induced melanoma growth requires the downstream target Microphthalmia-associated transcription factor. J Cell Biol 158:1079–1087

Wilson A, Radtke F (2006) Multiple functions of Notch signaling in self-renewing organs and cancer. FEBS Lett 580:2860–2868

Wu M, Hemesath TJ, Takemoto CM, Horstmann MA, Wells AG, Price ER, Fisher DZ, Fisher DE (2000) c-Kit triggers dual phosphorylations, which couple activation and degradation of the essential melanocyte factor Mi. Genes Dev 14:301–312

Xie S, Price JE, Luca M, Jean D, Ronai Z, Bar-Eli M (1997) Dominant-negative CREB inhibits tumor growth and metastasis of human melanoma cells. Oncogene 15:2069–2075

Xie TX, Wei D, Liu M, Gao AC, Ali-Osman F, Sawaya R, Huang S (2004) Stat3 activation regulates the expression of matrix metalloproteinase-2 and tumor invasion and metastasis. Oncogene 23:3550–3560

Xu Q, Briggs J, Park S, Niu G, Kortylewski M, Zhang S, Gritsko T, Turkson J, Kay H, Semenza GL, Cheng JQ, Jove R, Yu H (2005) Targeting Stat3 blocks both HIF-1 and VEGF expression induced by multiple oncogenic growth signaling pathways. Oncogene 24:5552–5560

Yamaguchi Y, Hearing VJ (2009) Physiological factors that regulate skin pigmentation. Biofactors 35:193–199

Yang J, Richmond A (2001) Constitutive IkappaB kinase activity correlates with nuclear factor-kappaB activation in human melanoma cells. Cancer Res 61:4901–4909

Yang J, Splittgerber R, Yull FE, Kantrow S, Ayers GD, Karin M, Richmond A (2010) Conditional ablation of Ikkb inhibits melanoma tumor development in mice. J Clin Invest 120:2563–2574

Yasumoto K, Yokoyama K, Shibata K, Tomita Y, Shibahara S (1994) Microphthalmia-associated transcription factor as a regulator for melanocyte-specific transcription of the human tyrosinase gene. Mol Cell Biol 14:8058–8070

Yokoyama S, Feige E, Poling LL, Levy C, Widlund HR, Khaled M, Kung AL, Fisher DE (2008) Pharmacologic suppression of MITF expression via HDAC inhibitors in the melanocyte lineage. Pigment Cell Melanoma Res 21:457–463

Yokoyama S, Woods SL, Boyle GM, Aoude LG, MacGregor S, Zismann V, Gartside M, Cust AE, Haq R, Harland M, Taylor JC, Duffy DL, Holohan K, Dutton-Regester K, Palmer JM, Bonazzi V, Stark MS, Symmons J, Law MH, Schmidt C, Lanagan C, O'Connor L, Holland EA, Schmid H, Maskiell JA, Jetann J, Ferguson M, Jenkins MA, Kefford RF, Giles GG, Armstrong BK, Aitken JF, Hopper JL, Whiteman DC, Pharoah PD, Easton DF, Dunning AM, Newton-Bishop JA, Montgomery GW, Martin NG, Mann GJ, Bishop DT, Tsao H, Trent JM, Fisher DE, Hayward NK, Brown KM (2011) A novel recurrent mutation in MITF predisposes to familial and sporadic melanoma. Nature 480:99–103

Yuan H, Corbi N, Basilico C, Dailey L (1995) Developmental-specific activity of the FGF-4 enhancer requires the synergistic action of Sox2 and Oct-3. Genes Dev 9:2635–2645

Zhu S, Wurdak H, Wang Y, Galkin A, Tao H, Li J, Lyssiotis CA, Yan F, Tu BP, Miraglia L, Walker J, Sun F, Orth A, Schultz PG, Wu X (2009) A genomic screen identifies TYRO3 as a MITF regulator in melanoma. Proc Natl Acad Sci U S A 106:17025–17030

Zhuang D, Mannava S, Grachtchouk V, Tang WH, Patil S, Wawrzyniak JA, Berman AE, Giordano TJ, Prochownik EV, Soengas MS, Nikiforov MA (2008) C-MYC overexpression is required for continuous suppression of oncogene-induced senescence in melanoma cells. Oncogene 27:6623–6634

Zilberberg A, Yaniv A, Gazit A (2004) The low density lipoprotein receptor-1, LRP1, interacts with the human frizzled-1 (HFz1) and down-regulates the canonical Wnt signaling pathway. J Biol Chem 279:17535–17542

MiRNAs in Malignant Melanoma

6

Maria Mione, Janika Liebig, Leonel Munoz, and Anja Bosserhoff

6.1 MiRNA Biogenesis and Function

6.1.1 Transcription of miRNA Genes and Processing in the Nucleus

MicroRNA genes are embedded in intergenic as well as intragenic regions of the human genome, encoding either a single miRNA species or a cluster of multiple miRNAs in a polycistronic manner (Lee et al. 2002). In the first step of miRNA expression, miRNA genes are transcribed into pri-miRNAs (primary miRNA transcripts; Fig. 6.1). In most cases, transcription is accomplished by RNA polymerase II, resulting in 5′-methyl-guanosine capped and polyadenylated pri-miRNAs, which contain local stem-loop structures and are up to several kilobases in length (Cai et al. 2004; Lee et al. 2004). Some specific miRNAs are initially transcribed by RNA polymerase III (Borchert et al. 2006). While still in the nucleus, the pri-miRNA is endonucleolytically cleaved by the so-called microprocessor complex composed of the RNAse III enzyme Drosha (RNASEN) and its co-factor DGCR8 [DiGeorge syndrome critical region on chromosome 8;

Maria Mione, Janika Liebig and Leonel Munoz contributed equally

M. Mione
ITG, Karlsruhe Institute of Technology, Eggestein-Leopoldshafen, Germany, and Cibio University of Trento, Trento, Italy

J. Liebig • A. Bosserhoff (✉)
Institute of Biochemistry (Emil-Fischer-Zentrum), University of Erlangen-Nürnberg, Fahrstr. 17, 91054 Erlangen, Germany
e-mail: anja.bosserhoff@fau.de

L. Munoz
ITG, Karlsruhe Institute of Technology, Eggestein-Leopoldshafen, Germany, and University of Valparaiso, Karlsruhe, Chile

A. Bosserhoff (ed.), *Melanoma Development*,
DOI 10.1007/978-3-319-41319-8_6

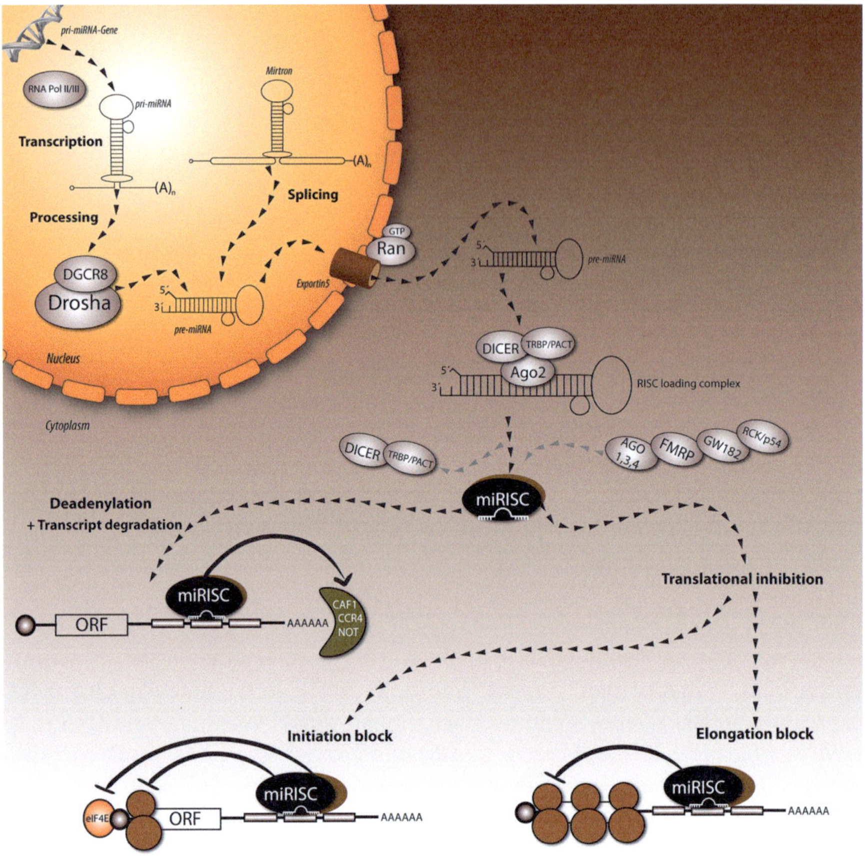

Fig. 6.1 Schematic overview of miRNA biogenesis and function. Please refer to Sect. 6.1 for detailed explanations on the molecular mechanisms involved in each step

also known as Pasha (Partner of Drosha) in *Drosophila melanogaster* and *C. elegans*] (Landthaler et al. 2004; Lee et al. 2003).

DGCR8 interacts with the ~33 bp stem-loop as well as with the adjacent unpaired flanking regions within the pri-miRNA, thus supporting Drosha-mediated cleavage in the stem region, about 11 bp away from the junction of ssRNA (single-stranded RNA) to dsRNA (double-stranded RNA) (Han et al. 2006; Zeng and Cullen 2005). The resulting pre-miRNA (~70 bp in length) is rapidly translocated to the cytoplasm via the Ran-GTP-dependent nuclear export factor exportin 5 (XPO5), a member of the nuclear transport receptor family (Kim 2004). Export of only correctly processed pre-miRNAs is ensured by recognition of the >14 bp dsRNA stem together with a short (1–8 nucleotides) 3′ overhang (Zeng and Cullen 2003). Exceptions to this rule have been reported, as in the case of cell adhesion complexes sequestering microprocessor components for the localized production of mature miRNAs from nuclear-exported pri-miRNAs (Kourtidis et al. 2015). Interestingly, a number of pre-miRNAs can be exported from the nucleus without undergoing processing by

Drosha. These so-called miRtrons are located in very short introns and are capable of forming a hairpin resembling pre-miRNA molecules after they were released from their host transcripts by splicing and debranching (Berezikov et al. 2007).

6.1.2 Cytoplasmic Processing and Modes of miRNA Mediated Gene Silencing

In the cytoplasm, maturation of pre-miRNAs occurs via a multi-enzyme complex called RISC (RNA induced silencing complex) loading complex (RLC). This RLC is composed of the RNase III enzyme Dicer, the double-stranded RNA-binding domain proteins TRBP (TAR RNA-binding protein) and PACT (protein activator of PKR), as well as AGO2 (Argonaute-2), which builds the core of the complex (Gregory et al. 2005; MacRae et al. 2008). TRBP and PACT facilitate Dicer-mediated cleavage of the pre-miRNA, which occurs near the terminal loop and results in an RNA duplex of ~22 nucleotides with two nucleotide overhangs on each 3′ terminus (Hutvagner et al. 2001; Knight and Bass 2001). In some cases, AGO2 – which exhibits robust RNaseH-like endonucleolytic activity – can support Dicer processing by cleaving the 3′ arm of specific pre-miRs (Diederichs and Haber 2007). Subsequently, Dicer and its interactors TRBP and PACT dissociate from the complex, and the miRNA duplex is separated into the guide strand (which is complementary to the target mRNAs and is thus functional in gene silencing) and the passenger strand (miRNA*), which usually gets degraded. It would appear that there is no universal helicase responsible for the unwinding of the miRNA duplex, but specific helicases may differentially regulate subgroups of miRNAs (Winter et al. 2009). In other cases, a helicase is not required at all for duplex unwinding (Pillai et al. 2005; Wu and Belasco 2005). The guide strand is characterized by the presence of a thermodynamically less stable base pair at the 5′ end of the duplex and is loaded onto the RISC complex after unwinding (Khvorova et al. 2003). Of note, miRNA* strands are not always simply by-products of miRNA biogenesis but are sometimes also acting as functional miRNAs on the miRISC (miRNA-containing RISC) (Chiang et al. 2010; Ghildiyal et al. 2010; Okamura et al. 2009). Nowadays, therefore the nomenclature changed to -5p or -3p miRNAs.

The assembly of the miRISC, also called miRNP (micro-ribonucleoprotein), is a dynamic process coupled with the preceding steps of pre-miRNA processing. Key components of the miRISC are proteins of the Argonaute (AGO) family, FMRP (fragile X mental retardation protein), and P-body components including GW182 and RCK/p54, which are essential for inducing miRNA-mediated gene repression (Filipowicz et al. 2008). Guided by the mature miRNA, the miRISC subsequently binds to target sequences in the 3′ untranslated regions (3′UTRs) of regulated transcripts, in order to inhibit their translation into functional proteins. To date, the general rules for the initial miRNA:mRNA interaction, which are fundamental for target recognition, are only incompletely determined experimentally and bioinformatically (Brennecke et al. 2005; Doench and Sharp 2004; Grimson et al. 2007; Lewis et al. 2005; Nielsen et al. 2007; Reyes Herrera and Ficarra 2012; Zheng et al. 2013; Peterson et al. 2014). In animals, miRNAs almost exclusively bind to their target mRNAs with imperfect complementarity. Nevertheless, an indispensible prerequisite for efficient transcript targeting is continuous base-pairing of miRNA nucleotides 2–8, which are called the miRNAs "seed-sequence" (Bartel 2009). It is actually this miRNA seed which is the major determinant of a miRNA's target repertoire. Nevertheless, apart from the miRNA seed sequence targets, mRNAs usually have multiple cis-elements in their 3′UTRs that can be bound by other trans-factors, namely, RNA binding proteins (RBPs) (reviewed by Ho and Marsden 2014). Different mechanisms of interplay between RBPs and miRNAs/RISC can determine a synergistic or a competing relationship with an mRNA, destabilizing or stabilizing its translation. When both kinds of molecules target the same cis-element, the mechanism may involve the interaction between the RBP and the miRNA or components of the RISC. When they bind different cis-elements, the effect is more likely to depend on which molecule binds first (influenced by subcellular localization of the process), the number of cis-element in the 3′UTR of a given mRNA, and the ability of one molecule to displace the other from the target. The RBP involved in mRNA stability can be classified according to their target sequences into AU-rich elements (ARE)-binding proteins, and pyrimidine (C/CU)-rich element binding proteins. In any case RBP-mediated degradation or translation is dependent on miRNA-containing RISC (Ho and Marsden 2014). These additional regulatory layers of mRNA fate stress the necessity of experimentally validating any bioinformatically predicted miRNA target, i.e., based purely upon complementary nucleotide sequence.

The resulting miRNA-induced posttranscriptional silencing of target genes is mediated either by destabilization of the corresponding mRNA (Behm-Ansmant et al. 2006b; Giraldez et al. 2006; Wu et al. 2006; Wu and Belasco 2005; Guo et al. 2010) or by repression of protein translation (Pillai et al. 2005; Standart and Jackson 2007), both pathways acting cooperatively but yet independently of each other. Current knowledge suggests that destabilization of target mRNAs starts with recruitment of the P-body component GW182 (glycine-tryptophan protein of 182 kDa) by Argonaute proteins (Till et al. 2007). GW182 subsequently mediates binding of the CAF1:CCR4:NOT1 deadenylase complex to the target mRNA. Deadenylation is then followed by removal of the 5′-methyl-guanosine cap via the DCP1:DCP2 decapping complex, ultimately leading to 5′→3′ exonucleolytic degradation of mRNA by exonuclease XRN1 (Behm-Ansmant et al. 2006a; Eulalio et al. 2007, 2009; reviewed by Hausser and Zavolan 2014). By contrast, there still is a lack of consensus concerning the mechanism(s) by which miRNAs induce repression of translation. While many experiments refer to the initiation of translation as a target for repression, there is also evidence that various post-initiation steps could be affected (reviewed by Chekulaeva and Filipowicz 2009). Present research aims to unravel whether miRNAs are actually capable of controlling translation by multiple mechanisms or if these discrepancies were due to different experimental approaches utilized in the past (Cannell et al. 2008; Kong et al. 2008). Figure 6.1 summarizes the mechanisms involved in miRNA biogenesis and function.

6.1.3 Regulation of miRNA Biogenesis, Function, and Decay

The general pathway of miRNA biogenesis and function – as well as the clearance of miRNAs through decay – is complicated by a large number of regulatory mechanisms, in which a vast quantity of yet unidentified proteins is likely to be involved. There may be specific alterations to the pathway for every individual miRNA or at least distinct subgroups of miRNAs (reviewed by Krol et al. 2010).

The expression of miRNAs can be regulated at the level of transcription (reviewed by Davis and Hata 2009; Turner and Slack 2009) or at various steps during the processing of the pri-miR into mature miRNA (reviewed by Davis and Hata 2009). The latter mechanism commonly involves the regulation of constituents of the miRNA processing machinery, like Drosha/DGCR8 (Han et al. 2009; Triboulet et al. 2009) and Dicer/TRBP (Chendrimada et al. 2005; Melo et al. 2009; Paroo et al. 2009). Additionally, accessory proteins can directly interact with miRNA precursors either repressing or stimulating their further processing (reviewed by Winter et al. 2009). By contrast, modulation of miRNA function is mainly based on mechanisms affecting proteins of the miRISC, predominantly AGO2 and GW182 (reviewed by Krol et al. 2010). With regard to melanoma, it has been suggested that the transcriptional regulation of Dicer by MITF might be a major determinant in melanocyte cell survival and differentiation (Levy et al. 2010a, b; please refer to Sect. 6.2 for detailed information). In addition, recent literature described the strong reduction of AGO2 expression in melanoma, influencing miRNA functionality (Voeller et al. 2013; Sand et al. 2012a). Further studies analyzed changes in expression level of Dicer, Drosha and additional processing enzymes (Jafari et al. 2013; Jafarnejad et al. 2013; Ma et al. 2011), but leave the definition of the role of these changes mainly open.

To date, little is known about the regulation of miRNA decay. Nevertheless, recent findings implicate that sequences present at the 3′ end of specific miRNAs or, more generally, enzyme catalyzed modifications to the 3′ end of miRNAs may determine the rate of miRNA clearance (Hwang et al. 2007; Jones et al. 2009; Katoh et al. 2009). Interestingly, degradation of mature miRNAs seems to depend on their activity. In the absence of its complementary targets, a miRNA may be specifically released from the miRISC. Thereby, its 5′ end gets accessible to the 5′ → 3′ exonuclease XRN-2, which subsequently degrades the miRNA (Chatterjee and Grosshans 2009).

These findings clearly show that miRNAs are not only active regulators of gene expression but are themselves subject to sophisticated control. Adding even more complexity, miRNAs have recently been shown to not exclusively repress gene expression but to conversely enhance translation of specific transcripts under certain cellular conditions – although these cases are still clearly the exception rather than the rule (Vasudevan et al. 2007, 2008).

New studies recently further showed an important role of RNA editing via adenosine deaminase acting on RNA (ADAR) enzymes in miR functions (Shoshan et al. 2015; Dietrich and Bosshoff 2015).

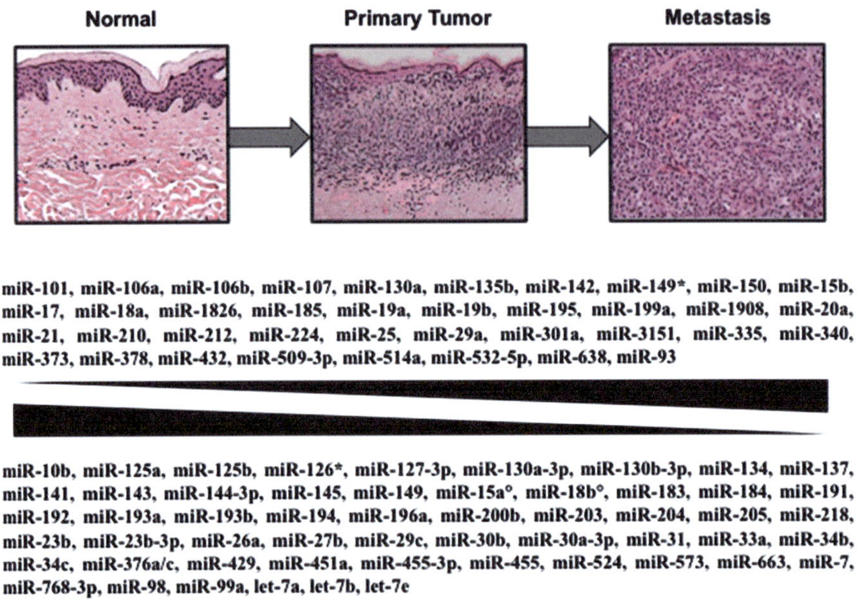

Fig. 6.2 Schematic overview of miRNAs deregulated during melanoma formation and progression (Reprinted from Mueller and Bosserhoff (2009), strongly modified. With kind permission from the *Br J Cancer*)

6.2 Impact of Specific miRNAs on Melanomagenesis

In contrast to other types of tumors, studies on the impact of specific miRNA species on melanomagenesis have not been conducted before the year 2008. Nevertheless, many miRNAs deregulated in melanoma cells compared to normal melanocytes have been characterized in regard to their target genes as well as their impact on melanoma cell function since then (Fig. 6.2 and Table 6.1). The following paragraph aims to integrate those findings in their meaningful context and to point out how miRNA-related research expanded our knowledge on the molecular mechanisms contributing to formation and progression of malignant melanoma. However, it cannot be comprehensive due to many new findings in the field. We try to integrate all miRs coming from arrays or miR sequencing approaches, which are confirmed by independent methods to be differentially expressed. However, based on multiple approaches published, we mainly focused on deregulated miRNAs, where functional consequences have been described.

6.2.1 Networking of miRNAs and MITF

It is not surprising that the very first miRNA identified to influence melanoma progression is involved in modulating the expression level of the key regulator of melanocyte cell fate—microphthalmia-associated transcription factor (MITF; see Chaps. 5 and 12). In their study, Bemis et al. (2008) set out to characterize an

Table 6.1 Summary of expression profiling as well as functional data available on miRNAs deregulated in melanoma cells

miRNA	Gain/loss in melanoma cells	Tissue/Cell line	Kind of evidence	Cause of loss/gain	Verified target(s) in MM	Reference(s)	Family/Cluster
miR-101	↑	Both	qRT-PCR, functional tests	Not yet determined	MITF, EZH2	(**80**)	miR-101 family
miR-106b	↑	Both	Microarray. qRT-PCR, functional tests	Not yet determined	CDKN1A	(**13**, **71**, **108**, **111**)	miR-17 family
mir-125a	↓	Both	Microarray, RT^2 Profiler Array, qRT-PCR	MAPK/ERK	LIN28B	(**13**, **17**, **108**, **144**)	miR-10 family
miR-125b	↓	Both	Microarray, qRT-PCR, functional tests	Hypermethylation, intracellular cAMP levels.	C-JUN, ITGA9, MAP3K11	(**38**, **49**, **56**, **58**, **104**, **108**, **140**, **141**)	miR-10 family
miR-126-3p & miR-126-5p	↓*	Both	Microarray, NGS, qRT-PCR, functional tests	TFAP2A level	ADAM9, MMP7	(**30**, **31**, **61**, **70**)	miR-126 family
miR-130a-3p	↓	Both	High-throughput RNA sequencing, qRT-PCR	Not yet determined	SMAD4°	(**22**)	miR-130 family
miR-130b-3p	↓(?)	Both	High-throughput RNA sequencing, qRT-PCR	Not yet determined	SMAD°	(**22**, **61**)	miR-130 family
miR-137	↓	Both	Microarray, qRT-PCR, functional tests	Amplification of a VNTR in the 5'UTR of the pri-miRNA	MITF, MET, YBX1, EZH2, CTBP1, PAK2	(**5**, **21**, **46**, **68**, **81**)	miR-137 family

(continued)

Table 6.1 (continued)

miRNA	Gain/loss in melanoma cells	Tissue/Cell line	Kind of evidence	Cause of loss/gain	Verified target(s) in MM	Reference(s)	Family/Cluster
miR-143	↓	Tissue	qRT-PCR, functional tests	Not yet determined	TCL1B	(**69**)	miR-143 family
miR-145	↓	Cell line	qRT-PCR, functional tests	Not yet determined	MYO5A, MYC°, FSCN1°	(**23**, **24**, **98**)	miR-145 family
miR-146a	↑	Both	Microarray, RT^2 Profiler Array, Small RNA profiling, qRT-PCR, functional tests	NRAS mutant (NRASQ61K), BRAF mutant (BRAFV600E), phosphorylation of myc by MAPK/ERK pathway, MITF level ?	NUMB	(**32**, **108**)	miR-146 family
	↓	Cell line	Microarray, qRT-PCR	MAPK/ERK, MITF level ?	Not yet determined	(**17**, **64**, **108**)	
miR-148a	↓*	Both	Microarray, RT^2 Profiler Array, qRT-PCR, functional tests	Hypermethylation	TGIF2, MITF	(**45**, **79**, **108**)	miR-148 family
miR-148b	↓*	Both	RT^2 Profiler Array, Microarray, qRT-PCR	MITF level, TFAP2A level	ALCAM, MITF	(**45**, **92**, **104**, **107**, **108**)	miR-148 family
miR-149*	↑	Both	qRT-PCR	p53 expression	GSK3A	(**55**)	miR-149 family
miR-15a	↓*	Tissue	qRT-PCR, functional tests	Not yet determined	IL-10RA	(**110**, **120**, **129**)	miR-15 family

miRNA	Gain/loss in melanoma cells	Tissue/Cell line	Kind of evidence	Cause of loss/gain	Verified target(s) in MM	Reference(s)	Family/Cluster
miR-155	↑	Tissue	RT^2 Profiler Array, qRT-PCR	IL1B	MITF, TYRP1	(**1**, **25**, **43**, **108**, **121**)	miR-155 family
	↓	Cell line	qRT-PCR, functional tests	Not yet determined	SKI	(**64**, **65**, **108**)	
miR-17	↑	Both	Microarray, qRT-PCR, functional tests	MAPK/ERK	ETV1, ADAR, LEF1, CCND1, CDKN1A	(**13**, **16**, **17**, **41**, **64**, **92**, **94**, **108**)	miR-17 family, miR-17-92 cluster
miR-18b	↓*	Both	Microarray, qRT-PCR, functional tests	Hypermethylation	MDM2	(**19**)	miR-17 family, miR-106-363 cluster
miR-182	↑	Both	Microarray, qRT-PCR, functional tests	Hypermethylation	MITF, FOXO3	(**74**, **122**)	miR-182 family
	↓	Both	Microarray	Not yet determined	Not yet determined	(**108**, **134**)	
miR-185	↑	Both	Microarray, qRT-PCR, functional tests	Not yet determined	IL10RA	(**92**, **108**, **129**)	miR-185 family
miR-19b	↑	Both	Microarray, qRT-PCR	MITF level	PITX1	(**92**, **103**, **104**, **108**)	miR-19 family, miR-17-92 cluster (19b-1), 106–363 cluster (19b-2)

(continued)

Table 6.1 (continued)

miRNA	Gain/loss in melanoma cells	Tissue/Cell line	Kind of evidence	Cause of loss/gain	Verified target(s) in MM	Reference(s)	Family/Cluster
miR-193b	↓	Both	Microarray, qRT-PCR, functional tests, Northern Blot	Not yet determined	CCND1, MCL1, STMN1	(**12**, **13**, **14**)	miR-193 family
miR-195	↑	Tissue	Taqman MicroRNA Assay, functional tests	Not yet determined	WEE1	(**6**)	miR-15 family
miR-196a	↓	Both	RT^2 Profiler Array, qRT-PCR, functional tests	Not yet determined	HOXB7, HOXC8	(**8**, **91**, **108**)	miR-196a family
miR-199a-3p	↑*	Both	Microarray, qRT-PCR, functional tests	Not yet determined	DNAJA4, MET	(**89**, **105**)	miR-199 family
miR-199a	↑	Both	Microarray, qRT-PCR, functional tests	Not yet determined	APOE, DNAJA4	(**105**)	miR-199 family
miR-1908	↑	Both	Microarray, qRT-PCR, functional tests	Not yet determined	APOE, DNAJA4	(**105**)	miR-1908 family
miR-20b	↑	Both	Microarray, qRT-PCR	MITF level ?	Not yet determined	(**92**, **104**, **134**)	miR-17 family, 106–363 Cluster
	↓	Cell line	Microarray	Not yet determined	F2R	(**114**)	
miR-200b	↓	Both	Microarray, qRT-PCR	Not yet determined	PTEN°, ZEB1°	(**57**, **115**, **134**)	miR-8 family

miRNA	Gain/loss in melanoma cells	Tissue/Cell line	Kind of evidence	Cause of loss/gain	Verified target(s) in MM	Reference(s)	Family/Cluster
miR-200c	↑	Cell line	qRT-PCR	Not yet determined	Not yet determined	(**26**, **92**)	miR-8 family
	↓	Both	Microarray, RT^2 Profiler Array, qRT-PCR, functional tests	Not yet determined	BMI1	(**76**, **108**, **128**, **134**)	
miR-203	↓	Both	Microarray, RT^2 Profiler Array, qRT-PCR, NGS, functional tests	Hypermethylation	E2F3, ZNF148, KIF5B, KIF2A, CREB1, VCAN, BMI1	(**9**, **11**, **61**, **96**, **97**, **99**, **100**, **108**, **134**)	miR-203 family
miR-205	↓	Both	Microarray, RT^2 Profiler Array, qRT-PCR, functional tests, NGS	Hypermethylation	E2F1, E2F5, MDM2	(**18**, **19**, **61**, **76**, **108**, **134**)	miR-205 family
miR-206	↓*	Tissue	Microarray, qRT-PCR, functional tests	Not yet determined	CDK4, CCND1, CCNC	(**36**, **127**)	miR-1 family
miR-21	↑	Both	Microarray, RT^2 Profiler Array, qRT-PCR, functional tests	MAPK/ERK, STAT3 activation	FBXO11, PTEN°, PDCD4°, BTG2°, TIMP3°	(**13**, **17**, **43**, **54**, **84**, **108**, **118**, **134**, **136**, **137**)	miR-21 family
miR-210	↑	Tissue	Microarray, RT^2 Profiler Array, qRT-PCR, functional tests	MAPK/ERK, HIF1A, HIF2A	MNT, PTPN1, HOXA1, TP53I11	(**17**, **101**, **108**, **117**, **143**)	miR-210 family

(continued)

Table 6.1 (continued)

miRNA	Gain/loss in melanoma cells	Tissue/Cell line	Kind of evidence	Cause of loss/gain	Verified target(s) in MM	Reference(s)	Family/Cluster
miR-211	↑	Both	Microarray, qRT-PCR	MITF level	IL-10RA	(**83**, **108**, **120**, **129**)	miR-204 family
	↓	Both	Microarray, NGS, qRT-PCR, functional tests	MITF level	RAB22A, AP1S2, SERINC3, M6PR, IGFBP5, PDE3A, SSRP1, SOX11, LIFR, SOX4, KCNMA1, TGFBR2, NGAT5, POU3F2, PRAME, NUAK1, IGF2R°, PDK4	(**4**, **7**, **10**, **13**, **61**, **66**, **83**, **86**, **88**, **113**, **134**)	
miR-214	↑	Both	Microarray, qRT-PCR, functional tests	Not yet determined	ITGA3, MET, TFAP2C, TFAP2A°, PAK2	(**106**, **107**, **121**)	miR-214 family
	↓	Tissue	RT^2 Profiler Array, qRT-PCR	Not yet determined	Not yet determined	(**13**, **77**, **108**)	
miR-218	↓	Both	RT^2 Profiler Array, qRT-PCR, functional tests	Not yet determined	MITF, KIAA1524, BMI1	(**44**, **108**, **133**, **142**)	miR-218 family
miR-22	↑	Tissue	Microarray, qRT-PCR	Not yet determined	Not yet determined	(**13**, **116**)	miR-22 family
	↓	Cell line	Microarray, qRT-PCR, functional tests	MAPK/ERK	LEF1, FOSL1, CDKN1A	(**17**)	

miRNA	Gain/loss in melanoma cells	Tissue/Cell line	Kind of evidence	Cause of loss/gain	Verified target(s) in MM	Reference(s)	Family/Cluster
miR-221	↑	Both	Microarray, qRT-PCR, functional tests, Northern Blot	HOXB7/PBX2, PLZF, hPNP^{old-35}, ADAR1	KIT, FOS, TFAP2A, CDKN1B	(**20**, **27**, **28**, **29**, **30**, **34**, **39**, **51**)	miR-221 family
	↓	Both	Microarray, qRT-PCR, functional tests	MITF/RBPJK, MAPK/ERK, hPNPase^{old-35}	TGFBR2, NFAT5	(**17**, **20**, **39**, **66**, **109**)	
miR-222	↑	Both	Microarray, qRT-PCR, functional tests, Northern Blot	HOXB7/PBX2, PLZF, hPNPold-35, ADAR1, Thr-38 phosphorylated Ets-1	ETS1, ICAM1, FOS, TFAP2A, CDKN1B	(**20**, **27**, **28**, **29**, **30**, **34**, **39**, **85**, **92**)	miR-221 family
	↓	Both	Microarray, qRT-PCR, Northern Blot	MITF/RBPJK, MAPK/ERK, ETS-1	ETS1	(**17**, **39**, **85**, **109**)	
miR-224	↑	Both	qRT-PCR, functional tests	E2F1, HIF1A	TXNIP	(**50**, **60**)	miR-224 family
	↓	Cell line	Microarray	Not yet determined	Not yet determined	(**108**, **134**)	
miR-25	↑	Both	Microarray, qRT-PCR	ERK dependent ?	PTEN°	(**15**, **57**, **108**)	miR-25 family
miR-26a	↓	Both	Microarray, NGS, qRT-PCR, functional tests	MAPK/ERK	BAG4, LIN28B, ZCCHC11	(**17**, **33**, **61**, **62**, **112**, **115**)	miR-26 family
miR-29a	↑	Tissue	RT^2 Profiler Array	STAT1	CDK6	(**108**, **119**)	miR-29 family

(continued)

Table 6.1 (continued)

miRNA	Gain/loss in melanoma cells	Tissue/Cell line	Kind of evidence	Cause of loss/gain	Verified target(s) in MM	Reference(s)	Family/Cluster
miR-29c	↓	Tissue	qRT-PCR	Hypermethylation	DNMT3A°, DNMT3B°, BCD276	(**95**, **132**)	miR-29 family
miR-30b	↑	Tissue	Microarray, qRT-PCR, functional tests	Not yet determined	GALNT7, GALNT1, SEMA3, CESLR3, TWF1	(**35**)	miR-30 family
	↓	Cell line	Microarray	MAPK/ERK	GALNT7	(**17**)	
miR-30d	↑	Tissue	Microarray, qRT-PCR, functional tests	Not yet determined	GALNT7, GALNT1, SEMA3, CESLR3, TWF1	(**35**)	miR-30 family
miR-31	↓	Both	Microarray, qRT-PCR, functional tests	Hypermethylation & EZH2-mediated histone H3K27 trimethylation	SRC, RAB27A, MAP3K14, MET, EZH2°	(**2**)	miR-31 family
miR-3151	↑	Tissue	qRT-PCR	BRAF	TP53	(**63**)	miR-3151 family
miR-33a	↓	Both	Microarray, qRT-PCR, functional tests	Not yet determined	HIF1A	(**146**)	miR-33 family
miR-338	↑	Tissue	Microarray, qRT-PCR	Aktivation of MAPK/ERK pathway	KIT°	(**51**, **53**)	miR-338 family
	↓	Tissue	qRT-PCR	Not yet determined	Not yet determined	(**10**, **109**)	

miRNA	Gain/loss in melanoma cells	Tissue/Cell line	Kind of evidence	Cause of loss/gain	Verified target(s) in MM	Reference(s)	Family/Cluster
miR-34a	↑	Tissue	RT^2 Profiler Array	CCL2	Not yet determined	(**108**, **130**)	miR-34 family
	↓	Both	Microarray, qRT-PCR, functional tests	Hypermethylation, B-Raf/MKK/ER, p53	FLOT2, ULBP2	(**17**, **42**, **47**, **48**, **73**, **78**, **117**, **135**)	
miR-34b	↓	Both	Microarray, qRT-PCR, functional tests	Hypermethylation, p53	MYC, CDK6, MET	(**47**, **79**, **87**, **89**, **135**)	miR-34 family
miR-34c	↓	Both	Microarray, qRT-PCR, functional tests	Hypermethylation, p53	E2F3, ULBP2, MET	(**47**, **48**, **79**, **89**, **116**, **135**)	miR-34 family
miR-340	↑	Cell line	qRT-PCR, functional tests	Not yet determined	Modulator of MAPK/ERK signaling, RHOA, MITF	(**40**, **52**, **126**)	miR-340 family
miR-365	↓*	Both	qRT-PCR, functional tests	Not yet determined	NRP1	(**3**)	miR-365 family
miR-376a	↓	Both	Microarray, qRT-PCR, functional tests	Epigenetic modifications (?)	IGF1R	(**108**, **138**)	miR-368 family
miR-376c	↓	Both	Microarray, qRT-PCR, functional tests	Epigenetic modifications (?)	IGF1R	(**108**, **138**)	miR-368 family

(continued)

Table 6.1 (continued)

miRNA	Gain/loss in melanoma cells	Tissue/Cell line	Kind of evidence	Cause of loss/gain	Verified target(s) in MM	Reference(s)	Family/Cluster
miR-377	↓*	Both	Microarray, qRT-PCR, functional tests	Epigenetic modifications (?)	E2F3, MAP3K7	(**138**, **139**)	miR-154 family
miR-425	↓*	Tissue	Microarray, qRT-PCR	Not yet determined	IGF1	(**72**, **110**)	miR-425 family
miR-432	↑	Tissue	qRT-PCR	Hypomethylation	ADAR	(**94**)	miR-432 family
miR-452	↑	Both	qRT-PCR, functional tests	E2F1	TXNIP	(**60**)	miR-452 family
miR-455-5p	↓	Both	Microarray, functional tests	Not yet determined	CPEB1	(**114**, **123**, **134**)	miR-455 family
miR-514a	↑	Both	Microarray, qRT-PCR, functional tests	Not yet determined	NF1	(**124**, **125**)	miR-506 family
miR-524-5p	↓	Both	Microarray, qRT-PCR, functional tests	Activity of the MAPK/ERK pathway	BRAF, MAPK1	(**77**)	miR-515 family
miR-532-5p	↑	Both	qRT-PCR, functional tests	Not yet determined	RUNX3°	(**59**)	miR-188 family
miR-573	↓	Both	qRT-PCR, functional tests	Not yet determined	MCAM	(**131**)	miR-573 family
miR-638	↑	Both	Microarray, qRT-PCR, functional tests	AP2A expression, Hypermethylation	TP53INP2	(**6**, **108**)	miR-638 family
miR-7	↓	Cell line	Microarray, qRT-PCR, functional tests	Not yet determined	IRS2	(**37**, **108**)	miR-7 family

miRNA	Gain/loss in melanoma cells	Tissue/Cell line	Kind of evidence	Cause of loss/gain	Verified target(s) in MM	Reference(s)	Family/Cluster
miR-768-3p	↓	Tissue	Microarray, functional tests	MAPK/ERK	elF4E	(**13**, **17**, **53**)	~
miR-9	↑	Tissue	Microarray, RT^2 Profiler Array, qRT-PCR	Not yet determined	Not yet determined	(**13**, **108**)	miR-9 family
	↓	Both	qRT-PCR, functional tests	Hypermethylation, Transcription factor YY1	NFKB1, RYBP	(**75**, **79**, **145**)	
miR-92a	↑*	Both	Microarray, qRT-PCR	MAPK/ERK	PTEN	(**13**, **17**, **57**, **64**, **92**, **108**)	miR-25 family, miR-17-92 cluster (miR-92a-1), miR-106-363 cluster (miR-92a-2)
miR-98	↓	Tissue	qRT-PCR, functional tests	Lin28b, NF-kB (IL-6 signalling)	IL6	(**67**)	let-7 family
let-7a	↓	Both	Microarray, RT^2 Profiler Array, qRT-PCR, Northern Blot, functional tests	Not yet determined	NRAS°, ITGB3	(**13**, **82**, **90**, **93**, **108**, **120**)	let-7 family
let-7b	↓	Tissue	Microarray, qRT-PCR, functional tests	Not yet determined	CCND1, CCND3°, CDK4°, CCNA°	(**13**, **120**)	let-7 family

Question marks in brackets indicate lack of compelling evidence. Due to space limitations, only miRNAs with confirmed targets were included. Please refer to Sects. 6.2 and 6.3 for details

↓*/↑*: One available publication shows contradictory results

Gene°: Gene is regulated directly or indirectly by the mentioned microRNA

(continued)

Table 6.1 (continued)

~: mir-768 overlaps an annotated snoRNA, HBII-239. Phylogenetic analysis show poor conservation of the reported mature miRNA sequence (miRBase)

(**1**) Arts et al. (2015), (**2**) Asangani et al. (2012), (**3**) Bai et al. (2015), (**4**) Bell et al. (2014), (**5**) Bemis et al. (2008), (**6**) Bhattacharya et al. (2013), (**7**) Boyle et al. (2011), (**8**) Braig et al. (2010), (**9**) Bu and Yang (2014), (**10**) Caramuta et al. (2010), (**11**) Chang et al. (2015), (**12**) Chen et al. (2013), (**13**) Chen et al. (2010), (**14**) Chen et al. (2011), (**15**) Ciuffreda et al. (2012), (**16**) Cohen et al. (2015), (**17**) Couts et al. (2013), (**18**) Dar et al. (2011), (**19**) Dar et al. (2013), (**20**) Das et al. (2010), (**21**) Deng et al. (2011), (**22**) Ding et al. (2015), (**23**) Dynoodt et al. (2013a), (**24**) Dynoodt et al. (2013b), (**25**) El Hajj et al. (2015), (**26**) Elson-Schwab et al. (2010), (**27**) Errico et al. (2013), (**28**) Felicetti et al. (2008a), (**29**) Felicetti et al. (2008b), (**30**) Felli et al. (2016), (**31**) Felli et al. (2013), (**32**) Forloni et al. (2014), (**33**) Fu et al. (2014), (**34**) Galore-Haskel et al. (2015), (**35**) Gaziel-Sovran et al. (2011), (**36**) Georgantas et al. (2013), (**37**) Giles et al. (2013), (**38**) Glud et al. (2010), (**39**) Golan et al. (2015), (**40**) Goswami et al. (2015), (**41**) Greenberg et al. (2014), (**42**) Greenberg et al. (2011), (**43**) Grignol et al. (2011), (**44**) Guo et al. (2014), (**45**) Haflidadottir et al. (2010), (**46**) Hao et al. (2015), (**47**) He et al. (2007), (**48**) Heinemann et al. (2012), (**49**) Holst et al. (2011), (**50**) Hwang et al. (2014), (**51**) Igoucheva and Alexeev (2009), (**52**) Jian et al. (2014), (**53**) Jiang et al. (2014), (**54**) Jiang et al. (2012), (**55**) Jin et al. (2011), (**56**) Kappelmann et al. (2013), (**57**) Karreth et al. (2011), (**58**) Kim et al. (2014a, b), (**59**) Kitago et al. (2009), (**60**) Knoll et al. (2014), (**61**) Kozubek et al. (2013), (**62**) Kwon et al. (2015), (**63**) Lankenau et al. (2014), (**64**) Levati et al. (2009), (**65**) Levati et al. (2011), (**66**) Levy et al. (2010a, b), (**67**) Li et al. (2014a, b), (**68**) Li (2016), (**69**) Li et al. (2014a, b), (**70**) Lin et al. (2015a), (**71**) Lin et al. (2015b), (**72**) Liu et al. (2015a, b), (**73**) Liu et al. (2015a, b), (**74**) Liu et al. (2013), (**75**) Liu et al. (2012a), (**76**) Liu et al. (2012b), (**77**) Liu et al. (2014), (**78**) Lodygin et al. (2008), (**79**) Lujambio et al. (2008), (**80**) Luo et al. (2013a), (**81**) Luo et al. (2013b), (**82**) Ma et al. (2009), (**83**) Margue et al. (2013), (**84**) Martin del Campo et al. (2015), (**85**) Mattia et al. (2011), (**86**) Mazar et al. (2010), (**87**) Mazar et al. (2011), (**88**) Mazar et al. (2016), (**89**) Migliore et al. (2008), (**90**) Mueller and Bosserhoff (2009), (**91**) Mueller and Bosserhoff (2011), (**92**) Mueller et al. (2009), (**93**) Muller and Bosserhoff (2008), (**94**) Nemlich et al. (2013), (**95**) Nguyen et al. (2011), (**96**) Noguchi et al. (2014a), (**97**) Noguchi et al. (2014b), (**98**) Noguchi et al. (2012a), (**99**) Noguchi et al. (2015), (**100**) Noguchi et al. (2012b), (**101**) Noman et al. (2012), (**102**) Nyholm et al. (2014), (**103**) Ohira et al. (2015), (**104**) Ozsolak et al. (2008), (**105**) Pencheva et al. (2012), (**106**) Penna et al. (2011), (**107**) Penna et al. (2013), (**108**) Philippidou et al. (2010), (**109**) Pinto et al. (2015), (**110**) Poliseno et al. (2012), (**111**) Prasad and Katiyar (2014), (**112**) Reuland et al. (2013), (**113**) Sakurai et al. (2011), (**114**) Saleiban et al. (2014), (**115**) Sand et al. (2012a, b), (**116**) Sand et al. (2013), (**117**) Satzger et al. (2010), (**118**) Satzger et al. (2012), (**119**) Schmitt et al. (2012), (**120**) Schultz et al. (2008), (**121**) Segura et al. (2010), (**122**) Segura et al. (2009), (**123**) Shoshan et al. (2015), (**124**) Stark et al. (2015a, b), (**125**) Streicher et al. (2012), (**126**) Strong et al. (2014), (**127**) Tian et al. (2015), (**128**) van Kempen et al. (2012), (**129**) Venza et al. (2015), (**130**) Vergani et al. (2016), (**131**) Wang et al. (2013a), (**132**) Wang et al. (2013b), (**133**) Wei et al. (2014), (**134**) Xu et al. (2012), (**135**) Yamazaki et al. (2012), (**136**) Yang et al. (2015), (**137**) Yang et al. (2011), (**138**) Zehavi et al. (2012), (**139**) Zehavi et al. (2015), (**140**) Zhang et al. (2014), (**141**) Zhang et al. (2015b), (**142**) Zhang et al. (2006), (**143**) Zhang et al. (2009), (**144**) Zhang et al. (2015c), (**145**) Zhao et al. (2015), (**146**) Zhou et al. (2015)

allele for melanoma susceptibility, previously determined to be located on chromosome 1p22 (Gillanders et al. 2003; Walker et al. 2004). It turned out that this genomic locus encodes a miRNA – miR-137 – capable of negatively regulating MITF expression (Bemis et al. 2008). Interestingly, the miR-137 primary transcript harbors a significantly higher number of a 15 bp VNTR (variable number of tandem repeats) in a subset of melanoma cell lines displaying high MITF expression than it does in melanoma cell lines displaying low levels of MITF. Those extra copies of the 15 bp VNTR alter the pri-miR-137 secondary structure in a way precluding its further processing into mature miR-137 (Bemis et al. 2008). Strikingly, the re-expression of functionally active miR-137 in those cell lines resulted in a decline of MITF levels.

As already suggested in the report cited above, it meanwhile turned out that several other miRNAs are involved in regulating MITF as well. Also based on a melanoma associated genomic aberration – amplification of chromosomal locus 7q31-34, which harbors the *c-MET* and *BRAF* oncogenes – Segura et al. (2009) detected enhanced expression of miR-182 in melanoma cell lines and tissue samples. MiR-182 levels increased with tumor progression and were additionally inversely correlated with the expression of MITF and FOXO3 (a transcription factor of the forkhead family). Both transcription factors were confirmed to be direct targets of miR-182. Furthermore, it was shown that for the expression of this miRNA the migration of melanoma cells in vitro as well as their metastatic potential in vivo, whereas silencing of miR-182 impedes melanoma cell invasion and triggers apoptosis (Segura et al. 2009). The stimulatory effect of miR-182 over-expression on melanoma cell migration was abolished by the concomitant over-expression of MITF or FOXO3, making those proteins the key mediators of miR-182's effects.

Interestingly, it has been reported that cancer cells can circumvent the miRNA-mediated regulation of oncogenes to which they are addicted, by expressing transcripts with shortened 3′UTRs (Mayr and Bartel 2009). Thereby, selective pressure favors cells that generate alternative transcripts of oncogenes missing the miRNA target sequence(s) in their 3′UTR. Prompted by those findings, Goswami et al. (2015) unraveled that a specific MITF isoform, harboring a shortened 3′UTR, is preferentially expressed by their set of melanoma cell lines in contrast to normal melanocytes. This alternative MITF transcript lacks the miR-137 and miR-182 binding sites but yet contains two target sequences for another miRNA, miR-340 (Goswami et al. 2015). The authors were able to show that miR-340 actually inhibits the expression of the alternative MITF transcript in their melanoma cells. Even more remarkable, a protein commonly over-expressed in melanoma termed CRD-BP (coding region determinant binding protein; Elcheva et al. 2008) is able to bind to the alternative MITF 3′UTR, thereby masking the miR-340 target sites and restoring MITF expression (Goswami et al. 2015). On a functional level, either the inhibition of miR-340 or the over-expression of CRD-BP resulted in a significantly enhanced ability of melanoma cells to form colonies in soft agar.

In addition to these findings, Haflidadottir et al. (2010) attempted to perform a comprehensive analysis on miRNA binding sites located in the MITF full length 3′UTR. Although not paying attention to a potential alternative 3′UTR shortening, they identified miR-148 and miR-101 as additional regulators of MITF expression in melanoma cell lines (Haflidadottir et al. 2010). In addition, miR-218, previously shown to be deregulated (Philippidou et al. 2010), miR-101, and miR-155 were revealed to directly modulate MITF expression (Guo et al. 2014; Luo et al. 2013a, b; Arts et al. 2015). Interestingly, miR-155, which is down-regulated in melanoma cells compared to melanocytes, is an example of a miRNA exerting a multilevel regulation over a signaling pathway, the WNT pathway, making it an attractive candidate as a therapeutic weapon. MiR-155 also interacts with the 3′UTR of the transcriptional regulator SKI, reducing its levels when exogenously expressed (Levati 2011). SKI is an important WNT/β-catenin inducer, leading to high MITF expression. Therefore, MITF should also be indirectly regulated by miRNAs that act upon WNT signaling, such as miR-155. Another indirect regulator of MITF is miR-203, which down-regulates MITF and its downstream effector Rab27a in melanoma cell lines by targeting its promoting transcription factor CREB1 (cAMP response element-binding protein 1) (Noguchi et al. 2014a, b).

MiRNAs can also mediate environmental effects via key transcription factors as MITF in melanocytes. Dynoodt et al. (2013a, b) observed a dramatic 15-fold decrease of miR-145 in UV-irradiated and forskolin treated mouse melanocytes. Over-expression or knockdown of this miRNA, respectively, decreased and increased the levels of MITF (among other proteins) and had a direct impact on the pigmentary process.

Taking all these findings into consideration, the question is how miRNA-mediated regulation impacts MITF expression in melanomagenesis. Reports on the role of MITF in formation and progression of malignant melanoma had initially been controversial. Nowadays, a model is proposed in which an intermediate level of MITF expression favors the proliferation and tumorigenic potential of melanoma cells, while a too high level results in cell cycle arrest and differentiation and a too low level results in cell cycle arrest and apoptosis (see Chaps. 4 and 5, and references therein). Although the expression of MITF has already been shown to be regulated through a plethora of mechanisms (including e.g., transcriptional control and post-translational modifications), miRNAs as well as 3′UTR binding proteins (acting as "target protectors") seem to represent an additional layer of complexity in adjusting MITF levels. Most likely, in melanoma cells the favored outcome "intermediate MITF level" can be achieved by the deregulation of every single wire (or a combination of several wires) in the MITF network. Hereby, the deregulation of miRNA-based mechanisms is one way to adjust MITF at the preferred level or to fine-tune it, respectively. This may also provide additional insights into melanoma's heterogeneity regarding MITF expression (reviewed by Bell and Levy 2011).

However, MITF is not only subject to regulation by miRNAs – vice versa, MITF regulates the expression of a subset of miRNAs in melanoma cell lines and may even influence global miRNA expression in cells of the melanocytic lineage. Ozsolak et al. (2008) identified the putative transcription start sites of as much as 175 miRNAs by combining nucleosome positioning patterns with chromatin immunoprecipitation (ChIP) screens for promoter signatures. This report significantly contributed to our current knowledge on the characteristics of miRNA promoters. Furthermore, the authors utilized the obtained data to identify a subset of 10 miRNAs and miRNA clusters, respectively, whose expression is MITF regulated by screening miRNA promoters for E-box elements (the binding sites for MITF in gene promoters; see Chap. 5). The cohort of miRNAs identified to be MITF transcriptional targets includes, e.g., miR-148b, miR-221/222, the miR-106a-363 cluster, miR-125, as well as several members of the let-7 family (Ozsolak et al. 2008). Interestingly, some of these miRNAs have already been proven to target genes playing a role in pigmentation and survival of melanocytes or to be involved in melanomagenesis. In melanocyte primary cultures, Wang et al. (2012) found 16 up-regulated and 6 down-regulated miRNAs through microarray profiling in MITF knocked-down (with siRNAs) melanocytes, compared to normal melanocytes. Using the TAM annotation method (Lu et al. 2010), they found that the miR-188 family was enriched, while the miR-221 family was depleted. Both groups of miRNAs were involved in cell-cycle, cell proliferation, and stem-cell regulation, and both groups were reported to be enriched in melanoma. Thus, the effects of MITF knockdown do not recapitulate the changes of microRNA expression reported in melanoma.

As miRNAs can be localized in introns of protein-coding genes, the expression of the protein and the miRNA are highly correlated. Noteworthy, intronic miR-211 was found responsible for the tumor suppressor effect attributed to its host gene, TRMP1 (Melastatin), upon MITF-promoted expression (Levy 2010; De Luca et al. 2015). MiR-211 contributes to melanoma cell adhesion by targeting NUAK1 (Bell et al. 2014), but as new targets for this miRNA emerge, its role in melanoma as a therapeutic target or as a biomarker has to be further characterized (Margue et al. 2013).

Additionally, Levy et al. (2010b) reported that MITF is able to transcriptionally regulate Dicer expression in melanocytes. Their study started with the observation that during melanocyte differentiation a population of miRNAs was up-regulated at the pre-miR level, whereas another population of miRNAs displayed stabile pre-miR but yet enhanced mature miRNA levels. Subsequently, it turned out that MITF is capable of inducing Dicer transcription by interacting with two E-box elements in the Dicer promoter, thus enforcing pre-miRNA processing (Levy et al. 2010a, b). Interestingly, melanocyte-specific knockout of Dicer in an in vivo mouse model resulted in a profound loss of both melanocyte stem cells and differentiated melanocytes. The authors assigned this impressive impact of Dicer on melanocyte survival to its ability to enhance the expression of miRNAs of the miR-17–92 cluster. Hereby, miR-17 targeting the pro-apoptotic Bim (Bcl-2 interacting mediator of cell death) protein may play a major role (Levy et al. 2010a, b) and further links the MITF-mediated regulation of Dicer to mechanisms involved in melanomagenesis.

Interestingly, further miRs regulating MITF were identified in the context of vitiligo and other pigmentation disorders. Here, miR-25 and miR-675 were proven to directly control MITF (Shi et al. 2016; Kim et al. 2014b).

These findings indicate that the melanocyte-specific transcription factor MITF might exert its powerful impact on pigmentation and lineage survival genes not only by direct transcriptional mechanisms but also that the effects of MITF are further enhanced by miRNAs as intermediates. Obviously, this will also enhance – or even potentiate – its oncogenic properties in melanoma formation and progression.

6.2.2 Oncogenic Role of miR-221/222 in Melanoma

Clustered on the X-chromosome, miR-221 and miR-222 are thought to be transcribed as a common precursor and to regulate overlapping or functionally related targets. Reports on an over-expression of these miRNAs in several types of tumors in which they regulate the expression of the c-KIT receptor tyrosine kinase (e.g., Felli et al. 2005; He et al. 2005; le Sage et al. 2007) led Felicetti et al. (2008b) to investigate a potential involvement of miR-221/222 in melanomagenesis (for further information on c-KIT in melanoma please refer to Chap. 7). They unraveled that loss of the tumor suppressive protein PLZF (promyelocytic leukemia zinc finger) leads to a stepwise up-regulation of miR-221/222 during melanoma progression (Felicetti et al. 2008a, b). These two miRNAs in turn are able to induce two distinct but functionally convergent oncogenic pathways by repressing c-KIT as well as $p27^{Kip1}$ (CDKN1B). In accordance, the over-expression of miR-221/222 in a moderately aggressive melanoma cell line resulted in an enhancement of proliferation rate, migratory and invasive potential, as well as anchorage-independent growth, paralleled by a significantly increased in vivo tumorigenicity (Felicetti et al. 2008a, b). Vice versa, the treatment of highly aggressive metastatic melanoma cells with inhibitory molecules (antagomiRs) against miR-221/222 not only caused obverse effects in vitro but – most strikingly – effectively inhibited in vivo tumor growth after bolus intratumor injection.

Expanding those findings, Igoucheva and Alexeev (2009) implicated that loss of c-KIT receptor expression in melanoma might be completely depending on miR-221/222 over-expression instead of being related to the down-regulation of the transcription factor AP-2 (see Chap. 5) as previously reported. This conclusion was drawn as there was no correlation detectable between AP-2 and c-KIT expression levels in their set of 27 melanoma cell lines but a strong inverse correlation of c-KIT and miR-221 expression levels was observed (Igoucheva and Alexeev 2009).

Including data generated in other tumor types, Howell et al. (2010) constructed an interesting network focusing on miR-221/222's regulatory effects in melanoma. It has been demonstrated that miR-221/222 regulate the expression of PTEN in aggressive non-small lung cancer and hepatocarcinoma cells (Garofalo et al. 2009). In the light of an increasingly important role of the AKT/PI3K pathway in melanomagenesis as well as a confusingly low rate of PTEN mutations detected in melanoma tissue samples (see Chap. 7), studies investigating a miRNA-mediated regulation of PTEN seem to be a promising option.

Additionally, Das et al. (2010) reported the existence of a $3' \rightarrow 5'$ exonuclease, human polynucleotide phosphorylase ($hPNPase^{old\text{-}35}$), specifically degrading mature miR-221 in melanoma cells. In response to the over-expression of $hPNPase^{old\text{-}35}$, the cellular miR-221 level decreased and its repressive impact on $p27^{Kip1}$ expression was abolished (Das et al. 2010). As $hPNPase^{old\text{-}35}$ is a type I interferon (IFN) inducible protein, the authors were able to unravel a pathway in which IFN-β-mediated growth arrest is based on induction of $hPNPase^{old\text{-}35}$, which subsequently degrades miR-221 and therefore triggers the up-regulation of $p27^{Kip1}$. Of note, $hPNPase^{old\text{-}35}$ had previously been shown to degrade c-Myc mRNA, thereby causing G_1 cell cycle arrest by $p27^{Kip1}$ activation involving another pathway (Sarkar et al. 2003, 2006).

Nevertheless, the over-expression of miR-221 in melanoma cells was sufficient to render them resistant against IFN-β-mediated growth arrest (Das et al. 2010).

In conclusion, miR-221/222 have already been established to be potent oncogenic miRNAs in melanoma. This is further supported by newer findings even suggesting miR-221/222 as potent tumor markers for melanoma (Inada et al. 2015; Felli et al. 2016). Several mechanisms are involved in regulating their expression, including transcriptional control by PLZF (Felicetti et al. 2008a, b) and MITF (Ozsolak et al. 2008), as well as positive and negative feedback loops involving their target genes (reviewed by Howell et al. 2010) and specific exonucleolytic degradation by hPNPase$^{old\text{-}35}$ (Das et al. 2010). Although the up-regulation of miR-221/222 may not be the sole cause for loss of c-KIT in melanoma cells, miRNA-mediated c-KIT repression could serve as an additional mechanism to escape c-KIT dependent apoptosis in a subset of melanomas harboring activating mutations in BRAF (Igoucheva and Alexeev 2009). Further, miR-221/222 over-expression may be responsible for resistance against IFN-β treatment (Becker et al. 2002) in at least some melanomas (Das et al. 2010).

6.2.3 Tumor-Suppressive Role of let-7 miRNA Family Members in Melanoma

One of the major breakthroughs regarding miRNAs in biomedical research took place in 2005 when Frank Slacks' group reported a causal link between the down-regulation of miRNA let-7 and the formation of lung cancer (Johnson et al. 2005). Thereby, the tumor-suppressive effect of let-7 miRNA family members in lung carcinomas is based on their potential to regulate the expression of the RAS oncogene. Strikingly, it meanwhile turned out that loss of the expression of at least some let-7 family members seems to be a common event in the progression of several types of human cancers (reviewed by Boyerinas et al. 2010–and that this is true for melanoma as well).

Performing an expression pattern analysis on 157 different miRNAs in laser-microdissected tissues comprising ten benign melanocytic nevi and ten primary melanomas, Schultz et al. (2008) found five members of the let-7 family (let-7a, let-7b, let-7d, let-7e, and let-7g) to be strongly down-regulated in the melanoma samples. Focusing only on let-7b in their subsequent experiments, they showed that introducing artificial let-7b molecules into melanoma cells decreased levels of a set of cell cycle regulators, in detail cyclins D1, D3, and A as well as cyclin-dependent kinase (CDK) 4 (Schultz et al. 2008). While the authors were able to give some evidence for a direct interaction of let-7b with the cyclin D1 3′UTR, they also point out that at least a few of the remaining let-7b effects described might be rather indirect. Nevertheless, the transfection of melanoma cell lines with artificial let-7b resulted in a reduced number of proliferating cells (less cells were detected to be in S-phase, accompanied with an increased number of cells in G_1) as well as a strong reduction of the cells' potential to form colonies in soft agar (Schultz et al. 2008).

Almost synchronously, Mueller and Bosserhoff (2008) reported loss of expression of a second member of the let-7 miRNA family – let-7a – to have a potent impact on the invasive potential of melanoma cells. Analyzing the regulation of integrin beta3 expression in detail, they found that (in contrast to other cell types) promoter-dependent mechanisms are only subsidiary in melanoma cells whereas the cellular let-7a level is the main determinant of integrin beta3 protein production (Muller and Bosserhoff 2008). Strikingly, the introduction of artificial let-7a molecules into a highly aggressive melanoma cell line lacking endogenous let-7a expression resulted in an about 75 % reduced invasive potential in vitro. Vice versa, blocking endogenous let-7a in otherwise normal melanocytes using anti-miRs was sufficient to induce migratory behavior in this cell-type (Muller and Bosserhoff 2008). The authors attributed these effects mainly to let-7a's impact on integrin beta3, as the up-regulation of the classical vitronectin receptor alphaVbeta3 has repeatedly been shown to be correlated with malignant potential and aggressive tumor growth in melanoma (Albelda et al. 1990; Danen et al. 1994, 1995; Van Belle et al. 1999). However, like presumably every miRNA known, let-7a targets a cohort of additional transcripts and this fact might strengthen or even potentiate its role in melanoma progression. Mueller and Bosserhoff (2008) highlight the suppression of N-Ras by let-7a, which they used to monitor the efficiency of let-7a transfection in their experiments. Although the significance of additional Ras knockdown is uncertain against the background of activating BRAF mutations, it might prove particularly effective in a subset of melanomas harboring activating mutations in N-Ras (see Chaps. 7 and 12).

Importantly, new sequencing studies helped to clearly differentiate the subforms of let-7 and revealed the regulation of all of these in melanoma (Kozubek et al. 2013; Qi et al. 2014).

Corroborating findings in other tumor types, members of the let-7 family of miRNAs take on a role as potent tumor suppressors in malignant melanoma as well. The complete set of let-7 target genes still remains to be established to identify the most important mediators of let-7's effects. Nevertheless, already at this point, the most intriguing fact about let-7 is its ability to interfere with constituents of several distinct pathways involved in malignant transformation of cells in general and in melanomagenesis in special.

6.2.4 Tumor-Suppressive Role of miR-196a in Melanoma

Another miRNA confirmed to act as a tumor suppressor in malignant melanoma cells is miR-196a. Thereby, it currently seems that this miRNA exerts much of its function by regulating the expression of at least two class I homeodomain containing transcription factors, HOX-B7 and HOX-C8 (Braig et al. 2010; Mueller and Bosserhoff 2010a).

The expression of miR-196a has been shown to be strongly reduced in melanoma cell lines as well as in a small set of tissue samples derived from primary cutaneous melanomas and melanoma metastases, respectively (Braig et al. 2010; Mueller and Bosserhoff 2010a). In line with general reports characterizing miR-196a as a potent regulator of HOX gene expression (e.g., Yekta et al. 2004), reduced miR-196a levels inversely correlate with strongly enhanced the expression of the HOX transcription factors HOX-B7 and HOX-C8 in melanoma cells (Braig et al. 2010; Mueller and Bosserhoff 2010a). 3′UTR reporter assays confirmed that miR-196a is actually capable to directly interact with the HOX-B7 (Braig et al. 2010) and HOX-C8 (Mueller and Bosserhoff 2010a) transcripts, thereby preventing their translation into protein.

Due to these efforts, Braig et al. (2010) were able to link loss of miR-196a to the over-expression of BMP4 (bone morphogenetic protein 4), an event strongly enhancing the migratory potential of melanoma cells (Hsu et al. 2005; Rothhammer et al. 2005, 2008). In their model proposed, diminished levels of miR-196a cause induction of the transcription factor HOX-B7, which in turn activates bFGF (basic fibroblast growth factor) production. In the end, this results in an enforced expression of BMP4, most likely mediated by transcription factors of the Ets family (Braig et al. 2010). Additionally, Mueller and Bosserhoff (2010a) demonstrated that miR-196a indirectly modulates the expression of several genes potentially involved in melanoma progression by regulating HOX-C8 levels. Many of the HOX-C8 target genes described in literature are related to oncogenic processes like cell adhesion, cytoskeleton remodeling, tumor formation, and invasive behavior of tumor cells (Lei et al. 2005, 2006). The authors demonstrated that at least three of them – *cadherin-11*, *calponin-1*, and *osteopontin* – appear to be deregulated in melanoma cells partially due to the over-expression of HOX-C8 (Mueller and Bosserhoff 2010a).

In the course of the studies cited, melanoma cell clones were generated, which stably re-express miR-196a at a level almost equal to that detected in normal melanocytes (Braig et al. 2010; Mueller and Bosserhoff 2010a). Remarkably, those cells were characterized by an about 50 % and 40 % reduction in their migratory (Braig et al. 2010) and invasive potential, respectively, as well as by diminished tumorigenicity after subcutaneous injection into nude mice as shown in a preliminary experimental setup (Mueller and Bosserhoff 2010a). Vice versa, the treatment of otherwise normal melanocytes with anti-miRs against miR-196a was sufficient to induce migratory behavior in this cell type (Braig et al. 2010).

As true for miR-221/222 and let-7, there is a need to extend the set of known, melanoma-relevant miR-196a target genes to eventually draw a complete picture of the molecules mediating this miRNAs' effects on melanomagenesis. This could be of importance as newer studies suggest a link of an SNP in miR196a to levels of intracellular reactive oxygen species and sensitivity to apoptotic signals (Huang et al. 2013). It also seems like the deregulation of HOX protein levels might well be worth a detailed examination as several studies clearly defined a link between aberrant *HOX* gene expression and cancer development (reviewed by Piérard and Piérard-Franchimont 2012; Shah and Sukumar 2010). Interestingly, a report highlighting miR-196 family members as metastasis suppressors in breast cancer (Li et al. 2010) additionally strengthens the tumor-suppressive role of miR-196a in malignant melanoma. By contrast, detection of increased miR-196a levels in other types of tumors when compared to their healthy biological correlates (e.g., Bloomston et al. 2007; Luthra et al. 2008; Maru et al. 2009; Schimanski et al. 2009) clearly point toward a tissue-specific role of this miRNA. Considering its targets, the *HOX* genes, as "tumor modulators" harboring the potential to act as both oncogenes and tumor suppressor genes depending on the respective tissue context (Abate-Shen 2002), seem to be rather plausible but add a further level of complexity to this area of research.

6.2.5 Tumor-Suppressive Role of the miR-34 Family in Melanoma

Recently, several reports conclusively demonstrated that the p53 tumor suppressor protein directly induces the expression of miR-34 miRNA family members and probably exerts a significant portion of its expansive impact on cell-cycle control and regulation of apoptosis through these mediators (reviewed by Hermeking 2010). Accordingly, the ectopic expression of miR-34 genes has profound effects on cell proliferation and survival causing cell-cycle arrest in G1 phase, inhibiting colony formation in soft agar, as well as inducing cellular senescence and apoptosis, respectively (Bommer et al. 2007; Chang et al. 2007; Corney et al. 2007; He et al. 2007; Raver-Shapira et al. 2007; Tarasov et al. 2007; Welch et al. 2007). Therefore, genes involved in cell-cycle regulation and apoptosis control are significantly enriched in the large set of confirmed miR-34 targets comprising *Bcl-2*, *CCND1*, *CCNE2*, *CDK2*, *CDK4*, *CREB*, *MET*, *MYC*, *SIRT1*, and many more (for a comprehensive list, see Hermeking 2010). Some of the studies defining this potent onco-suppressive role of miR-34 members in various tumor entities also include data regarding melanoma (Lodygin et al. 2008; Lujambio et al. 2008; Migliore et al. 2008). Newer data revealed miR-34a/c to regulate the NK2D ligand ULBP2 and thereby modulate tumor cell recognition by NK cells (Heinemann et al. 2012). The following paragraph aims to summarize these findings and recombine them with results generated in other cancer types to present a perspective on the possibly far-reaching but yet underestimated influence of miR-34 on melanomagenesis.

In humans, the miRNAs of the miR-34 family are encoded by two different loci with one locus encoding miR-34a and the other locus encoding a common precursor for miR-34b/c. The high similarity shared by all three mature miR-34 forms generates points to an overlapping although not completely identical repertoire of target transcripts. Lodygin et al. (2008) demonstrated that the expression of miR-34a is commonly silenced in a variety of tumors as a consequence of promoter hypermethylation. This is also true for melanoma cells as 19 of 44 (43.2 %) investigated melanoma cell lines as well as 20 of 32 (62.5 %) primary melanomas investigated displayed hypermethylation of the miR-34a promoter resulting in loss of miR-34a pri-miRNA expression (Lodygin et al. 2008). CpG methylation presumably occurs at a region 100–500 bp upstream of the miR-34a transcription start site which also includes the p53 binding site. By contrast, normal melanocytes derived from two different donors did not display miR-34a promoter methylation, implicating that this mechanism represents a tumor-specific event. Interestingly, miR-34a is encoded at chromosome 1p36 – a chromosomal locus repeatedly described to harbor a gene for melanoma susceptibility, which surprisingly has not been identified to date (e.g.,

Ng et al. 2008; Poetsch et al. 2003). LOH for 1p36 had been detected in 77% of nodular melanomas, 86 % of metastatic melanomas, but only 20% of superficially spreading melanomas (Poetsch et al. 2003). Additionally, in neuroblastoma, a correlation between 1p36 loss and miR-34a down-regulation had been confirmed (Wei et al. 2008). It is therefore tempting to speculate, that in melanoma cells either loss of 1p36, hypermethylation of the miR-34a promoter or a combination of both mechanisms may result in loss of miR-34a and its tumor-suppressive function.

CpG island methylation had also been found to be the cause for silencing of miR-34b/c in melanoma and several other types of cancer (Kozaki et al. 2008; Lujambio et al. 2008; Toyota et al. 2008). Thereby, the study of Lujambio et al. (2008) strikingly unraveled a highly significant correlation between miR-34b/c promoter hypermethylation and the presence of lymph node metastases in a panel of melanoma tissue samples. A report published by Migliore et al. (2008) implicates that this might be due to the release of c-MET expression from miR-34b/c-mediated repression. Performing a bioinformatical search for miRNAs targeting c-MET they found miR-34b/c as well as miR-199* to be able to suppress c-MET production and therefore the ability of cancer cells to respond to HGF (hepatocyte growth factor) stimulation – even if they harbored c-MET gene amplification or over-expression resulting in high levels of constitutively active receptor (Migliore et al. 2008). In their study, melanoma-derived primary cells expressed only limited amounts of miR-34c (and therefore possibly also of miR-34b). The transfection of synthetic miR-34b/c molecules into these cells led to the down-regulation of c-MET expression as well as to impairment of c-MET-mediated motility in vitro (Migliore et al. 2008). The MET oncogene encodes a tyrosine kinase receptor which upon activation by binding its ligand HGF (also called scatter factor) activates a complex biological program which in the end results in invasive growth and metastatic dissemination of tumor cells (Birchmeier et al. 2003). In melanoma, the over-expression of c-MET has repeatedly been reported and its transcriptional activation had been linked to increased levels of SOX10, PAX3, and MITF whereas loss of Plexin B1 prevents suppression of c-MET activation by absent receptor–receptor interactions (e.g., Cruz et al. 2003; Kiriakidou et al. 2004; Mascarenhas et al. 2010; Puri et al. 2007). It is known from other tumor types that c-MET expression can also be induced during hypoxia (through binding of HIF-1α to the MET promoter; Pennacchietti et al. 2003) or activation of several oncogenes including *Ets* family members (Gambarotta et al. 1996; Ivan et al. 1997; Webb et al. 1998). While HGF is a paracrine mitogen for normal melanocytes, most melanoma cells gain the potential to produce HGF themselves thereby establishing sustained autocrine stimulation of the receptor (Li et al. 2001). Notably, correlations between c-MET expression and the metastatic potential of melanoma cells as well as patient survival have been described (Barnhill and Mihm 1993; Natali et al. 1993; Slominski et al. 2001).

These findings implicate that the loss of expression of miR-34 family members – potentially caused by multiple mechanisms (including aberrant methylation and chromosomal aberrations) – might be a central event in the progression of primary melanomas on to invasive and metastatic disease. They may additionally shed new light on the controversially disputed role of p53 in melanomagenesis. Whereas silencing of p53 is acknowledged to be one of the most influential events in the formation of virtually all tumor types, its role in melanoma has been neglected due to a low frequency of missense mutations detected (0–10 %; reviewed by Box and Terzian 2008). However, as indicated by several studies performed in animal models, the impact of p53 on melanomagenesis should be revisited; e.g., Terzian et al. (2010) recently demonstrated that high levels of p53 prevent the conversion of nevi into malignant and metastatic melanomas. Some of the conflicting effects observed might be explained by alterations in the expression of miR-34 family members impairing p53's ability to maintain its tumor suppressive function in advanced melanomas. That is, their rapidly growing *TP-ras0/+* tumors (Terzian et al. 2010) might overcome the tumor-suppressive effect of high-level stabilized wild-type p53 by losing miR-34 expression. In summary, these observations might also harbor some exciting insights into a key aspect contributing to the pronounced chemotherapy resistance of melanoma (Soengas and Lowe 2003) as loss of miR-34 expression had been linked to resistance against apoptosis induced by p53 activating agents (Zenz et al. 2009; Yamasaki et al. 2012).

6.2.6 Other miRNAs with a Functional Impact on Melanomagenesis

6.2.6.1 MiR-193b

Profiling the expression of 470 miRNAs in a set of formalin-fixed paraffin-embedded (FFPE) specimens derived from eight benign nevi and eight metastatic melanomas, Chen et al. (2010) detected 31 miRNAs to be differentially expressed in the melanoma samples (13 up-regulated, 18 down-regulated miRNAs). The authors selected the miRNA most strongly down-regulated, miR-193b, for a more detailed functional analysis. The introduction of artificial miR-193b molecules into three different melanoma cell lines resulted in a reduction of their proliferative capacity of between 30 and 60 % marked by an increased number of cells in G1 phase whereas the fractions of cells detected to be in S phase or G2 phase decreased (Chen et al. 2010). Combining whole genome cDNA microarray profiling and bioinformatic miRNA target prediction the authors identified cyclin D1 (CCND1) as a potential target for miR-193b. Subsequent 3′UTR reporter assays confirmed miR-193b to be a further miRNA targeting CCND1 in melanoma – in addition to let-7b (see above). The same group followed up the finding on the deregulation of miR-193b and revealed Stathmin1, a regulator of microtubule dynamics, and MCL1 (myeloid cell leukemia sequence 1) to be a direct target (Chen et al. 2013).

6.2.6.2 miR-532-5p

Members of the Runt-related (RUNX) family of transcription factors function as scaffolds interacting with co-regulatory factors often involved in tissue differentiation (Javed et al. 2005). Driven by findings on a tumor-suppressive role of RUNX3 in several types of tumors, Kitago et al. (2009) detected a significant down-regulation of this transcription factor on mRNA level in their set of 82 primary melanomas and 41 melanoma metastases as compared to 12 normal skin samples. Thereby, RUNX3 down-regulation displayed a nonlinear association with AJCC stage of the tumors with AJCC stage IV classified metastatic melanomas showing an even stronger reduction of RUNX3 expression compared to primary tumors. Interestingly, multivariate analysis revealed that the down-regulation of RUNX3 mRNA was related to disease outcome in those patients (Kitago et al. 2009). In contrast to tumors derived from other tissues (Ito 2004), loss of RUNX3 expression was not due to promoter hypermethylation in the melanoma samples but seems to be associated with increased expression of miR-532-5p. Kitago et al. (2009) detected this miRNA to be significantly over-expressed in their metastatic cell lines compared to melanocytes as well as in the metastatic melanoma samples compared to primary tumors pointing toward an enforced expression of miR-532-5p as progression to metastatic disease occurs. While the transfection of anti-miRs against miR-532-5p into a metastatic melanoma cell line resulted in the increased expression of RUNX3 on mRNA and protein level, a direct interaction of the miRNA with a target site in the RUNX3 3′UTR has not yet been confirmed. Another interesting fact is that miR-532-5p is actually encoded at Xp11.23 which is located next to Xp11.3 – the genomic locus encoding miR-221/222 (see above).

6.2.6.3 miR-155

Levati et al. (2009) analyzed several miRNAs known to be involved in oncogenic processes for their expression in a panel of melanoma cell lines. In the majority of cell lines used, they detected an enhanced expression of miRNAs belonging to the miR-17-92 cluster – miR-17-5p, miR-18a, miR-20a, and miR-92a – as well as a diminished expression of miR-146a, miR-146b, and miR-155 compared to normal melanocytes (Levati et al. 2009). As miR-155 down-regulation was most prominent, the authors decided to examine this miRNA's impact on melanoma cell function. The transfection of artificial miR-155 molecules into melanoma cells inhibited proliferation by between 30 and 98 % in 12 out of 13 cell lines tested. Subsequent experiments performed in four of the cell lines implicated that this impairment of melanoma cell proliferation was at least partly based on induction of apoptosis in miR-155 transfected cells, further they revealed the regulation of the transcriptional repressor SKI (Levati et al. 2009; Levati et al. 2011). Reports on other types of tumors point towards a tissue-specific function of miR-155 ascribing the latter oncogenic as well as a tumor-suppressive potential depending on cellular context (e.g., Gartel and Kandel 2008; Volinia et al. 2006). The functional impact of miR-155 down-regulation on melanomagenesis remains to be defined as it appears to be only weakly expressed already in normal melanocytes. MiR-155 was recently shown to regulate MITF (Arts et al. 2015; see Sect. 6.2.1) and TYRP1 (El Hajj et al. 2015) shedding some light on its potential function. In addition, miR-155 was associated with patient outcome and might therefore be of prognostic potential (Jayawardana et al. 2015).

6.2.6.4 miR-210

Zhang and co-workers reported a correlation between elevated pri-miR-210 levels in melanoma tissues and shorter metastasis-free survival of the patients in Kaplan–Meier analysis (Zhang et al. 2009). MiR-210 is the miRNA species most prominently induced during hypoxia (reviewed by Huang et al. 2010). In their study, Zhang et al. (2009) demonstrated that the over-expression of this miRNA overrides hypoxia-induced cell-cycle arrest by indirectly activating the cell cycle and metabolic regulator MYC via repression of its antagonist MNT in several tumor cell lines. It was therefore hypothesized that miR-210 is involved in the regulation of mitochondrial biogenesis and central carbon metabolism to adapt tumor cells to hypoxic episodes and to further provide them a competitive advantage in developing tumors once normal oxygen levels are restored (Morrish 2009). Hypoxia and HIF signaling have also been shown to be implicated in melanomagenesis and melanoma metastasis (reviewed by Bedogni and Powell 2009), especially as a potential constitutive HIF-1 activity has been described for melanoma (Kuphal et al. 2010). Unfortunately, besides the Kaplan–Meier analysis cited above, no data regarding melanoma cells is provided by Zhang and colleagues which performed all their experiments in cell lines derived from other tumor types. However, Satzger et al. (2010) detected significantly enhanced the expression of miR-210 in 16 primary melanoma samples as compared to 11 melanocytic nevi investigated. miR-210 expression did not correlate with recurrence-free survival or overall survival in an extended set of 112 primary tumors (Satzger et al. 2010). Additionally, considering a currently disputed bipolar effect of hypoxia and miR-210 on tumorigenesis and a modulation of tumor cell susceptibility to lysis by antigen-specific cytotoxic T cells (Huang et al. 2009; Noman et al. 2012), a lot more research will be necessary to define the specific impact of miR-210 on the progression of this disease. Recently, miR-210 was clearly associated with early recurrence and may be useful as a diagnostic marker (Ono et al. 2015).

6.2.6.5 miR-125b

Several studies revealed a strong downregulation of miR-125b expression in melanoma (Glud et al. 2010). Based on these studies, multiple effects on melanoma cells have been shown, for example, Kappelmann et al. (2013) described a regulation of c-Jun by miR-125b. Here, the regulative effect can only be found on protein level hinting at a post-transcriptional regulation by modulation translation of c-Jun. Further, Mixed linked kinase 3 (MLK3) was proven to be regulated by miR-125b and thereby induced in melanoma, supporting cell growth and invasion (Zhang et al. 2014). Nyholm et al. (2014) could implicate miR-125b in the induction of senescence, thereby further confirming that the lack of miR-125b in melanoma is implicated in tumor development.

6.2.6.6 miR-21

A recent review by Melnik (2015) summarized the importance of miR-21 in melanoma. In contrast to most described and previously analyzed miRs, miR-21 is upregulated in melanoma and associated with progression (Grignol et al. 2011; Satzger et al. 2012). A functionally regulation of melanoma cell apoptosis but also a probably even more important regulating of invasive processes were demonstrated (Satzger et al. 2012; Yang et al. 2015; Martin del Campo et al. 2015). Here, FBXO11 and TIMP3 were shown to be direct targets of miR-21. Interestingly, NRAS and BRAF mutations are associated with miR-21 induction (Melnik 2015).

6.2.6.7 Additional Deregulated miRNAs

In Table 6.1, all miRNAs are listed, where deregulation was confirmed by more than one group and target genes have been identified. Additionally, miR-101, miR-106a, miR-106b, miR-107, miR-130a, miR-135b, miR-142, miR-149*, miR-150, miR-15b, miR-17, miR-18a, miR-1826, miR-185, miR-19a, miR-19b, miR-195, miR-199a, miR-1908, miR-20a, miR-21, miR-210, miR-212, miR-224, miR-25, miR-29a, miR-301a, miR-3151, miR-335, miR-340, miR-373, miR-378, miR-432, miR-509-3p, miR-514a, miR-532-5p, miR-638, miR-93 were described as upregulated and miR-10b, miR-125a, miR-125b, miR-126*, miR-127-3p, miR-130a-3p, miR-130b-3p, miR-134, miR-137, miR-141, miR-143, miR-144-3p, miR-145, miR-149, miR-183, miR-184, miR-191, miR-192, miR-193a, miR-193b, miR-194, miR-196a, miR-200b, miR-203, miR-204, miR-205, miR-218, miR-23b, miR-23b-3p, miR-26a, miR-27b, miR-29c, miR-30b, miR-30a-3p, miR-31, miR-33a, miR-34b, miR-34c, miR-376a/c, miR-429, miR-451a, miR-455-3p, miR-455, miR-524, miR-573, miR-663, miR-7, miR-768-3p, miR-98, miR-99a, let-7a, let-7b, and let-7e were downregulated in melanoma (see also Fig. 6.2).

6.3 Lessons to Learn from miRNA Expression Profiling in Malignant Melanoma

In addition to analyses focusing upon the functional impact of single miRNA species on melanoma progression, several studies performing global miRNA expression profiling or determining expression patterns of miRNA subsets in melanoma cell lines and tissue samples have been conducted. In the beginning, this topic was only addressed as a part of large scale profiling studies in which few melanoma samples had been included (Blower et al. 2007; Gaur et al. 2007; Lu et al. 2005; Zhang et al. 2006; reviewed by Mueller and Bosserhoff 2009). Therefore, it had been difficult to deduce information on alterations in the miRNA profile of melanoma cells clearly distinguishing them from normal melanocytes with only these data published.

From 2008 on, research specifically aimed to identify differences in the miRNA expression patterns of normal melanocytes, nevi, and melanoma cells. The objective was to either identify single deregulated miRNAs as targets for in-depth functional characterization (Chen et al. 2010; Molnar et al. 2008; Mueller et al. 2009; Philippidou et al. 2010; Schultz et al. 2008) or to identify potential melanoma biomarkers (Caramuta et al. 2010; Glud et al. 2009; Jukic et al. 2010; Leidinger et al. 2010; Liu et al. 2009; Ma et al. 2009; Segura et al. 2010). Further, some groups analyzed limited sets of miRNAs already known to be involved in tumorigenic mechanisms to confirm their deregulated expression in melanoma as well (Levati et al. 2009; Satzger et al. 2010). Another experimental approach utilized next generation sequencing to potentially identify the complete miRNAome of the melanocytic lineage (Stark et al. 2010; discussed in detail in Mueller and Bosserhoff 2010b). The data obtained during these studies can be exploited in different ways. On the one hand, the deregulated expression of miRNAs that had already been functionally characterized in melanoma before can be confirmed in larger sets of cell lines or tissue samples, as well as new candidates for functional analysis can be identified depending on the degree of deregulation detected. On the other hand, miRNA classifiers suited for diagnostic and/or prognostic purposes could be created–based less presumably on a single miRNA but rather on a larger set of miRNAs. Ding et al. (2015) focused on 21 miRNAs that were up-regulated and 42 that were down-regulated in a metastatic as well as in a nonmetastatic melanoma cell line compared to a melanocyte cell line. These included miR-148-3p, miR-129-5p, miR-34-5p, miR-363-3p, and miR-374b-5p, and the networks constructed for their putative target genes were related with cell morphology, cell development, and DNA replication. They also discovered a novel miRNA to be annotated (Ding 2015). Nevertheless, Kozubek et al. (2013) observed a consistent lower expression of miR-203, miR-204-5p, miR-205-5p, miR-211-5p, miR-23b-3p, miR-26a-5p, and miR-26b-5p in human melanoma biopsies compared to nevi. Furthermore, miR-211-5p expression levels could accurately distinguish invasive melanoma, in situ melanoma, and dysplastic nevi from common nevi in a discovery cohort using Next Generation Sequencing, (NGS) and in an independent validation cohort using qRT-PCR. Importantly, this signature differed significantly from the one discriminating between melanoma cell lines and melanocytes (Kozubek 2013), stressing the importance and feasibility of this approach with archived FFPE specimens matched to invaluable clinical information. The Cancer Genome Atlas (TCGA, http://cancergenome.nih.gov/) has recently released data on microRNA expression in melanoma, which, together with the genomic alterations through DNA, RNA, and protein-based analysis of 333 primary and/or metastatic melanomas, has allowed classification of cutaneous melanomas into four categories (TCGA network 2015).

6.3.1 Confirmation of Deregulated Expression of Single miRNAs and Identification of New miRNA Candidates for Functional Characterization

The mis-expression of many of the miRNAs discussed in Sect. 6.2 was confirmed in independent sample sets during profiling studies highlighting their importance in melanoma progression (data included in Table 6.1). For example, down-modulation of let-7a in melanoma tissues has repeatedly been detected. In summary, those findings point to a model in which normal skin melanocytes as well as benign nevi show the high expression of let-7a which then successively gets diminished during melanoma progression with melanoma metastases displaying the lowest let-7a levels (Chen et al. 2010; Glud et al. 2009; Ma et al. 2009; Philippidou et al. 2010). Further, a reduced expression of let-7b (Chen et al. 2010) and miR-196a (Caramuta et al. 2010; Philippidou et al. 2010) as well as an enhanced expression of miR-221/222 (Mueller et al. 2009; Philippidou et al. 2010) has concurrently been observed in different sets of melanoma cell lines and tissue samples. These are examples of positive correlations, indicating that miRNA profiling studies can clearly be utilized to support and strengthen findings obtained during functional studies, which are usually performed in vitro in rather small sets of cell lines. However, microarray data should be taken into account with care unless validated by qRT-PCR or Northern blotting.

Although consistent results have been obtained in regard to specific and prominent aberrations in miRNA expression, there are also some discrepancies, and the overall correlation between independent miRNA profiling studies in melanoma is rather poor. For instance, Caramuta et al. (2010) reported let-7b to be up-regulated in their melanoma specimens and Satzger et al. (2010) did not find miR-222 significantly up-regulated in their set of tissue samples. Further, Caramuta et al. (2010) detected reduced levels of miR-15b in melanoma cells – in sharp contrast to Satzger and co-workers (2010) who detected miR-15b to be strongly up-regulated (see below). Adding to the confusion, a highly pronounced variation was observed in the expression levels of single miRNAs between melanoma cell lines and tissue samples, respectively (Caramuta et al. 2010; Philippidou et al. 2010; Satzger et al. 2010). As an example, Segura et al. (2010) found the expression of miR-155 rather up-regulated in melanoma lesions compared to benign nevi, which is in stark contrast to the functional report published by Levati et al. (2009) (see above). This caveat might be resolved by the findings from Philippidou et al. (2010) who detected miR-155 to be down-regulated in melanoma cell lines compared to normal melanocytes, but up-regulated when comparing melanoma tissue samples to benign nevi.

This, among other things, indicates that the interpretation of data obtained during miRNA profiling studies is heavily depending on the type of sample used as baseline control. As isolated melanocytes show, a high degree of variation in their miRNA expression profiles dependent not only on donor source but also on passage number (as already known from their cDNA and protein profiles), each study should include an extended set of melanocytes derived from different donors and intervals of propagation in cell culture should be adequately limited. Interestingly, the miRNA profiles generated from tissue samples seem between independent studies than do expression profiles generated from cell lines (e.g., Philippidou et al. 2010, compared to Glud et al. 2009). However, when analyzing tissue specimens most commonly benign nevi are used as baseline control and therefore serve as biological correlate for melanoma cells. Undoubtedly, nevi cells cannot be considered equivalent to normal skin melanocytes as they already harbor potentially malignant genetic alterations rendering them abnormal by definition (for a detailed discussion, see Mueller and Bosserhoff 2010b). Additionally, tissue samples are prone to contamination by nonmelanocytic cells derived from the surrounding tumor stroma. Therefore, microdissection should be established a standard in sample preparation in order to obtain reliable results.

Of note, not only the baseline control will influence interpretation of miRNA profiling data but so will data processing. Although challenging, a consensus must be aspired on normalization of miRNA microarray data as well as on a common stable reference gene for qRT-PCR based miRNA profiling methods (reviewed by Meyer et al. 2010). Moreover, as NGS setups find their way into everyday laboratory use (see also Stark et al. 2010, and related discussion by Mueller and Bosserhoff 2010b) the general debate on the best method for miRNA expression profiling is fueled further (reviewed by Git et al. 2010).

The high variability observed in the profiling studies cited above indicates that miRNAs consistently detected to be deregulated in independent sample sets might be best candidates to actually playing a central role in melanomagenesis. Indeed, some miRNAs meet this claim. The most prominent example is miR-17-5p, which together with other members of the well-characterized oncogenic miR-17-92 cluster (reviewed by Olive et al. 2010) has been reported to be up-regulated in melanoma cells (Chen et al. 2010; Levati et al. 2009; Mueller et al. 2009; Philippidou et al. 2010). Interestingly, Levy et al. (2010a, b) recently hypothesized that miR-17-mediated suppression of the proapoptotic BIM protein may play a significant role in survival of melanocytic cells in the absence of Bcl-2. Further, reduced expression of miR-200 family members which play a major role in epithelial-to-mesenchymal transition (reviewed by Bracken et al. 2009) had concordantly been demonstrated by several groups indicating a role of these miRNAs in the progression to advanced melanoma as well (Chen et al. 2010; Philippidou et al. 2010; Schultz et al. 2008). The down-regulation of miR-194 (Caramuta et al. 2010; Mueller et al. 2009) and miR-211 (Caramuta et al. 2010; Chen et al. 2010; Jukic et al. 2010) as well as the up-regulation of miR-210 (Caramuta et al. 2010; Philippidou et al. 2010) and miR-373 (Mueller et al. 2009; Philippidou et al. 2010) are further examples for deregulated expression of miRNAs not yet analyzed for their specific functions in malignant melanoma. Thereby, the role of miR-373 in melanoma might be more sophisticated than in other types of tumors (Mueller et al. 2009; Satzger et al. 2010).

This implicates that a lot more miRNAs might be functionally involved in the formation and progression of malignant melanoma than the few we started to analyze in detail so far. Fortunately, a reasonable amount of miRNA profiling data are now available to support the identification of candidate miRNAs for future functional validation. Nevertheless, for every single miRNA, it remains to be elucidated if its deregulated expression really is a defect driving melanoma progression or if it just has to be considered a passenger defect not reflective of the fundamental molecular mechanisms underlying tumorigenesis.

6.3.2 Identification of miRNA Biomarkers Suitable for Diagnostics and Prognostics in Melanoma

In the beginnings of cancer-related miRNA research, groundbreaking publications demonstrated that (1) many miRNAs are encoded at genomic loci matching to fragile sites or regions associated with cancers (Calin et al. 2004) as well as that (2) miRNA expression profiles reflect the developmental lineage and the differentiation state of solid tumors (Lu et al. 2005; Volinia et al. 2006). Strikingly, poorly differentiated tumors can be successfully classified by their miRNA expression profile, in contrast to their mRNA profile – leading Rosenfeld and colleagues to construct a 48 miRNA classifier capable to determine the origin of metastatic tumors of unknown primary origin with high accuracy (Gaur et al. 2007; Lu et al. 2005; Rosenfeld et al. 2008). With regard to melanoma, these studies unrevealed that 85.9 % of genomic loci harboring one or more of 283 examined miRNA genes exhibited DNA copy number alterations and that some of these changes were specific to this tumor type (Zhang et al. 2006). In addition, a set of 15 miRNAs expressed at significantly different levels separated the eight melanoma cell lines included in the NCI-60 panel from the other cancer cell lines investigated (Gaur et al. 2007). Taken together, these findings paved the way to explore the potential of miRNA expression profiling to identify miRNA biomarkers with a diagnostic and/or prognostic value in malignant melanoma.

Fortunately, in accordance to other tumor tissues, FFPE specimens derived from melanocytic lesions are suitable starting material for miRNA expression profiling (Glud et al. 2009; Liu et al. 2009; Ma et al. 2009). In the light of a very limited availability of fresh-frozen melanoma samples (due to therapeutic guidelines requiring microscopic analysis of the whole primary tumor to determine histopathological prognostic parameters, including Breslow thickness), as well as of the large quantity of archival material stored in pathological institutes worldwide this really opens avenues for miRNA biomarker discovery. First interesting results already point out that miRNA profiles actually do harbor the potential to be utilized in diagnostics and prognostics of melanoma in the future. In this way, Satzger and colleagues (2010) found significant association of high miR-15b expression with poor recurrence-free survival and overall survival in Kaplan–Meier analysis of a total of 128 melanoma patients (median follow-up 43.1 months). They also showed that the up-regulation of miR-15b was a statistically significant independent parameter of disease-free survival and overall survival in multivariate Cox analysis in addition to Breslow thickness and ulceration of the primary tumor (Satzger et al. 2010). In addition, Caramuta et al. (2010) described low levels of miR-191 and high levels of miR-193b in melanoma lymph node metastases to be associated with shorter survival after diagnosis of metastatic dissemination into the regional lymph nodes analyzing 16 melanoma patients.

In contrast to these studies focusing on single miRNA markers associated with melanoma survival, Segura et al. (2010) constructed a miRNA classifier consisting of six miRNAs (miR-150, miR-342-3p, miR-455-3p, miR-145, miR-155, and miR-497) indicative for melanoma prognosis. Based on this classifier, they were able to predict post-recurrence survival in their set of 59 FFPE melanoma metastases (derived from patients with detailed clinical follow-up) with an estimated accuracy of about 80 %. Notably, the miRNA classifier was also able to significantly risk-stratify stage III melanoma patients into "better" and "worse" prognostic categories based on survival probability in contrast to the AJCC standard classification system (stages IIIB and IIIC; Segura et al. 2010, detailed discussion in Mueller and Bosserhoff 2010b). Pointing towards clinical application by using three retrospective cohorts (training, validation cohorts profiled with miRNA arrays and an independent cohort assessed through qPCR), Hanniford et al. (2015) identified a miRNA classifier in primary melanoma tumors. The classifier consists of a four miRNA signature including miR-150-5p, miR-15b-5p, miR-16-5p, and miR-374-3p, which, combined with the current clinicopathological staging system, could increase the prognostic value for the risk of developing brain metastasis of the clinicopathological staging alone. Interestingly, miR-150-5p, which was less abundant in primary melanomas that metastasized to the brain, correlated with tumor infiltrating lymphocytes, reflecting tumor-tissue-specific miRNA signature, as opposed to just a cancer-cell-specific signature, putting forward a new advantage of approaches profiling miRNAs from human FFPE samples (Hanniford 2015).

In the era of personalized medicine, miRNA classifiers may represent good prognosis markers and can help in decision making. Pinto et al. compared BRAF mutated versus BRAF nonmutated melanoma patients, finding that miR-192 exhibited a higher expression in BRAF-mutated patients compared to a panel of 15 other miRNAs. This high expression, together with miR-193*, and low expression of miR-132 was associated with worse clinical outcome (Pinto et al. 2015).

6.3.3 Circulating miRNA in Melanoma

While the reports cited above rely on miRNA expression profiling in tissue samples, Leidinger et al. (2010) analyzed blood cell miRNA profiles in 35 melanoma patients and 20 healthy control individuals. Utilizing a subset of 16 significantly regulated miRNAs, they were able to separate melanoma patients from healthy individuals with an accuracy of 97.4 %, a specificity of 95 % and a sensitivity of 98.9 % (Leidinger et al. 2010). This study provides first evidence that miRNA expression profiles generated from peripheral blood cells could be engaged to distinguish patients suffering melanoma from healthy individuals in a noninvasive routine diagnostic approach. In 2008, Mitchell et al. made an important breakthrough when they made a comparative profiling of circulating miRNAs extracted from plasma and serum samples. Furthermore, they were able to detect specific miRNAs in circulation from a murine prostate tumor xenograft model and to find circulating miRNAs which can be used to distinguish between healthy and prostate cancer patients (Mitchell et al. 2008). Having demonstrated that miRNAs were degraded when exposed to RNases present in blood plasma and serum, one of the most intriguing questions regarded the mechanism through which miRNAs could be stably detected in samples after at least 24 h at room temperature or after repeated freezing and thawing cycles.

To date, there are three stabilizing mechanisms for circulating miRNAs. These are (1) exosome-transported miRNAs (Valadi et al. 2007; Hunter et al. 2008), (2) HDL-transported miRNAs (Vickers et al. 2011), and (3) miRNA–protein complexes, where AGO2 appears to play a central role, raising the hypothesis that cells release functional miRNA-induced silencing complexes (miRISC) into the circulation (Arroyo et al. 2011). Although most of the efforts have been directed towards the structural and functional characterization of exosomes (which are also loaded with functional mRNA and proteins), the group headed by Muneesh Tewari has more recently generated strong evidence showing that the exosomal fraction of miRNA represents around 15 % of the total circulating miRNA, being the great majority of these molecules in the vesicle-free (i.e., miRNA-protein complexes) compartment (Arroyo et al. 2011; Chevillet et al. 2014). Moreover, these mechanisms are not mutually exclusive, and, as their roles and mechanisms are progressively understood, they open new avenues for diagnostic and therapeutic clinical use.

In brief, miR-320 and miR-150 were found particularly abundant in exosomes from cells of different types (normal and cancer cells) (Zhang et al. 2015). MiR-451 is abundant in exosomes derived from non-cancer cells, while miR-214 and miR-155 are enriched in exosomes derived from tumor cell lines or peripheral blood of cancer patients (Zhang et al., 2015). Further, miR-17, miR-19a, miR-21, miR-126, and miR-149, were found at significantly higher levels in plasma exosomes derived from a cohort of metastatic melanoma patients compared to a cohort of healthy controls, a cohort of nonrecurrent treated familial melanoma patients carriers of mutated CDKN2A/p16, and a cohort of carriers of the same mutation that had no evidence of disease (Pfeffer et al. 2015).

Stark et al. (2015b) tested a panel of seven miRNAs in blood samples of stage III and IV melanoma patients compared to controls that detected the presence of melanoma with a sensitivity of 93 % and a specificity of at least 82 %. This panel was found to be a better predictor for progression recurrence and survival than current serological clinical markers (Stark et al. 2015a, b). In a broader approach, Margue et al. (2015) used qRT-PCR arrays to compare the serum miRNomes of 52 melanoma patients with 30 healthy volunteers, and the serum profiles with tissue miRNA profiles. They found miR-30b-5p, miR-3754a-5p, among others, to be exclusively expressed in tissue samples, while miR-3201 and miR-122-5p had a higher expression in serum samples. Importantly, the serum miRNome could distinguish only later stage melanoma patients from healthy volunteers, raising doubts about circulating miRNAs as early diagnostic biomarkers, while establishing an important database platform as a reference for further studies (Margue 2015).

As true as for other cancers where tumor markers for early neoplastic transformation remain to be discovered, melanoma biomarkers distinguishing between nevi and early melanoma are urgently needed – especially considering the ability to metastasize a very early event in the progression of malignant melanoma. MicroRNA biomarkers hopefully not only suite this purpose but may also be utilized for separating primary melanomas which will lead (or have already led) to metastasis from nonmetastasizing tumors. Regarding prognostic applications of miRNAs, a central goal has to be the identification of miRNA classifiers (which are representative of molecular biomarkers in general) that can subsequently be incorporated into established staging systems relying solely on morphological criteria. In the end, this will hopefully allow better separation of patients into treatment groups, based on their risk and prognosis. Thereby, patients responsive to one kind of adjuvant treatment could be identified while nonresponders could be spared negative effects of treatment. However, for prognostic as well as diagnostic applications, large-scale studies in comprehensive sets of tissue or blood samples (for which detailed clinical data have to be available) are needed ultimately to prove the usefulness of single miRNAs or miRNA classifiers which already have been proposed as melanoma biomarkers to date. Taken together, although miRNA analysis is unlikely to replace the existing tools for tumor diagnosis and management (like immunohistological staining or established serum marker-proteins), miRNA biomarkers promise huge benefits if used to complement established methodologics.

6.3.4 MiRs as Therapeutical Targets or Therapeutic Options

The unique features of miRNAs and the increasing evidence of their role in disease have stimulated the biotechnology industry to develop miRNA targeting strategies or use synthetic miRNAs as therapeutic agents. MiRNAs are often conserved among species in sequence and function, which makes them particularly attractive for the development and testing of anti-miR drugs. The success of antisense technologies in research has paved the way to the development of anti-miRs, using specific chemistries to increase stability and pharmacokinetics (reviewed by van Rooij et al. 2012). Anti-miRs are modified antisense oligonucleotides targeting a mature miRNA through complementary sequence. An anti-miR should be cell-permeable, stable in the circulation and have high specificity to the target microRNA. The most successful anti-miRs are based on LNA (Locked Nucleic Acid) chemistry, one of them, the antagomiR Miravirsen, targeting miR-122, has reached phase II clinical trial in patients infected with Hepatitis C virus (HCV) (https://www.clinicaltrials.gov/ct2/results?term=Miravirsen&Search=Search). In addition, synthetic microRNAs, called mimics or mimetics, are being designed to use them as weapons against specific gene products. These are usually RNA duplexes carrying specific modifications that will increase their stability and cell permeability. These modifications include linkers, such as cholesterol or nanoparticles (reviewed by Esau and Monia 2007). To increase tissue or cell specificity and prevent side-effects due to general uptake, delivery in viral vectors, such as the AAV has been used. Specificity is achieved via different virus serotypes with tissue tropism, or tissue-specific promoters.

Only a few of these microRNA therapeutic agents have reached clinical trials, among them MRX34, mimicking the tumor suppressor miR-34, is being tested in a phase I trial in different cancers including metastatic melanoma (https://www.clinicaltrials.gov/ct2/show/NCT01829971?term=mirna+therapeutics&rank=115). In summary, there is great hope that the success of these clinical trials will boost further development from the pharmacological industry.

Conclusion

Undoubtedly, a sense of euphoria encases the scientific community when considering future therapeutic and biomarker applications based on miRNAs. This attitude is strengthened as first diagnostic kits (Asuragen Inc.; Rosetta

Genomics) made their way into commercial application and a first miRNA-based drug entered phase IIa clinical trials in the USA and Europe (Santaris Pharma A/S) – with some equally promising miRNA therapeutics subjected to tests in preclinical studies (Regulus Therapeutics Inc.; Mirna Therapeutics Inc.). While we successfully demonstrated that miRNAs are new players in melanomagenesis, we are yet far away from a complete understanding of the impact those tiny molecules exert on formation and progression of this malignancy. Expanding our knowledge on melanoma-relevant miRNAs will be an indispensable prerequisite to develop therapeutic approaches based on miRNA to eventually allow the effective treatment of melanoma patients in the future. Nevertheless, already at this point it seems like miRNAs could at least fill some of the gaps in our yet limited knowledge of the molecular mechanisms underlying this deadly disease. A beginning has been made – a long but promising way is still ahead.

References

Albelda SM, Mette SA, Elder DE, Stewart R, Damjanovich L, Herlyn M, Buck CA (1990) Integrin distribution in malignant melanoma: association of the beta 3 subunit with tumor progression. Cancer Res 50:6757–6764

Arroyo JD, Chevillet JR, Kroh EM, Ruf IK, Pritchard CC, Gibson DF, Mitchell PS, Bennett CF, Pogosova-Agadjanyan EL, Stirewalt DL, Tait JF, Tewari M (2011) Argonaute2 complexes carry a population of circulating microRNAs independent of vesicles in human plasma. Proc Natl Acad Sci U S A 108:5003–5008

Arts N, Cané S, Hennequart M, Lamy J, Bommer G, Van den Eynde B, De Plaen E (2015) microRNA-155, induced by interleukin-1ß, represses the expression of microphthalmia-associated transcription factor (MITF-M) in melanoma cells. PLoS One 10:e0122517

Asangani IA, Harms PW, Dodson L, Pandhi M, Kunju LP, Maher CA, Fullen DR, Johnson TM, Giordano TJ, Palanisamy N, Chinnaiyan AM (2012) Genetic and epigenetic loss of microRNA-31 leads to feed-forward expression of EZH2 in melanoma. Oncotarget 3:1011–1025

Bai J, Zhang Z, Li X, Liu H (2015) MicroRNA-365 inhibits growth, invasion and metastasis of malignant melanoma by targeting NRP1 expression. Cancer Biomark 15:599–608

Barnhill RL, Mihm MC Jr (1993) The histopathology of cutaneous malignant melanoma. Semin Diagn Pathol 10:47–75

Bartel DP (2009) MicroRNAs: target recognition and regulatory functions. Cell 136:215–233

Becker JC, Terheyden P, Kampgen E, Wagner S, Neumann C, Schadendorf D, Steinmann A, Wittenberg G, Lieb W, Brocker EB (2002) Treatment of disseminated ocular melanoma with sequential fotemustine, interferon alpha, and interleukin 2. Br J Cancer 87:840–845

Bedogni B, Powell MB (2009) Hypoxia, melanocytes and melanoma—survival and tumor development in the permissive microenvironment of the skin. Pigment Cell Melanoma Res 22:166–174

Behm-Ansmant I, Rehwinkel J, Doerks T, Stark A, Bork P, Izaurralde E (2006a) mRNA degradation by miRNAs and GW182 requires both CCR4:NOT deadenylase and DCP1:DCP2 decapping complexes. Genes Dev 20:1885–1898

Behm-Ansmant I, Rehwinkel J, Izaurralde E (2006b) MicroRNAs silence gene expression by repressing protein expression and/or by promoting mRNA decay. Cold Spring Harb Symp Quant Biol 71(523–30):523–530

Bell RE, Levy C (2011) The three M's: melanoma, microphthalmia-associated transcription factor and microRNA. Pigment Cell Melanoma Res 24:1088–1106
Bell RE, Khaled M, Netanely D, Schubert S, Golan T, Buxbaum A, Janas MM, Postolsky B, Goldberg MS, Shamir R, Levy C (2014) Transcription factor/microRNA axis blocks melanoma invasion program by miR-211 targeting NUAK1. J Invest Dermatol 134:441–451
Bemis LT, Chen R, Amato CM, Classen EH, Robinson SE, Coffey DG, Erickson PF, Shellman YG, Robinson WA (2008) MicroRNA-137 targets microphthalmia-associated transcription factor in melanoma cell lines. Cancer Res 68:1362–1368
Berezikov E, Chung WJ, Willis J, Cuppen E, Lai EC (2007) Mammalian mirtron genes. Mol Cell 28:328–336
Bhattacharya A, Schmitz U, Wolkenhauer O, Schonherr M, Raatz Y, Kunz M (2013) Regulation of cell cycle checkpoint kinase WEE1 by miR-195 in malignant melanoma. Oncogene 32:3175–3183
Birchmeier C, Birchmeier W, Gherardi E, Vande Woude GF (2003) Met, metastasis, motility and more. Nat Rev Mol Cell Biol 4:915–925
Bloomston M, Frankel WL, Petrocca F, Volinia S, Alder H, Hagan JP, Liu CG, Bhatt D, Taccioli C, Croce CM (2007) MicroRNA expression patterns to differentiate pancreatic adenocarcinoma from normal pancreas and chronic pancreatitis. JAMA 297:1901–1908
Blower PE, Verducci JS, Lin S, Zhou J, Chung JH, Dai Z, Liu CG, Reinhold W, Lorenzi PL, Kaldjian EP, Croce CM, Weinstein JN, Sadee W (2007) MicroRNA expression profiles for the NCI-60 cancer cell panel. Mol Cancer Ther 6:1483–1491
Bommer GT, Gerin I, Feng Y, Kaczorowski AJ, Kuick R, Love RE, Zhai Y, Giordano TJ, Qin ZS, Moore BB, MacDougald OA, Cho KR, Fearon ER (2007) p53-mediated activation of miRNA34 candidate tumor-suppressor genes. Curr Biol 17:1298–1307
Borchert GM, Lanier W, Davidson BL (2006) RNA polymerase III transcribes human microRNAs. Nat Struct Mol Biol 13:1097–1101
Box NF, Terzian T (2008) The role of p53 in pigmentation, tanning and melanoma. Pigment Cell Melanoma Res 21:525–533
Boyerinas B, Park SM, Hau A, Murmann AE, Peter ME (2010) The role of let-7 in cell differentiation and cancer. Endocr Relat Cancer 17:F19–F36
Boyle GM, Woods SL, Bonazzi VF, Stark MS, Hacker E, Aoude LG, Dutton-Regester K, Cook AL, Sturm RA, Hayward NK (2011) Melanoma cell invasiveness is regulated by miR-211 suppression of the BRN2 transcription factor. Pigment Cell Melanoma Res 24:525–537
Bracken CP, Gregory PA, Khew-Goodall Y, Goodall GJ (2009) The role of microRNAs in metastasis and epithelial-mesenchymal transition. Cell Mol Life Sci 66:1682–1699
Braig S, Mueller DW, Rothhammer T, Bosserhoff AK (2010) MicroRNA miR-196a is a central regulator of HOX-B7 and BMP4 expression in malignant melanoma. Cell Mol Life Sci 67:3535–3548
Brennecke J, Stark A, Russell RB, Cohen SM (2005) Principles of microRNA-target recognition. PLoS Biol 3:e85
Bu P, Yang P (2014) MicroRNA-203 inhibits malignant melanoma cell migration by targeting versican. Exp Ther Med 8:309–315
Cai X, Hagedorn CH, Cullen BR (2004) Human microRNAs are processed from capped, polyadenylated transcripts that can also function as mRNAs. RNA 10:1957–1966
Calin GA, Sevignani C, Dumitru CD, Hyslop T, Noch E, Yendamuri S, Shimizu M, Rattan S, Bullrich F, Negrini M, Croce CM (2004) Human microRNA genes are frequently located at fragile sites and genomic regions involved in cancers. Proc Natl Acad Sci U S A 101:2999–3004
Cannell IG, Kong YW, Bushell M (2008) How do microRNAs regulate gene expression? Biochem Soc Trans 36:1224–1231
Caramuta S, Egyhazi S, Rodolfo M, Witten D, Hansson J, Larsson C, Lui WO (2010) MicroRNA expression profiles associated with mutational status and survival in malignant melanoma. J Invest Dermatol 130:2062–2070
Chang TC, Wentzel EA, Kent OA, Ramachandran K, Mullendore M, Lee KH, Feldmann G, Yamakuchi M, Ferlito M, Lowenstein CJ, Arking DE, Beer MA, Maitra A, Mendell JT (2007)

Transactivation of miR-34a by p53 broadly influences gene expression and promotes apoptosis. Mol Cell 26:745–752

Chang X, Sun Y, Han S, Zhu W, Zhang H, Lian S (2015) MiR-203 inhibits melanoma invasive and proliferative abilities by targeting the polycomb group gene BMI1. Biochem Biophys Res Commun 456:361–366

Chatterjee S, Grosshans H (2009) Active turnover modulates mature microRNA activity in *Caenorhabditis elegans*. Nature 461:546–549

Chekulaeva M, Filipowicz W (2009) Mechanisms of miRNA-mediated post-transcriptional regulation in animal cells. Curr Opin Cell Biol 21:452–460

Chen J, Feilotter HE, Pare GC, Zhang X, Pemberton JG, Garady C, Lai D, Yang X, Tron VA (2010) MicroRNA-193b represses cell proliferation and regulates cyclin D1 in melanoma. Am J Pathol 176:2520–2529

Chen J, Zhang X, Lentz C, Abi-Daoud M, Pare GC, Yang X, Feilotter HE, Tron VA (2011) miR-193b Regulates Mcl-1 in Melanoma. Am J Pathol 179:2162–2168

Chen J, Abi-Daoud M, Wang A, Yang X, Zhang X, Feilotter HE, Tron VA (2013) Stathmin 1 is a potential novel oncogene in melanoma. Oncogene 32:1330–1337

Chendrimada TP, Gregory RI, Kumaraswamy E, Norman J, Cooch N, Nishikura K, Shiekhattar R (2005) TRBP recruits the Dicer complex to Ago2 for microRNA processing and gene silencing. Nature 436:740–744

Chevillet JR, Kang Q, Ruf IK, Briggs HA, Vojtech LN, Hughes SM, Cheng HH, Arroyo JD, Meredith EK, Gallichotte EN, Pogosova-Agadjanyan EL, Morrissey C, Stirewalt DL, Hladik F, Yu EY, Higano CS, Tewari M (2014) Quantitative and stoichiometric analysis of the microRNA content of exosomes. Proc Natl Acad Sci U S A 111:14888–14893

Chiang HR, Schoenfeld LW, Ruby JG, Auyeung VC, Spies N, Baek D, Johnston WK, Russ C, Luo S, Babiarz JE, Blelloch R, Schroth GP, Nusbaum C, Bartel DP (2010) Mammalian microRNAs: experimental evaluation of novel and previously annotated genes. Genes Dev 24:992–1009

Ciuffreda L, Di Sanza C, Incani UC, Eramo A, Desideri M, Biagioni F, Passeri D, Falcone I, Sette G, Bergamo P (2012) The mitogen-activated protein kinase (MAPK) cascade controls phosphatase and tensin homolog (PTEN) expression through multiple mechanisms. J Mol Med 90:667–679

Cohen R, Greenberg E, Nemlich Y, Schachter J, Markel G (2015) miR-17 regulates melanoma cell motility by inhibiting the translation of ETV1. Oncotarget 6:19006–19016

Corney DC, Flesken-Nikitin A, Godwin AK, Wang W, Nikitin AY (2007) MicroRNA-34b and MicroRNA-34c are targets of p53 and cooperate in control of cell proliferation and adhesion-independent growth. Cancer Res 67:8433–8438

Couts KL, Anderson EM, Gross MM, Sullivan K, Ahn NG (2013) Oncogenic B-Raf signaling in melanoma cells controls a network of microRNAs with combinatorial functions. Oncogene 32:1959–1970

Cruz J, Reis-Filho JS, Silva P, Lopes JM (2003) Expression of c-met tyrosine kinase receptor is biologically and prognostically relevant for primary cutaneous malignant melanomas. Oncology 65:72–82

Danen EH, Ten Berge PJ, Van Muijen GN, Van't Hof-Grootenboer a, Brocker EB, Ruiter DJ (1994) Emergence of alpha 5 beta 1 fibronectin- and alpha v beta 3 vitronectin-receptor expression in melanocytic tumour progression. Histopathology 24:249–256

Danen EH, Jansen KF, Van Kraats AA, Cornelissen IM, Ruiter DJ, Van Muijen GN (1995) Alpha v-integrins in human melanoma: gain of alpha v beta 3 and loss of alpha v beta 5 are related to tumor progression in situ but not to metastatic capacity of cell lines in nude mice. Int J Cancer 61:491–496

Dar AA, Majid S, de Semir D, Nosrati M, Bezrookove V, Kashani-Sabet M (2011) miRNA-205 suppresses melanoma cell proliferation and induces senescence via regulation of E2F1 protein. J Biol Chem 286:16606–16614

Dar AA, Majid S, Rittsteuer C, de Semir D, Bezrookove V, Tong S, Nosrati M, Sagebiel R, Miller JR 3rd, Kashani-Sabet M (2013) The role of miR-18b in MDM2-p53 pathway signaling and melanoma progression. J Natl Cancer Inst 105:433–442

Das SK, Sokhi UK, Bhutia SK, Azab B, Su ZZ, Sarkar D, Fisher PB (2010) Human polynucleotide phosphorylase selectively and preferentially degrades microRNA-221 in human melanoma cells. Proc Natl Acad Sci U S A 107:11948–11953

Davis BN, Hata A (2009) Regulation of MicroRNA biogenesis: a miRiad of mechanisms. Cell Commun Signal 7:18

De Luca T, Pelosi A, Trisciuoglio D, D'Aguanno S, Desideri M, Farini V, Di Martile M, Bellei B, Tupone MG, Candiloro A, Regazzo G, Rizzo MG (2015) Del Bufalo D (2015) miR-211 and MITF Modulation by Bcl-2 Protein in Melanoma Cells. Mol Carcinog. doi:10.1002/mc.22437

Deng Y, Deng H, Bi F, Liu J, Bemis LT, Norris D, Wang XJ, Zhang Q (2011) MicroRNA-137 targets carboxyl-terminal binding protein 1 in melanoma cell lines. Int J Biol Sci 7:133–137

Diederichs S, Haber DA (2007) Dual role for argonautes in microRNA processing and posttranscriptional regulation of microRNA expression. Cell 131:1097–1108

Dietrich P, Bosserhoff AK (2015) Modifying microRNAs – another piece of the melanoma puzzle. Pigment Cell Melanoma Res 28:488–489

Ding N, Wang S, Yang Q, Li Y, Cheng H, Wang J, Wang D, Deng Y, Yang Y, Hu S, Zhao H, Fang X (2015) Deep sequencing analysis of microRNA expression in human melanocyte and melanoma cell lines. Gene 572:135–145

Doench JG, Sharp PA (2004) Specificity of microRNA target selection in translational repression. Genes Dev 18:504–511

Dynoodt P, Mestdagh P, Van Peer G, Vandesompele J, Goossens K, Peelman LJ, Geusens B, Speeckaert RM, Lambert JL, Van Gele MJ (2013a) Identification of miR-145 as a key regulator of the pigmentary process. J Invest Dermatol 133:201–209

Dynoodt P, Speeckaert R, De Wever O, Chevolet I, Brochez L, Lambert J, Van Gele M (2013b) miR-145 overexpression suppresses the migration and invasion of metastatic melanoma cells. Int J Oncol 42:1443–1451

El Hajj P, Gilot D, Migault M, Theunis A, van Kempen LC, Salés F, Fayyad-Kazan H, Badran B, Larsimont D, Awada A, Bachelot L, Galibert MD, Ghanem G, Journe F (2015) SNPs at miR-155 binding sites of TYRP1 explain discrepancy between mRNA and protein and refine TYRP1 prognostic value in melanoma. Br J Cancer 113:91–98

Elcheva I, Tarapore RS, Bhatia N, Spiegelman VS (2008) Overexpression of mRNA-binding protein CRD-BP in malignant melanomas. Oncogene 27:5069–5074

Elson-Schwab I, Lorentzen A and Marshall CJ (2010) MicroRNA-200 family members differentially regulate morphological plasticity and mode of melanoma cell invasion. PLoS One 4;5(10). pii: e13176.

Errico MC, Felicetti F, Bottero L, Mattia G, Boe A, Felli N, Petrini M, Bellenghi M, Pandha HS, Calvaruso M, Tripodo C, Colombo MP, Morgan R, Care A (2013) The abrogation of the HOXB7/PBX2 complex induces apoptosis in melanoma through the miR-221&222-c-FOS pathway. Int J Cancer 133:879–892

Esau CC, Monia BP (2007) Therapeutic potential for microRNAs. Adv Drug Deliv Rev 59:101–114

Eulalio A, Rehwinkel J, Stricker M, Huntzinger E, Yang SF, Doerks T, Dorner S, Bork P, Boutros M, Izaurralde E (2007) Target-specific requirements for enhancers of decapping in miRNA-mediated gene silencing. Genes Dev 21:2558–2570

Eulalio A, Huntzinger E, Nishihara T, Rehwinkel J, Fauser M, Izaurralde E (2009) Deadenylation is a widespread effect of miRNA regulation. RNA 15:21–32

Felicetti F, Errico MC, Bottero L, Segnalini P, Stoppacciaro A, Biffoni M, Felli N, Mattia G, Petrini M, Colombo MP, Peschle C, Care A (2008a) The promyelocytic leukemia zinc finger-microRNA-221/-222 pathway controls melanoma progression through multiple oncogenic mechanisms. Cancer Res 68:2745–2754

Felicetti F, Errico MC, Segnalini P, Mattia G, Care A (2008b) MicroRNA-221 and −222 pathway controls melanoma progression. Expert Rev Anticancer Ther 8:1759–1765

Felli N, Fontana L, Pelosi E, Botta R, Bonci D, Facchiano F, Liuzzi F, Lulli V, Morsilli O, Santoro S, Valtieri M, Calin GA, Liu CG, Sorrentino A, Croce CM, Peschle C (2005) MicroRNAs 221 and 222 inhibit normal erythropoiesis and erythroleukemic cell growth via kit receptor down-modulation. Proc Natl Acad Sci U S A 102:18081–18086

Felli N, Felicetti F, Lustri AM, Errico MC, Bottero L, Cannistraci A, De Feo A, Petrini M, Pedini F, Biffoni M, Alvino E, Negrini M, Ferracin M, Mattia G, Care A (2013) miR-126&126* restored expressions play a tumor suppressor role by directly regulating ADAM9 and MMP7 in melanoma. PLoS One 8:e56824

Felli N, Errico MC, Pedini F, Petrini M, Puglisi R, Bellenghi M, Boe A, Felicetti F, Mattia G, De Feo A, Bottero L, Tripodo C, Carè A (2016) AP2α controls the dynamic balance between miR-126&126* and miR-221&222 during melanoma progression. Oncogene 35(23):3016–3026

Filipowicz W, Bhattacharyya SN, Sonenberg N (2008) Mechanisms of post-transcriptional regulation by microRNAs: are the answers in sight? Nat Rev Genet 9:102–114

Forloni M, Dogra SK, Dong Y, Conte D Jr, Ou J, Zhu LJ, Deng A, Mahalingam M, Green MR, Wajapeyee N (2014) miR-146a promotes the initiation and progression of melanoma by activating Notch signaling. Elife 3:e01460

Friedman RC, Farh KK, Burge CB, Bartel DP (2009) Most mammalian mRNAs are conserved targets of microRNAs. Genome Res 19:92–105

Fu X, Meng Z, Liang W, Tian Y, Wang X, Han W, Lou G, Wang X, Lou F, Yen Y, Yu H, Jove R, Huang W (2014) miR-26a enhances miRNA biogenesis by targeting Lin28B and Zcchc11 to suppress tumor growth and metastasis. Oncogene 33:4296–4306

Galore-Haskel G, Nemlich Y, Greenberg E, Ashkenazi S, Hakim M, Itzhaki O, Shoshani N, Shapira-Fromer R, Ben-Ami E, Ofek E, Anafi L, Besser MJ, Schachter J, Markel G (2015) A novel immune resistance mechanism of melanoma cells controlled by the ADAR1 enzyme. Oncotarget 6:28999–29015

Gambarotta G, Boccaccio C, Giordano S, Ando M, Stella MC, Comoglio PM (1996) Ets up-regulates MET transcription. Oncogene 13:1911–1917

Garofalo M, Di Leva G, Romano G, Nuovo G, Suh SS, Ngankeu A, Taccioli C, Pichiorri F, Alder H, Secchiero P, Gasparini P, Gonelli A, Costinean S, Acunzo M, Condorelli G, Croce CM (2009) miR-221&222 regulate TRAIL resistance and enhance tumorigenicity through PTEN and TIMP3 downregulation. Cancer Cell 16:498–509

Gartel AL, Kandel ES (2008) miRNAs: little known mediators of oncogenesis. Semin Cancer Biol 18:103–110

Gaur A, Jewell DA, Liang Y, Ridzon D, Moore JH, Chen C, Ambros VR, Israel MA (2007) Characterization of microRNA expression levels and their biological correlates in human cancer cell lines. Cancer Res 67:2456–2468

Gaziel-Sovran A, Segura MF, Di Micco R, Collins MK, Hanniford D, Vega-Saenz de Miera E, Rakus JF, Dankert JF, Shang S, Kerbel RS, Bhardwaj N, Shao Y, Darvishian F, Zavadil J, Erlebacher A, Mahal LK, Osman I, Hernando E (2011) miR-30b/30d regulation of GalNAc transferases enhances invasion and immunosuppression during metastasis. Cancer Cell 20:104–118

Georgantas RW, Streicher K, Luo X, Zhu W, Liu Z, Brohawn P, Morehouse C, Higgs BW, Richman L, Jallal B (2013) Effect of microRNA-206 on G1 arrest by inhibition of CDK4, cyclin C, and cyclin D in melanoma cells. J Clin Oncol 31:e20047

Ghildiyal M, Xu J, Seitz H, Weng Z, Zamore PD (2010) Sorting of *Drosophila* small silencing RNAs partitions microRNA* strands into the RNA interference pathway. RNA 16:43–56

Giles KM, Brown RA, Epis MR, Kalinowski FC, Leedman PJ (2013) miRNA-7-5p inhibits melanoma cell migration and invasion. Biochem Biophys Res Commun 430:706–710

Gillanders E, Juo SH, Holland EA, Jones M, Nancarrow D, Freas-Lutz D, Sood R, Park N, Faruque M, Markey C, Kefford RF, Palmer J, Bergman W, Bishop DT, Tucker MA, Bressac-de Paillerets B, Hansson J, Stark M, Gruis N, Bishop JN, Goldstein AM, Bailey-Wilson JE, Mann GJ, Hayward N, Trent J (2003) Localization of a novel melanoma susceptibility locus to 1p22. Am J Hum Genet 73:301–313

Giraldez AJ, Mishima Y, Rihel J, Grocock RJ, van Dongen S, Inoue K, Enright AJ, Schier AF (2006) Zebrafish MiR-430 promotes deadenylation and clearance of maternal mRNAs. Science 312:75–79

Git A, Dvinge H, Salmon-Divon M, Osborne M, Kutter C, Hadfield J, Bertone P, Caldas C (2010) Systematic comparison of microarray profiling, real-time PCR, and next-generation sequencing technologies for measuring differential microRNA expression. RNA 16:991–1006

Glud M, Klausen M, Gniadecki R, Rossing M, Hastrup N, Nielsen FC, Drzewiecki KT (2009) MicroRNA expression in melanocytic nevi: the usefulness of formalin-fixed, paraffin-embedded material for miRNA microarray profiling. J Invest Dermatol 129:1219–1224

Glud M, Rossing M, Hother C, Holst L, Hastrup N, Nielsen FC, Gniadecki R, Drzewiecki KT (2010) Downregulation of miR-125b in metastatic cutaneous malignant melanoma. Melanoma Res 20:479–484

Golan T, Messer AR, Amitai-Lange A, Melamed Z, Ohana R, Bell RE, Kapitansky O, Lerman G, Greenberger S, Khaled M (2015) Interactions of melanoma cells with distal keratinocytes trigger metastasis via notch signaling inhibition of MITF. Mol Cell 59:664–676

Goswami S, Tarapore RS, Poenitzsch Strong AM, TeSlaa JJ, Grinblat Y, Setaluri V, Spiegelman VS (2015) MicroRNA-340-mediated degradation of microphthalmia-associated transcription factor (MITF) mRNA is inhibited by coding region determinant-binding protein (CRD-BP). J Biol Chem 290:384–395

Greenberg E, Hershkovitz L, Itzhaki O, Hajdu S, Nemlich Y, Ortenberg R, Gefen N, Edry L, Modai S, Keisari Y, Besser MJ, Schachter J, Shomron N, Markel G (2011) Regulation of cancer aggressive features in melanoma cells by microRNAs. PLoS One 6:e18936

Greenberg E, Hajdu S, Nemlich Y, Cohen R, Itzhaki O, Jacob-Hirsch J, Besser MJ, Schachter J, Markel G (2014) Differential regulation of aggressive features in melanoma cells by members of the miR-17-92 complex. Open Biol 4:140030

Gregory RI, Chendrimada TP, Cooch N, Shiekhattar R (2005) Human RISC couples microRNA biogenesis and posttranscriptional gene silencing. Cell 123:631–640

Griffiths-Jones S, Saini HK, van Dongen S, Enright AJ (2008) miRBase: tools for microRNA genomics. Nucleic Acids Res 36:D154–D158

Grignol V, Fairchild ET, Zimmerer JM, Lesinski GB, Walker MJ, Magro CM, Kacher JE, Karpa VI, Clark J, Nuovo G, Lehman A, Volinia S, Agnese DM, Croce CM, Carson WE 3rd (2011) miR-21 and miR-155 are associated with mitotic activity and lesion depth of borderline melanocytic lesions. Br J Cancer 105:1023–1029

Grimson A, Farh KK, Johnston WK, Garrett-Engele P, Lim LP, Bartel DP (2007) MicroRNA targeting specificity in mammals: determinants beyond seed pairing. Mol Cell 27:91–105

Guo H, Ingolia NT, Weissman JS, Bartel DP (2010) Mammalian microRNAs predominantly act to decrease target mRNA levels. Nature 466:835–840

Guo J, Zhang JF, Wang WM, Cheung FW, Lu YF, Ng CF, Kung HF, Liu WK (2014) MicroRNA-218 inhibits melanogenesis by directly suppressing microphthalmia-associated transcription factor expression. RNA Biol 11:732–741

Haflidadottir BS, Bergsteinsdottir K, Praetorius C, Steingrimsson E (2010) miR-148 regulates Mitf in melanoma cells. PLoS One 5:e11574

Han J, Lee Y, Yeom KH, Nam JW, Heo I, Rhee JK, Sohn SY, Cho Y, Zhang BT, Kim VN (2006) Molecular basis for the recognition of primary microRNAs by the Drosha-DGCR8 complex. Cell 125:887–901

Han J, Pedersen JS, Kwon SC, Belair CD, Kim YK, Yeom KH, Yang WY, Haussler D, Blelloch R, Kim VN (2009) Posttranscriptional crossregulation between Drosha and DGCR8. Cell 136:75–84

Hanniford D, Zhong J, Koetz L, Gaziel-Sovran A, Lackaye DJ, Shang S, Pavlick A, Shapiro R, Berman R, Darvishian F, Shao Y, Osman I, Hernando E (2015) A miRNA-based signature detected in primary melanoma tissue predicts development of brain metastasis. Clin Cancer Res 21:4903–4912

Hao S, Luo C, Abukiwan A, Wang G, He J, Huang L, Weber CE, Lv N, Xiao X, Eichmuller SB, He D (2015) miR-137 inhibits proliferation of melanoma cells by targeting PAK2. Exp Dermatol 24:947–952

Hausser J, Zavolan M (2014) Identification and consequences of miRNA–target interactions — beyond repression of gene expression. Nat Rev Genet 15:599–612

He H, Jazdzewski K, Li W, Liyanarachchi S, Nagy R, Volinia S, Calin GA, Liu CG, Franssila K, Suster S, Kloos RT, Croce CM, de la Chapelle CA (2005) The role of microRNA genes in papillary thyroid carcinoma. Proc Natl Acad Sci U S A 102:19075–19080

He L, He X, Lim LP, de Stanchina E, Xuan Z, Liang Y, Xue W, Zender L, Magnus J, Ridzon D, Jackson AL, Linsley PS, Chen C, Lowe SW, Cleary MA, Hannon GJ (2007) A microRNA component of the p53 tumour suppressor network. Nature 447:1130–1134

Heinemann A, Zhao F, Pechlivanis S, Eberle J, Steinle A, Diederichs S, Schadendorf D, Paschen A (2012) Tumor suppressive microRNAs miR-34a/c control cancer cell expression of ULBP2, a stress-induced ligand of the natural killer cell receptor NKG2D. Cancer Res 72:460–471

Hermeking H (2010) The miR-34 family in cancer and apoptosis. Cell Death Differ 17:193–199

Ho JJ, Marsden PA (2014) Competition and collaboration between RNA-binding proteins and microRNAs. Wiley Interdiscip Rev RNA 5:69–86

Holst LM, Kaczkowski B, Glud M, Futoma-Kazmierczak E, Hansen LF, Gniadecki R (2011) The microRNA molecular signature of atypic and common acquired melanocytic nevi: differential expression of miR-125b and let-7c. Exp Dermatol 20:278–280

Howell PM, Li X, Riker AI, Xi Y (2010) MicroRNA in melanoma. Ochsner J 10:83–92

Hsu MY, Rovinsky S, Penmatcha S, Herlyn M, Muirhead D (2005) Bone morphogenetic proteins in melanoma: angel or devil? Cancer Metastasis Rev 24:251–263

Huang X, Ding L, Bennewith KL, Tong RT, Welford SM, Ang KK, Story M, Le QT, Giaccia AJ (2009) Hypoxia-inducible mir-210 regulates normoxic gene expression involved in tumor initiation. Mol Cell 35:856–867

Huang X, Le QT, Giaccia AJ (2010) MiR-210—micromanager of the hypoxia pathway. Trends Mol Med 16:230–237

Huang Y, Yi X, Jian Z, Wei C, Li S, Cai C, Zhang P, Li K, Guo S, Liu L, Shi Q, Gao T, Li C (2013) A single-nucleotide polymorphism of miR-196a-2 and vitiligo: an association study and functional analysis in a Han Chinese population. Pigment Cell Melanoma Res 26(3):338–347

Hunter MP, Ismail N, Zhang X, Aguda BD, Lee EJ, Yu L, Xiao T, Schafer J, Lee ML, Schmittgen TD, Nana-Sinkam SP, Jarjoura D, Marsh CB (2008) Detection of microRNA Expression in Human Peripheral Blood Microvesicles. PLoS One 3:e3694

Hutvagner G, McLachlan J, Pasquinelli AE, Balint E, Tuschl T, Zamore PD (2001) A cellular function for the RNA-interference enzyme Dicer in the maturation of the let-7 small temporal RNA. Science 293:834–838

Hwang HW, Wentzel EA, Mendell JT (2007) A hexanucleotide element directs microRNA nuclear import. Science 315:97–100

Hwang HW, Baxter LL, Loftus SK, Cronin JC, Trivedi NS, Borate B, Pavan WJ (2014) Distinct microRNA expression signatures are associated with melanoma subtypes and are regulated by HIF1A. Pigment Cell Melanoma Res 27:777–787

Igoucheva O, Alexeev V (2009) MicroRNA-dependent regulation of cKit in cutaneous melanoma. Biochem Biophys Res Commun 379:790–794

Inada T, Fukushima S, Murai M, Jinnin M, Miyashita A, Nakahara S, Yamashita J, Aoi J, Masuguchi S, Ihn H (2015) Hair shaft miRNA-221 levels as a new tumor marker of malignant melanoma. J Dermatol 42:198–201

Ito Y (2004) Oncogenic potential of the RUNX gene family: "overview". Oncogene 23:4198–4208

Ivan M, Bond JA, Prat M, Comoglio PM, Wynford-Thomas D (1997) Activated ras and ret oncogenes induce over-expression of c-met (hepatocyte growth factor receptor) in human thyroid epithelial cells. Oncogene 14:2417–2423

Jafari N, Dogaheh HP, Bohlooli S, Oyong GG, Shirzad Z, Alibeiki F, Asl SH, Zargar SJ (2013) Expression levels of microRNA machinery components Drosha, Dicer and DGCR8 in human (AGS, HepG2, and KEYSE-30) cancer cell lines. Int J Clin Exp Med 6:269–274

Jafarnejad SM, Sjoestroem C, Martinka M, Li G (2013) Expression of the RNase III enzyme DROSHA is reduced during progression of human cutaneous melanoma. Mod Pathol 26:902–910

Javed A, Barnes GL, Pratap J, Antkowiak T, Gerstenfeld LC, van Wijnen AJ, Stein JL, Lian JB, Stein GS (2005) Impaired intranuclear trafficking of Runx2 (AML3/CBFA1) transcription factors in breast cancer cells inhibits osteolysis in vivo. Proc Natl Acad Sci U S A 102:1454–1459

Jayawardana K, Schramm SJ, Tembe V, Mueller S, Thompson JF, Scolyer RA, Mann GJ, Yang JY (2015) Identification, review and systematic cross-validation of microRNA prognostic signatures in metastatic melanoma. J Invest Dermatol. doi: 10.1038/jid.2015.355

Jian Q, An Q, Zhu D, Hui K, Liu Y, Chi S, Li C (2014) MicroRNA 340 Is involved in UVB-induced dendrite formation through the regulation of RhoA expression in melanocytes. Mol Cell Biol 34:3407–3420

Jiang L, Lv X, Li J, Li J, Li X, Li W, Li Y (2012) The status of microRNA-21 expression and its clinical significance in human cutaneous malignant melanoma. Acta Histochem 114:582–588

Jiang CC, Croft A, Tseng HY, Guo ST, Jin L, Hersey P, Zhang XD (2014) Repression of microRNA-768-3p by MEK/ERK signalling contributes to enhanced mRNA translation in human melanoma. Oncogene 33:2577–2588

Jin L, Hu WL, Jiang CC, Wang JX, Han CC, Chu P, Zhang LJ, Thorne RF, Wilmott J, Scolyer RA, Hersey P, Zhang XD, Wu M (2011) MicroRNA-149*, a p53-responsive microRNA, functions as an oncogenic regulator in human melanoma. Proc Natl Acad Sci U S A 108:15840–15845

Jones MR, Quinton LJ, Blahna MT, Neilson JR, Fu S, Ivanov AR, Wolf DA, Mizgerd JP (2009) Zcchc11-dependent uridylation of microRNA directs cytokine expression. Nat Cell Biol 11:1157–1163

Jukic DM, Rao UN, Kelly L, Skaf JS, Drogowski LM, Kirkwood JM, Panelli MC (2010) MicroRNA profiling analysis of differences between the melanoma of young adults and older adults. J Transl Med 8:27

Kappelmann M, Kuphal S, Meister G, Vardimon L, Bosserhoff AK (2013) MicroRNA miR-125b controls melanoma progression by direct regulation of c-Jun protein expression. Oncogene 32:2984–2991

Karreth FA, Tay Y, Perna D, Ala U, Tan SM, Rust AG, DeNicola G, Webster KA, Weiss D, Perez-Mancera PA, Krauthammer M, Halaban R, Provero P, Adams DJ, Tuveson DA, Pandolfi PP (2011) In vivo identification of tumor- suppressive PTEN ceRNAs in an oncogenic BRAF-induced mouse model of melanoma. Cell 147:382–395

Katoh T, Sakaguchi Y, Miyauchi K, Suzuki T, Kashiwabara S, Baba T, Suzuki T (2009) Selective stabilization of mammalian microRNAs by 3′ adenylation mediated by the cytoplasmic poly(A) polymerase GLD-2. Genes Dev 23:433–438

Khvorova A, Reynolds A, Jayasena SD (2003) Functional siRNAs and miRNAs exhibit strand bias. Cell 115:209–216

Kim VN (2004) MicroRNA precursors in motion: exportin-5 mediates their nuclear export. Trends Cell Biol 14:156–159

Kim KH, Bin BH, Kim J, Dong SE, Park PJ, Choi H, Kim BJ, Yu SJ, Kang H, Kang HH, Cho EG, Lee TR (2014a) Novel inhibitory function of miR-125b in melanogenesis. Pigment Cell Melanoma Res 27:140–144

Kim NH, Choi SH, Kim CH, Lee CH, Lee TR, Lee AY (2014b) Reduced MiR-675 in exosome in H19 RNA-related melanogenesis via MITF as a direct target. J Invest Dermatol 134:1075–1082

Kiriakidou M, Nelson PT, Kouranov A, Fitziev P, Bouyioukos C, Mourelatos Z, Hatzigeorgiou A (2004) A combined computational-experimental approach predicts human microRNA targets. Genes Dev 18:1165–1178

Kitago M, Martinez SR, Nakamura T, Sim MS, Hoon DS (2009) Regulation of RUNX3 tumor suppressor gene expression in cutaneous melanoma. Clin Cancer Res 15:2988–2994

Knight SW, Bass BL (2001) A role for the RNase III enzyme DCR-1 in RNA interference and germ line development in *Caenorhabditis elegans*. Science 293:2269–2271

Knoll S, Furst K, Kowtharapu B, Schmitz U, Marquardt S, Wolkenhauer O, Martin H, Putzer BM (2014) E2F1 induces miR-224/452 expression to drive EMT through TXNIP downregulation. EMBO Rep 15:1315–1329

Kong YW, Cannell IG, de Moor CH, Hill K, Garside PG, Hamilton TL, Meijer HA, Dobbyn HC, Stoneley M, Spriggs KA, Willis AE, Bushell M (2008) The mechanism of micro-RNA-mediated translation repression is determined by the promoter of the target gene. Proc Natl Acad Sci U S A 105:8866–8871

Kourtidis A, Ngok SP, Pulimeno P, Feathers RW, Carpio LR, Baker TR, Carr JM, Yan IK, Borges S, Perez EA, Storz P, Copland JA, Patel T, Thompson EA, Citi S, Anastasiadis PZ (2015) Distinct E-cadherin-based complexes regulate cell behaviour through miRNA processing or Src and p120 catenin activity. Nat Cell Biol 17:1145–1157

Kozaki K, Imoto I, Mogi S, Omura K, Inazawa J (2008) Exploration of tumor-suppressive microRNAs silenced by DNA hypermethylation in oral cancer. Cancer Res 68:2094–2105

Kozomara A, Griffiths-Jones S (2014) miRBase: annotating high confidence microRNAs using deep sequencing data. Nucleic Acids Res 42(Database issue):D68–D73

Kozubek J, Ma Z, Fleming E, Duggan T, Wu R, Shin DG, Dadras SS (2013) In-depth characterization of microRNA transcriptome in melanoma. PLoS One 8:e72699

Krek A, Grun D, Poy MN, Wolf R, Rosenberg L, Epstein EJ, MacMenamin P, da Piedade I, Gunsalus KC, Stoffel M, Rajewsky N (2005) Combinatorial microRNA target predictions. Nat Genet 37:495–500

Krol J, Loedige I, Filipowicz W (2010) The widespread regulation of microRNA biogenesis, function and decay. Nat Rev Genet 11:597–610

Kuphal S, Winklmeier A, Warnecke C, Bosserhoff AK (2010) Constitutive HIF-1 activity in malignant melanoma. Eur J Cancer 46:1159–1169

Kwon Y, Kim Y, Eom S, Kim M, Park D, Kim H, Noh K, Lee H, Lee YS, Choe J, Kim YM, Jeoung D (2015) MicroRNA-26a/-26b-COX-2-MIP-2 loop regulates allergic inflammation and allergic inflammation-promoted enhanced tumorigenic and metastatic potential of cancer cells. J Biol Chem 290:14245–14266

Landthaler M, Yalcin A, Tuschl T (2004) The human DiGeorge syndrome critical region gene 8 and Its D. melanogaster homolog are required for miRNA biogenesis. Curr Biol 14:2162–2167

Lankenau M, Patel R, Markowitz J, Carson WE, de la Chapelle A, Eisfeld A-K (2014) Overexpression of miR-3151 leads to direct deregulation of the TP53 pathway and is associated with BRAF mutations in malignant melanoma. Cancer Res 74:4790

le Sage C, Nagel R, Egan DA, Schrier M, Mesman E, Mangiola A, Anile C, Maira G, Mercatelli N, Ciafre SA, Farace MG, Agami R (2007) Regulation of the p27(Kip1) tumor suppressor by miR-221 and miR-222 promotes cancer cell proliferation. EMBO J 26:3699–3708

Lee RC, Feinbaum RL, Ambros V (1993) The *C. elegans* heterochronic gene lin-4 encodes small RNAs with antisense complementarity to lin-14. Cell 75:843–854

Lee Y, Jeon K, Lee JT, Kim S, Kim VN (2002) MicroRNA maturation: stepwise processing and subcellular localization. EMBO J 21:4663–4670

Lee Y, Ahn C, Han J, Choi H, Kim J, Yim J, Lee J, Provost P, Radmark O, Kim S, Kim VN (2003) The nuclear RNase III Drosha initiates microRNA processing. Nature 425:415–419

Lee Y, Kim M, Han J, Yeom KH, Lee S, Baek SH, Kim VN (2004) MicroRNA genes are transcribed by RNA polymerase II. EMBO J 23:4051–4060

Lee YS, Kim HK, Chung S, Kim KS, Dutta A (2005) Depletion of human micro-RNA miR-125b reveals that it is critical for the proliferation of differentiated cells but not for the down-regulation of putative targets during differentiation. J Biol Chem 280:16635–16641

Lei H, Wang H, Juan AH, Ruddle FH (2005) The identification of Hoxc8 target genes. Proc Natl Acad Sci U S A 102:2420–2424

Lei H, Juan AH, Kim MS, Ruddle FH (2006) Identification of a Hoxc8-regulated transcriptional network in mouse embryo fibroblast cells. Proc Natl Acad Sci U S A 103:10305–10309

Leidinger P, Keller A, Borries A, Reichrath J, Rass K, Jager SU, Lenhof HP, Meese E (2010) High-throughput miRNA profiling of human melanoma blood samples. BMC Cancer 10:262

Levati L, Alvino E, Pagani E, Arcelli D, Caporaso P, Bondanza S, Di Leva G, Ferracin M, Volinia S, Bonmassar E, Croce CM, D'Atri S (2009) Altered expression of selected microRNAs in melanoma: antiproliferative and proapoptotic activity of miRNA-155. Int J Oncol 35:393–400

Levati L, Pagani E, Romani S, Castiglia D, Piccinni E, Covaciu C, Caporaso P, Bondanza S, Antonetti FR, Bonmassar E, Martelli F, Alvino E, D'Atri S (2011) MicroRNA-155 targets the SKI gene in human melanoma cell lines. Pigment Cell Melanoma Res 24:538–550
Levy C, Khaled M, Iliopoulos D, Janas MM, Schubert S, Pinner S, Chen PH, Li S, Fletcher AL, Yokoyama S, Scott KL, Garraway LA, Song JS, Granter SR, Turley SJ, Fisher DE, Novina CD (2010a) Intronic miR-211 assumes the tumor suppressive function of its host gene in melanoma. Mol Cell 40:841–849
Levy C, Khaled M, Robinson KC, Veguilla RA, Chen PH, Yokoyama S, Makino E, Lu J, Larue L, Beermann F, Chin L, Bosenberg M, Song JS, Fisher DE (2010b) Lineage-specific transcriptional regulation of DICER by MITF in melanocytes. Cell 141:994–1005
Lewis BP, Burge CB, Bartel DP (2005) Conserved seed pairing, often flanked by adenosines, indicates that thousands of human genes are microRNA targets. Cell 120:15–20
Li N (2016) Low expression of Mir-137 predicts poor prognosis in cutaneous melanoma patients. Med Sci Monit 22:140–144
Li G, Schaider H, Satyamoorthy K, Hanakawa Y, Hashimoto K, Herlyn M (2001) Downregulation of E-cadherin and Desmoglein 1 by autocrine hepatocyte growth factor during melanoma development. Oncogene 20:8125–8135
Li Y, Zhang M, Chen H, Dong Z, Ganapathy V, Thangaraju M, Huang S (2010) Ratio of miR-196s to HOXC8 messenger RNA correlates with breast cancer cell migration and metastasis. Cancer Res 70:7894–7904
Li F, Li XJ, Qiao L, Shi F, Liu W, Li Y, Dang YP, Gu WJ, Wang XG, Liu W (2014a) miR-98 suppresses melanoma metastasis through a negative feedback loop with its target gene IL-6. Exp Mol Med 46:e116
Li R, Zhang L, Jia L, Duan Y, Li Y, Wang J, Bao L, Sha N (2014b) MicroRNA-143 targets Syndecan-1 to repress cell growth in melanoma. PLoS One 9:e94855
Lim LP, Lau NC, Garrett-Engele P, Grimson A, Schelter JM, Castle J, Bartel DP, Linsley PS, Johnson JM (2005) Microarray analysis shows that some microRNAs downregulate large numbers of target mRNAs. Nature 433:769–773
Lin N, Zhou Y, Lian X, Tu Y (2015a) Down-regulation of tissue microRNA-126 was associated with poor prognosis in patients with cutaneous melanoma. Int J Clin Exp Med 8:4297–4301
Lin N, Zhou Y, Lian X, Tu Y (2015b) Expression of microRNA-106b and its clinical significance in cutaneous melanoma. Genet Mol Res 14:16379–16385
Liu A, Tetzlaff MT, Vanbelle P, Elder D, Feldman M, Tobias JW, Sepulveda AR, Xu X (2009) MicroRNA expression profiling outperforms mRNA expression profiling in formalin-fixed paraffin-embedded tissues. Int J Clin Exp Pathol 2:519–527
Liu S, Kumar SM, Lu H, Liu A, Yang R, Pushparajan A, Guo W, Xu X (2012a) MicroRNA-9 up-regulates E-cadherin through inhibition of NF-kappaB1-Snail1 pathway in melanoma. J Pathol 226:61–72
Liu S, Tetzlaff MT, Cui R, Xu X (2012b) miR-200c inhibits melanoma progression and drug resistance through down-regulation of BMI-1. Am J Pathol 181:1823–1835
Liu S, Howell PM, Riker AI (2013) Up-regulation of miR-182 expression after epigenetic modulation of human melanoma cells. Ann Surg Oncol 20:1745–1752
Liu SM, Lu J, Lee HC, Chung FH, Ma N (2014) miR-524-5p suppresses the growth of oncogenic BRAF melanoma by targeting BRAF and ERK2. Oncotarget 5:9444–9459
Liu P, Hu Y, Ma L, Du M, Xia L, Hu Z (2015a) miR-425 inhibits melanoma metastasis through repression of PI3K-Akt pathway by targeting IGF-1. Biomed Pharmacother 75:51–57
Liu R, Xie H, Luo C, Chen Z, Zhou X, Xia K, Chen X, Zhou M, Cao P, Cao K, Zhou J (2015b) Identification of FLOT2 as a novel target for microRNA-34a in melanoma. J Cancer Res Clin Oncol 141:993–1006
Lodygin D, Tarasov V, Epanchintsev A, Berking C, Knyazeva T, Korner H, Knyazev P, Diebold J, Hermeking H (2008) Inactivation of miR-34a by aberrant CpG methylation in multiple types of cancer. Cell Cycle 7:2591–2600
Lu J, Getz G, Miska EA, Alvarez-Saavedra E, Lamb J, Peck D, Sweet-Cordero A, Ebert BL, Mak RH, Ferrando AA, Downing JR, Jacks T, Horvitz HR, Golub TR (2005) MicroRNA expression profiles classify human cancers. Nature 435:834–838

Lu M, Shi B, Wang J, Cao Q, Cui Q (2010) TAM: a method for enrichment and depletion analysis of a microRNA category in a list of microRNAs. BMC Bioinf 11:419

Lujambio A, Calin GA, Villanueva A, Ropero S, Sanchez-Cespedes M, Blanco D, Montuenga LM, Rossi S, Nicoloso MS, Faller WJ, Gallagher WM, Eccles SA, Croce CM, Esteller M (2008) A microRNA DNA methylation signature for human cancer metastasis. Proc Natl Acad Sci U S A 105:13556–13561

Luo C, Merz PR, Chen Y, Dickes E, Pscherer A, Schadendorf D, Eichmüller SB (2013a) MiR-101 inhibits melanoma cell invasion and proliferation by targeting MITF and EZH2. Cancer Lett 341:240–247

Luo C, Tetteh PW, Merz PR, Dickes E, Abukiwan A, Hotz-Wagenblatt A, Holland-Cunz S, Sinnberg T, Schittek B, Schadendorf D, Diederichs S, Eichmuller SB (2013b) miR-137 inhibits the invasion of melanoma cells through downregulation of multiple oncogenic target genes. J Invest Dermatol 133:768–775

Luthra R, Singh RR, Luthra MG, Li YX, Hannah C, Romans AM, Barkoh BA, Chen SS, Ensor J, Maru DM, Broaddus RR, Rashid A, Albarracin CT (2008) MicroRNA-196a targets annexin A1: a microRNA-mediated mechanism of annexin A1 downregulation in cancers. Oncogene 27:6667–6678

Ma Z, Lui WO, Fire A, Dadras SS (2009) Profiling and discovery of novel miRNAs from formalin-fixed, paraffin-embedded melanoma and nodal specimens. J Mol Diagn 11:420–429

Ma Z, Swede H, Cassarino D, Fleming E, Fire A, Dadras SS (2011) Up-regulated Dicer expression in patients with cutaneous melanoma. PLoS One 6(6):e20494

MacRae IJ, Ma E, Zhou M, Robinson CV, Doudna JA (2008) In vitro reconstitution of the human RISC-loading complex. Proc Natl Acad Sci U S A 105:512–517

Margue C, Philippidou D, Reinsbach SE, Schmitt M, Behrmann I, Kreis S (2013) New target genes of MITF-induced microRNA-211 contribute to melanoma cell invasion. PLoS One 8:e73473

Margue C, Reinsbach S, Philippidou D, Beaume N, Walters C, Schneider JG, Nashan D, Behrmann I, Kreis S (2015) Comparison of a healthy miRNome with melanoma patient miRNomes: are microRNAs suitable serum biomarkers for cancer? Oncotarget 6:12110–12127

Martin del Campo SE, Latchana N, Levine KM, Grignol VP, Fairchild ET, Jaime-Ramirez AC, Dao TV, Karpa VI, Carson M, Ganju A, Chan AN, Carson WE 3rd (2015) MiR-21 enhances melanoma invasiveness via inhibition of tissue inhibitor of metalloproteinases 3 expression: in vivo effects of MiR-21 inhibitor. PLoS One 10:e0115919

Maru DM, Singh RR, Hannah C, Albarracin CT, Li YX, Abraham R, Romans AM, Yao H, Luthra MG, Anandasabapathy S, Swisher SG, Hofstetter WL, Rashid A, Luthra R (2009) MicroRNA-196a is a potential marker of progression during Barrett's metaplasia-dysplasia-invasive adenocarcinoma sequence in esophagus. Am J Pathol 174:1940–1948

Mascarenhas JB, Littlejohn EL, Wolsky RJ, Young KP, Nelson M, Salgia R, Lang D (2010) PAX3 and SOX10 activate MET receptor expression in melanoma. Pigment Cell Melanoma Res 23:225–237

Mattia G, Errico MC, Felicetti F, Petrini M, Bottero L, Tomasello L, Romania P, Boe A, Segnalini P, Di Virgilio A, Colombo MP, Care A (2011) Constitutive activation of the ETS-1-miR-222 circuitry in metastatic melanoma. Pigment Cell Melanoma Res 24:953–965

Mayr C, Bartel DP (2009) Widespread shortening of 3′UTRs by alternative cleavage and polyadenylation activates oncogenes in cancer cells. Cell 138:673–684

Mazar J, DeYoung K, Khaitan D, Meister E, Almodovar A, Goydos J, Ray A, Perera RJ (2010) The regulation of miRNA-211 expression and its role in melanoma cell invasiveness. PLoS One 5:e13779

Mazar J, Khaitan D, DeBlasio D, Zhong C, Govindarajan SS, Kopanathi S, Zhang S, Ray A, Perera RJ (2011) Epigenetic regulation of microRNA genes and the role of miR-34b in cell invasion and motility in human melanoma. PLoS One 6:e24922

Mazar J, Qi F, Lee B, Marchica J, Govindarajan S, Shelley J, Li J-L, Ray A, Perera RJ (2016) miR-211 functions as a metabolic switch in human melanoma cells. Mol Cell Biol 00762–15

Melnik BC (2015) MiR-21: an environmental driver of malignant melanoma? J Transl Med 13:202

Melo SA, Ropero S, Moutinho C, Aaltonen LA, Yamamoto H, Calin GA, Rossi S, Fernandez AF, Carneiro F, Oliveira C, Ferreira B, Liu CG, Villanueva A, Capella G, Schwartz S Jr, Shiekhattar R, Esteller M (2009) A TARBP2 mutation in human cancer impairs microRNA processing and DICER1 function. Nat Genet 41:365–370

Meyer SU, Pfaffl MW, Ulbrich SE (2010) Normalization strategies for microRNA profiling experiments: a "normal" way to a hidden layer of complexity? Biotechnol Lett 32:1777–1788

Migliore C, Petrelli A, Ghiso E, Corso S, Capparuccia L, Eramo A, Comoglio PM, Giordano S (2008) MicroRNAs impair MET-mediated invasive growth. Cancer Res 68:10128–10136

Mione M, Bosserhoff A (2015) MicroRNAs in melanocyte and melanoma biology. Pigment Cell Melanoma Res 28:340–354

Mirnezami AH, Pickard K, Zhang L, Primrose JN, Packham G (2009) MicroRNAs: key players in carcinogenesis and novel therapeutic targets. Eur J Surg Oncol 35:339–347

Mitchell PS, Parkin RK, Kroh EM, Fritz BR, Wyman SK, Pogosova-Agadjanyan EL, Peterson A, Noteboom J, O'Briant KC, Allen A, Lin DW, Urban N, Drescher CW, Knudsen BS, Stirewalt DL, Gentleman R, Vessella RL, Nelson PS, Martin DB, Tewari M (2008) Circulating microRNAs as stable blood-based markers for cancer detection. Proc Natl Acad Sci U S A 105:10513–10518

Molnar V, Tamasi V, Bakos B, Wiener Z, Falus A (2008) Changes in miRNA expression in solid tumors: an miRNA profiling in melanomas. Semin Cancer Biol 18:111–122

Morrish F (2009) micRo-manageMeNT of MYC during hypoxia. Cell Cycle 8:2865

Mueller DW, Bosserhoff AK (2009) Role of miRNAs in the progression of malignant melanoma. Br J Cancer 101:551–556

Mueller DW, Bosserhoff AK (2010a) MicroRNA miR-196a controls melanoma-associated genes by regulating HOX-C8 expression. Int J Cancer 129(5):1064–1074

Mueller DW, Bosserhoff AK (2010b) The evolving concept of "melano-miRs"-microRNAs in melanomagenesis. Pigment Cell Melanoma Res 23:620–626

Mueller DW, Rehli M, Bosserhoff AK (2009) miRNA expression profiling in melanocytes and melanoma cell lines reveals miRNAs associated with formation and progression of malignant melanoma. J Invest Dermatol 129:1740–1751

Muller DW, Bosserhoff AK (2008) Integrin beta 3 expression is regulated by let-7a miRNA in malignant melanoma. Oncogene 27:6698–6706

Natali PG, Nicotra MR, Di Renzo MF, Prat M, Bigotti A, Cavaliere R, Comoglio PM (1993) Expression of the c-Met/HGF receptor in human melanocytic neoplasms: demonstration of the relationship to malignant melanoma tumour progression. Br J Cancer 68:746–750

Nemlich Y, Greenberg E, Ortenberg R, Besser MJ, Barshack I, Jacob-Hirsch J, Jacoby E, Eyal E, Rivkin L, Prieto VG, Chakravarti N, Duncan LM, Kallenberg DM, Galun E, Bennett DC, Amariglio N, Bar-Eli M, Schachter J, Rechavi G, Markel G (2013) MicroRNA-mediated loss of ADAR1 in metastatic melanoma promotes tumor growth. J Clin Invest 123:2703–2718

Ng D, Yang XR, Tucker MA, Goldstein AM (2008) Mutation screening of CHD5 in melanoma-prone families linked to 1p36 revealed no deleterious coding or splice site changes. BMC Res Notes 1:86

Nguyen T, Kuo C, Nicholl MB, Sim MS, Turner RR, Morton DL, Hoon DS (2011) Downregulation of microRNA-29c is associated with hypermethylation of tumor-related genes and disease outcome in cutaneous melanoma. Epigenetics 6:388–394

Nielsen CB, Shomron N, Sandberg R, Hornstein E, Kitzman J, Burge CB (2007) Determinants of targeting by endogenous and exogenous microRNAs and siRNAs. RNA 13:1894–1910

Noguchi S, Mori T, Hoshino Y, Yamada N, Nakagawa T, Sasaki N, Akao Y, Maruo K (2012a) Comparative study of anti-oncogenic microRNA-145 in canine and human malignant melanoma. J Vet Med Sci 74:1–8

Noguchi S, Mori T, Otsuka Y, Yamada N, Yasui Y, Iwasaki J, Kumazaki M, Maruo K, Akao Y (2012b) Anti-oncogenic microRNA-203 induces senescence by targeting E2F3 protein in human melanoma cells. J Biol Chem 287:11769–11777

Noguchi S, Kumazaki M, Mori T, Baba K, Okuda M, Mizuno T and Akao Y (2014) Analysis of microRNA-203 function in CREB/MITF/RAB27a pathway: comparison between canine and human melanoma cells. Vet Comp Oncol. doi: 10.1111/vco.12118.

Noguchi S, Kumazaki M, Yasui Y, Mori T, Yamada N, Akao Y (2014b) MicroRNA-203 regulates melanosome transport and tyrosinase expression in melanoma cells by targeting kinesin superfamily protein 5b. J Invest Dermatol 134:461–469

Noguchi S, Mori T, Nakagawa T, Itamoto K, Haraguchi T, Mizuno T (2015) DNA methylation contributes toward silencing of antioncogenic microRNA-203 in human and canine melanoma cells. Melanoma Res 25:390–398

Noman MZ, Buart S, Romero P, Ketari S, Janji B, Mari B, Mami-Chouaib F, Chouaib S (2012) Hypoxia-inducible miR-210 regulates the susceptibility of tumor cells to lysis by cytotoxic T cells. Cancer Res 72:4629–4641

Nyholm AM, Lerche CM, Manfé V, Biskup E, Johansen P, Morling N, Thomsen BM, Glud M, Gniadecki R (2014) MiR-125b induces cellular senescence in malignant melanoma. BMC Dermatol 14:8

Ohira T, Naohiro S, Nakayama Y, Osaki M, Okada F, Oshimura M, Kugoh H (2015) MiR-19b regulates hTERT mRNA expression through targeting PITX1 mRNA in melanoma cells. Sci Rep 5:8201

Okamura K, Liu N, Lai EC (2009) Distinct mechanisms for microRNA strand selection by *Drosophila argonautes*. Mol Cell 36:431–444

Olive V, Jiang I, He L (2010) mir-17-92, a cluster of miRNAs in the midst of the cancer network. Int J Biochem Cell Biol 42:1348–1354

Ono S, Oyama T, Lam S, Chong K, Foshag LJ, Hoon DS (2015) A direct plasma assay of circulating microRNA-210 of hypoxia can identify early systemic metastasis recurrence in melanoma patients. Oncotarget 6:7053–7064

Ozsolak F, Poling LL, Wang Z, Liu H, Liu XS, Roeder RG, Zhang X, Song JS, Fisher DE (2008) Chromatin structure analyses identify miRNA promoters. Genes Dev 22:3172–3183

Paroo Z, Ye X, Chen S, Liu Q (2009) Phosphorylation of the human microRNA-generating complex mediates MAPK/Erk signaling. Cell 139:112–122

Pasquinelli AE, Reinhart BJ, Slack F, Martindale MQ, Kuroda MI, Maller B, Hayward DC, Ball EE, Degnan B, Muller P, Spring J, Srinivasan A, Fishman M, Finnerty J, Corbo J, Levine M, Leahy P, Davidson E, Ruvkun G (2000) Conservation of the sequence and temporal expression of let-7 heterochronic regulatory RNA. Nature 408:86–89

Pencheva N, Tran H, Buss C, Huh D, Drobnjak M, Busam K, Tavazoie SF (2012) Convergent multi-miRNA targeting of ApoE drives LRP1/LRP8-dependent melanoma metastasis and angiogenesis. Cell 151:1068–1082

Penna E, Orso F, Cimino D, Tenaglia E, Lembo A, Quaglino E, Poliseno L, Haimovic A, Osella-Abate S, De Pitta C, Pinatel E, Stadler MB, Provero P, Bernengo MG, Osman I, Taverna D (2011) microRNA-214 contributes to melanoma tumour progression through suppression of TFAP2C. EMBO J 30:1990–2007

Penna E, Orso F, Cimino D, Vercellino I, Grassi E, Quaglino E, Turco E, Taverna D (2013) miR-214 coordinates melanoma progression by upregulating ALCAM through TFAP2 and miR-148b downmodulation. Cancer Res 73:4098–4111

Pennacchietti S, Michieli P, Galluzzo M, Mazzone M, Giordano S, Comoglio PM (2003) Hypoxia promotes invasive growth by transcriptional activation of the met protooncogene. Cancer Cell 3:347–361

Peterson SM, Thompson JA, Ufkin ML, Sathyanarayana P, Liaw L, Congdon CB (2014) Common features of microRNA target prediction tools. Front Genet 18:5–23

Pfeffer SR, Grossmann KF, Cassidy PB, Yang CH, Fan M, Kopelovich L, Leachman SA, Pfeffer LM (2015) Detection of exosomal miRNAs in the plasma of melanoma patients. J Clin Med 4:2012–2027

Philippidou D, Schmitt M, Moser D, Margue C, Nazarov PV, Muller A, Vallar L, Nashan D, Behrmann I, Kreis S (2010) Signatures of microRNAs and selected microRNA target genes in human melanoma. Cancer Res 70:4163–4173

Piérard GE, Piérard-Franchimont C (2012) HOX gene aberrant expression in skin melanoma: a review. J Skin Cancer 2012:707260
Pillai RS, Bhattacharyya SN, Artus CG, Zoller T, Cougot N, Basyuk E, Bertrand E, Filipowicz W (2005) Inhibition of translational initiation by Let-7 MicroRNA in human cells. Science 309:1573–1576
Pinto R, Strippoli S, De Summa S, Albano A, Azzariti A, Guida G, Popescu O, Lorusso V, Guida M, Tommasi S (2015) MicroRNA expression in BRAF-mutated and wild- type metastatic melanoma and its correlation with response duration to BRAF inhibitors. Expert Opin Ther Targets 19:1027–1035
Poetsch M, Dittberner T, Woenckhaus C (2003) Microsatellite analysis at 1p36.3 in malignant melanoma of the skin: fine mapping in search of a possible tumour suppressor gene region. Melanoma Res 13:29–33
Poliseno L, Haimovic A, Segura MF, Hanniford D, Christos PJ, Darvishian F, Wang J, Shapiro RL, Pavlick AC, Berman RS, Hernando E, Zavadil J, Osman I (2012) Histology-specific microRNA alterations in melanoma. J Invest Dermatol 132:1860–1868
Prasad R, Katiyar SK (2014) Down-regulation of miRNA-106b inhibits growth of melanoma cells by promoting G1-phase cell cycle arrest and reactivation of p21/WAF1/Cip1 protein. Oncotarget 5:10636–10649
Puri N, Ahmed S, Janamanchi V, Tretiakova M, Zumba O, Krausz T, Jagadeeswaran R, Salgia R (2007) c-Met is a potentially new therapeutic target for treatment of human melanoma. Clin Cancer Res 13:2246–2253
Qi M, Huang X, Zhou L, Zhang J (2014) Identification of differentially expressed microRNAs in metastatic melanoma using next-generation sequencing technology. Int J Mol Med 33:1117–1121
Raver-Shapira N, Marciano E, Meiri E, Spector Y, Rosenfeld N, Moskovits N, Bentwich Z, Oren M (2007) Transcriptional activation of miR-34a contributes to p53-mediated apoptosis. Mol Cell 26:731–743
Reinhart BJ, Slack FJ, Basson M, Pasquinelli AE, Bettinger JC, Rougvie AE, Horvitz HR, Ruvkun G (2000) The 21-nucleotide let-7 RNA regulates developmental timing in *Caenorhabditis elegans*. Nature 403:901–906
Reuland SN, Smith SM, Bemis LT, Goldstein NB, Almeida AR, Partyka KA, Marquez VE, Zhang Q, Norris DA, Shellman YG (2013) MicroRNA-26a is strongly downregulated in melanoma and induces cell death through repression of silencer of death domains (SODD). J Invest Dermatol 133:1286–1293
Reyes-Herrera PH, Ficarra E (2012) One decade of development and evolution of microRNA target prediction algorithms. Genomics Proteomics Bioinformatics 10:254–263
Rosenfeld N, Aharonov R, Meiri E, Rosenwald S, Spector Y, Zepeniuk M, Benjamin H, Shabes N, Tabak S, Levy A, Lebanony D, Goren Y, Silberschein E, Targan N, Ben Ari A, Gilad S, Sion-Vardy N, Tobar A, Feinmesser M, Kharenko O, Nativ O, Nass D, Perelman M, Yosepovich A, Shalmon B, Polak-Charcon S, Fridman E, Avniel A, Bentwich I, Bentwich Z, Cohen D, Chajut A, Barshack I (2008) MicroRNAs accurately identify cancer tissue origin. Nat Biotechnol 26:462–469
Rothhammer T, Poser I, Soncin F, Bataille F, Moser M, Bosserhoff AK (2005) Bone morphogenic proteins are overexpressed in malignant melanoma and promote cell invasion and migration. Cancer Res 65:448–456
Rothhammer T, Braig S, Bosserhoff AK (2008) Bone morphogenetic proteins induce expression of metalloproteinases in melanoma cells and fibroblasts. Eur J Cancer 44:2526–2534
Sakurai E, Maesawa C, Shibazaki M, Yasuhira S, Oikawa H, Sato M, Tsunoda K, Ishikawa Y, Watanabe A, Takahashi K, Akasaka T, Masuda T (2011) Downregulation of microRNA-211 is involved in expression of preferentially expressed antigen of melanoma in melanoma cells. Int J Oncol 39:665–672
Saleiban A, Faxalv L, Claesson K, Jonsson JI, Osman A (2014) miR-20b regulates expression of proteinase-activated receptor-1 (PAR-1) thrombin receptor in melanoma cells. Pigment Cell Melanoma Res 27:431–441

Sand M, Skrygan M, Georgas D, Arenz C, Gambichler T, Sand D, Altmeyer P, Bechara FG (2012a) Expression levels of the microRNA maturing microprocessor complex component DGCR8 and the NA-induced silencing complex (RISC) components argonaute-1, argonaute-2, PACT, TARBP1, and TARBP2 in epithelial skin cancer. Mol Carcinog 51(11):916–922

Sand M, Skrygan M, Georgas D, Sand D, Gambichler T, Altmeyer P, Bechara FG (2012b) The miRNA machinery in primary cutaneous malignant melanoma, cutaneous malignant melanoma metastases and benign melanocytic nevi. Cell Tissue Res 350:119–126

Sand M, Skrygan M, Sand D, Georgas D, Gambichler T, Hahn SA, Altmeyer P, Bechara FG (2013) Comparative microarray analysis of microRNA expression profiles in primary cutaneous malignant melanoma, cutaneous malignant melanoma metastases, and benign melanocytic nevi. Cell Tissue Res 351:85–98

Sarkar D, Leszczyniecka M, Kang DC, Lebedeva IV, Valerie K, Dhar S, Pandita TK, Fisher PB (2003) Down-regulation of Myc as a potential target for growth arrest induced by human polynucleotide phosphorylase (hPNPaseold-35) in human melanoma cells. J Biol Chem 278:24542–24551

Sarkar D, Park ES, Fisher PB (2006) Defining the mechanism by which IFN-beta dowregulates c-myc expression in human melanoma cells: pivotal role for human polynucleotide phosphorylase (hPNPaseold-35). Cell Death Differ 13:1541–1553

Satzger I, Mattern A, Kuettler U, Weinspach D, Voelker B, Kapp A, Gutzmer R (2010) MicroRNA-15b represents an independent prognostic parameter and is correlated with tumor cell proliferation and apoptosis in malignant melanoma. Int J Cancer 126:2553–2562

Satzger I, Mattern A, Kuettler U, Weinspach D, Niebuhr M, Kapp A, Gutzmer R (2012) microRNA-21 is upregulated in malignant melanoma and influences apoptosis of melanocytic cells. Exp Dermatol 21:509–514

Schimanski CC, Frerichs K, Rahman F, Berger M, Lang H, Galle PR, Moehler M, Gockel I (2009) High miR-196a levels promote the oncogenic phenotype of colorectal cancer cells. World J Gastroenterol 15:2089–2096

Schmitt MJ, Philippidou D, Reinsbach SE, Margue C, Wienecke-Baldacchino A, Nashan D, Behrmann I, Kreis S (2012) Interferon-gamma-induced activation of Signal Transducer and Activator of Transcription 1 (STAT1) up-regulates the tumor suppressing microRNA-29 family in melanoma cells. Cell Commun Signal 10:41

Schultz J, Lorenz P, Gross G, Ibrahim S, Kunz M (2008) MicroRNA let-7b targets important cell cycle molecules in malignant melanoma cells and interferes with anchorage-independent growth. Cell Res 18:549–557

Segura MF, Hanniford D, Menendez S, Reavie L, Zou X, Alvarez-Diaz S, Zakrzewski J, Blochin E, Rose A, Bogunovic D, Polsky D, Wei J, Lee P, Belitskaya-Levy I, Bhardwaj N, Osman I, Hernando E (2009) Aberrant miR-182 expression promotes melanoma metastasis by repressing FOXO3 and microphthalmia-associated transcription factor. Proc Natl Acad Sci U S A 106:1814–1819

Segura MF, Belitskaya-Levy I, Rose AE, Zakrzewski J, Gaziel A, Hanniford D, Darvishian F, Berman RS, Shapiro RL, Pavlick AC, Osman I, Hernando E (2010) Melanoma MicroRNA signature predicts post-recurrence survival. Clin Cancer Res 16:1577–1586

Shah N, Sukumar S (2010) The Hox genes and their roles in oncogenesis. Nat Rev Cancer 10:361–371

Shi Q, Zhang W, Guo S, Jian Z, Li S, Li K, Ge R, Dai W, Wang G, Gao T, Li C (2016) Oxidative stress-induced overexpression of miR-25: the mechanism underlying the degeneration of melanocytes in vitiligo. Cell Death Differ 23(3):496–508

Shoshan E, Mobley AK, Braeuer RR, Kamiya T, Huang L, Vasquez ME, Salameh A, Lee HJ, Kim SJ, Ivan C, Velazquez-Torres G, Nip KM, Zhu K, Brooks D, Jones SJ, Birol I, Mosqueda M, Wen YY, Eterovic AK, Sood AK, Hwu P, Gershenwald JE, Robertson AG, Calin GA, Markel G, Fidler IJ, Bar-Eli M (2015) Reduced adenosine-to-inosine miR-455-5p editing promotes melanoma growth and metastasis. Nat Cell Biol 17:311–321

Slack FJ, Basson M, Liu Z, Ambros V, Horvitz HR, Ruvkun G (2000) The lin-41 RBCC gene acts in the *C. elegans* heterochronic pathway between the let-7 regulatory RNA and the LIN-29 transcription factor. Mol Cell 5:659–669

Slominski A, Wortsman J, Carlson AJ, Matsuoka LY, Balch CM, Mihm MC (2001) Malignant melanoma. Arch Pathol Lab Med 125:1295–1306

Soengas MS, Lowe SW (2003) Apoptosis and melanoma chemoresistance. Oncogene 22:3138–3151

Standart N, Jackson RJ (2007) MicroRNAs repress translation of m7G ppp-capped target mRNAs in vitro by inhibiting initiation and promoting deadenylation. Genes Dev 21:1975–1982

Stark MS, Tyagi S, Nancarrow DJ, Boyle GM, Cook AL, Whiteman DC, Parsons PG, Schmidt C, Sturm RA, Hayward NK (2010) Characterization of the melanoma miRNAome by deep sequencing. PLoS One 5:e9685

Stark MS, Bonazzi VF, Boyle GM, Palmer JM, Symmons J, Lanagan CM, Schmidt CW, Herington AC, Ballotti R, Pollock PM, Hayward NK (2015a) miR-514a regulates the tumour suppressor NF1 and modulates BRAFi sensitivity in melanoma. Oncotarget 6:17753–17763

Stark MS, Klein K, Weide B, Haydu LE, Pflugfelder A, Tang YH, Palmer JM, Whiteman DC, Scolyer RA, Mann GJ, Thompson JF, Long GV, Barbour AP, Soyer HP, Garbe C, Herington A, Pollock PM, Hayward NK (2015b) The prognostic and predictive value of melanoma-related microRNAs using tissue and serum: a MicroRNA expression analysis. EBioMedicine 2:671–680

Streicher KL, Zhu W, Lehmann KP, Georgantas RW, Morehouse CA, Brohawn P, Carrasco RA, Xiao Z, Tice DA, Higgs BW, Richman L, Jallal B, Ranade K, Yao Y (2012) A novel oncogenic role for the miRNA-506-514 cluster in initiating melanocyte transformation and promoting melanoma growth. Oncogene 31:1558–1570

Strong AMP, Setaluri V, Spiegelman VS (2014) microRNA-340 as a modulator of RAS–RAF–MAPK signaling in melanoma. Arch Biochem Biophys 563:118–124

Tarasov V, Jung P, Verdoodt B, Lodygin D, Epanchintsev A, Menssen A, Meister G, Hermeking H (2007) Differential regulation of microRNAs by p53 revealed by massively parallel sequencing: miR-34a is a p53 target that induces apoptosis and G1-arrest. Cell Cycle 6:1586–1593

Terzian T, Torchia EC, Dai D, Robinson SE, Murao K, Stiegmann RA, Gonzalez V, Boyle GM, Powell MB, Pollock P, Lozano G, Robinson WA, Roop DR, Box NF (2010) p53 prevents progression of nevi to melanoma predominantly through cell cycle regulation. Pigment Cell Melanoma Res 23(6):781–794

The Cancer Genome Atlas Network (2015) Genomic classification of cutaneous melanoma. Cell 161:1681–1696

Tian R, Liu T, Qiao L, Gao M, Li J (2015) Decreased serum microRNA-206 level predicts unfavorable prognosis in patients with melanoma. Int J Clin Exp Pathol 8:3097–3103

Till S, Lejeune E, Thermann R, Bortfeld M, Hothorn M, Enderle D, Heinrich C, Hentze MW, Ladurner AG (2007) A conserved motif in Argonaute-interacting proteins mediates functional interactions through the Argonaute PIWI domain. Nat Struct Mol Biol 14:897–903

Toyota M, Suzuki H, Sasaki Y, Maruyama R, Imai K, Shinomura Y, Tokino T (2008) Epigenetic silencing of microRNA-34b/c and B-cell translocation gene 4 is associated with CpG island methylation in colorectal cancer. Cancer Res 68:4123–4132

Triboulet R, Chang HM, Lapierre RJ, Gregory RI (2009) Post-transcriptional control of DGCR8 expression by the microprocessor. RNA 15:1005–1011

Turner MJ, Slack FJ (2009) Transcriptional control of microRNA expression in C. elegans: promoting better understanding. RNA Biol 6:49–53

Valadi H, Ekström K, Bossios A, Sjöstrand M, Lee JJ, Lötvall JO (2007) Exosome-mediated transfer of mRNAs and microRNAs is a novel mechanism of genetic exchange between cells. Nat Cell Biol 9:654–659

Van Belle PA, Elenitsas R, Satyamoorthy K, Wolfe JT, Guerry D, Schuchter L, Van Belle TJ, Albelda S, Tahin P, Herlyn M, Elder DE (1999) Progression-related expression of beta3 integrin in melanomas and nevi. Hum Pathol 30:562–567 van Kempen LC, van den Hurk K, Lazar V, Michiels S, Winnepenninckx V, Stas M, Spatz A, van den Oord JJ (2012) Loss of microRNA-200a and c, and microRNA-203 expression at the invasive front of primary cutaneous melanoma is associated with increased thickness and disease progression. Virchows Arch 461:441–448

Van Rooij E, Purcell AL, Levin AA (2012) Developing microRNA therapeutics. Circ Res 110:496–507

Vasudevan S, Tong Y, Steitz JA (2007) Switching from repression to activation: microRNAs can up-regulate translation. Science 318:1931–1934

Vasudevan S, Tong Y, Steitz JA (2008) Cell-cycle control of microRNA-mediated translation regulation. Cell Cycle 7:1545–1549

Venza I, Visalli M, Beninati C, Benfatto S, Teti D, Venza M (2015) IL-10Ralpha expression is post-transcriptionally regulated by miR-15a, miR-185, and miR-211 in melanoma. BMC Med Genomics 8:81

Vergani E, Di Guardo L, Dugo M, Rigoletto S, Tragni G, Ruggeri R, Perrone F, Tamborini E, Gloghini A, Arienti F, Vergani B, Deho P, De Cecco L, Vallacchi V, Frati P, Shahaj E, Villa A, Santinami M, De Braud F, Rivoltini L, Rodolfo M (2016) Overcoming melanoma resistance to vemurafenib by targeting CCL2-induced miR-34a, miR-100 and miR-125b. Oncotarget 7(4):4428–4441

Vickers KC, Palmisano BT, Shoucri BM, Shamburek RD, Remaley AT (2011) MicroRNAs are transported in plasma and delivered to recipient cells by high-density lipoproteins. Nat Cell Biol 13:423–433

Visone R, Croce CM (2009) MiRNAs and cancer. Am J Pathol 174:1131–1138

Voeller D, Reinders J, Meister G, Bosserhoff AK (2013) Strong reduction of AGO2 expression in melanoma and cellular consequences. Br J Cancer 109:3116–3124

Volinia S, Calin GA, Liu CG, Ambs S, Cimmino A, Petrocca F, Visone R, Iorio M, Roldo C, Ferracin M, Prueitt RL, Yanaihara N, Lanza G, Scarpa A, Vecchione A, Negrini M, Harris CC, Croce CM (2006) A microRNA expression signature of human solid tumors defines cancer gene targets. Proc Natl Acad Sci U S A 103:2257–2261

Walker GJ, Indsto JO, Sood R, Faruque MU, Hu P, Pollock PM, Duray P, Holland EA, Brown K, Kefford RF, Trent JM, Mann GJ, Hayward NK (2004) Deletion mapping suggests that the 1p22 melanoma susceptibility gene is a tumor suppressor localized to a 9-Mb interval. Genes Chromosomes Cancer 41:56–64

Wang P, Li Y, Hong W, Zhen J, Ren J, Li Z, Xu A (2012) The changes of microRNA expression profiles and tyrosinase related proteins in MITF knocked down melanocytes. Mol Biosyst 8:2924–2931

Wang HF, Chen H, Ma MW, Wang JA, Tang TT, Ni LS, Yu JL, Li YZ, Bai BX (2013a) miR-573 regulates melanoma progression by targeting the melanoma cell adhesion molecule. Oncol Rep 30:520–526

Wang J, Chong KK, Nakamura Y, Nguyen L, Huang SK, Kuo C, Zhang W, Yu H, Morton DL, Hoon DS (2013b) B7-H3 associated with tumor progression and epigenetic regulatory activity in cutaneous melanoma. J Invest Dermatol 133:2050–2058

Webb CP, Taylor GA, Jeffers M, Fiscella M, Oskarsson M, Resau JH, Vande Woude GF (1998) Evidence for a role of Met-HGF/SF during ras-mediated tumorigenesis/metastasis. Oncogene 17:2019–2025

Wei JS, Song YK, Durinck S, Chen QR, Cheuk AT, Tsang P, Zhang Q, Thiele CJ, Slack A, Shohet J, Khan J (2008) The MYCN oncogene is a direct target of miR-34a. Oncogene 27:5204–5213

Wei Y, Du Y, Chen X, Li P, Wang Y, Zang W, Zhao L, Li Z, Zhao G (2014) Expression patterns of microRNA-218 and its potential functions by targeting CIP2A and BMI1 genes in melanoma. Tumour Biol 35:8007–8015

Welch C, Chen Y, Stallings RL (2007) MicroRNA-34a functions as a potential tumor suppressor by inducing apoptosis in neuroblastoma cells. Oncogene 26:5017–5022

Wightman B, Ha I, Ruvkun G (1993) Posttranscriptional regulation of the heterochronic gene lin-14 by lin-4 mediates temporal pattern formation in *C. elegans*. Cell 75:855–862

Winter J, Jung S, Keller S, Gregory RI, Diederichs S (2009) Many roads to maturity: microRNA biogenesis pathways and their regulation. Nat Cell Biol 11:228–234

Wu L, Belasco JG (2005) Micro-RNA regulation of the mammalian lin-28 gene during neuronal differentiation of embryonal carcinoma cells. Mol Cell Biol 25:9198–9208

Wu L, Fan J, Belasco JG (2006) MicroRNAs direct rapid deadenylation of mRNA. Proc Natl Acad Sci U S A 103:4034–4039

Xu Y, Brenn T, Brown ER, Doherty V, Melton DW (2012) Differential expression of microRNAs during melanoma progression: miR-200c, miR-205 and miR-211 are downregulated in melanoma and act as tumour suppressors. Br J Cancer 106:553–561

Yamazaki H, Chijiwa T, Inoue Y, Abe Y, Suemizu H, Kawai K, Wakui M, Furukawa D, Mukai M, Kuwao S, Saegusa M, Nakamura M (2012) Overexpression of the miR-34 family suppresses invasive growth of malignant melanoma with the wild-type p53 gene. Exp Ther Med 3:793–796

Yang CH, Yue J, Pfeffer SR, Handorf CR, Pfeffer LM (2011) MicroRNA miR-21 regulates the metastatic behavior of B16 melanoma cells. J Biol Chem 286:39172–39178

Yang CH, Pfeffer SR, Sims M, Yue J, Wang Y, Linga VG, Paulus E, Davidoff AM, Pfeffer LM (2015) The oncogenic microRNA-21 inhibits the tumor suppressive activity of FBXO11 to promote tumorigenesis. J Biol Chem 290:6037–6046

Yekta S, Shih IH, Bartel DP (2004) MicroRNA-directed cleavage of HOXB8 mRNA. Science 304:594–596

Zehavi L, Avraham R, Barzilai A, Bar-Ilan D, Navon R, Sidi Y, Avni D, Leibowitz-Amit R (2012) Silencing of a large microRNA cluster on human chromosome 14q32 in melanoma: biological effects of mir-376a and mir-376c on insulin growth factor 1 receptor. Mol Cancer 11:44

Zehavi L, Schayek H, Jacob-Hirsch J, Sidi Y, Leibowitz-Amit R, Avni D (2015) MiR-377 targets E2F3 and alters the NF-kB signaling pathway through MAP3K7 in malignant melanoma. Mol Cancer 14:68

Zeng Y, Cullen BR (2003) Sequence requirements for micro RNA processing and function in human cells. RNA 9:112–123

Zeng Y, Cullen BR (2005) Efficient processing of primary microRNA hairpins by Drosha requires flanking nonstructured RNA sequences. J Biol Chem 280:27595–27603

Zenz T, Mohr J, Eldering E, Kater AP, Buhler A, Kienle D, Winkler D, Durig J, van Oers MH, Mertens D, Dohner H, Stilgenbauer S (2009) miR-34a as part of the resistance network in chronic lymphocytic leukemia. Blood 113:3801–3808

Zhang L, Huang J, Yang N, Greshock J, Megraw MS, Giannakakis A, Liang S, Naylor TL, Barchetti A, Ward MR, Yao G, Medina A, O'brien-Jenkins A, Katsaros D, Hatzigeorgiou A, Gimotty PA, Weber BL, Coukos G (2006) microRNAs exhibit high frequency genomic alterations in human cancer. Proc Natl Acad Sci U S A 103:9136–9141

Zhang Z, Sun H, Dai H, Walsh RM, Imakura M, Schelter J, Burchard J, Dai X, Chang AN, Diaz RL, Marszalek JR, Bartz SR, Carleton M, Cleary MA, Linsley PS, Grandori C (2009) MicroRNA miR-210 modulates cellular response to hypoxia through the MYC antagonist MNT. Cell Cycle 8:2756–2768

Zhang J, Lu L, Xiong Y, Qin W, Zhang Y, Qian Y, Jiang H, Liu W (2014) MLK3 promotes melanoma proliferation and invasion and is a target of microRNA-125b. Clin Exp Dermatol 39:376–384

Zhang J, Li S, Li L, Li M, Guo C, Yao J, Mi S (2015a) Exosome and exosomal microRNA: trafficking, sorting, and function. Genomics Proteomics Bioinformatics 13:17–24

Zhang J, Na S, Liu C, Pan S, Cai J, Qiu J (2015b) MicroRNA-125b suppresses the epithelial-mesenchymal transition and cell invasion by targeting ITGA9 in melanoma. Tumour Biol. 2016;37(5):5941–9

Zhang Z, Zhang S, Ma P, Jing Y, Peng H, Gao WQ, Zhuang G (2015c) Lin28B promotes melanoma growth by mediating a microRNA regulatory circuit. Carcinogenesis 36:937–945

Zhao G, Li Q, Wang A, Jiao J (2015) YY1 regulates melanoma tumorigenesis through a miR-9 ~ RYBP axis. J Exp Clin Cancer Res 34:1

Zheng H, Fu R, Wang J-T, Liu O, Chen H, Jiang SW (2013) Advances in the techniques for the prediction of microRNA targets. Int J Mol Sci 14:8179–8187

Zhou J, Xu D, Xie H, Tang J, Liu R, Li J, Wang S, Chen X, Su J, Zhou X, Xia K, He Q, Chen J, Xiong W, Cao P, Cao K (2015) miR-33a functions as a tumor suppressor in melanoma by targeting HIF-1alpha. Cancer Biol Ther 16:846–855

Altered Signal Transduction Pathways in Melanoma

7

Yann Cheli, Eric Lau, and Ze'ev A. Ronai

7.1 Introduction

Signal transduction pathways are central to all cellular biological processes, as they provide the link between extracellular or intracellular stimuli and an array of regulatory proteins, including protein kinases, ubiquitin ligases, and transcription factors. Given this, it is not surprising that signal transduction pathways are often deregulated in cancer. Indeed, melanoma is a paradigm for rewired signaling because most critical mutations discovered in this tumor type are centered around relatively few major signaling cues, the most significant of which are the mitogen-activated protein kinase (MAPK) and phosphatidylinositol-3-kinase (PI3K) pathways. Both pathways contain regulatory components with catalytic activities, making them the preferred targets for therapy. Here, we summarize our current understanding of the major deregulated signaling pathways in melanoma and the implications of such deregulation for tumor biology.

7.1.1 Extracellular Receptors

Among the receptors reported to be deregulated in melanoma are numerous membrane-bound G protein-coupled receptors and receptor tyrosine kinases (RTKs), including MC1R (melanocortin 1 receptor), c-Kit (mast/stem cell growth factor receptor), c-Met (hepatocyte growth factor receptor), IGFR (insulin-like

Y. Cheli • E. Lau
Tumor Initiation and Maintenance Program, Cancer Center, Sanford Burnham Prebys Medical Discovery Institute, La Jolla, CA 92037, USA

Z.A. Ronai (✉)
Sanford Burnham Prebys Medical Discovery Institute,
10901 North Torrey Pines Road, La Jolla, CA 92037, USA
e-mail: zeev@ronailab.net

A. Bosserhoff (ed.), *Melanoma Development*,
DOI 10.1007/978-3-319-41319-8_7

growth factor receptor), and Frizzled (WNT receptor). Deregulation of other RTKs, including AXL, epidermal growth factor receptor (EGFR), fibroblast growth factor receptor (FGFR), and vascular endothelial growth factor receptor (VEGFR), has also been implicated in the resistance of melanomas to certain treatments such as BRAF inhibitors (BRAFi) (Fargnoli et al. 2010; Landi et al. 2006; Mattei et al. 1994; Topcu-Yilmaz et al. 2010; van Ginkel et al. 2004).

7.1.1.1 MC1R

MC1R is a melanocyte-specific G protein-coupled receptor that binds to α-melanocyte-stimulating hormone (α-MSH, Fig. 7.1). MC1R–α-MSH interactions play a central role in the regulation of both pigmentation, by inducing generation of eumelanin and cAMP, and melanocyte proliferation (Hunt et al. 1995; Mountjoy et al. 1992; Robinson and Healy 2002; Suzuki et al. 1996).

MC1R exhibits genetic variance, with mutations at the hot spot residues R151C, R160W, and D294H being the most significant. The mutations reduce receptor function and result in a phenotype of fair, freckled skin and red hair (Kadekaro et al. 2003). Stimulation of MC1R by α-MSH normally potentiates p16INK4A tumor suppressor activity after UV exposure (Pavey et al. 2002); these specific mutations are associated with reduced UV-induced DNA damage repair efficiency and increased melanoma risk (Scott et al. 2002; Song et al. 2009). In contrast, overexpression of MC1R variants has been shown to render cells insensitive to α-MSH-mediated suppression of cell proliferation (Robinson and Healy 2002), suggesting that polymorphic variants of MC1R may enhance melanoma susceptibility or progression by attenuating p16INK4A function, at least in part.

Although MC1R is neither genetically nor epigenetically silenced (Kim et al. 2008a), expression of the functionally impaired variants compromises receptor activity and correlates with increased melanoma risk (Landi et al. 2006). Carriers of MC1R variants who have mutations in CDK2NA also have a higher melanoma risk (Fargnoli et al. 2010). Notably, germline mutations of MC1R are associated with an increased incidence of BRAF mutations in melanoma (Landi et al. 2006). Likewise, inactivation of MC1R in the $Braf^{V600E}$:$Pten^{-/-}$ mouse melanoma model increases the incidence of melanoma independently of UV radiation (Mitra et al. 2012).

Mutation of G proteins themselves, in particular the α-subunit of G(q) (GNAQ), may induce alterations in early melanoma lesions (Kusters-Vandevelde et al. 2010; Lamba et al. 2010; Van Raamsdonk et al. 2009). GNAQ is mutated within a RAS-like domain at position Q209L, which renders the protein constitutively active and amplifies PKC and MAPK signaling. Accordingly, overexpression of the GNAQ Q209L mutant is sufficient to confer anchorage independence and increase the tumorigenicity of immortalized melanocytes.

7.1.1.2 Receptor Tyrosine Kinases

Many cell surface receptors for growth factors, hormones, and cytokines are RTKs. Ligand binding activates the intrinsic RTK enzymatic activity, often by autophosphorylation, with subsequent phosphorylation of tyrosine residues on many substrates, including PLCγ, PI3K, and MAPK, which drive cell proliferation

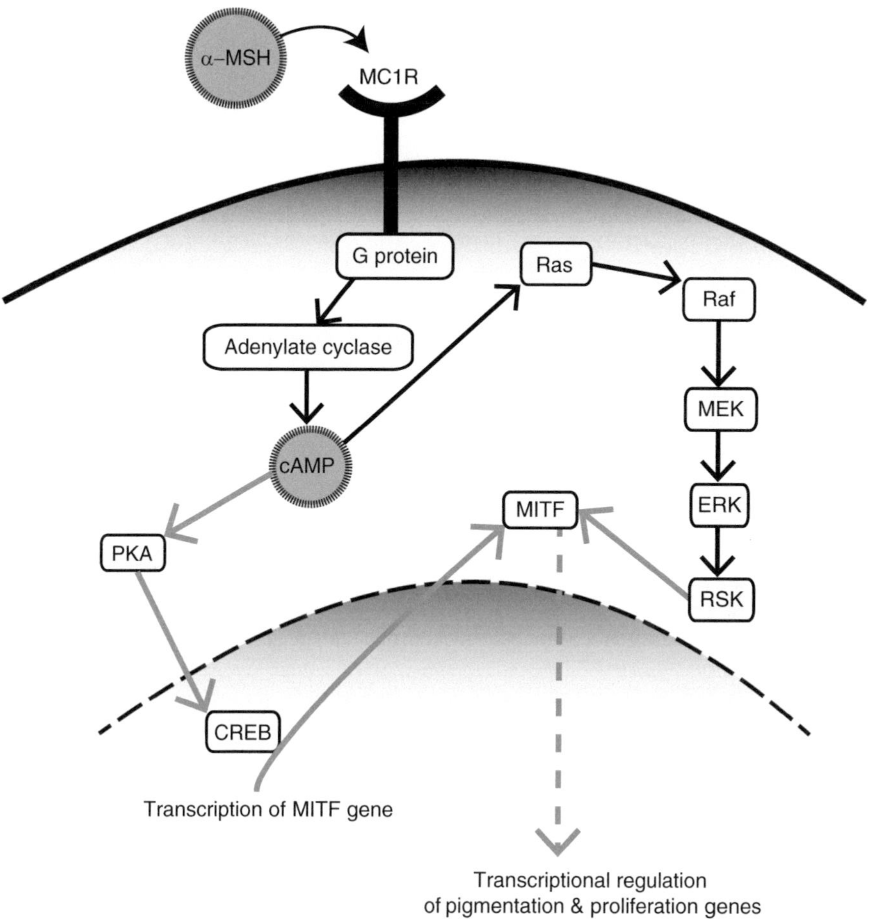

Fig. 7.1 α-MSH and MC1R receptor signaling. Binding of α-melanocyte stimulating hormone (*α-MSH*) to its cognate receptor melanocortin-1 receptor (*MC1R*) activates G protein-coupled adenylate cyclase and increases cytoplasmic cAMP levels. cAMP initiates a cascade that sequentially activates protein kinase A (*PKA*), CREB, and transcription of MITF. In parallel, cAMP activates the RAS–RAF–MAPK–RSK cascade, which results in MITF activation. MITF then modulates the transcription of downstream pigmentation and proliferation genes. Branches of this signaling pathway that are upregulated in melanoma are indicated in *black*. The *dashed arrow* indicates modulation of transcriptional programming by MITF to favor tumorigenesis

differentiation, survival, and cell migration. Among the growth factor RTKs deregulated in melanoma are AXL, EGFR, c-Kit, c-Met, and IGFR, which bind to growth arrest-specific 6 (Gas6), epidermal growth factor (EGF), stem cell factor (SCF), hepatocyte growth factor (HGF), and insulin-like growth factor (IGF), respectively (Fig. 7.2). Ligand binding by these receptors activates the downstream RAS–RAF–MEK–MAPK and PI3K–AKT signaling pathways independently of any existing MAPK pathway mutations and promotes cell survival and proliferation. Changes in

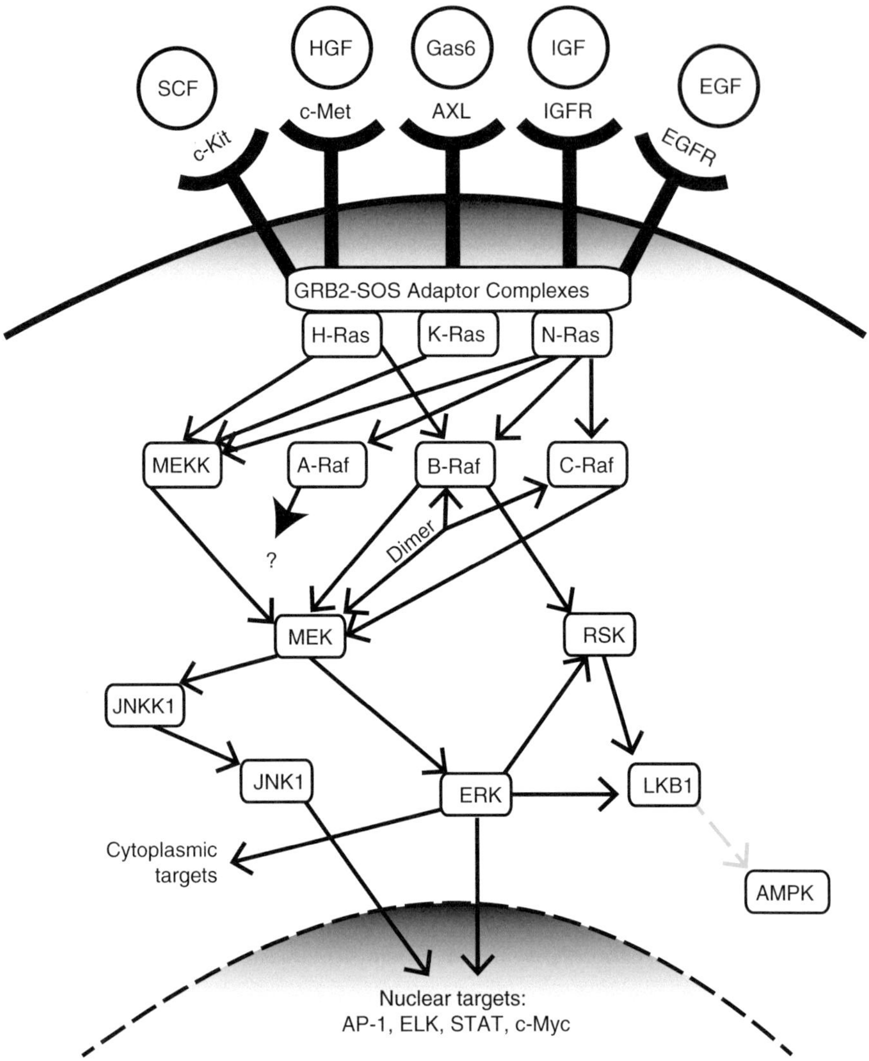

Fig. 7.2 Growth factor receptors and MAPK signaling. Membrane-bound growth factor receptors (*c-Kit, c-Met, IGFR, AXL, EGFR*) generally signal inwards through adaptor complexes containing proteins, such as GRB-SOS, which recruit the RAS family members HRAS, KRAS, or NRAS for activation. In melanoma, NRAS is the most commonly mutated protein and plays a predominant role in activation of the downstream effector kinases, RAF and MEKK. The RAF family of effector kinases includes A-, B-, and CRAF. Although signaling through ARAF has been less studied, in melanoma, it appears that BRAF- and CRAF-mediated signaling predominate. BRAF and CRAF activate downstream MEKK, MEK, and RSK. MEK activation leads to further downstream activation of JNKK1–JNK1 and ERK, as well as their cytoplasmic or nuclear transcriptional targets. Together, BRAF and ERK activate RSK to suppress LKB1, which would otherwise activate AMPK. In melanoma, this arm of AMPK activation, which normally regulates cell growth and survival, is downregulated (*gray dashed arrow*). Branches of the MAPK pathway that are upregulated in melanoma appear in *black*

the expression of these receptors have been implicated in several tumor types; in melanoma, altered expression has not been observed uniformly but may be associated with specific phases of tumor development.

7.1.1.3 AXL

AXL RTK is ubiquitously expressed in epithelial, mesenchymal, and hematopoietic tumors, and in the corresponding non-transformed cells. AXL was discovered in patients with chronic myeloproliferative disorder, and has since been implicated in the proliferation and drug resistance of numerous cancers, including melanoma (Paccez et al. 2014).

AXL is upregulated in ocular melanomas and melanoma cell lines, where it promotes cell proliferation and confers a survival advantage under serum starvation conditions (van Ginkel et al. 2004). Increased AXL expression is also found in both NRAS- or BRAF-mutated tumors, although the incidence is higher in NRAS mutant melanomas. Of interest, AXL expression inversely correlates with melanoma differentiation and microphthalmia-associated transcription factor (MITF) expression (Muller et al. 2014), and the combination of low MITF and high AXL expression is associated with a highly invasive phenotype. Pharmacological AXL inhibitors attenuate but do not abolish the invasive phenotype (Sensi et al. 2011), indicating a role for other RTKs and/or signaling pathways in the invasive phenotype. In response to chemotherapy, a subset of tumor cells that exhibit a senescence phenotype show elevated production and secretion of cytokines (Ohanna et al. 2011), with concomitant activation of STAT3 and AXL and increased migration and invasion properties in surrounding cells (Ohanna et al. 2013).

Lastly, a major clinical obstacle in melanoma therapy is the acquisition of resistance to either BRAFi or MEKi. The mechanisms underlying such resistance include upregulation of AXL, among many RTKs, which coincides with low levels of MITF and activation of NF-kB and JAK1 (Konieczkowski et al. 2014). Accordingly, treatment of resistant melanomas with a pharmacological inhibitor of AXL augments the effect of the BRAFi or MEKi and enhances cell death (Muller et al. 2014).

7.1.1.4 EGFR

EGFR is a transmembrane receptor for members of the EGF family of growth factors. Increased expression or mutation of the EGFR gene is commonly seen in a number of tumor types, including colorectal, breast, and non-small cell lung cancers, where it is thought to serve as an oncogenic driver.

EGFR upregulation has been implicated as a mechanism of therapy resistance for several tumor types, including melanoma. Consistent with this, co-administration of BRAFi and EGFRi appears to attenuate ERK activity and sensitizes resistant melanomas to BRAFi or MEKi inhibition (Girotti et al. 2013). The resistance of $BRAF^{V600E}$ mutant colorectal cancer to BRAFi therapy has also been associated with high EGFR expression, which enables reactivation of ERK via RAS and CRAF to bypass BRAF inhibition (Corcoran et al. 2012).

Elevated EGFR expression, as observed in resistant melanoma, has been linked to SOX10 and MITF expression (Ji et al. 2015). Furthermore, EGFR upregulation is often accompanied by upregulation of other RTKs that are associated with SOX10 and TGF-β signaling, including platelet-derived growth factor receptor β (Sun et al. 2014).

Interestingly, SOX10 was also found to regulate the expression of the ubiquitin ligase RNF125, which controls JAK1 stability through ubiquitin–proteasome-dependent degradation. BRAFi-resistant melanomas exhibit downregulation of SOX10 and concomitant inhibition of RNF125 expression. Consequently, JAK1 stability and availability increase, and the expression of several RTKs, including EGFR and AXL, is stimulated. As might be expected, inhibition of JAK1 effectively reduces the expression of RTKs and overcomes the resistance of melanomas to BRAFi (Kim et al. 2015).

7.1.1.5 c-Kit

c-Kit expression is apparent in early or radial growth phase melanomas. Although the penetrance appears to be low, a c-Kit-activating mutation, L576P, has been reported in melanoma (Antonescu et al. 2007; Rivera et al. 2008; Willmore-Payne et al. 2006). Interestingly, however, downregulation of c-Kit expression is associated with melanoma progression (Giehl et al. 2007; Janku et al. 2005; Montone et al. 1997; Natali et al. 1992). These observations suggest that upregulation of c-Kit and its ligand SCF may be required to establish the primary lesions, but that continued expression of c-Kit is not needed for invasion and metastasis. The disparity of mutations in or altered expression of c-Kit among different melanomas was initially overlooked in clinical trials of c-Kit-specific inhibitors. In more recent trials, clinical efficacy has been observed when patient cohorts harboring c-Kit mutations were treated with the highly selective pharmacological inhibitor, Gleevec (Terheyden et al. 2010). How inhibition of c-Kit contributes to melanoma progression remains an important topic for investigation. The c-Kit ligand SCF is a keratinocyte-secreted factor, and it has been proposed that downregulation of c-Kit in melanoma cells may allow them to escape SCF-induced cell death. Indeed, *in vitro* studies have shown that re-expression of c-Kit in metastatic melanoma sensitizes the cells to SCF-mediated apoptosis and reduces their tumorigenic and metastatic potential in vivo (Bar-Eli 1997; Huang et al. 1996; Willmore-Payne et al. 2005).

Although the mechanism by which c-Kit is downregulated during melanoma progression remains unclear, a recent study found that downregulation may be epigenetically linked to expression of microRNAs (miRNAs) (see also Chap. 6), specifically miR-221 and miR-222, which were shown to suppress expression of both c-Kit and p27Kip (Felicetti et al. 2008).

7.1.1.6 c-Met

c-Met-dependent signaling is amplified in melanoma, although genetic mutations or modifications that result in aberrant activation of c-Met do not appear to be common. Two c-Met mutations, N948S and R988C, have been identified in melanoma cell lines and tumor tissues and shown to activate c-Met signaling through several downstream effectors, including MITF, tyrosinase, and AKT and its effectors (Chin et al. 2006; Puri et al. 2007). However, c-Met upregulation has also been observed in melanoma, particularly in the later stages of disease (Natali et al. 1993). This has been suggested to play a role in metastasis, especially in the liver (Rusciano et al. 1995). Genetic amplification and activation of c-Met concomitant with Src activation has been reported in BRAFi-resistant melanoma cells; accordingly, genetic or pharmacological inhibition of c-Met attenuated the proliferation and invasion of the BRAFi-resistant cells (Vergani et al. 2011).

c-Met upregulation can be induced by a number of mechanisms. One is via MITF, which is induced by MC1R–α-MSH signaling, as mentioned above (Rouzaud et al. 2006; Rusciano et al. 1999). Indeed, impaired MC1R function, which is frequently observed in melanoma, is indicative of deregulated c-Met at both the genetic and protein levels.

The ubiquitin ligase skeletotrophin is another protein implicated in the regulation of c-Met. In melanoma, expression of skeletotrophin is lost due to increased SNAIL-mediated transcriptional repression. Re-expression of skeletotrophin impairs the invasive capacity of melanoma cells *in vitro*, and this correlates with a reduction in c-Met mRNA transcripts (Takeuchi et al. 2006). MicroRNAs have been shown to contribute to increased c-Met levels in melanoma. miR-34a is normally expressed in melanocytes but is downregulated in melanoma. Here too, re-expression of miR-34a *in vitro* reduces c-Met expression and suppresses the growth, migration, and invasive capacities of melanoma cells (Yan et al. 2009).

7.1.1.7 IGFR1

IGF1R is another growth factor receptor that is upregulated in progressively malignant melanoma (Mallikarjuna et al. 2006). In early melanoma lesions, IGF1R appears to enhance cellular growth and survival by promoting MAPK- and ß-catenin-dependent signaling pathways; however, IGF1R-dependent stimulation of these two pathways may be dispensable in later stage melanomas where other oncogenes are constitutively activated (Satyamoorthy et al. 2001).

Upregulation of IGF1R is associated with both malignant progression and resistance to apoptotic stimuli. Antisense-mediated inhibition of IGF1R is sufficient to inhibit the growth of mouse melanoma cells in nude mice (Resnicoff et al. 1994), and monoclonal antibody-targeted inhibition of IGF1R in human melanoma cells similarly inhibits their growth and invasion in xenograft mouse models (Maloney et al. 2003). Furthermore, disruption of IGF1R can sensitize melanoma cells to TRAIL-induced apoptosis (Karasic et al. 2010) and increase radiosensitivity of melanoma by impairing the ATM-mediated DNA damage response (Macaulay et al. 2001). Moreover, inhibition of IGF1R is sufficient to suppress growth of human melanomas harboring the $BRAF^{V600E}$ mutation (discussed further below), indicating that IGF1R inhibition can override signaling events that circumvent the known IGF1R effector, the RAS-MAPK signaling axis (Yeh et al. 2006). High levels of IGF1R have been reported in BRAFi-resistant cells, and have been implicated in upregulation of the PI3K pathway (Villanueva et al. 2010).

7.2 Cellular Kinases and Transcription Factors

7.2.1 WNT–ß-catenin

The WNT–ß-catenin signaling pathway plays an important regulatory role in melanocyte development and is deregulated in melanoma (see also Chap. 5). WNT is a

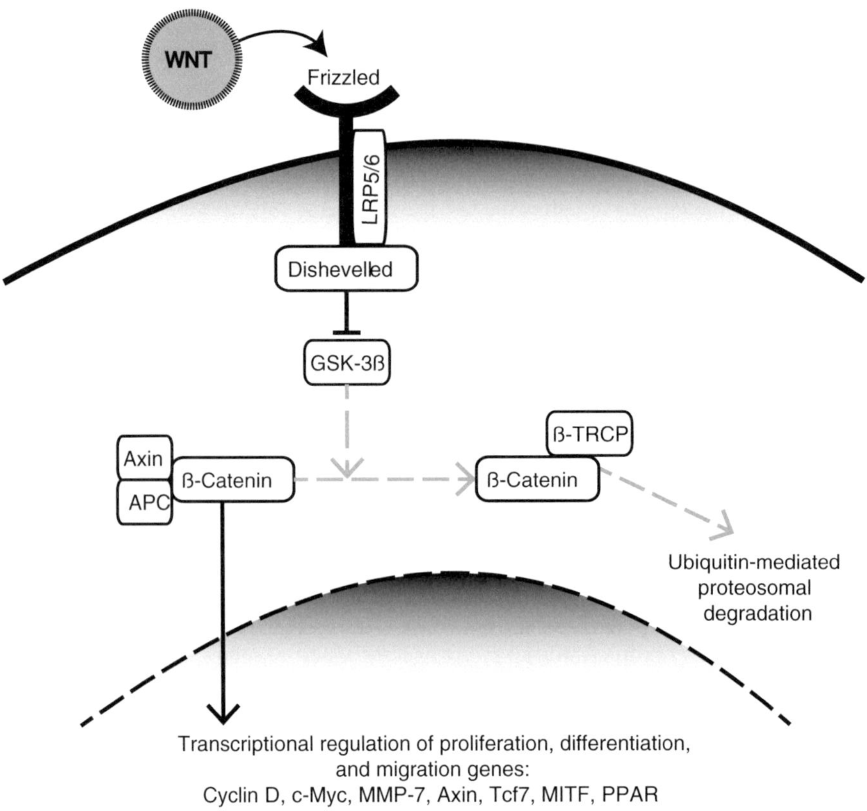

Fig. 7.3 WNT signaling pathway. Binding of WNT to its cognate receptor Frizzled and co-receptor LRP5/6 results in inactivation of GSK3ß via Dishevelled. Inactivation of Dishevelled stabilizes ß-catenin by releasing it from its degradation complex, which includes Axin and APC. Under non-stimulated conditions, ß-catenin is bound by ß-TRCP, which facilitates its ubiquitination and subsequent proteasomal degradation. Stabilized ß-catenin is then imported into the nucleus to facilitate transcriptional regulation of proliferation, differentiation, and migration genes. Branches of this signaling pathway that are upregulated in melanoma are indicated in *black*; downregulated branches are indicated by *dashed gray arrows*

secreted ligand for the membrane receptor, Frizzled (Fig. 7.3), and WNT binding activates the cytoplasmic Frizzled effector, Dishevelled. Consequently, Dishevelled inhibits GSK3ß–Axin–APC-mediated degradation of ß-catenin, stabilizing its levels and allowing nuclear import to execute its transcriptional functions. Activation of the WNT–ß-catenin pathway facilitates ß-catenin-mediated upregulation of MITF, which promotes melanocyte differentiation and development (Dorsky et al. 2000; Takeda et al. 2000). MITF can itself bind to ß-catenin, thereby tilting the transcriptional activity towards MITF targets and generating a positive feedback loop (Schepsky et al. 2006).

As expected, melanomas harboring activating ß-catenin mutations also have increased MITF levels (Doglioni et al. 2003). In turn, MITF upregulation has been shown to increase multivesicular body synthesis and consequently WNT signaling, allowing the cells to enter a proliferative stage (Ploper et al. 2015). Interestingly, ß-catenin also upregulates the transcription factor Brn-2, which transcriptionally represses Mitf and simultaneously enhances invasive melanoma behavior. Brn-2 expression also characterizes distinct subsets of MITF-negative melanoma cells (Goodall et al. 2008). The implications of MITF heterogeneity within the same and different tumors is the subject of intense investigation.

WNT–ß-catenin signaling is upregulated in melanoma, and although only ~3 % of melanoma biopsies harbor ß-catenin mutations, ~30 % of human melanomas exhibit increased nuclear localization of ß-catenin (Larue and Delmas 2006). Increased WNT signaling directly upregulates Mitf and Brn-2 expression, with concomitant suppression of p16INK4A transcription; these changes act in concert to drive melanoma growth and proliferation (Delmas et al. 2007; Goodall et al. 2004a; Widlund et al. 2002). Nuclear localization of ß-catenin is observed in melanomas carrying mutant phosphatase and tensin homolog (PTEN) phosphatase and has been implicated in melanomagenesis by cooperating with $NRAS^{Q61K}$ to increase caveolin-dependent transcriptional activity. This effectively bypasses the senescence phenotype elicited by mutant NRAS alone and promotes metastasis, in part by internalization of E-cadherin (Conde-Perez et al. 2015).

Interestingly, the functional role of WNT signaling in melanoma development varies with the specific WNT isoform. WNT3, an activator of the canonical WNT signaling axis, is anti-tumorigenic and its expression correlates with primary/nevi lesions and decreased proliferation of tumor models *in vitro* and *in vivo*. Furthermore, WNT3 expression correlates with upregulation of genes controlling melanocyte development and differentiation, including *Axin*, *Tcf7*, and *Mitf* (Chien et al. 2009). In contrast, WNT5A, which activates the non-canonical WNT signaling axis, appears to antagonize the transcriptional effects of WNT3A. Indeed, WNT5A is pro-tumorigenic, cooperating with other signaling pathways (e.g., PKC) to enhance the metastatic and invasive behavior of melanoma cells, which most likely occurs through its known function in the re-distribution of adhesion receptors (Weeraratna et al. 2002; Witze et al. 2008). Consistent with this, WNT5A-positive melanoma tumors appear to exhibit increased invasiveness and decreased proliferation compared with WNT5A-negative but MITF- and Melan-A-positive tumors, supporting a model of proliferative vs invasive phenotype switching during tumor progression (Eichhoff et al. 2010). Of note, increased WNT5A expression was also seen in tumors with acquired BRAFi resistance, and its inhibition re-sensitized tumors to BRAFi and reduced their proliferation, in part via attenuation of p-AKT activity (Anastas et al. 2014).

Melanomas with activated WNT–β-catenin signaling have a strong immunosuppressive effect on dendritic cells and cytotoxic T lymphocytes, mediated by increased IL-10 secretion and reduced IFN-γ secretion by the T cells. In this regard, it is interesting to note that activated WNT–β-catenin signaling has been linked with resistance to immunotherapy (Spranger et al. 2015; Yaguchi et al. 2012).

7.2.2 MAPK Signaling Axis

Alterations in the expression or activity of AXL, EGFR, MC1R, c-Kit, c-Met, IGFR, and WNT are examples of the most external layers of perturbed signaling cues that promote melanoma formation and progression. Several of the signaling pathways downstream of these receptors are themselves deregulated in melanoma.

The majority of melanomas display deregulated MAPK signaling due to mutations in the NRAS or BRAF genes. As a consequence, the downstream kinases and transcription factors are rendered constitutively active, regardless of aberrations upstream of NRAS or BRAF. In this section, we review our current understanding of alterations in the MAPK signaling axis and the implications for melanoma development or progression.

The MAPK pathway is coupled to upstream membrane receptors by the RAS family of small G proteins; HRAS, KRAS, and NRAS (Bos 1989; Dhillon et al. 2007). In non-transformed cells, the RAS proteins are responsive to activation by c-Kit, c-Met, IGFR, and WNT, for example, and transduce activating signals through interplay with the RAF family of effector serine/threonine kinases; ARAF, BRAF, and CRAF. Signals are then transduced by sequential activation of a cascade of MAP kinases: MEK, MEKK, and finally, ERK (Fig. 7.2). Of these proteins, NRAS and BRAF are the most commonly mutated in melanoma, with ~15 % and more than 50 % of melanomas harboring NRAS and BRAF mutations, respectively (Davies et al. 2002; Fecher et al. 2007). Further downstream, MEK mutations have also been reported, particularly in the context of acquired resistance to chemotherapy. For instance, MEK1 mutations occur at low incidence overall, but they are most frequently reported following BRAFi therapy and confer resistance to MEKi and BRAFi (Emery et al. 2009; Murugan et al. 2009).

While most melanoma-associated mutations in NRAS occur at amino acid 61, BRAF deregulation is attributed to mutations at several hotspots, most prominently V600E, resulting in a constitutively active kinase (Wan et al. 2004). Indeed, the catalytic activity of $BRAF^{V600E}$ was calculated to be ~10-fold higher than that of wild-type BRAF (Brummer et al. 2006). While mutant BRAF and NRAS share some downstream effectors, most notably ERK, they each also activate unique downstream components. As illustrated in Fig. 7.2, BRAF activity also affects MEK–ERK kinases and RSK. These kinases in turn suppress the activity of the LKB1–AMPK signaling pathway, thereby promoting melanoma proliferation (Esteve-Puig et al. 2009; Zheng et al. 2009). As a result of their unique contributions to signaling, BRAF and NRAS mutants have distinct characteristics with respect to melanoma development and progression.

As noted above, ERK is the downstream kinase most commonly affected by NRAS and BRAF mutations in melanoma, and constitutive or super-activation of ERK perturbs critical regulators of cellular behavior. For example, $BRAF^{V600E}$ antagonizes apoptosis via ERK-dependent inhibition of the apoptotic proteins Bad, Bim, and PUMA, and upregulation of anti-apoptotic proteins such as Mcl-1 (Jiang et al. 2008; Sheridan et al. 2008; Wang et al. 2007b). Enhanced ERK activation also alters cell cycle control and proliferation by suppressing the negative cell cycle regulator p27/Kip1 (Kortylewski et al. 2001) and, importantly, by modulating the expression of melanocyte MITF isoforms and inducing the M-MITF 6a isoform (Primot et al. 2010; Wellbrock et al. 2008). MAPK/ERK activation can further enhance the proliferative capacity of melanoma cells by promoting upregulation of other transcription factors such as c-Jun and Brn-2, either by increasing their stability (c-Jun) or increasing their expression (Brn-2) (Goodall et al. 2004a, b; Lopez-Bergami et al. 2007). Mutant BRAF-mediated ERK signaling also impinges on invasive cellular behaviors resulting from changes in growth or invasion regulatory proteins such as Plexin B or matrix metalloproteinase-1 (Argast et al. 2009; Huntington et al. 2004). Indeed, activation of the RAS–RAF–MAPK–ERK pathway has been implicated in immune evasion by modulating the production of immunosuppressive cytokines such as IL-6, IL-10, and VEGF by melanoma cells (Sumimoto et al. 2006).

Constitutive upregulation of ERK signaling results in rewiring of signaling pathways, a common occurrence in many tumors, including melanoma. For example, rewired ERK signaling causes constitutive activation of c-Jun via two complementary pathways. ERK-mediated upregulation of RSK–CREB increases c-Jun transcription, whereas ERK-mediated phosphorylation of GSK3ß inhibits its ability to phosphorylate c-Jun on residue 243, which is required for targeting of c-Jun for ubiquitination and degradation by FBW7 (Nateri et al. 2004; Wei et al. 2005), thereby resulting in increased c-Jun stability (Lopez-Bergami et al. 2007). In turn, c-Jun induces transcription of a large set of targets genes that include cell cycle regulators such as Cyclin D as well as components of other signaling pathways. One is the PKC adaptor protein RACK1, which potentiates both PKC and JNK signaling. As a result, RACK1–PKC signaling increases JNK activity and further activates its substrates, including c-Jun, thus enforcing a feed-forward signaling pathway. Another c-Jun transcriptional target implicated in melanoma development is the kinase PDK1, which activates AKT. The c-Jun-mediated increase in PDK1 transcription, and thus activation of both the AKT and PKC pathways. Inhibition of c-Jun effectively attenuates melanoma development in a xenograft mouse model, and this can be rescued by re-expression of PDK1 (Lopez-Bergami et al. 2010). Thus, ERK signaling causes activation of the JNK, PKC, PDK1, and AKT pathways, representing a paradigm for rewired signaling.

Constitutive activation of MAPK itself is sufficient for transformation of immortalized melanocytes through elevation of angiogenic and invasive behavior secondary to upregulation of VEGF and MMP-2 (Govindarajan et al. 2003). However, synergistic crosstalk between upregulated MAPK signaling and other major signaling axes (e.g., PI3K–AKT–MTOR), can further promote additional tumorigenic behaviors such as the enhanced proliferation observed in uveal melanoma (Babchia et al. 2010).

Upregulated or constitutive activation of the MAPK signaling cascade correlates with poor clinical outcome (Houben et al. 2004), which is commonly attributed to activating mutations at different branch points along the signaling pathway. Thus, HRAS and KRAS mutations appear to correlate with benign Spitz nevi and primary lesions, whereas NRAS is most frequently mutated in primary and metastatic melanoma and is characteristic of chronically sun-exposed lesions (Ball et al. 1994; Jafari et al. 1995; Jiveskog et al. 1998; Shukla et al. 1989; van Dijk et al. 2005; van Elsas et al. 1995). Immediately downstream of the RAS proteins are the RAF kinases, of which BRAF is the most frequently mutated (specifically $BRAF^{V600E}$) in melanoma. The more dominant oncogenic role of BRAF compared with ARAF and CRAF is most likely due to its higher kinase activity (Emuss et al. 2005; Lee et al. 2005). Although BRAF germline mutations have been reported, they are not common in familial melanoma (Lang et al. 2003), suggesting that BRAF mutations occur during melanoma development. Interestingly, $BRAF^{V600E}$ and NRAS mutations appear to be mutually exclusive in melanoma; a phenomenon that may be influenced by type and site of origin of the melanoma tumor. For example, BRAF mutation does not appear to correlate with the degree of sun exposure, as is the case for NRAS mutations (Davies et al. 2002). Interestingly, NRAS mutations induce a switch in the dominant usage of RAF isoforms from BRAF to CRAF (Dumaz et al. 2006).

Mutant BRAF is also found in congenital nevi and other non-malignant lesions, where it is associated with upregulation of senescence markers such as senescence-associated ß-galactosidase (SA-ß-gal) and mosaic p16INK4A induction (Michaloglou et al. 2005). Indeed, mutations of NRAS and BRAF (V600E) alone can promote cellular senescence *in vitro*, which not only illustrates oncogene-induced senescence but also highlights the need for other oncogenic events to drive tumor progression (see also Chaps. 4, 5, and 11). Nevertheless, ERK activity does not always correlate with BRAF activation, most likely due to variations in the functional status of ERK phosphatases. It has been proposed that some ERK phosphatases might be less active in malignant than non-malignant cells, although it is not yet clear whether and how ERK phosphatases might be deregulated in melanoma. In this regard, BRAF mutation alone is insufficient to transform melanocytes, and secondary mutations that confer uncontrolled cell cycle progression are required. The notion that BRAF acts cooperatively to induce melanoma development is supported by observations in zebrafish, where mutant BRAF promotes nevi development but additional oncogenic changes, such as loss of p53, can promote progression to invasive lesions (Patton et al. 2005).

Other secondary mutations that can support uncontrolled proliferation include p16INK4A and p19INK4D (see cell cycle section). Although it is unclear what role p16INK4A may play in BRAF-driven senescence, loss of p16INK4A can facilitate melanoma tumor formation driven by mutant RAS (Ackermann et al. 2005; Chin et al. 1997). Interestingly, cooperative stabilization of ß-catenin results in silencing of p16INK4A, and in combination with mutant NRAS, this is sufficient to promote melanoma progression (Delmas et al. 2007). Additional signaling mechanisms that contribute to oncogene-induced senescence and earlier barriers to melanoma progression continue to be identified. For example, early oncogene-induced activation of the ER stress-activated unfolded protein response was found to halt tumorigenesis independently of conventional senescence mechanisms (Denoyelle et al. 2006).

Although epigenetic perturbations that promote activation of these pathways remain largely obscure, the mutational status of melanoma tumors is known to correlate with some characteristic epigenetic profiles. For example, melanomas with BRAF mutations exhibit changes in several miRNAs, such as downregulation of miR-193a, miR-338, and miR-565, and upregulation of miR-191 (Caramuta et al. 2010). A further level of complexity is suggested by the finding that pseudogene transcripts can act as false miRNA "decoy" targets (a.k.a., competitive endogenous RNAs), thereby absorbing and nullifying the function of miRNAs targeting specific endogenous transcripts (Chen 2010; Poliseno et al. 2010; Karreth et al. 2015). Such regulation has been demonstrated for PTEN and BRAF and may effectively alter the expression of other genes that are central to the control of melanoma development. As increasing effort is devoted to sequencing the melanoma genome, a wealth of pseudogenes contributing to different stages of melanoma biology are expected to be identified (Pleasance et al. 2010).

7.2.3 PTEN–PI3K–AKT

The phosphatidylinositol-3-kinase–AKT (PI3K–AKT) pathway is also frequently deregulated in melanoma (Inoue-Narita et al. 2008; Robertson 2005), although the mechanisms underlying the deregulation of many components remain largely elusive. Like the MAPK pathway, the PI3K pathway is an effector signaling cascade positioned downstream of the membrane receptors described earlier, including c-Met and IGFR1. PI3K converts phosphatidylinositol-4,5 bisphosphate (PIP2), located on the cytoplasmic face of the plasma membrane, into the secondary lipid signaling molecule, phosphatidylinositol-3,4,5 trisphosphate (PIP3). In turn, PIP3 activates the downstream effector AKT/protein kinase B. The three members of the AKT family of serine/threonine kinases (AKT1, AKT2, and AKT3) have well-characterized prosurvival functions (Datta et al. 1999; Madhunapantula and Robertson 2009) (Fig. 7.4), with AKT3 appearing to be the isoform most affected in melanoma.

One mechanism by which AKT signaling is enhanced is via deregulation of PIP2 processing by perturbation of inositol polyphosphate 4-phosphatase type II (Gewinner et al. 2009). However, upregulation of AKT activity in melanoma can largely be attributed to deregulation of its negative regulator, PTEN (Parmiter et al. 1988). Although loss of PTEN protein is prevalent in melanoma (Chudnovsky et al. 2005), deregulation by mutation accounts for only a small fraction of melanomas with deregulated PTEN. Accordingly, while PTEN is commonly mutated in melanoma cell lines, such genetic mutations are rare in actual tumor samples, particularly those of metastatic grade (Goel et al. 2006; Pollock et al. 2002; Wu et al. 2003). These observations indicate that downregulation or loss of PTEN in patient's tumors results from additional transcriptional and post-translational modifications, with the latter being the most common. Although not shown yet in melanoma, the ubiquitin ligase NEDD-4, which targets PTEN for destruction, is upregulated in numerous cancer types, including gastric and colorectal cancers (Kim et al. 2008b; Trotman et al. 2007; Wang et al. 2007a). Oncogenic deregulation of PTEN also occurs via Fyn-related kinase (FRK, previously known as RAK), which is overexpressed in melanoma and numerous other cancers. FRK phosphorylates PTEN, thereby abrogating its interaction with NEDD-4 and increasing its availability (Brauer and Tyner 2009; Yim et al. 2009).

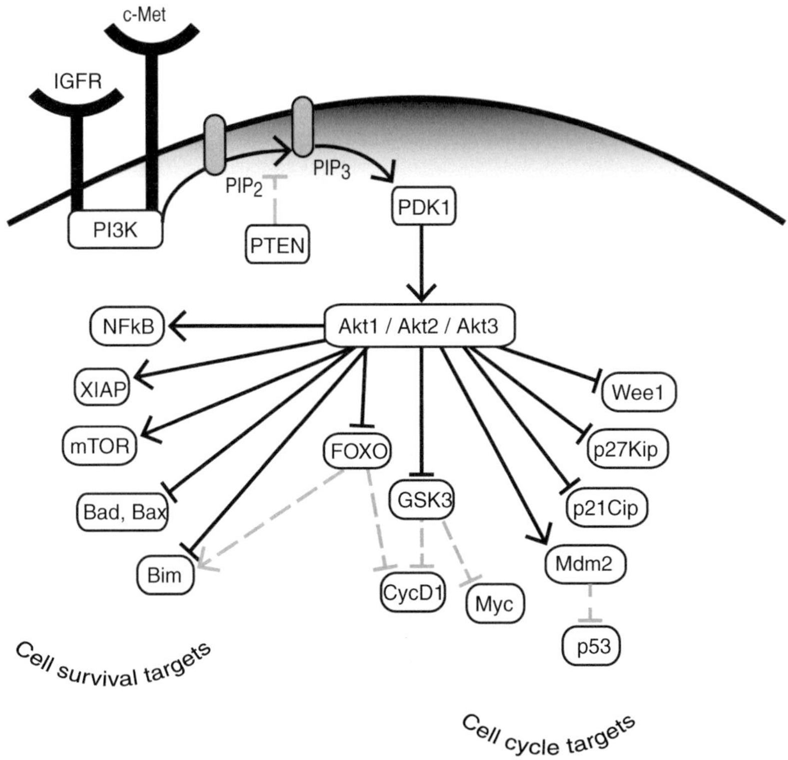

Fig. 7.4 AKT signaling. Various membrane-bound growth factor receptors (c-Met and IGFR) signal inwards via PI3K, which phosphorylates PIP_2 to produce the secondary messenger molecule PIP_3. PIP_3 then functions to activate PDK1, which in turn activates AKT family kinases (*AKT1, AKT2*, and *AKT3*). AKT is a widely recognized pro-survival effector kinase that acts by upregulating or activating numerous cell survival-related proteins, such as NF-kB, XIAP, and mTOR, and inhibiting cell death-related proteins such as Bad, Bax, and Bim (see also Chap. 10). AKT also inhibits transcription factors, such as FOXO, which contribute to cell death or cell cycle arrest. AKT promotes cell cycle progression by inhibiting cell cycle inhibitors, including Wee1, p21Kip, p21Cip, and p53 (via activation of *Mdm2*), and relieving Cyclin D1 and Myc from suppression by GSK3. Branches of the AKT pathway that are upregulated in melanoma appear in *black*; down-regulated branches appear in *dashed gray*

Other forms of epigenetic silencing of PTEN include promoter methylation, which is observed in up to 62% of patients with metastatic melanoma (Mirmohammadsadegh et al. 2006). In effect, loss of PTEN promotes an excess of PIP3 and activation of AKT and its downstream targets, resulting in increased growth and survival of melanoma. Notably, activated AKT which is affected by deregulated PTEN is inversely correlated with a positive clinical outcome for melanoma patients (Dai et al. 2005).

In addition to loss of PTEN, direct changes to AKT family members can modulate the PI3K pathway in melanoma. Of the three AKT isoforms, AKT3 is specifically and significantly upregulated in sporadic melanoma tumors, particularly those of metastatic grade (Robertson 2005; Stahl et al. 2004). Although AKT3 upregulation has mainly been attributed directly to an increase in genomic copy number, a recent report has identified a novel activating mutation of AKT3 (E17K) in some melanoma cases (Davies et al. 2008). Targeted siRNA-mediated silencing of AKT3 is sufficient to suppress melanoma progression and induce cell death, emphasizing the oncogenic potential of deregulated AKT3 activation.

AKT signaling affects numerous cellular process: it influences cell cycle dynamics through regulation of the G1/S phase regulator Cyclin D3 (Spofford et al. 2006); affects cell growth, metabolism, and proliferation via control of VEGF expression and interplay with mTOR and the TORC1 and TORC2 complexes (Bhaskar and Hay 2007; Govindarajan et al. 2007; Levine et al. 2006); contributes to invasive behavior by NF-kB-mediated regulation of matrix metalloproteinase-2 and -9 (Kim et al. 2001); and suppresses apoptosis by inhibiting the expression of pro-apoptotic proteins such as Bad and caspase-9 (Cardone et al. 1998; Datta et al. 1997). Each of these AKT effects can be attenuated or suppressed by the antagonistic function of PTEN. Importantly, deregulation of the ERK–c-Jun signaling axis in melanoma leads to c-Jun-mediated transcriptional upregulation of PDK1, further enhancing AKT activation (Lopez-Bergami et al. 2010). PDK1 has also been demonstrated to make critical AKT-independent contributions to tumorigenesis via activation of its substrate SGK3/CISK; this has been shown for breast cancer, among others (Vasudevan et al. 2009).

Recent studies using genetic melanoma models have substantiated the role of PDK1 in the development and progression of melanoma. Thus, melanocyte-specific inactivation of PDK1 in the $Braf^{V600E}$::$Pten^{-/-}$ mouse model delayed the formation of tumors and largely abolished the metastatic lesions commonly seen in this model. Consistent with these findings, examination of melanoma tissue microarrays revealed upregulation of PDK1 in primary melanomas compared with nevi (Scortegagna et al. 2014). Further dissection of the pathways underlying the PDK1 effects on melanoma development identified a role for the PDK1 substrate SGK3. Indeed, inhibition of SGK3 partially phenocopied the changes seen upon PDK1 inhibition. Interestingly, a synthetic lethal screen for kinases that may synergize with PDK1 in eliciting these effects identified PI3K, suggesting that concerted inhibition of the PI3K–PDK1 axis alone may suffice to inhibit growth of BRAF-mutant melanomas (Scortegagna et al. 2014, 2015).

7.3 Cell Cycle Regulation

Malignant melanoma cells are highly proliferative and often exhibit genomic instability (Hazan et al. 2002; Henrique et al. 2000; Satoh et al. 2000; Soyer 1991; Steinbeck et al. 1996; Urso et al. 1992). Such an aggressive proliferative state results from the specific expansion of transformed cells with imbalanced signal transduction favoring proliferation while deregulating normal replicative senescence and apoptotic signaling (Bennett 2008). Accordingly, the stringent cell cycle regulatory mechanisms that govern cell proliferation in normal skin tissues are frequently impaired during melanoma development. For instance, proper function of the G1/S checkpoint that restricts cell cycle progression is often lost in melanoma (Sauroja

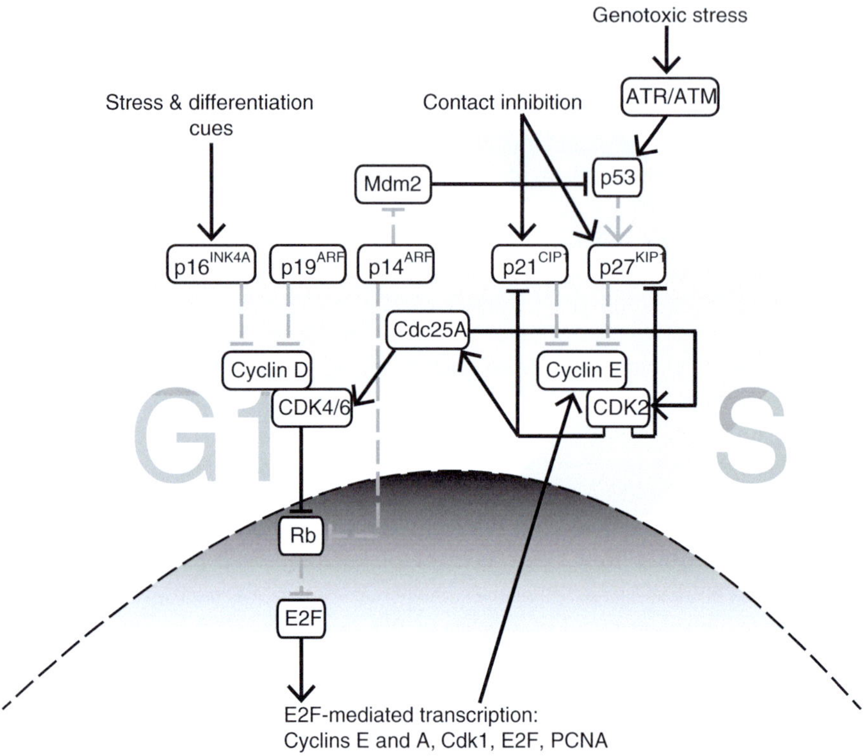

Fig. 7.5 Cell cycle control. In melanoma, loss of CDK2NA compromises major branch points in the regulatory pathways governing G1/S progression. Loss of p16INK4A, p19ARF, and p14ARF causes deregulation of Cyclin D/CDK4/6 and subsequent deregulation of Rb and p53 function, thereby promoting enhanced E2F transcriptional activity and cell cycle progression. Loss of function of other cell cycle inhibitors, such as p21CIP1 and p27KIP1, results in enhanced Cyclin E/CDK2 activity, which positively feeds back on itself and on CDK4/6 via CDC25. Branches of the cell cycle regulation that are upregulated in melanoma appear in *black*; downregulated branches appear in *dashed gray*

et al. 2000). Similar perturbations in signaling can be traced to specific familial mutations or epigenetic dysregulation that result in the downregulation of tumor suppressor genes that negatively regulate the cell cycle or the upregulation of oncogenic genes that promote cell cycle progression.

Patients afflicted with familial melanoma commonly exhibit conserved mutations in 9p21, a chromosomal locus associated with deregulation of cell cycle control. The 9p21 locus comprises the CDK2NA gene, which encodes p16INK4A and its alternate reading frames p14ARF and p19ARF. These proteins negatively regulate cell cycle progression and contribute to senescence through their control of cell cycle-promoting proteins such as Cyclin D and E and the transcription factor E2F1 (Fig. 7.5) (Bandyopadhyay and Medrano 2000; Ranade et al. 1995). Furthermore, p16INK4A binds to and inhibits the cell cycle-promoting kinase CDK4, with concomitant effects on Rb and its control of E2F in the cell cycle. Germline mutations in CDK2NA have been reported in melanoma (Koh et al. 1995; Ranade et al. 1995) and result in amplified CDK4-mediated signaling, thereby perturbing normal cell cycle control. The increased CDK4 activity observed in melanoma can also result from mutations in the CDK4 gene (Chudnovsky et al. 2005). These perturbations impair proper cell cycle control and appropriate entry of melanocytes into senescence (Bandyopadhyay and Medrano 2000; Haferkamp et al. 2008; Rane et al. 2002).

Mutational perturbation of the alternate reading frame gene product p14ARF also promotes cellular proliferation. Indeed, mutation of ARF has been demonstrated to synergize with RAS mutations in promoting melanoma tumor development (Ha et al. 2007). p14ARF normally contributes to p53 function by targeting and suppressing the p53 negative regulator, Mdm2. Thus, although mutations in p53 are relatively rare in melanoma, its activity can be downregulated by the increased Mdm2 levels induced by mutational silencing of ARF (Freedberg et al. 2008). Of note, there have been few reports on upregulation of Mdm2 or downregulation of p53 expression or activity in melanoma (Bardeesy et al. 2001) (see also Chap. 4). Hence, the precise contribution of p53 to melanoma development remains unclear. Among the possibilities currently being explored is that p53 is partially inactivated, impairing its ability to control cell cycle arrest or apoptotic cues in melanoma.

Enhanced proliferation of melanoma cells can also be elicited by alterations in other negative regulators of cell cycle progression, including Rb. Notably, Rb is silenced in melanoma (Yang et al. 2005) as a result of nonsense mutations or of inactivating phosphorylation of the translated protein (Bartkova et al. 1996; Brantley and Harbour 2000). Loss of Rb function can also contribute to abrogation of melanocyte senescence (Haferkamp et al. 2008).

In addition to genetic mutations, alterations in the epigenetic regulation of core cell cycle and proliferation genes also contribute to melanoma development and progression. Direct modification of chromatin structure, such as by aberrant promoter hypermethylation, results in the CDK2NA silencing reported in multiple melanoma types (Straume et al. 2002; van der Velden et al. 2001). CDKN2A silencing can also be achieved via upregulation of repressor proteins. One example in melanoma is overexpression of the CDKN2A transcriptional repressor Id1 (Healey et al. 2010). Suppression of p16INK4A in melanoma is also mediated by ß-catenin (Delmas et al. 2007). The histone methyltransferase EZH2 has been implicated in the epigenetic repression of the CDK2NA locus and is upregulated in melanoma via a non-canonical NF-kB pathway. Inhibition of this pathway promotes senescence by inducing re-expression of p16INK and p21 (De Donatis et al. 2016).

Recent studies have highlighted the role played by miRNAs in the epigenetic control of melanoma progression (Jukic et al. 2010). Several miRNAs that suppress proliferation are downregulated during melanoma progression, including miR-let-7 and miR-34a. miR-let-7 targets numerous cell cycle proteins, including Cyclin D1/D3/A, and is expressed at lower levels in melanoma compared with nevi (Schultz et al. 2008). Expression of miR-34a, a transcriptional target of p53, is sufficient to induce G1 arrest/senescence and can act as a tumor suppressor by targeting c-Met. However, in melanoma, miR-34a is silenced by aberrant CpG promoter methylation

(Lodygin et al. 2008), which derepresses the cell cycle proteins Rb, CDC2, and E2F3, among others (Satzger et al. 2010; Yan et al. 2009). Deregulation of other miRNAs, including miR-210 and miR-15b, have been demonstrated to promote melanoma tumorigenesis (Satzger et al. 2010; Zhang et al. 2009) (see also the section on miRNAs and melanoma).

7.4 Therapeutic Targets

The MAPK–MEK–ERK and PTEN–P13K–AKT pathways are recognized to be critical determinants of melanoma development and progression, and an intensive effort is under way to develop inhibitors of components of these pathways (Madhunapantula and Robertson 2009; Meier et al. 2005; Russo et al. 2009). A series of specific inhibitors of $BRAF^{V600E}$ showed impressive results in early clinical trials (Kumar et al. 2004). However, the initial success was tempered by the high incidence of therapy-resistant tumors, limiting the effectiveness of these specific drugs (Flaherty et al. 2010). In recent years, extensive work on the molecular basis for this resistance has pointed to diverse mechanisms, most of which cause amplification of the downstream MAPK signaling pathway and bypass the effects of the BRAFi. One emerging approach to overcome resistance is the use of immunotherapeutic drugs that do not directly target the tumor per se, but instead unleash the anti-tumor immune response. Among these therapies are antibodies to CTLA-4 and PD-1, which overcome the drug-resistant tumor phenotype by blocking inhibitory immune checkpoints. These agents have recently been assessed as first-line therapy or as combination therapies with selective BRAFi or MEKi (Larkin et al. 2015; Menzies and Long 2013).

7.4.1 Overcoming Resistance to Targeted Therapies

To date, the use of single agents as first-line therapy has demonstrated only limited clinical efficacy. This disappointing outcome has been attributed to the unexpected plasticity of tumors, as reflected by their ability to adapt to harsh growth conditions and become resistant to initially effective drugs. The mechanisms for achieving resistance largely center on signal transduction pathways that have been rewired, either by genetic mutation or alteration in epigenetic control (Smalley et al. 2009; Emery et al. 2009).

Although BRAF inhibitors suppress tumor growth, the effect is transient, and the tumor cells eventually develop one or more "salvage" mechanisms that bypass BRAF or MEK inhibition. Such mechanisms include upregulation of activated CRAF activity (Gollob et al. 2006; Hatzivassiliou et al. 2010; Kaplan et al. 2011; Montagut et al. 2008; Paraiso et al. 2010; Tsai et al. 2008; Wellbrock and Hurlstone 2010); mutation of NRAS, which leads to CRAF activation and bypasses BRAF inhibition (Nazarian et al. 2010); upregulation of COT, which activates ERK in a MEK-dependent and RAF-independent manner (Johannessen et al. 2010); and upregulation of RTKs (Nazarian et al. 2010) (see section 7.1.1.2 on RTKs).

Melanomas may also develop resistance to BRAF-targeting therapies via upregulation of AKT3-dependent mechanisms (Shao and Aplin 2010), which is consistent with the reported cooperation between mutant BRAF and active AKT (Dankort et al. 2009). Additionally, resistance to BRAFi can be achieved by alternative splicing of BRAF (Wellbrock et al. 2004), which results in a protein lacking the RAS-binding domain due to a silent mutation in intron 8 (Salton et al. 2015). This BRAF isoform dimerizes even in the presence of low levels of RAS, conferring drug resistance through reactivation of the ERK pathway.

Combined targeting of MEK and BRAF results in additive and synergistic effects on progression-free survival of melanoma patients, with a 67 % response rate and 93 % overall survival at 6 months (Flaherty et al. 2012a; Flaherty et al. 2012b). Nevertheless, resistance to MEKi emerges through the same mechanisms seen in BRAFi resistance, including increased CRAF activity and mutation of both NRAS and MEK1 (Greger et al. 2012).

Most tumor resistance mechanisms result in increased activity of the translation initiation complex, which supports the translation of cancer-driving genes such as oncogenes and cell cycle/DNA damage response genes. Hence, partial disruption of the eIF4F complex is a potential therapeutic strategy for drug-resistant tumors, including melanoma. In support of this approach, recent studies have demonstrated efficacy in overcoming melanoma resistance to therapy by targeting eIF4F with silvestrol and several flavaglines (Boussemart et al. 2014), and by targeting a key component of the eIF4F complex, eIF4G1, with the small molecule SBI-756 (Feng et al. 2015).

7.4.2 Immunotherapy

A great deal of effort has been devoted to the use of immune-based therapies to overcome drug resistance in melanoma (Hu-Lieskovan et al. 2014; Vanneman and Dranoff 2012), but the success rate has been low and pronounced toxicity has been observed in most cases. The notion that the immune system could be manipulated to enable a global attack on tumors was initially met with skepticism, largely due to fears that uncontrolled activation would lead to autoimmunity. However, the pioneering work of Drs. Allison and Honjo introduced the immune checkpoint molecules, CTLA-4 and PD-1, respectively, as new paradigms for cancer immunotherapy (Leach et al. 1996; Okazaki et al. 2013; Peggs et al. 2006). Targeting of CTLA-4 circumvents downregulation of T-cell proliferation, whereas PD-1 blockade is likely to affect both activation of T cells and the direct anti-tumor activity of effector T cells.

Clinical trials with anti-CTLA-4 antibodies have shown unexpected success, with an overall response rate of about 20 %, albeit with notable toxicity (Attia et al. 2005; Hodi et al. 2010). Clinical trials with anti-PD-1 antibodies have achieved greater response rates (30–40 %) and significant increases in patient survival (Topalian et al. 2014). More recently, combination therapy with anti-CTLA-4 and anti-PD-1 achieved about 60 % response rate and 79 % 2-year survival rate (Topalian et al. 2014). Other ongoing work includes the evaluation of combination therapies of immune checkpoint blockers with BRAFi or MEKi, which have shown promising results in pre-clinical experiments (Hu-Lieskovan et al. 2015).

7.5 Epilogue

Our understanding of the mechanisms underlying the development, progression, and drug resistance of melanoma has increased significantly in recent years. At the same time, we have come to appreciate that a major obstacle to achieving sustained therapeutic responses is the innate plasticity of tumor cells, which allows them to adapt to harsh conditions, withstand therapy, and acquire metastatic ability. This means that the rewired signaling observed in tumor cells could be further changed by the tumor microenvironment or by stress imposed by the chemotherapeutic drugs. Thus, we must divert from our current approach to cancer therapy—more intense targeting of a mutated pathway—to find new therapeutic modalities. These include fine-tuning the immune checkpoint machinery to enable a concerted immune attack on the tumor, and targeting the central mechanisms that provide a global advantage to the tumors. Among the latter mechanisms are the translation initiation complex and the unfolded protein response, which are cardinal nodes for tumor-driving genes and may offer a more global approach to targeting the plastic tumor. These molecular hubs have already garnered attention and we may expect an exciting new cadre of modulators to reach clinical evaluation in the coming years.

References

Ackermann J, Frutschi M, Kaloulis K, McKee T, Trumpp A, Beermann F (2005) Metastasizing melanoma formation caused by expression of activated N-RasQ61K on an INK4a-deficient background. Cancer Res 65:4005–4011

Anastas JN, Kulikauskas RM, Tamir T, Rizos H, Long GV, von Euw EM, Yang PT, Chen HW, Haydu L, Toroni RA et al (2014) WNT5A enhances resistance of melanoma cells to targeted BRAF inhibitors. J Clin Invest 124:2877–2890

Antonescu CR, Busam KJ, Francone TD, Wong GC, Guo T, Agaram NP, Besmer P, Jungbluth A, Gimbel M, Chen CT et al (2007) L576P KIT mutation in anal melanomas correlates with KIT protein expression and is sensitive to specific kinase inhibition. Int J Cancer 121:257–264

Argast GM, Croy CH, Couts KL, Zhang Z, Litman E, Chan DC, Ahn NG (2009) Plexin B1 is repressed by oncogenic B-Raf signaling and functions as a tumor suppressor in melanoma cells. Oncogene 28:2697–2709

Attia P, Phan GQ, Maker AV, Robinson MR, Quezado MM, Yang JC, Sherry RM, Topalian SL, Kammula US, Royal RE et al (2005) Autoimmunity correlates with tumor regression in patients with metastatic melanoma treated with anti-cytotoxic T-lymphocyte antigen-4. J Clin Oncol 23:6043–6053

Babchia N, Calipel A, Mouriaux F, Faussat AM, Mascarelli F (2010) The PI3K/Akt and mTOR/P70S6K signaling pathways in human uveal melanoma cells: interaction with B-Raf/ERK. Invest Ophthalmol Vis Sci 51:421–429

Ball NJ, Yohn JJ, Morelli JG, Norris DA, Golitz LE, Hoeffler JP (1994) Ras mutations in human melanoma: a marker of malignant progression. J Invest Dermatol 102:285–290

Bandyopadhyay D, Medrano EE (2000) Melanin accumulation accelerates melanocyte senescence by a mechanism involving p16INK4a/CDK4/pRB and E2F1. Ann N Y Acad Sci 908:71–84
Bardeesy N, Bastian BC, Hezel A, Pinkel D, DePinho RA, Chin L (2001) Dual inactivation of RB and p53 pathways in RAS-induced melanomas. Mol Cell Biol 21:2144–2153
Bar-Eli M (1997) Molecular mechanisms of melanoma metastasis. J Cell Physiol 173:275–278
Bartkova J, Lukas J, Guldberg P, Alsner J, Kirkin AF, Zeuthen J, Bartek J (1996) The p16-cyclin D/Cdk4-pRb pathway as a functional unit frequently altered in melanoma pathogenesis. Cancer Res 56:5475–5483
Bennett DC (2008) How to make a melanoma: what do we know of the primary clonal events? Pigment Cell Melanoma Res 21:27–38
Bhaskar PT, Hay N (2007) The two TORCs and Akt. Dev Cell 12:487–502
Bos JL (1989) ras oncogenes in human cancer: a review. Cancer Res 49:4682–4689
Boussemart L, Malka-Mahieu H, Girault I, Allard D, Hemmingsson O, Tomasic G, Thomas M, Basmadjian C, Ribeiro N, Thuaud F et al (2014) eIF4F is a nexus of resistance to anti-BRAF and anti-MEK cancer therapies. Nature 513:105–109
Brantley MA Jr, Harbour JW (2000) Inactivation of retinoblastoma protein in uveal melanoma by phosphorylation of sites in the COOH-terminal region. Cancer Res 60:4320–4323
Brauer PM, Tyner AL (2009) RAKing in AKT: a tumor suppressor function for the intracellular tyrosine kinase FRK. Cell Cycle 8:2728–2732
Brummer T, Martin P, Herzog S, Misawa Y, Daly RJ, Reth M (2006) Functional analysis of the regulatory requirements of B-Raf and the B-Raf(V600E) oncoprotein. Oncogene 25:6262–6276
Caramuta S, Egyhazi S, Rodolfo M, Witten D, Hansson J, Larsson C, Lui WO (2010) MicroRNA expression profiles associated with mutational status and survival in malignant melanoma. J Invest Dermatol 130:2062–2070
Cardone MH, Roy N, Stennicke HR, Salvesen GS, Franke TF, Stanbridge E, Frisch S, Reed JC (1998) Regulation of cell death protease caspase-9 by phosphorylation. Science 282:1318–1321
Chen M (2010) Smoke and miRrors: pseudogenes tricking miRNAs. Pigment Cell Melanoma Res 23(5):583–584
Chien AJ, Moore EC, Lonsdorf AS, Kulikauskas RM, Rothberg BG, Berger AJ, Major MB, Hwang ST, Rimm DL, Moon RT (2009) Activated Wnt/beta-catenin signaling in melanoma is associated with decreased proliferation in patient tumors and a murine melanoma model. Proc Natl Acad Sci U S A 106:1193–1198
Chin L, Pomerantz J, Polsky D, Jacobson M, Cohen C, Cordon-Cardo C, Horner JW 2nd, DePinho RA (1997) Cooperative effects of INK4a and ras in melanoma susceptibility in vivo. Genes Dev 11:2822–2834
Chin L, Garraway LA, Fisher DE (2006) Malignant melanoma: genetics and therapeutics in the genomic era. Genes Dev 20:2149–2182
Chudnovsky Y, Adams AE, Robbins PB, Lin Q, Khavari PA (2005) Use of human tissue to assess the oncogenic activity of melanoma-associated mutations. Nat Genet 37:745–749
Conde-Perez A, Gros G, Longvert C, Pedersen M, Petit V, Aktary Z, Viros A, Gesbert F, Delmas V, Rambow F et al (2015) A caveolin-dependent and PI3K/AKT-independent role of PTEN in beta-catenin transcriptional activity. Nat Commun 6:8093
Corcoran RB, Ebi H, Turke AB, Coffee EM, Nishino M, Cogdill AP, Brown RD, Della Pelle P, Dias-Santagata D, Hung KE et al (2012) EGFR-mediated re-activation of MAPK signaling contributes to insensitivity of BRAF mutant colorectal cancers to RAF inhibition with vemurafenib. Cancer Discov 2:227–235
Dai DL, Martinka M, Li G (2005) Prognostic significance of activated Akt expression in melanoma: a clinicopathologic study of 292 cases. J Clin Oncol 23:1473–1482
Dankort D, Curley DP, Cartlidge RA, Nelson B, Karnezis AN, Damsky WE Jr, You MJ, DePinho RA, McMahon M, Bosenberg M (2009) Braf(V600E) cooperates with Pten loss to induce metastatic melanoma. Nat Genet 41:544–552
Datta SR, Dudek H, Tao X, Masters S, Fu H, Gotoh Y, Greenberg ME (1997) Akt phosphorylation of BAD couples survival signals to the cell-intrinsic death machinery. Cell 91:231–241

Datta SR, Brunet A, Greenberg ME (1999) Cellular survival: a play in three Akts. Genes Dev 13:2905–2927

Davies H, Bignell GR, Cox C, Stephens P, Edkins S, Clegg S, Teague J, Woffendin H, Garnett MJ, Bottomley W et al (2002) Mutations of the BRAF gene in human cancer. Nature 417:949–954

Davies MA, Stemke-Hale K, Tellez C, Calderone TL, Deng W, Prieto VG, Lazar AJ, Gershenwald JE, Mills GB (2008) A novel AKT3 mutation in melanoma tumours and cell lines. Br J Cancer 99:1265–1268

De Donatis GM, Pape EL, Pierron A, Cheli Y, Hofman V, Hofman P, Allegra M, Zahaf K, Bahadoran P, Rocchi S et al (2016) NF-kB2 induces senescence bypass in melanoma via a direct transcriptional activation of EZH2. Oncogene 35(21):2735–2745

Delmas V, Beermann F, Martinozzi S, Carreira S, Ackermann J, Kumasaka M, Denat L, Goodall J, Luciani F, Viros A et al (2007) Beta-catenin induces immortalization of melanocytes by suppressing p16INK4a expression and cooperates with N-Ras in melanoma development. Genes Dev 21:2923–2935

Denoyelle C, Abou-Rjaily G, Bezrookove V, Verhaegen M, Johnson TM, Fullen DR, Pointer JN, Gruber SB, Su LD, Nikiforov MA et al (2006) Anti-oncogenic role of the endoplasmic reticulum differentially activated by mutations in the MAPK pathway. Nat Cell Biol 8:1053–1063

Dhillon AS, Hagan S, Rath O, Kolch W (2007) MAP kinase signalling pathways in cancer. Oncogene 26:3279–3290

Doglioni C, Piccinin S, Demontis S, Cangi MG, Pecciarini L, Chiarelli C, Armellin M, Vukosavljevic T, Boiocchi M, Maestro R (2003) Alterations of beta-catenin pathway in non-melanoma skin tumors: loss of alpha-ABC nuclear reactivity correlates with the presence of beta-catenin gene mutation. Am J Pathol 163:2277–2287

Dorsky RI, Raible DW, Moon RT (2000) Direct regulation of nacre, a zebrafish MITF homolog required for pigment cell formation, by the Wnt pathway. Genes Dev 14:158–162

Dumaz N, Hayward R, Martin J, Ogilvie L, Hedley D, Curtin JA, Bastian BC, Springer C, Marais R (2006) In melanoma, RAS mutations are accompanied by switching signaling from BRAF to CRAF and disrupted cyclic AMP signaling. Cancer Res 66:9483–9491

Eichhoff OM, Zipser MC, Xu M, Weeraratna AT, Mihic D, Dummer R, Hoek KS (2010) The immunohistochemistry of invasive and proliferative phenotype switching in melanoma: a case report. Melanoma Res 20:349–355

Emery CM, Vijayendran KG, Zipser MC, Sawyer AM, Niu L, Kim JJ, Hatton C, Chopra R, Oberholzer PA, Karpova MB et al (2009) MEK1 mutations confer resistance to MEK and B-RAF inhibition. Proc Natl Acad Sci U S A 106:20411–20416

Emuss V, Garnett M, Mason C, Marais R (2005) Mutations of C-RAF are rare in human cancer because C-RAF has a low basal kinase activity compared with B-RAF. Cancer Res 65:9719–9726

Esteve-Puig R, Canals F, Colome N, Merlino G, Recio JA (2009) Uncoupling of the LKB1-AMPKalpha energy sensor pathway by growth factors and oncogenic BRAF. PLoS One 4:e4771

Fargnoli MC, Gandini S, Peris K, Maisonneuve P, Raimondi S (2010) MC1R variants increase melanoma risk in families with CDKN2A mutations: a meta-analysis. Eur J Cancer 46:1413–1420

Fecher LA, Cummings SD, Keefe MJ, Alani RM (2007) Toward a molecular classification of melanoma. J Clin Oncol 25:1606–1620

Felicetti F, Errico MC, Segnalini P, Mattia G, Care A (2008) MicroRNA-221 and −222 pathway controls melanoma progression. Expert Rev Anticancer Ther 8:1759–1765

Feng Y, Pinkerton A, Hulea L, Zhang T, Davies M, Grotegut S, Cheli Y, Yin H, Lau E, Kim H et al (2015) SBI-0640756 attenuates the growth of clinically unresponsive melanomas by disrupting the eIF4F translation initiation complex. Cancer Res 75(24):5211–5218

Flaherty KT, Puzanov I, Kim KB, Ribas A, McArthur GA, Sosman JA, O'Dwyer PJ, Lee RJ, Grippo JF, Nolop K et al (2010) Inhibition of mutated, activated BRAF in metastatic melanoma. N Engl J Med 363:809–819

Flaherty KT, Infante JR, Daud A, Gonzalez R, Kefford RF, Sosman J, Hamid O, Schuchter L, Cebon J, Ibrahim N et al (2012a) Combined BRAF and MEK inhibition in melanoma with BRAF V600 mutations. N Engl J Med 367:1694–1703

Flaherty KT, Robert C, Hersey P, Nathan P, Garbe C, Milhem M, Demidov LV, Hassel JC, Rutkowski P, Mohr P et al (2012b) Improved survival with MEK inhibition in BRAF-mutated melanoma. N Engl J Med 367:107–114

Freedberg DE, Rigas SH, Russak J, Gai W, Kaplow M, Osman I, Turner F, Randerson-Moor JA, Houghton A, Busam K et al (2008) Frequent p16-independent inactivation of p14ARF in human melanoma. J Natl Cancer Inst 100:784–795

Gewinner C, Wang ZC, Richardson A, Teruya-Feldstein J, Etemadmoghadam D, Bowtell D, Barretina J, Lin WM, Rameh L, Salmena L, Pandolfi PP and Cantley LC. (2009) Evidence that inositol polyphosphate 4-phosphatase type II is a tumor suppressor that inhibits PI3K signaling. Cancer Cell 16(2):115–125

Giehl KA, Nagele U, Volkenandt M, Berking C (2007) Protein expression of melanocyte growth factors (bFGF, SCF) and their receptors (FGFR-1, c-kit) in nevi and melanoma. J Cutan Pathol 34:7–14

Girotti MR, Pedersen M, Sanchez-Laorden B, Viros A, Turajlic S, Niculescu-Duvaz D, Zambon A, Sinclair J, Hayes A, Gore M et al (2013) Inhibiting EGF receptor or SRC family kinase signaling overcomes BRAF inhibitor resistance in melanoma. Cancer Discov 3:158–167

Goel VK, Lazar AJ, Warneke CL, Redston MS, Haluska FG (2006) Examination of mutations in BRAF, NRAS, and PTEN in primary cutaneous melanoma. J Invest Dermatol 126:154–160

Gollob JA, Wilhelm S, Carter C, Kelley SL (2006) Role of Raf kinase in cancer: therapeutic potential of targeting the Raf/MEK/ERK signal transduction pathway. Semin Oncol 33:392–406

Goodall J, Martinozzi S, Dexter TJ, Champeval D, Carreira S, Larue L, Goding CR (2004a) Brn-2 expression controls melanoma proliferation and is directly regulated by beta-catenin. Mol Cell Biol 24:2915–2922

Goodall J, Wellbrock C, Dexter TJ, Roberts K, Marais R, Goding CR (2004b) The Brn-2 transcription factor links activated BRAF to melanoma proliferation. Mol Cell Biol 24:2923–2931

Goodall J, Carreira S, Denat L, Kobi D, Davidson I, Nuciforo P, Sturm RA, Larue L, Goding CR (2008) Brn-2 represses microphthalmia-associated transcription factor expression and marks a distinct subpopulation of microphthalmia-associated transcription factor-negative melanoma cells. Cancer Res 68:7788–7794

Govindarajan B, Bai X, Cohen C, Zhong H, Kilroy S, Louis G, Moses M, Arbiser JL (2003) Malignant transformation of melanocytes to melanoma by constitutive activation of mitogen-activated protein kinase kinase (MAPKK) signaling. J Biol Chem 278:9790–9795

Govindarajan B, Sligh JE, Vincent BJ, Li M, Canter JA, Nickoloff BJ, Rodenburg RJ, Smeitink JA, Oberley L, Zhang Y et al (2007) Overexpression of Akt converts radial growth melanoma to vertical growth melanoma. J Clin Invest 117:719–729

Greger JG, Eastman SD, Zhang V, Bleam MR, Hughes AM, Smitheman KN, Dickerson SH, Laquerre SG, Liu L, Gilmer TM (2012) Combinations of BRAF, MEK, and PI3K/mTOR inhibitors overcome acquired resistance to the BRAF inhibitor GSK2118436 dabrafenib, mediated by NRAS or MEK mutations. Mol Cancer Ther 11:909–920

Ha L, Ichikawa T, Anver M, Dickins R, Lowe S, Sharpless NE, Krimpenfort P, Depinho RA, Bennett DC, Sviderskaya EV et al (2007) ARF functions as a melanoma tumor suppressor by inducing p53-independent senescence. Proc Natl Acad Sci U S A 104:10968–10973

Haferkamp S, Becker TM, Scurr LL, Kefford RF, Rizos H (2008) p16INK4a-induced senescence is disabled by melanoma-associated mutations. Aging Cell 7:733–745

Hatzivassiliou G, Song K, Yen I, Brandhuber BJ, Anderson DJ, Alvarado R, Ludlam MJ, Stokoe D, Gloor SL, Vigers G et al (2010) RAF inhibitors prime wild-type RAF to activate the MAPK pathway and enhance growth. Nature 464:431–435

Hazan C, Melzer K, Panageas KS, Li E, Kamino H, Kopf A, Cordon-Cardo C, Osman I, Polsky D (2002) Evaluation of the proliferation marker MIB-1 in the prognosis of cutaneous malignant melanoma. Cancer 95:634–640

Healey MA, Deaton SL, Alder JK, Winnepenninckx V, Casero RA Jr, Herman JG (2010) Id1 overexpression is independent of repression and epigenetic silencing of tumor suppressor genes in melanoma. Epigenetics 5:410–421

Henrique R, Azevedo R, Bento MJ, Domingues JC, Silva C, Jeronimo C (2000) Prognostic value of Ki-67 expression in localized cutaneous malignant melanoma. J Am Acad Dermatol 43:991–1000

Hodi FS, O'Day SJ, McDermott DF, Weber RW, Sosman JA, Haanen JB, Gonzalez R, Robert C, Schadendorf D, Hassel JC et al (2010) Improved survival with ipilimumab in patients with metastatic melanoma. N Engl J Med 363:711–723

Houben R, Becker JC, Kappel A, Terheyden P, Brocker EB, Goetz R, Rapp UR (2004) Constitutive activation of the Ras-Raf signaling pathway in metastatic melanoma is associated with poor prognosis. J Carcinog 3:6

Huang S, Luca M, Gutman M, McConkey DJ, Langley KE, Lyman SD, Bar-Eli M (1996) Enforced c-KIT expression renders highly metastatic human melanoma cells susceptible to stem cell factor-induced apoptosis and inhibits their tumorigenic and metastatic potential. Oncogene 13:2339–2347

Hu-Lieskovan S, Robert L, Homet Moreno B, Ribas A (2014) Combining targeted therapy with immunotherapy in BRAF-mutant melanoma: promise and challenges. J Clin Oncol 32:2248–2254

Hu-Lieskovan S, Mok S, Homet Moreno B, Tsoi J, Robert L, Goedert L, Pinheiro EM, Koya RC, Graeber TG, Comin-Anduix B et al (2015) Improved antitumor activity of immunotherapy with BRAF and MEK inhibitors in BRAF(V600E) melanoma. Sci Transl Med 7:279ra241

Hunt G, Kyne S, Wakamatsu K, Ito S, Thody AJ (1995) Nle4DPhe7 alpha-melanocyte-stimulating hormone increases the eumelanin:phaeomelanin ratio in cultured human melanocytes. J Invest Dermatol 104:83–85

Huntington JT, Shields JM, Der CJ, Wyatt CA, Benbow U, Slingluff CL Jr, Brinckerhoff CE (2004) Overexpression of collagenase 1 (MMP-1) is mediated by the ERK pathway in invasive melanoma cells: role of BRAF mutation and fibroblast growth factor signaling. J Biol Chem 279:33168–33176

Inoue-Narita T, Hamada K, Sasaki T, Hatakeyama S, Fujita S, Kawahara K, Sasaki M, Kishimoto H, Eguchi S, Kojima I et al (2008) Pten deficiency in melanocytes results in resistance to hair graying and susceptibility to carcinogen-induced melanomagenesis. Cancer Res 68:5760–5768

Jafari M, Papp T, Kirchner S, Diener U, Henschler D, Burg G, Schiffmann D (1995) Analysis of ras mutations in human melanocytic lesions: activation of the ras gene seems to be associated with the nodular type of human malignant melanoma. J Cancer Res Clin Oncol 121:23–30

Janku F, Novotny J, Julis I, Julisova I, Pecen L, Tomancova V, Kocmanova G, Krasna L, Krajsova I, Stork J et al (2005) KIT receptor is expressed in more than 50% of early-stage malignant melanoma: a retrospective study of 261 patients. Melanoma Res 15:251–256

Ji Z, Erin Chen Y, Kumar R, Taylor M, Jenny Njauw CN, Miao B, Frederick DT, Wargo JA, Flaherty KT, Jonsson G et al (2015) MITF modulates therapeutic resistance through EGFR signaling. J Invest Dermatol 135:1863–1872

Jiang CC, Lucas K, Avery-Kiejda KA, Wade M, deBock CE, Thorne RF, Allen J, Hersey P, Zhang XD (2008) Up-regulation of Mcl-1 is critical for survival of human melanoma cells upon endoplasmic reticulum stress. Cancer Res 68:6708–6717

Jiveskog S, Ragnarsson-Olding B, Platz A, Ringborg U (1998) N-ras mutations are common in melanomas from sun-exposed skin of humans but rare in mucosal membranes or unexposed skin. J Invest Dermatol 111:757–761

Johannessen CM, Boehm JS, Kim SY, Thomas SR, Wardwell L, Johnson LA, Emery CM, Stransky N, Cogdill AP, Barretina J et al (2010) COT drives resistance to RAF inhibition through MAP kinase pathway reactivation. Nature 468:968–972

Jukic DM, Rao UN, Kelly L, Skaf JS, Drogowski LM, Kirkwood JM, Panelli MC (2010) Microrna profiling analysis of differences between the melanoma of young adults and older adults. J Transl Med 8:27

Kadekaro AL, Kanto H, Kavanagh R, Abdel-Malek ZA (2003) Significance of the melanocortin 1 receptor in regulating human melanocyte pigmentation, proliferation, and survival. Ann N Y Acad Sci 994:359–365

Kaplan FM, Shao Y, Mayberry MM, Aplin AE (2011) Hyperactivation of MEK-ERK1/2 signaling and resistance to apoptosis induced by the oncogenic B-RAF inhibitor, PLX4720, in mutant N-RAS melanoma cells. Oncogene 30(3):366–371

Karasic TB, Hei TK, Ivanov VN (2010) Disruption of IGF-1R signaling increases TRAIL-induced apoptosis: a new potential therapy for the treatment of melanoma. Exp Cell Res 316:1994–2007

Karreth FA, Reschke M, Ruocco A, Ng C, Chapuy B, Leopold V, Sjoberg M, Keane TM, Verma A, Ala U et al (2015) The BRAF pseudogene functions as a competitive endogenous RNA and induces lymphoma in vivo. Cell 161:319–332

Kim D, Kim S, Koh H, Yoon SO, Chung AS, Cho KS, Chung J (2001) Akt/PKB promotes cancer cell invasion via increased motility and metalloproteinase production. FASEB J 15:1953–1962

Kim RD, Curtin JA, Bastian BC (2008a) Lack of somatic alterations of MC1R in primary melanoma. Pigment Cell Melanoma Res 21:579–582

Kim SS, Yoo NJ, Jeong EG, Kim MS, Lee SH (2008b) Expression of NEDD4-1, a PTEN regulator, in gastric and colorectal carcinomas. APMIS 116:779–784

Kim H, Frederick DT, Levesque MP, Cooper ZA, Feng Y, Krepler C, Brill L, Samuels Y, Hayward NK, Perlina A et al (2015) Downregulation of the ubiquitin ligase RNF125 underlies resistance of melanoma cells to BRAF inhibitors via JAK1 deregulation. Cell Rep 11:1458–1473

Koh J, Enders GH, Dynlacht BD, Harlow E (1995) Tumour-derived p16 alleles encoding proteins defective in cell-cycle inhibition. Nature 375:506–510

Konieczkowski DJ, Johannessen CM, Abudayyeh O, Kim JW, Cooper ZA, Piris A, Frederick DT, Barzily-Rokni M, Straussman R, Haq R et al (2014) A melanoma cell state distinction influences sensitivity to MAPK pathway inhibitors. Cancer Discov 4:816–827

Kortylewski M, Heinrich PC, Kauffmann ME, Bohm M, MacKiewicz A, Behrmann I (2001) Mitogen-activated protein kinases control p27/Kip1 expression and growth of human melanoma cells. Biochem J 357:297–303

Kumar R, Angelini S, Snellman E, Hemminki K (2004) BRAF mutations are common somatic events in melanocytic nevi. J Invest Dermatol 122:342–348

Kusters-Vandevelde HV, Klaasen A, Kusters B, Groenen PJ, van Engen-van Grunsven IA, van Dijk MR, Reifenberger G, Wesseling P, Blokx WA (2010) Activating mutations of the GNAQ gene: a frequent event in primary melanocytic neoplasms of the central nervous system. Acta Neuropathol 119(3):317–323

Lamba S, Felicioni L, Buttitta F, Bleeker FE, Malatesta S, Corbo V, Scarpa A, Rodolfo M, Knowles M, Frattini M et al (2010) Mutational profile of GNAQQ209 in human tumors. PLoS One 4:e6833

Landi MT, Bauer J, Pfeiffer RM, Elder DE, Hulley B, Minghetti P, Calista D, Kanetsky PA, Pinkel D, Bastian BC (2006) MC1R germline variants confer risk for BRAF-mutant melanoma. Science 313:521–522

Lang J, Boxer M, MacKie R (2003) Absence of exon 15 BRAF germline mutations in familial melanoma. Hum Mutat 21:327–330

Larkin J, Chiarion-Sileni V, Gonzalez R, Grob JJ, Cowey CL, Lao CD, Schadendorf D, Dummer R, Smylie M, Rutkowski P et al (2015) Combined Nivolumab and Ipilimumab or Monotherapy in Untreated Melanoma. N Engl J Med 373:23–34

Larue L, Delmas V (2006) The WNT/Beta-catenin pathway in melanoma. Front Biosci 11:733–742

Leach DR, Krummel MF, Allison JP (1996) Enhancement of antitumor immunity by CTLA-4 blockade. Science 271:1734–1736

Lee JW, Soung YH, Kim SY, Park WS, Nam SW, Min WS, Kim SH, Lee JY, Yoo NJ, Lee SH (2005) Mutational analysis of the ARAF gene in human cancers. APMIS 113:54–57
Levine AJ, Feng Z, Mak TW, You H, Jin S (2006) Coordination and communication between the p53 and IGF-1-AKT-TOR signal transduction pathways. Genes Dev 20:267–275
Lodygin D, Tarasov V, Epanchintsev A, Berking C, Knyazeva T, Korner H, Knyazev P, Diebold J, Hermeking H (2008) Inactivation of miR-34a by aberrant CpG methylation in multiple types of cancer. Cell Cycle 7:2591–2600
Lopez-Bergami P, Huang C, Goydos JS, Yip D, Bar-Eli M, Herlyn M, Smalley KS, Mahale A, Eroshkin A, Aaronson S et al (2007) Rewired ERK-JNK signaling pathways in melanoma. Cancer Cell 11:447–460
Lopez-Bergami P, Kim H, Dewing A, Goydos J, Aaronson S, Ronai Z (2010) c-Jun regulates phosphoinositide-dependent kinase 1 transcription: implication for Akt and protein kinase C activities and melanoma tumorigenesis. J Biol Chem 285:903–913
Macaulay VM, Salisbury AJ, Bohula EA, Playford MP, Smorodinsky NI, Shiloh Y (2001) Downregulation of the type 1 insulin-like growth factor receptor in mouse melanoma cells is associated with enhanced radiosensitivity and impaired activation of Atm kinase. Oncogene 20:4029–4040
Madhunapantula SV, Robertson GP (2009) The PTEN-AKT3 signaling cascade as a therapeutic target in melanoma. Pigment Cell Melanoma Res 22:400–419
Mallikarjuna K, Pushparaj V, Biswas J, Krishnakumar S (2006) Expression of insulin-like growth factor receptor (IGF-1R), c-Fos, and c-Jun in uveal melanoma: an immunohistochemical study. Curr Eye Res 31:875–883
Maloney EK, McLaughlin JL, Dagdigian NE, Garrett LM, Connors KM, Zhou XM, Blattler WA, Chittenden T, Singh R (2003) An anti-insulin-like growth factor I receptor antibody that is a potent inhibitor of cancer cell proliferation. Cancer Res 63:5073–5083
Mattei S, Colombo MP, Melani C, Silvani A, Parmiani G, Herlyn M (1994) Expression of cytokine/growth factors and their receptors in human melanoma and melanocytes. Int J Cancer 56:853–857
Meier F, Schittek B, Busch S, Garbe C, Smalley K, Satyamoorthy K, Li G, Herlyn M (2005) The RAS/RAF/MEK/ERK and PI3K/AKT signaling pathways present molecular targets for the effective treatment of advanced melanoma. Front Biosci 10:2986–3001
Menzies AM, Long GV (2013) New combinations and immunotherapies for melanoma: latest evidence and clinical utility. Ther Adv Med Oncol 5:278–285
Michaloglou C, Vredeveld LC, Soengas MS, Denoyelle C, Kuilman T, van der Horst CM, Majoor DM, Shay JW, Mooi WJ, Peeper DS (2005) BRAFE600-associated senescence-like cell cycle arrest of human naevi. Nature 436:720–724
Mirmohammadsadegh A, Marini A, Nambiar S, Hassan M, Tannapfel A, Ruzicka T, Hengge UR (2006) Epigenetic silencing of the PTEN gene in melanoma. Cancer Res 66:6546–6552
Mitra D, Luo X, Morgan A, Wang J, Hoang MP, Lo J, Guerrero CR, Lennerz JK, Mihm MC, Wargo JA et al (2012) An ultraviolet-radiation-independent pathway to melanoma carcinogenesis in the red hair/fair skin background. Nature 491:449–453
Montagut C, Sharma SV, Shioda T, McDermott U, Ulman M, Ulkus LE, Dias-Santagata D, Stubbs H, Lee DY, Singh A et al (2008) Elevated CRAF as a potential mechanism of acquired resistance to BRAF inhibition in melanoma. Cancer Res 68:4853–4861
Montone KT, van Belle P, Elenitsas R, Elder DE (1997) Proto-oncogene c-kit expression in malignant melanoma: protein loss with tumor progression. Mod Pathol 10:939–944
Mountjoy KG, Robbins LS, Mortrud MT, Cone RD (1992) The cloning of a family of genes that encode the melanocortin receptors. Science 257:1248–1251
Muller J, Krijgsman O, Tsoi J, Robert L, Hugo W, Song C, Kong X, Possik PA, Cornelissen-Steijger PD, Foppen MH et al (2014) Low MITF/AXL ratio predicts early resistance to multiple targeted drugs in melanoma. Nat Commun 5:5712
Murugan AK, Dong J, Xie J, Xing M (2009) MEK1 mutations, but not ERK2 mutations, occur in melanomas and colon carcinomas, but none in thyroid carcinomas. Cell Cycle 8:2122–2124

Natali PG, Nicotra MR, Winkler AB, Cavaliere R, Bigotti A, Ullrich A (1992) Progression of human cutaneous melanoma is associated with loss of expression of c-kit proto-oncogene receptor. Int J Cancer 52:197–201

Natali PG, Nicotra MR, Di Renzo MF, Prat M, Bigotti A, Cavaliere R, Comoglio PM (1993) Expression of the c-Met/HGF receptor in human melanocytic neoplasms: demonstration of the relationship to malignant melanoma tumour progression. Br J Cancer 68:746–750

Nateri AS, Riera-Sans L, Da Costa C, Behrens A (2004) The ubiquitin ligase SCFFbw7 antagonizes apoptotic JNK signaling. Science 303:1374–1378

Nazarian R, Shi H, Wang Q, Kong X, Koya RC, Lee H, Chen Z, Lee MK, Attar N, Sazegar H et al (2010) Melanomas acquire resistance to B-RAF(V600E) inhibition by RTK or N-RAS upregulation. Nature 468:973–977

Ohanna M, Giuliano S, Bonet C, Imbert V, Hofman V, Zangari J, Bille K, Robert C, Bressac-de Paillerets B, Hofman P et al (2011) Senescent cells develop a PARP-1 and nuclear factor-{kappa}B-associated secretome (PNAS). Genes Dev 25:1245–1261

Ohanna M, Cheli Y, Bonet C, Bonazzi VF, Allegra M, Giuliano S, Bille K, Bahadoran P, Giacchero D, Lacour JP et al (2013) Secretome from senescent melanoma engages the STAT3 pathway to favor reprogramming of naive melanoma towards a tumor-initiating cell phenotype. Oncotarget 4:2212–2224

Okazaki T, Chikuma S, Iwai Y, Fagarasan S, Honjo T (2013) A rheostat for immune responses: the unique properties of PD-1 and their advantages for clinical application. Nat Immunol 14:1212–1218

Paccez JD, Vogelsang M, Parker MI, Zerbini LF (2014) The receptor tyrosine kinase Axl in cancer: biological functions and therapeutic implications. Int J Cancer 134:1024–1033

Paraiso KH, Fedorenko IV, Cantini LP, Munko AC, Hall M, Sondak VK, Messina JL, Flaherty KT, Smalley KS (2010) Recovery of phospho-ERK activity allows melanoma cells to escape from BRAF inhibitor therapy. Br J Cancer 102:1724–1730

Parmiter AH, Balaban G, Clark WH Jr, Nowell PC (1988) Possible involvement of the chromosome region 10q24----q26 in early stages of melanocytic neoplasia. Cancer Genet Cytogenet 30:313–317

Patton EE, Widlund HR, Kutok JL, Kopani KR, Amatruda JF, Murphey RD, Berghmans S, Mayhall EA, Traver D, Fletcher CD et al (2005) BRAF mutations are sufficient to promote nevi formation and cooperate with p53 in the genesis of melanoma. Curr Biol 15:249–254

Pavey SJ, Cummings MC, Whiteman DC, Castellano M, Walsh MD, Gabrielli BG, Green A, Hayward NK (2002) Loss of p16 expression is associated with histological features of melanoma invasion. Melanoma Res 12:539–547

Peggs KS, Quezada SA, Korman AJ, Allison JP (2006) Principles and use of anti-CTLA4 antibody in human cancer immunotherapy. Curr Opin Immunol 18:206–213

Pleasance ED, Cheetham RK, Stephens PJ, McBride DJ, Humphray SJ, Greenman CD, Varela I, Lin ML, Ordonez GR, Bignell GR et al (2010) A comprehensive catalogue of somatic mutations from a human cancer genome. Nature 463:191–196

Ploper D, Taelman VF, Robert L, Perez BS, Titz B, Chen HW, Graeber TG, von Euw E, Ribas A, De Robertis EM (2015) MITF drives endolysosomal biogenesis and potentiates Wnt signaling in melanoma cells. Proc Natl Acad Sci U S A 112:E420–E429

Poliseno L, Salmena L, Zhang J, Carver B, Haveman WJ, Pandolfi PP (2010) A coding-independent function of gene and pseudogene mRNAs regulates tumour biology. Nature 465:1033–1038

Pollock PM, Walker GJ, Glendening JM, Que Noy T, Bloch NC, Fountain JW, Hayward NK (2002) PTEN inactivation is rare in melanoma tumours but occurs frequently in melanoma cell lines. Melanoma Res 12:565–575

Primot A, Mogha A, Corre S, Roberts K, Debbache J, Adamski H, Dreno B, Khammari A, Lesimple T, Mereau A et al (2010) ERK-regulated differential expression of the Mitf 6a/b splicing isoforms in melanoma. Pigment Cell Melanoma Res 23:93–102

Puri N, Ahmed S, Janamanchi V, Tretiakova M, Zumba O, Krausz T, Jagadeeswaran R, Salgia R (2007) c-Met is a potentially new therapeutic target for treatment of human melanoma. Clin Cancer Res 13:2246–2253

Ranade K, Hussussian CJ, Sikorski RS, Varmus HE, Goldstein AM, Tucker MA, Serrano M, Hannon GJ, Beach D, Dracopoli NC (1995) Mutations associated with familial melanoma impair p16INK4 function. Nat Genet 10:114–116

Rane SG, Cosenza SC, Mettus RV, Reddy EP (2002) Germ line transmission of the Cdk4(R24C) mutation facilitates tumorigenesis and escape from cellular senescence. Mol Cell Biol 22:644–656

Resnicoff M, Coppola D, Sell C, Rubin R, Ferrone S, Baserga R (1994) Growth inhibition of human melanoma cells in nude mice by antisense strategies to the type 1 insulin-like growth factor receptor. Cancer Res 54:4848–4850

Rivera RS, Nagatsuka H, Gunduz M, Cengiz B, Gunduz E, Siar CH, Tsujigiwa H, Tamamura R, Han KN, Nagai N (2008) C-kit protein expression correlated with activating mutations in KIT gene in oral mucosal melanoma. Virchows Arch 452:27–32

Robertson GP (2005) Functional and therapeutic significance of Akt deregulation in malignant melanoma. Cancer Metastasis Rev 24:273–285

Robinson SJ, Healy E (2002) Human melanocortin 1 receptor (MC1R) gene variants alter melanoma cell growth and adhesion to extracellular matrix. Oncogene 21:8037–8046

Rouzaud F, Costin GE, Yamaguchi Y, Valencia JC, Berens WF, Chen KG, Hoashi T, Bohm M, Abdel-Malek ZA, Hearing VJ (2006) Regulation of constitutive and UVR-induced skin pigmentation by melanocortin 1 receptor isoforms. FASEB J 20:1927–1929

Rusciano D, Lorenzoni P, Burger MM (1995) Expression of constitutively activated hepatocyte growth factor/scatter factor receptor (c-met) in B16 melanoma cells selected for enhanced liver colonization. Oncogene 11:1979–1987

Rusciano D, Lorenzoni P, Burger MM (1999) Regulation of c-met expression in B16 murine melanoma cells by melanocyte stimulating hormone. J Cell Sci 112(Pt 5):623–630

Russo AE, Torrisi E, Bevelacqua Y, Perrotta R, Libra M, McCubrey JA, Spandidos DA, Stivala F, Malaponte G (2009) Melanoma: molecular pathogenesis and emerging target therapies (review). Int J Oncol 34:1481–1489

Salton M, Kasprzak WK, Voss T, Shapiro BA, Poulikakos PI, Misteli T (2015) Inhibition of vemurafenib-resistant melanoma by interference with pre-mRNA splicing. Nat Commun 6:7103

Satoh S, Hashimoto-Tamaoki T, Furuyama J, Mihara K, Namba M, Kitano Y (2000) High frequency of tetraploidy detected in malignant melanoma of Japanese patients by fluorescence in situ hybridization. Int J Oncol 17:707–715

Satyamoorthy K, Li G, Vaidya B, Patel D, Herlyn M (2001) Insulin-like growth factor-1 induces survival and growth of biologically early melanoma cells through both the mitogen-activated protein kinase and beta-catenin pathways. Cancer Res 61:7318–7324

Satzger I, Mattern A, Kuettler U, Weinspach D, Voelker B, Kapp A, Gutzmer R (2010) MicroRNA-15b represents an independent prognostic parameter and is correlated with tumor cell proliferation and apoptosis in malignant melanoma. Int J Cancer 126:2553–2562

Sauroja I, Smeds J, Vlaykova T, Kumar R, Talve L, Hahka-Kemppinen M, Punnonen K, Jansen CT, Hemminki K, Pyrhonen S (2000) Analysis of G(1)/S checkpoint regulators in metastatic melanoma. Genes Chromosomes Cancer 28:404–414

Schepsky A, Bruser K, Gunnarsson GJ, Goodall J, Hallsson JH, Goding CR, Steingrimsson E, Hecht A (2006) The microphthalmia-associated transcription factor Mitf interacts with beta-catenin to determine target gene expression. Mol Cell Biol 26:8914–8927

Schultz J, Lorenz P, Gross G, Ibrahim S, Kunz M (2008) MicroRNA let-7b targets important cell cycle molecules in malignant melanoma cells and interferes with anchorage-independent growth. Cell Res 18:549–557

Scortegagna M, Ruller C, Feng Y, Lazova R, Kluger H, Li JL, De SK, Rickert R, Pellecchia M, Bosenberg M et al (2014) Genetic inactivation or pharmacological inhibition of Pdk1 delays development and inhibits metastasis of Braf(V600E)::Pten(−/−) melanoma. Oncogene 33:4330–4339

Scortegagna M, Lau E, Zhang T, Feng Y, Sereduk C, Yin H, De SK, Meeth K, Platt JT, Langdon CG et al (2015) PDK1 and SGK3 contribute to the growth of BRAF-mutant melanomas and are potential therapeutic targets. Cancer Res 75:1399–1412

Scott MC, Wakamatsu K, Ito S, Kadekaro AL, Kobayashi N, Groden J, Kavanagh R, Takakuwa T, Virador V, Hearing VJ et al (2002) Human melanocortin 1 receptor variants, receptor function and melanocyte response to UV radiation. J Cell Sci 115:2349–2355

Sensi M, Catani M, Castellano G, Nicolini G, Alciato F, Tragni G, De Santis G, Bersani I, Avanzi G, Tomassetti A et al (2011) Human cutaneous melanomas lacking MITF and melanocyte differentiation antigens express a functional Axl receptor kinase. J Invest Dermatol 131:2448–2457

Shao Y, Aplin AE (2010) Akt3-mediated resistance to apoptosis in B-RAF-targeted melanoma cells. Cancer Res 70:6670–6681

Sheridan C, Brumatti G, Martin SJ (2008) Oncogenic B-RafV600E inhibits apoptosis and promotes ERK-dependent inactivation of Bad and Bim. J Biol Chem 283:22128–22135

Shukla VK, Hughes DC, Hughes LE, McCormick F, Padua RA (1989) ras mutations in human melanotic lesions: K-ras activation is a frequent and early event in melanoma development. Oncogene Res 5:121–127

Smalley KS, Nathanson KL, Flaherty KT (2009) Genetic subgrouping of melanoma reveals new opportunities for targeted therapy. Cancer Res 69:3241–3244

Song X, Mosby N, Yang J, Xu A, Abdel-Malek Z, Kadekaro AL (2009) alpha-MSH activates immediate defense responses to UV-induced oxidative stress in human melanocytes. Pigment Cell Melanoma Res 22:809–818

Soyer HP (1991) Ki 67 immunostaining in melanocytic skin tumors. Correlation with histologic parameters. J Cutan Pathol 18:264–272

Spofford LS, Abel EV, Boisvert-Adamo K, Aplin AE (2006) Cyclin D3 expression in melanoma cells is regulated by adhesion-dependent phosphatidylinositol 3-kinase signaling and contributes to G1-S progression. J Biol Chem 281:25644–25651

Spranger S, Bao R, Gajewski TF (2015) Melanoma-intrinsic beta-catenin signalling prevents anti-tumour immunity. Nature 523:231–235

Stahl JM, Sharma A, Cheung M, Zimmerman M, Cheng JQ, Bosenberg MW, Kester M, Sandirasegarane L, Robertson GP (2004) Deregulated Akt3 activity promotes development of malignant melanoma. Cancer Res 64:7002–7010

Steinbeck ZR, Heselmeyer KM, Gerlach B, Bjornhagen V, Auer GU (1996) Diagnostic impact of nuclear DNA content and proliferative activity in benign and malignant melanocytic lesions. Melanoma Res 6:37–43

Straume O, Smeds J, Kumar R, Hemminki K, Akslen LA (2002) Significant impact of promoter hypermethylation and the 540 C>T polymorphism of CDKN2A in cutaneous melanoma of the vertical growth phase. Am J Pathol 161:229–237

Sumimoto H, Imabayashi F, Iwata T, Kawakami Y (2006) The BRAF-MAPK signaling pathway is essential for cancer-immune evasion in human melanoma cells. J Exp Med 203:1651–1656

Sun C, Wang L, Huang S, Heynen GJ, Prahallad A, Robert C, Haanen J, Blank C, Wesseling J, Willems SM et al (2014) Reversible and adaptive resistance to BRAF(V600E) inhibition in melanoma. Nature 508:118–122

Suzuki I, Cone RD, Im S, Nordlund J, Abdel-Malek ZA (1996) Binding of melanotropic hormones to the melanocortin receptor MC1R on human melanocytes stimulates proliferation and melanogenesis. Endocrinology 137:1627–1633

Takeda K, Yasumoto K, Takada R, Takada S, Watanabe K, Udono T, Saito H, Takahashi K, Shibahara S (2000) Induction of melanocyte-specific microphthalmia-associated transcription factor by Wnt-3a. J Biol Chem 275:14013–14016

Takeuchi T, Adachi Y, Sonobe H, Furihata M, Ohtsuki Y (2006) A ubiquitin ligase, skeletrophin, is a negative regulator of melanoma invasion. Oncogene 25:7059–7069

Terheyden P, Houben R, Pajouh P, Thorns C, Zillikens D, Becker JC (2010) Response to imatinib mesylate depends on the presence of the V559A-mutated KIT oncogene. J Invest Dermatol 130:314–316

Topalian SL, Sznol M, McDermott DF, Kluger HM, Carvajal RD, Sharfman WH, Brahmer JR, Lawrence DP, Atkins MB, Powderly JD et al (2014) Survival, durable tumor remission, and long-term safety in patients with advanced melanoma receiving nivolumab. J Clin Oncol 32:1020–1030

Topcu-Yilmaz P, Kiratli H, Saglam A, Soylemezoglu F, Hascelik G (2010) Correlation of clinicopathological parameters with HGF, c-Met, EGFR, and IGF-1R expression in uveal melanoma. Melanoma Res 20:126–132

Trotman LC, Wang X, Alimonti A, Chen Z, Teruya-Feldstein J, Yang H, Pavletich NP, Carver BS, Cordon-Cardo C, Erdjument-Bromage H et al (2007) Ubiquitination regulates PTEN nuclear import and tumor suppression. Cell 128:141–156

Tsai J, Lee JT, Wang W, Zhang J, Cho H, Mamo S, Bremer R, Gillette S, Kong J, Haass NK et al (2008) Discovery of a selective inhibitor of oncogenic B-Raf kinase with potent antimelanoma activity. Proc Natl Acad Sci U S A 105:3041–3046

Urso C, Bondi R, Balzi M, Scubla E, Mauri P, Becciolini A, Tarocchi S, Vallecchi C (1992) Cell kinetics of melanocytes in common and dysplastic nevi and in primary and metastatic cutaneous melanoma. Pathol Res Pract 188:323–329

van der Velden PA, Metzelaar-Blok JA, Bergman W, Monique H, Hurks H, Frants RR, Gruis NA, Jager MJ (2001) Promoter hypermethylation: a common cause of reduced p16(INK4a) expression in uveal melanoma. Cancer Res 61:5303–5306

van Dijk MC, Bernsen MR, Ruiter DJ (2005) Analysis of mutations in B-RAF, N-RAS, and H-RAS genes in the differential diagnosis of Spitz nevus and spitzoid melanoma. Am J Surg Pathol 29:1145–1151

van Elsas A, Zerp S, van der Flier S, Kruse-Wolters M, Vacca A, Ruiter DJ, Schrier P (1995) Analysis of N-ras mutations in human cutaneous melanoma: tumor heterogeneity detected by polymerase chain reaction/single-stranded conformation polymorphism analysis. Recent Results Cancer Res 139:57–67

van Ginkel PR, Gee RL, Shearer RL, Subramanian L, Walker TM, Albert DM, Meisner LF, Varnum BC, Polans AS (2004) Expression of the receptor tyrosine kinase Axl promotes ocular melanoma cell survival. Cancer Res 64:128–134

Van Raamsdonk CD, Bezrookove V, Green G, Bauer J, Gaugler L, O'Brien JM, Simpson EM, Barsh GS, Bastian BC (2009) Frequent somatic mutations of GNAQ in uveal melanoma and blue naevi. Nature 457:599–602

Vanneman M, Dranoff G (2012) Combining immunotherapy and targeted therapies in cancer treatment. Nat Rev Cancer 12:237–251

Vasudevan KM, Barbie DA, Davies MA, Rabinovsky R, McNear CJ, Kim JJ, Hennessy BT, Tseng H, Pochanard P, Kim SY et al (2009) AKT-independent signaling downstream of oncogenic PIK3CA mutations in human cancer. Cancer Cell 16:21–32

Vergani E, Vallacchi V, Frigerio S, Deho P, Mondellini P, Perego P, Cassinelli G, Lanzi C, Testi MA, Rivoltini L et al (2011) Identification of MET and SRC activation in melanoma cell lines showing primary resistance to PLX4032. Neoplasia 13:1132–1142

Villanueva J, Vultur A, Lee JT, Somasundaram R, Fukunaga-Kalabis M, Cipolla AK, Wubbenhorst B, Xu X, Gimotty PA, Kee D et al (2010) Acquired resistance to BRAF inhibitors mediated by a RAF kinase switch in melanoma can be overcome by cotargeting MEK and IGF-1R/PI3K. Cancer Cell 18:683–695

Wan PT, Garnett MJ, Roe SM, Lee S, Niculescu-Duvaz D, Good VM, Jones CM, Marshall CJ, Springer CJ, Barford D et al (2004) Mechanism of activation of the RAF-ERK signaling pathway by oncogenic mutations of B-RAF. Cell 116:855–867

Wang X, Trotman LC, Koppie T, Alimonti A, Chen Z, Gao Z, Wang J, Erdjument-Bromage H, Tempst P, Cordon-Cardo C et al (2007a) NEDD4-1 is a proto-oncogenic ubiquitin ligase for PTEN. Cell 128:129–139

Wang YF, Jiang CC, Kiejda KA, Gillespie S, Zhang XD, Hersey P (2007b) Apoptosis induction in human melanoma cells by inhibition of MEK is caspase-independent and mediated by the Bcl-2 family members PUMA, Bim, and Mcl-1. Clin Cancer Res 13:4934–4942

Weeraratna AT, Jiang Y, Hostetter G, Rosenblatt K, Duray P, Bittner M, Trent JM (2002) Wnt5a signaling directly affects cell motility and invasion of metastatic melanoma. Cancer Cell 1:279–288

Wei W, Jin J, Schlisio S, Harper JW, Kaelin WG Jr (2005) The v-Jun point mutation allows c-Jun to escape GSK3-dependent recognition and destruction by the Fbw7 ubiquitin ligase. Cancer Cell 8:25–33

Wellbrock C, Hurlstone A (2010) BRAF as therapeutic target in melanoma. Biochem Pharmacol 80:561–567

Wellbrock C, Karasarides M, Marais R (2004) The RAF proteins take centre stage. Nat Rev Mol Cell Biol 5:875–885

Wellbrock C, Rana S, Paterson H, Pickersgill H, Brummelkamp T, Marais R (2008) Oncogenic BRAF regulates melanoma proliferation through the lineage specific factor MITF. PLoS One 3:e2734

Widlund HR, Horstmann MA, Price ER, Cui J, Lessnick SL, Wu M, He X, Fisher DE (2002) Beta-catenin-induced melanoma growth requires the downstream target Microphthalmia-associated transcription factor. J Cell Biol 158:1079–1087

Willmore-Payne C, Holden JA, Tripp S, Layfield LJ (2005) Human malignant melanoma: detection of BRAF- and c-kit-activating mutations by high-resolution amplicon melting analysis. Hum Pathol 36:486–493

Willmore-Payne C, Holden JA, Hirschowitz S, Layfield LJ (2006) BRAF and c-kit gene copy number in mutation-positive malignant melanoma. Hum Pathol 37:520–527

Witze ES, Litman ES, Argast GM, Moon RT, Ahn NG (2008) Wnt5a control of cell polarity and directional movement by polarized redistribution of adhesion receptors. Science 320:365–369

Wu H, Goel V, Haluska FG (2003) PTEN signaling pathways in melanoma. Oncogene 22:3113–3122

Yaguchi T, Goto Y, Kido K, Mochimaru H, Sakurai T, Tsukamoto N, Kudo-Saito C, Fujita T, Sumimoto H, Kawakami Y (2012) Immune suppression and resistance mediated by constitutive activation of Wnt/beta-catenin signaling in human melanoma cells. J Immunol 189:2110–2117

Yan D, Zhou X, Chen X, Hu DN, Dong XD, Wang J, Lu F, Tu L, Qu J (2009) MicroRNA-34a inhibits uveal melanoma cell proliferation and migration through downregulation of c-Met. Invest Ophthalmol Vis Sci 50:1559–1565

Yang G, Rajadurai A, Tsao H (2005) Recurrent patterns of dual RB and p53 pathway inactivation in melanoma. J Invest Dermatol 125:1242–1251

Yeh AH, Bohula EA, Macaulay VM (2006) Human melanoma cells expressing V600E B-RAF are susceptible to IGF1R targeting by small interfering RNAs. Oncogene 25:6574–6581

Yim EK, Peng G, Dai H, Hu R, Li K, Lu Y, Mills GB, Meric-Bernstam F, Hennessy BT, Craven RJ et al (2009) Rak functions as a tumor suppressor by regulating PTEN protein stability and function. Cancer Cell 15:304–314

Zhang Z, Sun H, Dai H, Walsh RM, Imakura M, Schelter J, Burchard J, Dai X, Chang AN, Diaz RL et al (2009) MicroRNA miR-210 modulates cellular response to hypoxia through the MYC antagonist MNT. Cell Cycle 8:2756–2768

Zheng B, Jeong JH, Asara JM, Yuan YY, Granter SR, Chin L, Cantley LC (2009) Oncogenic B-RAF negatively regulates the tumor suppressor LKB1 to promote melanoma cell proliferation. Mol Cell 33:237–247

Proteases in Melanoma

8

Paola Zigrino and Cornelia Mauch

8.1 Introduction

Activity of proteolytic enzymes expressed by tumor cells is involved in sustaining cellular growth and invasion. In addition, cross-communication of tumor cells and the stromal compartment, thereby including cellular and structural components, further contributes to cancer progression. Such interactions are particularly important for the dissociation of tumor cells from the primary tumor, the invasion of the surrounding connective tissue, and the penetration of vessel walls. While tumor cells invade and degrade the neighboring stroma, they generate a permissive microenvironment convenient for their growth, migration, and metastatic spread.

The tumor stroma, including that of melanoma, is composed of matrix proteins and a rich cellular population that includes fibroblasts, smooth muscle cells, endothelial cells, dendritic cells, macrophages, and other inflammatory cells. Several molecular modifications of the microenvironment occur by the activity of tumor cells or by stimulated stromal cells and include release of matrix or cell surface-bound factors, bioactive matrix fragments as well as cell–cell and cell–matrix contacts (see also Chap. 14). All these events are controlled by the activity of several proteolytic enzymes produced by either tumor or stromal cells (Fig. 8.1). The major proteases involved in these processes are classified into serine-, cysteine-, aspartyl-, and metalloproteinases according to structural characteristics of their active enzymatic center. In this review, we will give an overview of the expression and activity of those enzymes that have been implicated in the development of malignant melanoma and their role in the pathogenesis of this disease.

P. Zigrino (✉) • C. Mauch
Department of Dermatology, University of Cologne,
Kerpener Strasse 62, 50937 Cologne, Germany
e-mail: paola.zigrino@uk-koeln.de

A. Bosserhoff (ed.), *Melanoma Development*,
DOI 10.1007/978-3-319-41319-8_8

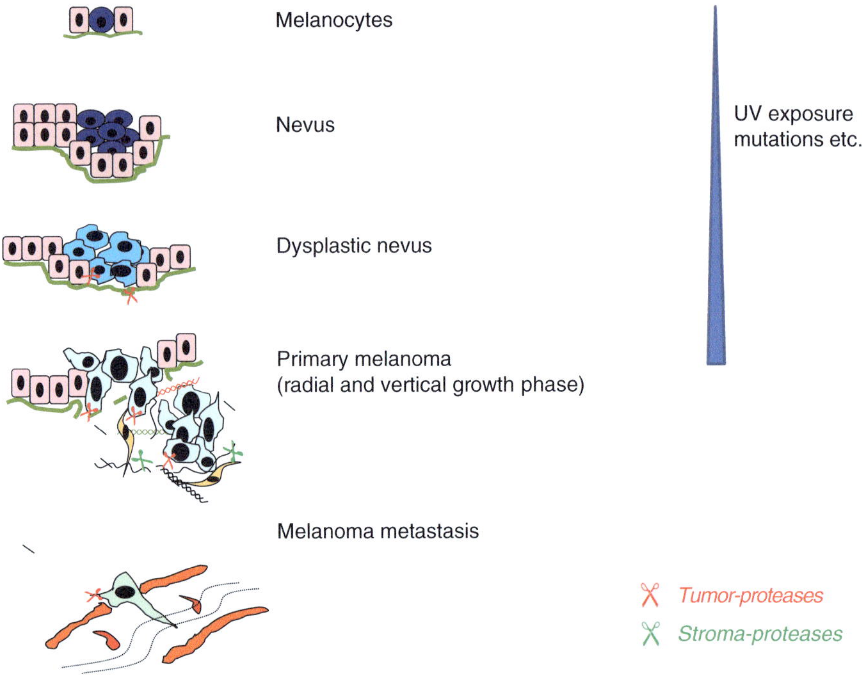

Fig. 8.1 Transformation of melanocytes or a nevus to melanoma. Benign transformation of melanocytes due to accumulation of mutations (e.g., upon UV exposure) into a nevus which progresses into a dysplastic nevus. The following step into a malignant radial and vertical growth melanoma is characterized by the activity of several proteolytic enzymes. Proteolytic enzymes either derived from tumor cells or activated stroma mediate cellular functions, leading to malignant cell progression through the tissue and contributes to the intravasation of melanoma cells into blood and lymph vessels

8.2 MMPs

Expression of matrix metalloproteinases (MMPs) in normal skin is almost undetectable; however, a low but constant expression of some MMPs is necessary for skin homeostasis. In normal skin, matrix remodeling occurs by a slow but continuous synthesis, constitutive degradation and reconstruction of matrix components. MMPs are strongly involved in the controlled degradation of connective tissue during wound repair, in the regulation of tissue architecture, and in embryonic development (reviewed in Page-McCaw et al. 2007).

Increased expression of MMPs has been observed in different malignancies and has been implicated in enhanced extracellular matrix (ECM) degradation. On the contrary, altered ECM deposition and degradation resulting from modifications of the endogenous tissue inhibitors of metalloproteinases (TIMPs) and collagenase expression such as during aging may lead to a higher cancer incidence (Lu et al.

2011) (see also Chap. 11). On a cellular level, once induced, MMPs may be either expressed on the cell surface, leading to pericellular proteolysis, or secreted, thus exerting their activity in the surrounding areas. Interestingly, membrane-associated proteases can also exert their activity in peritumoral areas as they can be associated and released through exosomes. This was observed in a proteomic profiling of exosomes derived from various melanoma cell lines. In this study, expression of MMP-14, ADAM-10, and also the inhibitor TIMP-3 was identified in these structures (Lazar et al. 2015).

In melanoma tissues, MMPs are mainly located at the tumor–stroma border and are produced by either tumor cells or stromal cells that are activated by tumor-derived soluble factors (Moro et al. 2014). In addition, growth factors and cytokines secreted by tumor-infiltrating inflammatory cells also modulate MMP expression in melanoma and stroma cells (Coussens et al. 2002).

In vitro and in vivo analysis have indicated an important role of the matrix itself for the induction of MMPs such as MMP-2/-9, and MMP-14 in invasive melanoma (Hofmann et al. 2000; Kurschat et al. 1999). Expression of MMP-14 was mainly localized in melanoma cells located at the invasive front of the tumor (Hofmann et al. 2000; Kurschat et al. 2002). This indicates that localization of both MMP-2 and MMP-14 at the interface between tumor and stroma may be required for enzyme activation and matrix degradation and highlights how the different cells cooperatively act to promote tumor progression. Indeed, the activity of MMP-2 in these peripheral areas of the tumors was suggested to be necessary to process collagen type I, to cleave fibronectin, and to promote adhesion and migration of melanoma cells (Jiao et al. 2012). Expression of the interstitial collagenases MMP-1 and −13, which are key enzymes in the cleavage of fibrillar collagens, was detected during the invasive vertical growth phase in melanoma cells thus indicating that this is a late event in melanocytic tumor progression (Airola et al. 1999). Expression of MMP-1 was also found in melanoma cells from radial growth phase (RGP) and lead to enhanced tumor growth and conferred metastatic capability in vivo (Blackburn et al. 2009). Interestingly, despite the fact that MMP-1 displays several promoter polymorphisms correlating with tumor ulceration status, it does not significantly associate with overall survival and other clinical factors (Liu et al. 2012; Wang et al. 2011).

However, even though the studies from Airola et al. (1999) show expression of both collagenolytic enzymes in tumor cells in vivo, several other in vivo and in vitro studies have indicated production of these enzymes primarily by peritumoral fibroblasts (Loffek et al. 2005; Uria et al. 1997; Wandel et al. 2000; Zigrino et al. 2009). We have recently shown that stromal expression of MMP-13 plays an important role in tumor growth of melanoma. Melanoma cells injected into the skin of MMP-13 depleted mice formed smaller tumors and developed fewer metastases as compared to wild type animals (Zigrino et al. 2009). Reduced tumor growth and metastasis is likely caused by the lack of peritumoral MMP-13, which is found to be strongly expressed in tumor-associated fibroblast-like cells. In addition, we and others could also show that MMP-13 modulates tumor vascularization by mediating the release of matrix-bound vascular endothelial growth factor (Lederle et al. 2010). In line with these data, MMP-13 has been associated with metastasis and poor survival in melanoma patients (Zhao et al. 2015). Interestingly, in this study, processing of laminin-332 or VE-cadherin by MMP-13 was shown to accelerate metastasis, but inhibited vasculogenic mimicry in vitro. Increased production of MMP-2 and MMP-14, and deposition of the γ2 chain of laminin 332 and/or its cleavage fragments have been observed in melanoma cells in vitro (Seftor et al. 2001). This process also likely contributes to tumor progression in vivo where the cleaved form of laminin 332 was found in tumors and in tissues undergoing remodeling but not in quiescent tissues (Lohi 2001; Patarroyo et al. 2002).

Besides MMP-13, several other MMPs were shown to contribute to both pro- and anti-angiogenic processes during tumor development. Recent studies have identified a novel mechanism by which MMP-1 promotes angiogenesis. MMP-1 proteolytically activates protease activated receptor-1 (PAR1), a thrombin receptor that is highly expressed in endothelial cells (Blackburn and Brinckerhoff 2008; Boire et al. 2005).

MMP-14 can facilitate endothelial cell migration and tube formation processes in vitro and in vivo (Chun et al. 2004; Mimura et al. 2009). In contrast, the anti-angiogenic activity of MMPs has been shown by MMP-12 and MMP-9 that hydrolyze plasminogen to form the angiogenesis inhibitor angiostatin (Patterson and Sang 1997; Raza et al. 2000). The importance of MMP-14 in invasive and angiogenic processes was recently highlighted by in vivo studies showing inhibition of human tumor xenograft upon supplying a specific antibody against active MMP-14 (Devy et al. 2009). Meanwhile, various endogenous angiogenesis inhibitors were identified which are released by MMP-mediated proteolytical cleavage of plasma proteins or ECM components, such as collagen XVIII for the generation of endostatins, perlecan for that of endorepellin, and collagen IV for the generation of tumstatin (Fjeldstad and Kolset 2005; Hamano and Kalluri 2005). Thus, the balance between MMP's pro- and anti-angiogenic activities and their tissue inhibitors is likely to dictate the outcome during tumor development. Apart from its role in angiogenesis, MMP-14 expression in melanoma cells was shown to be important for the processing of Notch1, which in turn sustains melanoma growth (Ma et al. 2014). As a feedback loop, Notch1 can drive furin expression thus leading to enhanced expression and activation of MMP-14 and ADAM-10 both contributing to melanoma development (Qiu et al. 2015). Most importantly, MMP-14 can negatively regulate transcription of the tumor suppressor SPRY4 via an MMP-2/RAC1 pathway and alter melanoma cell motility, even though it is unclear whether proteolytic activity is required for this event (Shaverdashvili et al. 2015). Two further membrane-associated MMPs, the MT2-MMP (MMP-15) and MT3-MMP (MMP-16) are increased in primary and metastatic melanoma cells. In addition, MMP-16 is overexpressed in human melanoma metastases and metastatic melanoma cell lines (Ohnishi et al. 2001). Interestingly, expression of MMP-16 is associated with rapid fibrin and poor collagen invasion, suggesting that MMP-16 might be important for infiltration of melanoma cells into the perivascular space which is frequently abundant with fibrin (Tatti et al. 2011). More recently, it has been shown that MMP-16 regulates expression of MMP-14 and L1CAM thereby supporting nodular-type growth of melanoma cells and steering the cell collectives into lymphatic vessels (Tatti et al. 2015). MT4-MMP (MMP-17) was shown to be highly expressed in two melanoma cell lines (A375 and G-361) as well as in normal skin, the precise role of MMP-17 expression has not been investigated thus far in the context of melanoma (Grant et al. 1999).

MMP-9 was also found to possess tumor-inhibiting activity. By grafting melanoma or lung carcinoma cells in either wild type or MMP-9 depleted animals it was demonstrated that this metalloproteinase functions as a metastasis suppressor but does not interfere with the growth of grafted tumors (Gutierrez-Fernandez et al. 2007). MMP-9 mediates the enzymatic cleavage of the basement membrane collagen type IV, generating the proteolytic fragment, tumstatin, that functions as an endogenous inhibitor of pathological angiogenesis and suppresses the activity of endothelial cells as well as growth of melanomas (Hamano and Kalluri 2005). In addition, using bone marrow transplantation in MMP-9 knockout mice with bone marrow-derived cells of MMP-9 control animals, peritumoral inflammatory cells were identified as the stromal source of MMP-9 during epithelial carcinogenesis and are required to sustain tumor growth (Coussens et al. 2000). Thus, to address the role of an MMP for tumor progression solely by expression studies may be insufficient, whereas addressing enzymatic activities may rule out the specific role of a proteolytic enzyme in pathological processes.

Another important role of MMPs is the shedding of cell surface receptors such as cleavage of E-cadherin (see also Chap. 9). Shedding of these cell–cell receptors has been shown to occur by the activity of MMP-7 and MMP-3, thereby regulating the invasive capacities of transformed or injured epithelial cells (McGuire et al. 2003; Noe et al. 2001). A significant increase in serum-soluble E-cadherin levels was detected in melanoma patients with advanced disease; thus suggesting that in melanoma, shedding, apart from transcriptional regulation of the receptor, contributes to render melanoma cells refractory to regulation mediated by keratinocytes (Billion et al. 2006; Hsu et al. 2000). Another example for MMP-mediated receptor shedding is that of CD44, known as the receptor for hyaluronan. Cleavage of CD44 by MMP-14 results in increased melanoma cell motility in vitro and likely plays a role for tumor progression in vivo (Kajita et al. 2001; Nakamura et al. 2004). Due to its structure as a transmembrane protein, MMP-14 was demonstrated to localize at specialized membrane areas such as lamellipodia. In agreement with this observation, high local concentrations of active MMP-14 on the cell membrane are believed to play an important role in cellular migration of melanoma cells (Friedl and Wolf 2008). It was also suggested that cancer cells may invade independently of protease activities employing an amoeboid-type of migration (Wolf et al. 2003). In amoeboid melanoma cells, this migratory "modus" would occur via regulation of actomyosin contraction by a proteolysis-independent mechanism mediated by MMP-9 (Orgaz et al. 2014). Interestingly, by using a zebrafish melanoma model, it could be shown that invasive cells switch from a protease-independent to an MMP-14-dependent invasion mode, which allows cooperative invasion of poorly invasive cells, thus preserving heterogeneity in the tumor (Chapman et al. 2014).

It is now generally accepted that MMPs may exert both pro- and anti-tumoral activities. Thus, despite their increased expression and correlation with advanced stages of tumors, caution must be taken in interpreting expression data solely. One example is the neutrophil collagenase, MMP-8. MMP-8 ablation in mice strongly increased the incidence of skin tumors. Notably, restoring the neutrophil pool by bone marrow transplantation re-established the natural protection against tumor development in male mice (Balbin et al. 2003). In addition, in high invasive breast cancer cells, transduction with MMP-8 decreased the metastatic performance in vitro and in vivo (Montel et al. 2004). A study by Palavalli et al. (2009) has identified 23% somatic mutations of MMPs in human melanoma, and five of these were found in the *MMP-8* gene associated with the loss of its enzymatic activity. Forced expression of the wild type gene resulted in reduced melanoma growth in vivo suggesting that this MMP is a tumor suppressor (Palavalli et al. 2009). Later, Debniak et al. (2011) suggested that *MMP-8* gene variation might be associated with an increased risk of malignant melanoma (Debniak et al. 2011).

8.3 ADAMs

ADAMs (a disintegrin and metalloproteinases) are likely to contribute to the proteolytic events necessary for tumor invasion and metastasis (Bergers and Coussens 2000; Schlondorff and Blobel 1999). Most of these proteins contain a metalloproteinase, a disintegrin, a cysteine-rich domain, and a transmembrane domain, some are also found as secreted proteins (Edwards et al. 2008). Based on their domain structure, these proteins can exert modulating effects on both the migratory behavior of tumor cells as well as on the proteolytic processes with regard to tumor invasion. In support of this, their overexpression has been detected in a variety of tumors (reviewed in Murphy 2008). Extensive expression analysis has been performed on breast and pancreatic carcinomas where expression of ADAM-9, −10, −12, and −15 have been reported to be increased (Murphy 2008). However, very limited information is available on the role of the different ADAM family members in the pathogenesis of melanoma. In our own studies, we found ADAM-9 being strongly expressed in primary melanomas and low in metastases (Zigrino et al. 2005). The importance of ADAM-9 in melanoma growth was further substantiated in animals depleted of ADAM-9 expression (Abety et al. 2012; Guaiquil et al. 2009). Moreover, down-regulation of ADAM-9 synthesis (by miR-126&126*) in the tumor cell but not in the stroma of the host, resulted in reduced melanoma growth and metastasis in nude mice (Felli et al. 2013). Presently, the contribution of this protease to development, invasion, and metastasis of melanoma is unclear. Another member, ADAM-10, was also found to be regulated in melanoma. However, opposite expression levels were detected at high amounts in metastases and at low levels in primary tumors (Lee et al. 2010). Although the exact role of ADAM-10 in tumorigenesis is not understood, the very recent identification of ADAM-10 mediated constitutive shedding of CD44 in human melanoma cells favors the idea that this protease facilitates melanoma cell proliferation (Anderegg et al. 2009). More recently, ADAM-10 has been correlated with poor progression-free survival of uveal melanoma patients. In vitro, despite cleaving the HGF receptor c-met, ADAM-10 also mediates HGF-induced uveal melanoma cell invasion (Gangemi et al. 2014).

In human tissues, ADAM-15 is expressed in melanocytes and endothelial cells of benign nevi and melanoma tissue; however, it is significantly downregulated in melanoma metastases compared to primary tumors (Ungerer et al. 2010). ADAM-15 overexpression in melanoma cells reduced invasion and growth in vitro, suggesting a tumor suppressor role for ADAM-15 in melanoma. Constitutive inactivation of ADAM-15 resulted in reduced growth and metastasis of injected melanoma cells to lungs and lymph nodes, thus suggesting a pro-metastatic role of ADAM-15 in melanoma when expressed by the host (Horiuchi et al. 2003; Schonefuss et al. 2012).

ADAM-8 has been recently described as a negative regulator of retinal vascularization and of growth of heterotopically injected B16F0 melanoma cells (Guaiquil et al. 2010) by modulating processing of several molecules involved in angiogenetic processes such as CD31, EphB4, and ephrinB2. However, in human melanoma, expression of this protease has not been investigated. Inactivation of ADAM-17 in endothelial cells significantly reduced pathological neovascularization in a mouse model for retinopathy of prematurity, and affected the growth of heterotopically injected murine melanoma cells. Surprisingly, differences in tumor growth could not be attributed to altered vascularization as no differences in CD31-positive tumor vessels were detected but rather hypothetically to the generation of factors from endothelial cells that contribute to tumor growth (Weskamp et al. 2010). However, all these data are derived from mouse models (see also Chap. 15) and whether these events may also be affected by these ADAMs during development of human melanoma is not clear yet.

Processes mediated by ADAM proteases may be relevant for melanoma growth and invasion, and these include shedding of ectodomains such as the epidermal growth factors. By shedding the ectodomains, soluble, diffusible factors are released and can carry out different biological functions as compared to their membrane-anchored protein form. An example is the EGF pathway, which is active in various cancer cell types and sustains their survival, proliferation, and motility (Edwards et al. 2008). One of the oldest examples for this is the release of the cytokine TNF-α from its inactive membrane-anchored form by ADAM-17 (Black and White 1998). In human melanoma, *ADAM-17* gene is strongly overexpressed in tumors with advanced stage and its expression correlates with the increased TNF-α expression in the blood of patients (Cireap and Narita 2013). Another shedding event relevant for cancer development is that of the ligands of the activating natural killer cell receptor, NKG2D, MHC class I chain-related molecule A and B (MICA and MICB). This shedding studied in vitro in cervix cancer cells is thought to be one of the mechanisms that promote resistance to the immunosurveillance by NK cells (Waldhauer et al., 2008). Another NK cell ligand, namely, B7-H6 is shed by ADAM-10 and −17 and, interestingly, levels of B7-H6 in blood from melanoma patients were found elevated (Schlecker et al. 2014). In other cancer cells, such as hepatocellular carcinoma, ADAM-9 was responsible for the shedding of MICA and treatment with anticancer drug Sorafenib, causing decreased expression of ADAM-9 followed by increased MICA expression at the cell surface (Kohga et al. 2010). Recently, shedding of the NKG2D ligand MICA was shown to be mediated by MMP-14 and to occur independently from ADAMs (Liu et al. 2010). Which protease is responsible for the shedding of these NKGD2 ligands is likely the result of the expression profile in the tumor cell type involved and needs further investigation.

Shedding of surface receptors mediating cellular interactions was demonstrated for ADAM proteases. E-, N-, and VE-cadherins are substrates for ADAM-10 (Reiss and Saftig 2009) and their shedding results in profound alterations in cellular interactions, migration, and cell proliferation. ADAM-10-mediated L1 release is involved in the motility and invasion of lymphoma, lung carcinoma, and melanoma cells (Gutwein et al. 2000; Lee et al. 2010).

Apart from modulating cell adhesion by shedding events, one important aspect of ADAMs is their direct involvement in mediating adhesive events through their adhesive domains. In vitro studies have shown that ADAM-15 interacts with $\alpha_v\beta_3$ and $\alpha_5\beta_1$ integrins (Nath et al. 1999), whereas ADAM-2 binds to $\alpha_6\beta_1$ integrin and ADAM-9 to $\alpha_6\beta_1$, $\alpha_v\beta_5$, and $\alpha_3\beta_1$ integrins (Almeida et al. 1995; Nath et al. 2000; Zhou et al. 2001). The interactions of ADAM proteases with cellular receptors have been proven to be of major importance in cell adhesion and fusion processes as for instance during spermatogenesis and myo- and osteogenesis (Edwards et al. 2008). In vitro studies have shown that ADAM-9 can mediate cell–cell interaction of fibroblasts and melanoma cells thereby lead synthesis of proteolytic enzymes in stromal cells (Zigrino et al. 2011). However, ADAM-9 can also be expressed in a soluble form. The secretion of a soluble splice variant of ADAM-9 by activated stromal cells is known to induce colon carcinoma cell invasion in vitro through binding to $\alpha_6\beta_4$ and $\alpha_2\beta_1$ integrins (Mazzocca et al. 2005). Recent studies have identified driver mutations in ADAMs, namely, ADAM-29 and −7, which often occur in melanoma and enhance cell migration or alter cell adhesive capacity (Wei et al. 2011). Nevertheless, limited information is available on the role of the different ADAM family members in the pathogenesis of melanoma.

8.4 ADAMTS

The ADAMTS (a disintegrin and metalloproteinase with thrombospondin motifs) have also been implicated in cancer development and progression (Rocks et al. 2008). These proteins are characterized by the presence of additional thrombospondin domains which are believed to function as a sulfated glycosaminoglycan binding domain (Tang 2001). High levels of ADAMTS transcripts were detected in tumor biopsies and cell lines from osteosarcoma and melanoma (Cal et al. 2002). ADAMTS-4 exists in three forms all co-expressed in human cancer tissues (Rao et al. 2013). ADAMTS-4 and its proteolytically active N-terminal autocatalytic fragment promoted B16 melanoma growth and angiogenesis in mice, whereas its catalytically inactive mutant increased tumor cell apoptosis (Rao et al. 2013). A single thrombospondin-type 1 repeat domain was essential and sufficient for the anti-tumorigenic activity displayed by the catalytically inactive ADAMTS-4 isoforms. Considering the diversity in the function of these various forms and their co-expression in the same tissue, it was suggested that a balance between pro- and anti-tumorigenic ADAMTS-4 isoforms would dictate the functional outcome (Rao et al. 2013). Overexpression of full-length ADAMTS-5 diminished angiogenesis, reduced proliferation, and increased apoptosis of tumor cells thus suppressing B16 melanoma growth in mice (Kumar et al. 2012). Finally, ADAMTS-18 was identified as a player in melanoma progression as mutations in the protein reduced growth-factor dependency of tumor cells, increased migration in vitro and led to increased metastasis in vivo (Wei et al. 2010).

The expression and activity of several ADAMTS proteins have not yet been carefully analyzed in melanoma. However, given the various functions attributed to these enzymes in the development of other diseases, their involvement in melanoma development is also conceivable.

8.5 Cathepsins

Cathepsins described in melanomas are both cysteine (B, H, K, and L) and aspartyl proteases (D and E). These enzymes are predominantly intracellularly localized within the lysosomal compartment. Some of these enzymes can be associated with the plasma membrane of melanoma cells in vitro or can be secreted from lysosomes upon cell contact with collagen type I (Klose et al. 2006; Moin et al. 1998). Frohlich et al. (2001) have analyzed the expression of cathepsins in normal skin, nevi, and melanoma samples to obtain information about their role and their regulation in melanoma. Activities and expression of the cathepsins B and L were found to be increased in all melanocytic lesions (Frohlich et al. 2001). In human melanoma and nevi, cathepsin B is prevalently expressed by melanoma cells, whereas cathepsin L is expressed by tumor-associated fibroblasts surrounding invading melanoma cells (Yin et al. 2012). In vitro, cathepsin B was shown to regulate expression/activity of TGF-β thereby leading to fibroblast activation and promotion of tumor invasion (Yin et al. 2012). In contrast, Humbert and Lebrun (2013) found that TGF-β strongly upregulated PAI-1 expression thus reducing plasmin activity and led to inhibition of invasion (Humbert and Lebrun 2013). The reasons for these discrepancies have not been addressed, but will need further clarifications.

Cathepsin H expression correlated inversely with the invasive potential of the lesion (Frohlich et al. 2001). The aspartyl protease cathepsin D has been detected in tumor cells as well as in the peritumoral stroma in melanoma (Kageshita et al. 1995). Expression of cathepsin D has also been inversely correlated with melanoma such that its expression is downregulated in melanoma cells as compared to melanocytes, thus suggesting a role for this enzyme in cellular transformation (Bernard et al. 2003). In vitro, cathepsin B activity was shown to be necessary for the invasion of dermal connective tissue by highly invasive melanoma cells (Dennhofer et al. 2003). Furthermore, forced expression of cathepsin L in human melanoma cells increased their metastatic potential thus increasing their tumorigenicity (Jean et al. 1996). Neutralization of cathepsin L in vivo by lentiviral transduction of melanoma cells with the anti-cathepsin L ScFv fusion protein resulted in inhibition of the tumorigenic and metastatic phenotype of human melanoma (Rousselet et al. 2004). In contrast, the work from Matarrese et al. (2010) showed that cathepsin B but not L and D inhibition by several targeting approaches could efficiently reduce tumor growth and metastatic potential of human melanoma cells in vitro and in vivo (Matarrese et al. 2010).

Another recently described cysteine protease expressed in melanoma is cathepsin K. This enzyme has been extensively studied during bone resorption processes where it mediates the degradation of various collagens (Bossard et al. 1996). Whereas cathepsin K is not expressed in normal skin, its expression has been localized in skin fibroblasts during scar formation (Runger et al. 2007). Cathepsin K has been detected in nevi and it is increased in human primary cutaneous melanoma and metastasis (Quintanilla-Dieck et al. 2008). A potential function ascribed to cathepsin K in melanoma cells is the intracellular degradation of collagen type IV (Quintanilla-Dieck et al. 2008).

8.6 Serine Proteases

Among the group of serine proteases involved in extracellular matrix degradation, plasmin, plasminogen activators, thrombin, cathepsin G, and elastases are of particular interest.

The serine protease plasmin can activate most proMMPs in vitro (Murphy et al. 1999). However, it has not been proven whether the function as proMMP activator is also fulfilled in vivo. Their proteolytic activity has also been shown towards extracellular matrix components and cell surface receptors thereby influencing the tumor microenvironment in multiple ways (Andreasen et al. 2000).

Release of elastin fragments by the serine protease elastase was shown to enhance melanoma cell invasion through type I collagen and increase angiogenesis by the induction of MMP-14 expression (Hornebeck et al. 2005). One hypothesis advanced by Antonicelli et al. is that these peptides could catalyze the vertical growth phase transition in melanoma through increased expression of MMP-2 and MMP-14 (Antonicelli et al. 2007). Plasminogen activation by the urokinase type (uPA) or the tissue type plasminogen activators (tPA) generates plasmin whose expression is associated with ECM degradation (Li and Wun 1998). Generated plasmin can also excise the angiostatin fragment from plasminogen thus regulating angiogenic processes. uPA is bound to the surface of tumor cells by means of a specific receptor (uPAR) and engagement of this receptor can act as a survival factor for melanoma by down-regulating p53 and therefore inducing an anti-apoptotic effect (Besch et al. 2007). uPA expression has been correlated with the ability of blue nevi to transform, as respective gene ablation in mice inhibited melanoma formation (Shapiro et al. 1996). A synergism between the uPA/uPAR system and MMP-9 was shown to mediate the IFN-γ- and TNF-α-induced invasive phenotype of murine melanoma cells (Bianchini et al. 2006). Increased uPA and MMP-2/-9 expression, accompanied by down-regulation of E-cadherin, was observed following overexpression of PKC-γ in mammary cells leading to acquired invasive abilities of those cells which became tumorigenic and able to spontaneously metastasize (Mazzoni et al. 2003). Overexpression of Hsp27 in the melanoma line A375 led to a reduced malignant phenotype by increased expression of E-cadherin and of both uPA and its inhibitor PAI-1 (Aldrian et al. 2003).

Human melanoma cells produce tPA which is bound to the cell surface (de Vries et al. 1996). In vivo, high tPA expression has been correlated with good prognosis (Ferrier et al. 2000). In these studies, lesions with more than 51% tPA-positive tumor cells were found to have the best prognosis, as compared to those with lower expression. Further, taking together tPA positivity, Breslow thickness, microscopic ulceration, and sex, showed that the extent of tPA tumor cell positivity was an independent prognostic factor for a distant metastasis-free interval and for the duration of survival (Ferrier et al. 2000). A potential reason for the better outcome is the generation of angiostatin, upon activation of plasmin and thereby cleavage of plasminogen, which may inhibit tumor-induced angiogenic processes.

Another serine protease that has also been investigated in melanoma is thrombin. Thrombin cleaves the N-terminus of protease-activated receptor-1 (PAR-1) that binds the receptor and activates signaling via G-proteins (Shapiro et al. 2000). PAR-1 can also be activated by ligands other than thrombin such as trypsin and plasmin (Kawabata and Kuroda 2000). PAR-1 is overexpressed predominantly in melanoma primary tumors and in metastatic lesions as compared with common melanocytic nevi (Massi et al. 2005). The importance of activating this pathway is described in a recent report from Melnikova et al. (2009). The authors showed that PAR-1 activation leads to the expression of melanoma cell adhesion molecule MCAM/MUC18 (MUC18) thereby mediating melanoma cell adhesion to microvascular endothelial cells, transendothelial migration, and ultimately, lung metastasis retention. The altered expression of a variety of kallikreins has also been associated with melanoma and among these increased hKLK7 was significantly associated with good prognosis and survival (Martins et al. 2011). However, KLK-7 mediated cleavage of midkine leads to reduced pro-proliferative and pro-migratory activity in melanoma cells in vitro (Yu et al. 2015). The apparent discrepancy with the in vivo human expression data may be explained in light of additional KLK-7 proteolytic activities towards, e.g., CYR61 and tenascin-C (Yu et al. 2015), which have not yet been investigated.

8.7 Summary

Although fundamental knowledge about the molecular processes of tumor progression has increased in recent years, the clinical application is still limited.

Concerns remain about the consequences of inhibiting the biological function of cell proteolytic enzymes. Several reports have contributed to gain knowledge of the regulation of proteases and their substrates and highlighted that this process is complex and multifactorial. Experimental evidence strongly suggests that proteases of the same class may display a dual function depending on the cellular source and act as both a tumor-promoter and suppressor. Further generation of mouse models for in vivo analysis of protease depletion, will help in clarifying the importance of their activity for physiology and pathology. In addition, for more specific targeting, a deeper knowledge of the proteolytic functions is needed and the field of degradomics has already started to uncover new proteases and physiological substrates. These studies identified new and known regulatory pathways that are controlled by proteolytic processing. The problematic for targeting of protease activity (e.g., of MMPs) in vivo has been further discussed by Dufour and Overall (2013).

The direct targeting of these proteases in a cell-specific manner with, for example, monoclonal antibodies or inactivating peptides, or the inhibition of the activity of their processed substrates may be developed as potentially useful therapeutic strategies.

Acknowledgments This work was supported by the Deutsche Forschungsgemeinschaft through the SFB829 and by the Melanoma Research Network of the Deutsche Krebshilfe (Melanoma Verbund).

References

Abety AN, Fox JW, Schonefuss A, Zamek J, Landsberg J, Krieg T, Blobel C, Mauch C, Zigrino P (2012) Stromal fibroblast-specific expression of ADAM-9 modulates proliferation and apoptosis in melanoma cells in vitro and in vivo. J Invest Dermatol 132:2451–2458

Airola K, Karonen T, Vaalamo M, Lehti K, Lohi J, Kariniemi AL, Keski-Oja J, Saarialho-Kere UK (1999) Expression of collagenases-1 and −3 and their inhibitors TIMP-1 and −3 correlates with the level of invasion in malignant melanomas. Br J Cancer 80:733–743

Aldrian S, Kindas-Mugge I, Trautinger F, Frohlich I, Gsur A, Herbacek I, Berger W, Micksche M (2003) Overexpression of Hsp27 in a human melanoma cell line: regulation of E-cadherin, MUC18/MCAM, and plasminogen activator (PA) system. Cell Stress Chaperones 8:249–257

Almeida EA, Huovila AP, Sutherland AE, Stephens LE, Calarco PG, Shaw LM, Mercurio AM, Sonnenberg A, Primakoff P, Myles DG, White JM (1995) Mouse egg integrin alpha 6 beta 1 functions as a sperm receptor. Cell 81:1095–1104

Anderegg U, Eichenberg T, Parthaune T, Haiduk C, Saalbach A, Milkova L, Ludwig A, Grosche J, Averbeck M, Gebhardt C, Voelcker V, Sleeman JP, Simon JC (2009) ADAM10 is the constitutive functional sheddase of CD44 in human melanoma cells. J Invest Dermatol 129:1471–1482

Andreasen PA, Egelund R, Petersen HH (2000) The plasminogen activation system in tumor growth, invasion, and metastasis. Cell Mole Life Sci CMLS 57:25–40

Antonicelli F, Bellon G, Debelle L, Hornebeck W (2007) Elastin-elastases and inflamm-aging. Curr Top Dev Biol 79:99–155

Balbin M, Fueyo A, Tester AM, Pendas AM, Pitiot AS, Astudillo A, Overall CM, Shapiro SD, Lopez-Otin C (2003) Loss of collagenase-2 confers increased skin tumor susceptibility to male mice. Nat Genet 35:252–257

Bergers G, Coussens LM (2000) Extrinsic regulators of epithelial tumor progression: metalloproteinases. Curr Opin Genet Dev 10:120–127

Bernard D, Mehul B, Thomas-Collignon A, Simonetti L, Remy V, Bernard MA, Schmidt R (2003) Analysis of proteins with caseinolytic activity in a human stratum corneum extract revealed a

yet unidentified cysteine protease and identified the so-called "stratum corneum thiol protease" as cathepsin l2. J Invest Dermatol 120:592–600
Besch R, Berking C, Kammerbauer C, Degitz K (2007) Inhibition of urokinase-type plasminogen activator receptor induces apoptosis in melanoma cells by activation of p53. Cell Death Differ 14:818–829
Bianchini F, D'Alessio S, Fibbi G, Del Rosso M, Calorini L (2006) Cytokine-dependent invasiveness in B16 murine melanoma cells: role of uPA system and MMP-9. Oncol Rep 15:709–714
Billion K, Ibrahim H, Mauch C, Niessen CM (2006) Increased soluble E-cadherin in melanoma patients. Skin Pharmacol Physiol 19:65–70
Black RA, White JM (1998) ADAMs: focus on the protease domain. Curr Opin Cell Biol 10:654–659
Blackburn JS, Brinckerhoff CE (2008) Matrix metalloproteinase-1 and thrombin differentially activate gene expression in endothelial cells via PAR-1 and promote angiogenesis. Am J Pathol 173:1736–1746
Blackburn JS, Liu I, Coon CI, Brinckerhoff CE (2009) A matrix metalloproteinase-1/protease activated receptor-1 signaling axis promotes melanoma invasion and metastasis. Oncogene 28:4237–4248
Boire A, Covic L, Agarwal A, Jacques S, Sherifi S, Kuliopulos A (2005) PAR1 is a matrix metalloprotease-1 receptor that promotes invasion and tumorigenesis of breast cancer cells. Cell 120:303–313
Bossard MJ, Tomaszek TA, Thompson SK, Amegadzie BY, Hanning CR, Jones C, Kurdyla JT, McNulty DE, Drake FH, Gowen M, Levy MA (1996) Proteolytic activity of human osteoclast cathepsin K. Expression, purification, activation, and substrate identification. J Biol Chem 271:12517–12524
Cal S, Obaya AJ, Llamazares M, Garabaya C, Quesada V, Lopez-Otin C (2002) Cloning, expression analysis, and structural characterization of seven novel human ADAMTSs, a family of metalloproteinases with disintegrin and thrombospondin-1 domains. Gene 283:49–62
Chapman A, Fernandez del Ama L, Ferguson J, Kamarashev J, Wellbrock C, Hurlstone A (2014) Heterogeneous tumor subpopulations cooperate to drive invasion. Cell Rep 8:688–695
Cireap N, Narita D (2013) Molecular Profiling of ADAM12 and ADAM17 Genes in Human Malignant Melanoma. Pathol Oncol Res 19(4):755–62
Coussens LM, Fingleton B, Matrisian LM (2002) Matrix metalloproteinase inhibitors and cancer: trials and tribulations. Science 295:2387–2392
Coussens LM, Tinkle CL, Hanahan D, Werb Z (2000) MMP-9 supplied by bone marrow-derived cells contributes to skin carcinogenesis. Cell 103:481–490
de Vries TJ, van Muijen GN, Ruiter DJ (1996) The plasminogen activation system in melanoma cell lines and in melanocytic lesions. Melanoma Res 6:79–88
Debniak T, Jakubowska A, Serrano-Fernandez P, Kurzawski G, Cybulski C, Chauhan SR, Laxton RC, Maleszka R, Lubinski J, Ye S (2011) Association of MMP8 gene variation with an increased risk of malignant melanoma. Melanoma Res 21:464–468
Dennhofer R, Kurschat P, Zigrino P, Klose A, Bosserhoff A, van Muijen G, Krieg T, Mauch C, Hunzelmann N (2003) Invasion of melanoma cells into dermal connective tissue in vitro: evidence for an important role of cysteine proteases. Int J cancer J Int Du cancer 106:316–323
Devy L, Huang L, Naa L, Yanamandra N, Pieters H, Frans N, Chang E, Tao Q, Vanhove M, Lejeune A, van Gool R, Sexton DJ, Kuang G, Rank D, Hogan S, Pazmany C, Ma YL, Schoonbroodt S, Nixon AE, Ladner RC, Hoet R, Henderikx P, Tenhoor C, Rabbani SA, Valentino ML, Wood CR, Dransfield DT (2009) Selective inhibition of matrix metalloproteinase-14 blocks tumor growth, invasion, and angiogenesis. Cancer Res 69:1517–1526
Dufour A, Overall CM (2013) Missing the target: matrix metalloproteinase antitargets in inflammation and cancer. Trends Pharmacol Sci 34:233–242
Edwards DR, Handsley MM, Pennington CJ (2008) The ADAM metalloproteinases. Mol Aspects Med 29:258–289
Felli N, Felicetti F, Lustri AM, Errico MC, Bottero L, Cannistraci A, De Feo A, Petrini M, Pedini F, Biffoni M, Alvino E, Negrini M, Ferracin M, Mattia G, Care A (2013) miR-126&126*

restored expressions play a tumor suppressor role by directly regulating ADAM9 and MMP7 in melanoma. PLoS One 8:e56824
Ferrier CM, Suciu S, van Geloof WL, Straatman H, Eggermont AM, Koops HS, Kroon BB, Lejeune FJ, Kleeberg UR, van Muijen GN, Ruiter DJ (2000) High tPA-expression in primary melanoma of the limb correlates with good prognosis. Br J Cancer 83:1351–1359
Fjeldstad K, Kolset SO (2005) Decreasing the metastatic potential in cancers–targeting the heparan sulfate proteoglycans. Curr Drug Targets 6:665–682
Friedl P, Wolf K (2008) Tube travel: the role of proteases in individual and collective cancer cell invasion. Cancer Res 68:7247–7249
Frohlich E, Schlagenhauff B, Mohrle M, Weber E, Klessen C, Rassner G (2001) Activity, expression, and transcription rate of the cathepsins B, D, H, and L in cutaneous malignant melanoma. Cancer 91:972–982
Gangemi R, Amaro A, Gino A, Barisione G, Fabbi M, Pfeffer U, Brizzolara A, Queirolo P, Salvi S, Boccardo S, Gualco M, Spagnolo F, Jager MJ, Mosci C, Rossello A, Ferrini S (2014) ADAM10 correlates with uveal melanoma metastasis and promotes in vitro invasion. Pigment Cell Melanoma Res 27:1138–1148
Grant GM, Giambernardi TA, Grant AM, Klebe RJ (1999) Overview of expression of matrix metalloproteinases (MMP-17, MMP-18, and MMP-20) in cultured human cells. Matrix Biol 18:145–148
Guaiquil V, Swendeman S, Yoshida T, Chavala S, Campochiaro PA, Blobel CP (2009) ADAM9 is involved in pathological retinal neovascularization. Mol Cell Biol 29:2694–2703
Guaiquil VH, Swendeman S, Zhou W, Guaiquil P, Weskamp G, Bartsch JW, Blobel CP (2010) ADAM8 is a negative regulator of retinal neovascularization and of the growth of heterotopically injected tumor cells in mice. J Mol Med (Berl) 88:497–505
Gutierrez-Fernandez A, Inada M, Balbin M, Fueyo A, Pitiot AS, Astudillo A, Hirose K, Hirata M, Shapiro SD, Noel A, Werb Z, Krane SM, Lopez-Otin C, Puente XS (2007) Increased inflammation delays wound healing in mice deficient in collagenase-2 (MMP-8). FASEB J 21:2580–2591
Gutwein P, Oleszewski M, Mechtersheimer S, Agmon-Levin N, Krauss K, Altevogt P (2000) Role of Src kinases in the ADAM-mediated release of L1 adhesion molecule from human tumor cells. J Biol Chem 275:15490–15497
Hamano Y, Kalluri R (2005) Tumstatin, the NC1 domain of alpha3 chain of type IV collagen, is an endogenous inhibitor of pathological angiogenesis and suppresses tumor growth. Biochem Biophys Res Commun 333:292–298
Hofmann UB, Westphal JR, Zendman AJ, Becker JC, Ruiter DJ, van Muijen GN (2000) Expression and activation of matrix metalloproteinase-2 (MMP-2) and its co-localization with membrane-type 1 matrix metalloproteinase (MT1-MMP) correlate with melanoma progression. J Pathol 191:245–256
Horiuchi K, Weskamp G, Lum L, Hammes HP, Cai H, Brodie TA, Ludwig T, Chiusaroli R, Baron R, Preissner KT, Manova K, Blobel CP (2003) Potential role for ADAM15 in pathological neovascularization in mice. Mol Cell Biol 23:5614–5624
Hornebeck W, Robinet A, Duca L, Antonicelli F, Wallach J, Bellon G (2005) The elastin connection and melanoma progression. Anticancer Res 25:2617–2625
Hsu MY, Meier FE, Nesbit M, Hsu JY, Van Belle P, Elder DE, Herlyn M (2000) E-cadherin expression in melanoma cells restores keratinocyte-mediated growth control and down-regulates expression of invasion-related adhesion receptors. Am J Pathol 156:1515–1525
Humbert L, Lebrun JJ (2013) TGF-beta inhibits human cutaneous melanoma cell migration and invasion through regulation of the plasminogen activator system. Cell Signal 25:490–500
Jean D, Bar-Eli M, Huang S, Xie K, Rodrigues-Lima F, Hermann J, Frade R (1996) A cysteine proteinase, which cleaves human C3, the third component of complement, is involved in tumorigenicity and metastasis of human melanoma. Cancer Res 56:254–258
Jiao Y, Feng X, Zhan Y, Wang R, Zheng S, Liu W, Zeng X (2012) Matrix metalloproteinase-2 promotes alphavbeta3 integrin-mediated adhesion and migration of human melanoma cells by cleaving fibronectin. PLoS One 7:e41591

Kageshita T, Yoshii A, Kimura T, Maruo K, Ono T, Himeno M, Nishimura Y (1995) Biochemical and immunohistochemical analysis of cathepsins B, H, L and D in human melanocytic tumours. Arch Dermatol Res 287:266–272

Kajita M, Itoh Y, Chiba T, Mori H, Okada A, Kinoh H, Seiki M (2001) Membrane-type 1 matrix metalloproteinase cleaves CD44 and promotes cell migration. J Cell Biol 153:893–904

Kawabata A, Kuroda R (2000) Protease-activated receptor (PAR), a novel family of G protein-coupled seven trans-membrane domain receptors: activation mechanisms and physiological roles. Jpn J Pharmacol 82:171–174

Klose A, Wilbrand-Hennes A, Zigrino P, Weber E, Krieg T, Mauch C, Hunzelmann N (2006) Contact of high-invasive, but not low-invasive, melanoma cells to native collagen I induces the release of mature cathepsin B. Int J Cancer J Int Du Cancer 118:2735–2743

Kohga K, Takehara T, Tatsumi T, Ishida H, Miyagi T, Hosui A, Hayashi N (2010) Sorafenib inhibits the shedding of major histocompatibility complex class I-related chain A on hepatocellular carcinoma cells by down-regulating a disintegrin and metalloproteinase 9. Hepatology 51:1264–1273

Kumar S, Sharghi-Namini S, Rao N, Ge R (2012) ADAMTS5 functions as an anti-angiogenic and anti-tumorigenic protein independent of its proteoglycanase activity. Am J Pathol 181:1056–1068

Kurschat P, Wickenhauser C, Groth W, Krieg T, Mauch C (2002) Identification of activated matrix metalloproteinase-2 (MMP-2) as the main gelatinolytic enzyme in malignant melanoma by in situ zymography. J Pathol 197:179–187

Kurschat P, Zigrino P, Nischt R, Breitkopf K, Steurer P, Klein CE, Krieg T, Mauch C (1999) Tissue inhibitor of matrix metalloproteinase-2 regulates matrix metalloproteinase-2 activation by modulation of membrane-type 1 matrix metalloproteinase activity in high and low invasive melanoma cell lines. J Biol Chem 274:21056–21062

Lazar I, Clement E, Ducoux-Petit M, Denat L, Soldan V, Dauvillier S, Balor S, Burlet-Schiltz O, Larue L, Muller C, Nieto L (2015) Proteome characterization of melanoma exosomes reveals a specific signature for metastatic cell lines. Pigment Cell Melanoma Res 28:464–475

Lederle W, Hartenstein B, Meides A, Kunzelmann H, Werb Z, Angel P, Mueller MM (2010) MMP13 as a stromal mediator in controlling persistent angiogenesis in skin carcinoma. Carcinogenesis 31:1175–1184

Lee SB, Schramme A, Doberstein K, Dummer R, Abdel-Bakky MS, Keller S, Altevogt P, Oh ST, Reichrath J, Oxmann D, Pfeilschifter J, Mihic-Probst D, Gutwein P (2010) ADAM10 is upregulated in melanoma metastasis compared with primary melanoma. J Invest Dermatol 130:763–773

Li A, Wun TC (1998) Proteolysis of tissue factor pathway inhibitor (TFPI) by plasmin: effect on TFPI activity. Thromb Haemost 80:423–427

Liu G, Atteridge CL, Wang X, Lundgren AD, Wu JD (2010) The membrane type matrix metalloproteinase MMP14 mediates constitutive shedding of MHC class I chain-related molecule A independent of A disintegrin and metalloproteinases. J Immunol 184:3346–3350

Liu H, Wei Q, Gershenwald JE, Prieto VG, Lee JE, Duvic M, Grimm EA, Wang LE (2012) Influence of single nucleotide polymorphisms in the MMP1 promoter region on cutaneous melanoma progression. Melanoma Res 22:169–175

Loffek S, Zigrino P, Angel P, Anwald B, Krieg T, Mauch C (2005) High invasive melanoma cells induce matrix metalloproteinase-1 synthesis in fibroblasts by interleukin-1alpha and basic fibroblast growth factor-mediated mechanisms. J Invest Dermatol 124:638–643

Lohi J (2001) Laminin-5 in the progression of carcinomas. Int J Cancer J Int Du Cancer 94:763–767

Lu P, Takai K, Weaver VM, Werb Z (2011) Extracellular matrix degradation and remodeling in development and disease. Cold Spring Harb Perspect Biol 3:1–25

Ma J, Tang X, Wong P, Jacobs B, Borden EC, Bedogni B (2014) Noncanonical activation of Notch1 protein by membrane type 1 matrix metalloproteinase (MT1-MMP) controls melanoma cell proliferation. J Biol Chem 289:8442–8449

Martins WK, Esteves GH, Almeida OM, Rezze GG, Landman G, Marques SM, Carvalho AF, LF LR, Duprat JP, Stolf BS (2011) Gene network analyses point to the importance of human tissue kallikreins in melanoma progression. BMC Med Genomics 4:76
Massi D, Naldini A, Ardinghi C, Carraro F, Franchi A, Paglierani M, Tarantini F, Ketabchi S, Cirino G, Hollenberg MD, Geppetti P, Santucci M (2005) Expression of protease-activated receptors 1 and 2 in melanocytic nevi and malignant melanoma. Hum Pathol 36:676–685
Matarrese P, Ascione B, Ciarlo L, Vona R, Leonetti C, Scarsella M, Mileo AM, Catricala C, Paggi MG, Malorni W (2010) Cathepsin B inhibition interferes with metastatic potential of human melanoma: an in vitro and in vivo study. Mol Cancer 9:207
Mazzocca A, Coppari R, De Franco R, Cho JY, Libermann TA, Pinzani M, Toker A (2005) A secreted form of ADAM9 promotes carcinoma invasion through tumor-stromal interactions. Cancer Res 65:4728–4738
Mazzoni E, Adam A, BaldeKier Joffe E, Aguirre-Ghiso JA (2003) Immortalized mammary epithelial cells overexpressing protein kinase C gamma acquire a malignant phenotype and become tumorigenic in vivo. Mol Cancer Res 1:776–787
McGuire JK, Li Q, Parks WC (2003) Matrilysin (matrix metalloproteinase-7) mediates E-cadherin ectodomain shedding in injured lung epithelium. Am J Pathol 162:1831–1843
Melnikova VO, Balasubramanian K, Villares GJ, Dobroff AS, Zigler M, Wang H, Petersson F, Price JE, Schroit A, Prieto VG, Hung MC, Bar-Eli M (2009) Crosstalk between protease-activated receptor 1 and platelet-activating factor receptor regulates melanoma cell adhesion molecule (MCAM/MUC18) expression and melanoma metastasis. J Biol Chem 284:28845–28855
Moin K, Cao L, Day NA, Koblinski JE, Sloane BF (1998) Tumor cell membrane cathepsin B. Biol Chem 379:1093–1099
Montel V, Kleeman J, Agarwal D, Spinella D, Kawai K, Tarin D (2004) Altered metastatic behavior of human breast cancer cells after experimental manipulation of matrix metalloproteinase 8 gene expression. Cancer Res 64:1687–1694
Moro N, Mauch C, Zigrino P (2014) Metalloproteinases in Melanoma. Eur J Cell Biol 93:23–29
Murphy G (2008) The ADAMs: signalling scissors in the tumour microenvironment. Nat Rev Cancer 8:929–941
Murphy G, Stanton H, Cowell S, Butler G, Knauper V, Atkinson S, Gavrilovic J (1999) Mechanisms for pro matrix metalloproteinase activation. APMIS Acta Pathologica Microbiologica Et Immunolog Scand 107:38–44
Nakamura H, Suenaga N, Taniwaki K, Matsuki H, Yonezawa K, Fujii M, Okada Y, Seiki M (2004) Constitutive and induced CD44 shedding by ADAM-like proteases and membrane-type 1 matrix metalloproteinase. Cancer Res 64:876–882
Nath D, Slocombe PM, Stephens PE, Warn A, Hutchinson GR, Yamada KM, Docherty AJ, Murphy G (1999) Interaction of metargidin (ADAM-15) with alphavbeta3 and alpha5beta1 integrins on different haemopoietic cells. J Cell Sci 112(Pt 4):579–587
Nath D, Slocombe PM, Webster A, Stephens PE, Docherty AJ, Murphy G (2000) Meltrin gamma(ADAM-9) mediates cellular adhesion through alpha(6)beta(1)integrin, leading to a marked induction of fibroblast cell motility. J Cell Sci 113(Pt 12):2319–2328
Noe V, Fingleton B, Jacobs K, Crawford HC, Vermeulen S, Steelant W, Bruyneel E, Matrisian LM, Mareel M (2001) Release of an invasion promoter E-cadherin fragment by matrilysin and stromelysin-1. J Cell Sci 114:111–118
Ohnishi Y, Tajima S, Ishibashi A (2001) Coordinate expression of membrane type-matrix metalloproteinases-2 and 3 (MT2-MMP and MT3-MMP) and matrix metalloproteinase-2 (MMP-2) in primary and metastatic melanoma cells. Eur J Dermatol 11:420–423
Orgaz JL, Pandya P, Dalmeida R, Karagiannis P, Sanchez-Laorden B, Viros A, Albrengues J, Nestle FO, Ridley AJ, Gaggioli C, Marais R, Karagiannis SN, Sanz-Moreno V (2014) Diverse matrix metalloproteinase functions regulate cancer amoeboid migration. Nat Commun 5:4255
Page-McCaw A, Ewald AJ, Werb Z (2007) Matrix metalloproteinases and the regulation of tissue remodelling. Nat Rev Mol Cell Biol 8:221–233

Palavalli LH, Prickett TD, Wunderlich JR, Wei X, Burrell AS, Porter-Gill P, Davis S, Wang C, Cronin JC, Agrawal NS, Lin JC, Westbroek W, Hoogstraten-Miller S, Molinolo AA, Fetsch P, Filie AC, O'Connell MP, Banister CE, Howard JD, Buckhaults P, Weeraratna AT, Brody LC, Rosenberg SA, Samuels Y (2009) Analysis of the matrix metalloproteinase family reveals that MMP8 is often mutated in melanoma. Nat Genet 41:518–520

Patarroyo M, Tryggvason K, Virtanen I (2002) Laminin isoforms in tumor invasion, angiogenesis and metastasis. Semin Cancer Biol 12:197–207

Patterson BC, Sang QA (1997) Angiostatin-converting enzyme activities of human matrilysin (MMP-7) and gelatinase B/type IV collagenase (MMP-9). J Biol Chem 272:28823–28825

Qiu H, Tang X, Ma J, Shaverdashvili K, Zhang K, Bedogni B (2015) Notch1 Autoactivation via Transcriptional Regulation of Furin, Which Sustains Notch1 Signaling by Processing Notch1-Activating Proteases ADAM10 and Membrane Type 1 Matrix Metalloproteinase. Mol Cell Biol 35:3622–3632

Quintanilla-Dieck MJ, Codriansky K, Keady M, Bhawan J, Runger TM (2008) Cathepsin K in melanoma invasion. J Invest Dermatol 128:2281–2288

Rao N, Ke Z, Liu H, Ho CJ, Kumar S, Xiang W, Zhu Y, Ge R (2013) ADAMTS4 and its proteolytic fragments differentially affect melanoma growth and angiogenesis in mice. Int J Cancer J Int Du Cancer 133:294–306

Raza SL, Nehring LC, Shapiro SD, Cornelius LA (2000) Proteinase-activated receptor-1 regulation of macrophage elastase (MMP-12) secretion by serine proteinases. J Biol Chem 275:41243–41250

Reiss K, Saftig P (2009) The "a disintegrin and metalloprotease" (ADAM) family of sheddases: physiological and cellular functions. Semin Cell Dev Biol 20:126–137

Rocks N, Paulissen G, El Hour M, Quesada F, Crahay C, Gueders M, Foidart JM, Noel A, Cataldo D (2008) Emerging roles of ADAM and ADAMTS metalloproteinases in cancer. Biochimie 90:369–379

Rousselet N, Mills L, Jean D, Tellez C, Bar-Eli M, Frade R (2004) Inhibition of tumorigenicity and metastasis of human melanoma cells by anti-cathepsin L single chain variable fragment. Cancer Res 64:146–151

Runger TM, Quintanilla-Dieck MJ, Bhawan J (2007) Role of cathepsin K in the turnover of the dermal extracellular matrix during scar formation. J Invest Dermatol 127:293–297

Schlecker E, Fiegler N, Arnold A, Altevogt P, Rose-John S, Moldenhauer G, Sucker A, Paschen A, von Strandmann EP, Textor S, Cerwenka A (2014) Metalloprotease-mediated tumor cell shedding of B7-H6, the ligand of the natural killer cell-activating receptor NKp30. Cancer Res 74:3429–3440

Schlondorff J, Blobel CP (1999) Metalloprotease-disintegrins: modular proteins capable of promoting cell-cell interactions and triggering signals by protein-ectodomain shedding. J Cell Sci 112(Pt 21):3603–3617

Schonefuss A, Abety AN, Zamek J, Mauch C, Zigrino P (2012) Role of ADAM-15 in wound healing and melanoma development. Exp Dermatol 21:437–442

Seftor RE, Seftor EA, Koshikawa N, Meltzer PS, Gardner LM, Bilban M, Stetler-Stevenson WG, Quaranta V, Hendrix MJ (2001) Cooperative interactions of laminin 5 gamma2 chain, matrix metalloproteinase-2, and membrane type-1-matrix/metalloproteinase are required for mimicry of embryonic vasculogenesis by aggressive melanoma. Cancer Res 61:6322–6327

Shapiro MJ, Weiss EJ, Faruqi TR, Coughlin SR (2000) Protease-activated receptors 1 and 4 are shut off with distinct kinetics after activation by thrombin. J Biol Chem 275:25216–25221

Shapiro RL, Duquette JG, Roses DF, Nunes I, Harris MN, Kamino H, Wilson EL, Rifkin DB (1996) Induction of primary cutaneous melanocytic neoplasms in urokinase-type plasminogen activator (uPA)-deficient and wild-type mice: cellular blue nevi invade but do not progress to malignant melanoma in uPA-deficient animals. Cancer Res 56:3597–3604

Shaverdashvili K, Zhang K, Osman I, Honda K, Jobava R, Bedogni B (2015) MT1-MMP dependent repression of the tumor suppressor SPRY4 contributes to MT1-MMP driven melanoma cell motility. Oncotarget 6(32):33512–22

Tang BL (2001) ADAMTS: a novel family of extracellular matrix proteases. Int J Biochem Cell Biol 33:33–44

Tatti O, Arjama M, Ranki A, Weiss SJ, Keski-Oja J, Lehti K (2011) Membrane-type-3 matrix metalloproteinase (MT3-MMP) functions as a matrix composition-dependent effector of melanoma cell invasion. PLoS One 6:e28325

Tatti O, Gucciardo E, Pekkonen P, Holopainen T, Louhimo R, Repo P, Maliniemi P, Lohi J, Rantanen V, Hautaniemi S, Alitalo K, Ranki A, Ojala PM, Keski-Oja J, Lehti K (2015) MMP16 Mediates a Proteolytic Switch to Promote Cell-Cell Adhesion, Collagen Alignment, and Lymphatic Invasion in Melanoma. Cancer Res 75:2083–2094

Ungerer C, Doberstein K, Burger C, Hardt K, Boehncke WH, Bohm B, Pfeilschifter J, Dummer R, Mihic-Probst D, Gutwein P (2010) ADAM15 expression is downregulated in melanoma metastasis compared to primary melanoma. Biochem Biophys Res Commun 401:363–369

Uria JA, Stahle-Backdahl M, Seiki M, Fueyo A, Lopez-Otin C (1997) Regulation of collagenase-3 expression in human breast carcinomas is mediated by stromal-epithelial cell interactions. Cancer Res 57:4882–4888

Wandel E, Grasshoff A, Mittag M, Haustein UF, Saalbach A (2000) Fibroblasts surrounding melanoma express elevated levels of matrix metalloproteinase-1 (MMP-1) and intercellular adhesion molecule-1 (ICAM-1) in vitro. Exp Dermatol 9:34–41

Wang LE, Huang YJ, Yin M, Gershenwald JE, Prieto VG, Lee JE, Duvic M, Grimm EA, Wei Q (2011) Promoter polymorphisms in matrix metallopeptidase 1 and risk of cutaneous melanoma. Eur J Cancer 47:107–115

Wei X, Moncada-Pazos A, Cal S, Soria-Valles C, Gartner J, Rudloff U, Lin JC, Rosenberg SA, Lopez-Otin C, Samuels Y (2011) Analysis of the disintegrin-metalloproteinases family reveals ADAM29 and ADAM7 are often mutated in melanoma. Hum Mutat 32:E2148–E2175

Wei X, Prickett TD, Viloria CG, Molinolo A, Lin JC, Cardenas-Navia I, Cruz P, Rosenberg SA, Davies MA, Gershenwald JE, Lopez-Otin C, Samuels Y (2010) Mutational and functional analysis reveals ADAMTS18 metalloproteinase as a novel driver in melanoma. Mole Cancer Research MCR 8:1513–1525

Weskamp G, Mendelson K, Swendeman S, Le Gall S, Ma Y, Lyman S, Hinoki A, Eguchi S, Guaiquil V, Horiuchi K, Blobel CP (2010) Pathological neovascularization is reduced by inactivation of ADAM17 in endothelial cells but not in pericytes. Circ Res 106:932–940

Wolf K, Mazo I, Leung H, Engelke K, von Andrian UH, Deryugina EI, Strongin AY, Brocker EB, Friedl P (2003) Compensation mechanism in tumor cell migration: mesenchymal-amoeboid transition after blocking of pericellular proteolysis. J Cell Biol 160:267–277

Yin M, Soikkeli J, Jahkola T, Virolainen S, Saksela O, Holtta E (2012) TGF-beta signaling, activated stromal fibroblasts, and cysteine cathepsins B and L drive the invasive growth of human melanoma cells. Am J Pathol 181:2202–2216

Yu Y, Prassas I, Dimitromanolakis A, Diamandis EP (2015) Novel Biological Substrates of Human Kallikrein 7 Identified through Degradomics. J Biol Chem 290:17762–17775

Zhao X, Sun B, Li Y, Liu Y, Zhang D, Wang X, Gu Q, Zhao J, Dong X, Liu Z, Che N (2015) Dual effects of collagenase-3 on melanoma: metastasis promotion and disruption of vasculogenic mimicry. Oncotarget 6:8890–8899

Zhou M, Graham R, Russell G, Croucher PI (2001) MDC-9 (ADAM-9/Meltrin gamma) functions as an adhesion molecule by binding the alpha(v)beta(5) integrin. Biochem Biophys Res Commun 280:574–580

Zigrino P, Kuhn I, Bauerle T, Zamek J, Fox JW, Neumann S, Licht A, Schorpp-Kistner M, Angel P, Mauch C (2009) Stromal expression of MMP-13 is required for melanoma invasion and metastasis. J Invest Dermatol 129:2686–2693

Zigrino P, Mauch C, Fox JW, Nischt R (2005) Adam-9 expression and regulation in human skin melanoma and melanoma cell lines. Int J Cancer J Int Du Cancer 116:853–859

Zigrino P, Nischt R, Mauch C (2011) The disintegrin-like and cysteine-rich domains of ADAM-9 mediate interactions between melanoma cells and fibroblasts. J Biol Chem 286:6801–6807

Cell–Cell Contacts in Melanoma and the Tumor Microenvironment

9

Silke Kuphal and Nikolas K. Haass

Abbreviations

CDH	Cadherin
Cx	Connexin(s)
Dsc 1–3	Desmocollin
Dsg	Desmoglein
GJ	Gap junction
GJIC	Gap junctional intercellular communication

9.1 Melanoma Microenvironment

This is an update of our previous reviews on this topic (Haass et al. 2004, 2005; Kuphal and Haass 2011; Brandner and Haass 2013).

The state of a cell – quiescence, proliferation, differentiation or cell death – is under normal conditions determined by homeostasis (Bissell and Radisky 2001). A symbiotic relationship between a melanocyte and approximately 36 associated

S. Kuphal (✉)
Friedrich-Alexander University of Erlangen-Nuremberg, Institute of Biochemistry and Molecular Medicine, Fahrstr 17, 91054 Erlangen, Germany
e-mail: silke.kuphal@fau.de

N.K. Haass
Centenary Institute of Cancer Medicine and Cell Biology, Newtown, NSW, Australia

Discipline of Dermatology, Faculty of Medicine, Central Clinical School, University of Sydney, Sydney, NSW, Australia

The University of Queensland, The University of Queensland Diamantina Institute, Translational Research Institute, 37 Kent St, Woolloongabba, Brisbane, QLD 4102, Australia
e-mail: n.haass1@uq.edu.au

A. Bosserhoff (ed.), *Melanoma Development*,
DOI 10.1007/978-3-319-41319-8_9

keratinocytes, which forms the epidermal melanin unit, maintains this homeostatic balance of the human epidermis (Fitzpatrick and Breathnach 1963; Jimbow et al. 1976). Within the *stratum basale*, the melanocytes keep a lifelong stable ratio of 1:5 with the keratinocytes (Fitzpatrick et al. 1979). This balance is maintained through regulated induction of melanocyte division coordinated through intercellular communication, which can be endocrine and paracrine via soluble factors and/or by direct contact via cell–cell and cell–matrix adhesion, or gap junctional intercellular communication (GJIC) (Haass et al. 2004, 2005). Dysregulation of this homeostasis may cause an imbalance of the epidermal melanin unit and trigger uncontrolled proliferation of the melanocytes, which may lead to the development of a nevus and/or a melanoma (Haass and Herlyn 2005).

Alterations in the interaction between neoplastic cells and their immediate microenvironment play a key role in these processes (Hanahan and Weinberg 2000, 2011; Park et al. 2000). The tumor microenvironment includes (1) the tumor stroma composed of fibroblasts, endothelial cells, immune cells, soluble molecules, and the extracellular matrix (ECM); (2) the tissue where the tumor had originated from; and (3) different sub-compartments within the tumor itself. Signals to and from the stroma via cell–cell and cell–matrix contact and/or via secretion of cytokines and growth factors may lead to a remodeling of the tumor microenvironment and consequently to promotion of melanoma development, growth, and metastasis by inducing angiogenesis, invasion, and migration (Villanueva and Herlyn 2008; Zigler et al. 2011). In addition to the interaction with the tumor stroma, primary melanoma progression as well as cutaneous melanoma metastases impact on the epidermal tumor microenvironment: the multilayered epithelium of the skin (Haass et al. 2010). Finally, different microenvironmental conditions within the tumor itself are created by differential access to nutrients and oxygen (Groebe and Mueller-Klieser 1991; Minchinton and Tannock 2006; Santiago-Walker et al. 2009; Haass et al. 2014; Haass 2015).

The microenvironment is not only important for the primary tumor, but also for colonization of a secondary organ. The "seed and soil" hypothesis implies that the metastatic process depends on the tumorigenic capacity of the cells and – again – on their interactions with the microenvironment (Fidler 2003).

9.2 Adherent Junction of Cadherins

Cross-talk between benign precursor cells, malignant cells, and surrounding host cells influences tumor development. Already in 1914, Theodor Boveri recognized the importance of changes in tumor cell adhesion for the development of cancer (Boveri 1914). Among the molecules involved in this intercellular communication are cadherins, which play a critical role for the homeostasis of normal skin and also during tumor formation and progression (Fig. 9.1). The identification of cadherins in the late 1970s and early 1980s was primarily motivated by an interest in understanding the mechanisms of cell adhesion during development (Franke 2009).

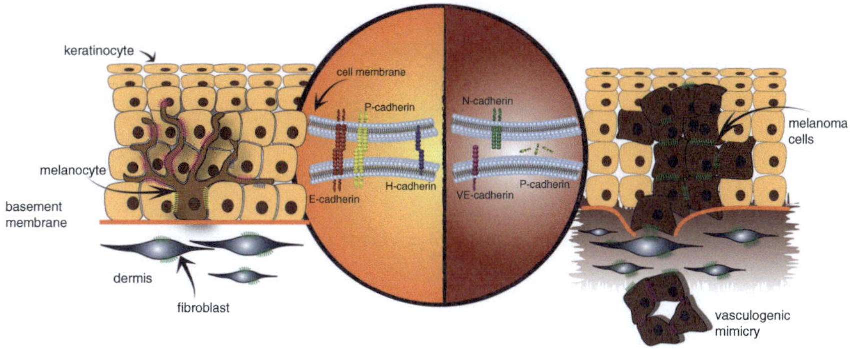

Fig 9.1 Overview of the cadherin repertoire in skin and melanoma (Illustration R.J. Bauer)

Cell–cell as well as cell–matrix adhesions are critical for cells and tissues to respond to mechanical stimuli from their environment. Both cell–cell and cell–matrix adhesions bear intrinsic mechanosensitivity, which allows them to promptly respond to stress and effectively propagate signals controlling cell shape and motility. This mechanosensitive response has been associated with pronounced changes in the size and molecular composition of specific adhesion sites and, consequently, the signals evoked by those adhesion sites. In polarized epithelia of vertebrates, the adherent junction is part of the tripartite junctional complex localized at the juxtaluminal region, which compromises the tight junction (TJ, see below), adherent junction (AJ), and desmosomes (macula adherens).

More than 80 proteins belong to the cadherin superfamily and are separated into the following "adherent junction" (AJ) subgroups in vertebrates:

1. Classical adhesive cadherins of type 1 (6 members) and type 2 (13 members), e.g., E-, N-, P-, R-, and VE-cadherin. The classical cadherin family comprises 19 members that share a common domain organization of five repetitive extracellular calcium-binding subdomains (Overduin et al. 1995). Most of these classical cell–cell adhesion molecules are connected to the actin filaments and microtubules of the cellular cytoskeleton via catenins. The four known catenins, alpha-, beta-, gamma (plakoglobin)-, and delta (p120)-catenin, are important regulatory elements either for sustained cell–cell adhesion or signaling cascades into the cell.
2. The "nonclassical" desmosomal cadherins, transmembrane proteins of desmosomes are, for example, desmocollin 1–3 (Dsc 1–3) and desmoglein 1–4 (Dsg 1–4). They are connected to intermediate filaments.
3. Finally, there are nonclassical cadherins, like the protocadherins (e.g., protocadherin 15, cadherin 23), H-cadherin, and cadherin-like molecules (e.g., Fat, Dachsous, Flamingo, or Ret) belonging to the cadherin superfamily.

The most important classical cell–cell adhesion molecules of the skin and during melanoma development are E (epithelial)-cadherin (CDH-1), N (neuronal)-cadherin (CDH-2), and P (placental)-cadherin (CDH-3), which belong to the group of calcium-dependent glycoproteins. Certainly, this group of classical adhesion molecules can be extended with atypical VE (vascular endothelial)-cadherin (CDH-5, CD144) and the nonclassical cadherin H (heart)-cadherin (T-cadherin, CDH-13) (Fig. 9.1). In normal epidermis, melanocytes and keratinocytes are mostly connected via E-cadherin, P-cadherin, and H-cadherin (Kuphal et al. 2009; Nishimura et al. 1999; Tang et al. 1994). Whereas melanocytes in the basal layer of the epidermis seem to contain predominantly E-cadherin and H-cadherin, those residing in hair follicles are rich in P-cadherin (Nishimura et al. 1999). In contrast, N-cadherin is expressed on fibroblasts and vascular endothelial cells of normal skin (Hsu et al. 1996).

9.2.1 Loss of E-Cadherin in Tumorigenesis

E-cadherin is the major cadherin in polarized epithelial cells. Furthermore, the crosstalk between melanocytes and keratinocytes mediated by E-cadherin plays an important role in human epidermis. The normal melanocytic phenotype and controlled proliferation of melanocytes are strictly regulated by keratinocytes via E-cadherin. The E-cadherin knockout mouse is lethal in early embryonic stages (Larue et al. 1994) supporting the finding that E-cadherin has an essential role in morpho- and organogenesis. In skin development, there is evidence that E- and P-cadherin play some role in guiding melanocyte precursor cells to their final destination in the epidermis (Nishimura et al. 1999).

Malignant transformation of melanocytes is frequently attended by loss of E-cadherin expression and induction of N-cadherin (Hsu et al. 1996). This leads to the loss of the regulatory dominance of keratinocytes over melanocytes. The degenerated melanocytes/melanoma cells express N-cadherin to get into contact to fibroblasts and vascular endothelial cells during migration and invasion into the tumor stroma, dermis, lymph, and blood vessels (Hsu et al. 2000) (Fig. 9.2). The switch of the cadherin class is an interesting phenomenon of melanoma cells and in epithelial–mesenchymal transition (EMT) in general.

However, immunohistochemical examination of primary melanomas and their metastases has revealed that a proportion of melanoma cells are still E-cadherin-positive and present little, if any, N-cadherin (Danen et al. 1996; Hsu et al. 1996; Sanders et al. 1999; Silye et al. 1998). Therefore, the cadherin switch as an obligatory prerequisite of malignant behavior is still controversial and might depend on the subtype of the melanoma examined. However, immunohistochemistry data could not show whether the expressed E-cadherin is really functionally active regarding adhesion or still possesses signaling function. The general consensus is that E-cadherin is a tumor invasion suppressor.

9.2.1.1 Regulators of E-Cadherin

The mechanism by which E-cadherin expression is lost during malignancy differs between tumor entities. Loss of E-cadherin function can be caused by various genetic or epigenetic mechanisms. In patients with diffuse gastric cancer and breast

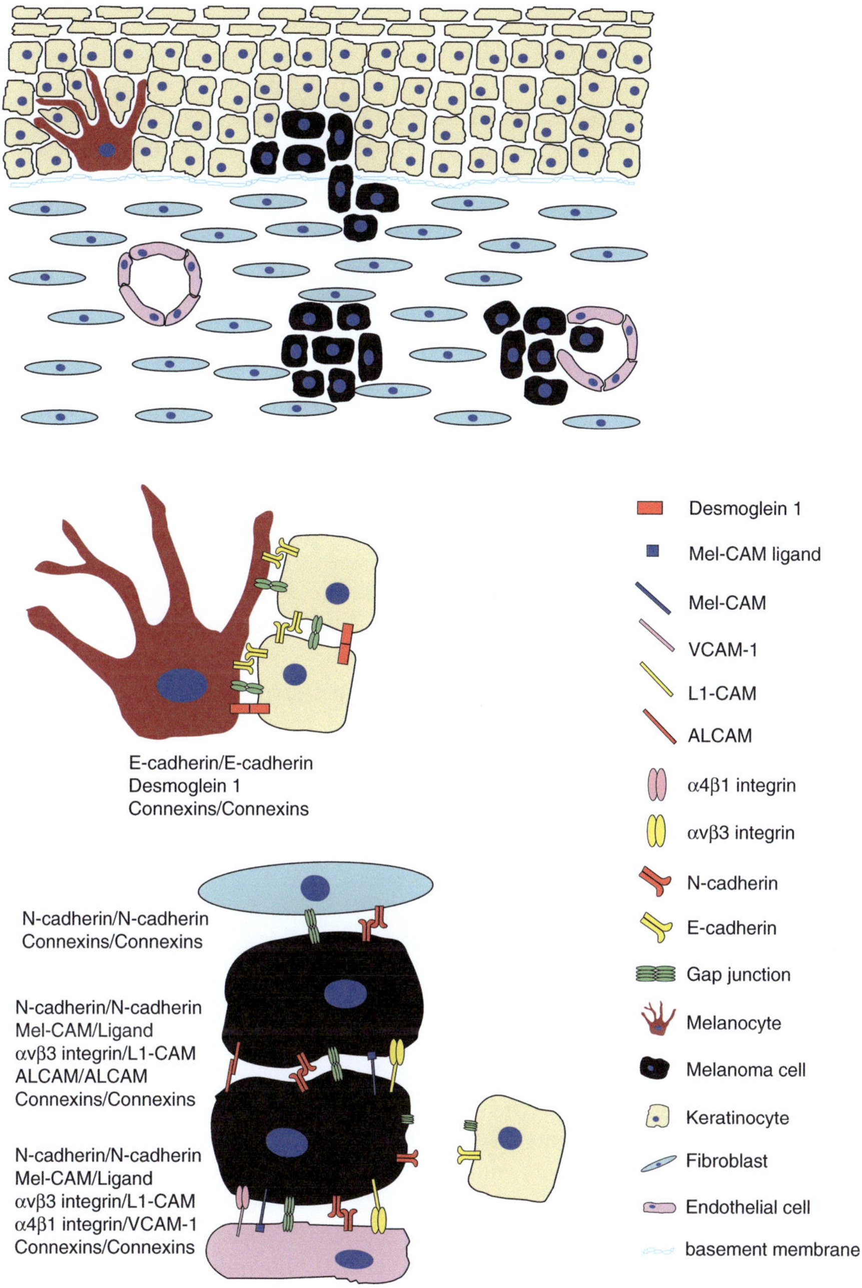

Fig. 9.2 (**a**) Cell–cell adhesion of melanocytes and melanoma cells. Melanocytes adhere to keratinocytes via E-cadherin and desmoglein, which enables them to communicate with each other through gap junctions with cells in their environment. (**b**) In melanoma cells, E-cadherin is downregulated. They interact with each other through N-cadherin, Mel-CAM/Mel-CAM ligand, αvβ3 integrin/L1-CAM, ALCAM, and connexins; with fibroblasts through N-cadherin and connexins; and with endothelial cells through N-cadherin, Mel-CAM/Mel-CAM ligand, αvβ3 integrin/L1-CAM, α4β1 integrin/VCAM-1, and connexins

cancer, the E-cadherin gene is mutated, leading to the expression of a nonfunctional protein (Strathdee 2002). The consequence is abnormal expression and abnormal subcellular localization of cadherin or the components of the cadherin-containing adhesion complex. Further, the *CDH-1* gene locus can be epigenetically silenced by hypermethylation, leading to downregulation of E-cadherin expression which is known from several cancer entities, e.g., hepatocellular carcinoma (Kanai et al. 1997), squamous cell carcinoma (Saito et al. 1998), and thyroid cancer (Graff et al. 1998).

In most cases, E-cadherin expression is downregulated at the transcriptional level. The zinc-finger containing transcriptional repressor Snail1, which is a master regulator of neural crest cell specification and melanocyte migration during development in vertebrates, is mainly responsible for the loss of E-cadherin in melanoma (Batlle et al. 2000; Poser et al. 2001). The level of Snail1 expression correlates directly with the loss of E-cadherin expression, and forces overexpression of Snail in primary melanocytes downregulates E-cadherin expression (Poser et al. 2001). Slug (Hajra et al. 2002; Bolós et al. 2003), Snail2, ZEB1 and ZEB2 (Eger et al. 2005; Caramel et al. 2013), and SIP1 (Comijn et al. 2001), also members of the zinc finger transcription factor family of Snail, are further regulators of E-cadherin in melanoma, as well as basic helix–loop–helix transcription factors E12/47 (Perez-Moreno et al. 2001) and Twist (Yang et al. 2004). Additionally, the T-box transcription factor Tbx3 is overexpressed in melanoma, which enhances melanoma invasiveness through prevention of E-cadherin expression (Rodriguez et al. 2008). Furthermore, within human melanoma lesions, GLI-2, a mediator of hedgehog signaling, is associated with loss of E-cadherin (Alexaki et al. 2010).

Proteolytic degradation of E-cadherin by matrix metalloproteinases (MMPs) is another mechanism by which E-cadherin-mediated cell–cell adhesion can be ablated. In this case, cell surface E-cadherin becomes soluble by cleavage of the extracellular domain, a process known as ectodomain shedding. For melanoma, Adam-10 is responsible for E-cadherin shedding (Billion et al. 2006) (see also Chap. 8).

A family of microRNAs, such as miR-200a, miR-200b, miR-200c, and miR-205 was reported to control the expression level of E-cadherin during the epithelial–mesenchymal transition. The microRNA targets the transcriptional repressors ZEB1 and ZEB2 of E-cadherin (Gregory et al. 2008; Hurteau et al. 2007). As one example for cancer, loss of miR-200c expression is significantly correlated with early stage T1 bladder tumor progression (Wiklund et al. 2011). Another miRNA, miR-373, induces expression of genes with complementary promoter sequences. It was found that miR-373 induces E-cadherin expression by recognizing a target site in the promoter of the *cdh-1* gene (Place et al. 2008). Liu et al. 2012 showed that miR-9 is downregulated in metastatic melanomas compared with primary melanomas. A tumor suppressor effect after re-expression of miR-9 in melanoma is mediated through its direct binding to sites within the NF-kB 3′-UTR, resulting in suppression of Snail1 and upregulation of E-cadherin. However, whether microRNAs are responsible for regulating cadherins directly and specifically in melanoma is still not known (see also Chap. 6).

9.2.2 Loss of P-Cadherin During Tumorigenesis

In human skin, P-cadherin is expressed mainly on cells of the epidermal basal layer (Furukawa et al. 1997) and those melanocytes residing in hair follicles (Nishimura et al. 1999). Concerning carcinogenesis, the effective role of P-cadherin remains an object of debate, since it can behave differently depending on the molecular context and tumor cell model studied. In melanoma cells, loss of full-length P-cadherin was reported (Bachmann et al. 2005; Van Marck et al. 2005; Jacobs et al. 2011). Therefore, P-cadherin has a similar tumor-suppressive behavior to E-cadherin. Additionally, a truncated 50 kDa form of the N-terminal part of P-cadherin was found, which appeared to be secreted from the melanoma cells. If this secreted form of P-cadherin is expressed from melanoma cells, it is responsible for cell migration and invasion (Bauer et al. 2005, 2006; Bauer and Bosserhoff 2006).

9.2.3 Loss of T-Cadherin During Tumorigenesis

T-cadherin (truncated-cadherin, cadherin 13, gene name *CDH13*) or H-cadherin, named for its strong expression in the heart, is an atypical member of the cadherin family, lacking the classical HisAlaVal recognition motif at its N-terminus, lacking the typical transmembrane and cytosolic domains and possessing a glycosylphosphatidylinositol moiety that anchors T-cadherin into the outer plasma membrane.

Immunohistochemistry of melanoma tissue samples showed positive T-cadherin staining of the endothelial cells. T-cadherin expression in endothelial cells was demonstrated to be redox sensitive (Joshi et al. 2008). The melanoma cells themselves showed loss of T-cadherin whereas healthy skin showed staining of melanocytes and keratinocytes of the basal layer of the epidermis. Loss of T-cadherin in melanoma is associated with migration and invasion of the cells (Kuphal et al. 2009). In general, the exact functional role and signaling of T-cadherin for melanoma cells itself and for the intratumoral angiogenesis are not clarified, so far. It was only shown that loss of T-cadherin in melanoma regulates AKT signaling and desensitizes for apoptosis (Bosserhoff et al. 2014). Also, a connection of loss of T-cadherin to tumor progression was speculated (Rubina et al. 2013) but not evidenced, until today.

9.2.4 N-Cadherin Expression During Tumorigenesis

N-cadherin plays a pivotal role in cell adhesion between melanoma cells and both dermal fibroblasts and vascular endothelial cells. During the cadherin class switch, loss of E-cadherin expression is accompanied by induced N-cadherin expression, which confers new adhesive properties on the cells (Fig. 9.2). The shift in cadherin profile during melanoma progression has been found not only in vitro but also in vivo (Hsu et al. 1996; Sanders et al. 1999). Experimentally, melanoma cell migration across fibroblasts is impaired upon addition of an N-cadherin neutralizing antibody (Li et al. 2001). The functional relevance of N-cadherin is to conduct migration and invasion of melanoma cells whereas N-cadherin expression correlates with progression to advanced-stage melanoma. The cell adhesion molecule N-cadherin has been suggested to represent a melanoma progression marker (Watson-Hurst and Becker 2006).

The switch of the cadherin class from E-cadherin to N-cadherin is directly connected. The transcriptional repressor Snail not only regulates E-cadherin repression but also represses the expression of the deubiquitinating enzyme CYLD. Loss of CYLD expression in melanoma in turn led to ubiquitination of Bcl-3 which is a transcriptional regulator of N-cadherin expression (Massoumi et al. 2009).

9.2.5 VE-Cadherin Expression During Tumorigenesis

The term *vasculogenic mimicry* describes the formation of vascular-like tubular structures and patterned networks through the connection of melanoma cells. The vascular structures are essential for the supply of the tumor. Several key molecules are responsible for the formation and maintenance of the tubular networks and these molecules are also often essential in normal blood vessels. One molecule expressed during vasculogenic mimicry of melanoma cells is VE-cadherin, previously considered to be endothelial cell specific. Analyzing VE-cadherin in detail demonstrated an interaction with EphrinA2 (EphA2), a tyrosine kinase. VE-cadherin engages the membrane-bound ligand of EphA2 and becomes phosphorylated on its tyrosines at the cytoplasmic domain. The mutual impact of VE-cadherin and EphA2 results in loosening of cell–cell adhesion and allowing for an increase in cell migration, invasion, and vasculogenic mimicry. Further studies describe the role of VE-cadherin for melanoma transendothelial migration. Here, p38 MAP kinase is necessary for increased VE-cadherin-mediated junction disassembly important for the migration processes of melanoma cells (Hendrix et al. 2001, 2003; Khanna et al. 2010).

9.2.6 FAT Expression During Tumorigenesis

FAT1, FAT2, FAT3, and FAT4 are human homologs of *Drosophila* Fat, which is involved in tumor suppression and planar cell polarity (PCP). FAT molecules belong to the cadherin-like protein family. FAT1 and FAT4 undergo the first proteolytic cleavage by Furin and are predicted to undergo the second cleavage by γ-secretase to release intracellular domain (ICD). Recently, it was shown using Northern blotting that human melanoma cell lines variably but universally express FAT1 and less commonly FAT2, FAT3, and FAT4. Both normal melanocytes and keratinocytes also express comparable FAT1 mRNA relative to melanoma cells. However, in melanoma cells, the non-cleaved proform of FAT1 is also expressed at the cell surface together with the furin-cleaved heterodimer. Moreover, furin-independent processing generates a potentially functional proteolytic product in melanoma cells, a persistent 65-kDa membrane-bound cytoplasmic fragment no longer in association with the extracellular fragment. In vitro localization studies of FAT1 showed that melanoma cells display high levels of cytosolic FAT1 protein. Such differences in protein distribution appear to reconcile with the different protein products generated by dual FAT1 processing. It was suggested that the uncleaved FAT1 could promote altered signaling, and the novel products of alternate processing provide a dominant negative function in melanoma (Sadeqzadeh et al. 2011). Among the human *FAT* gene family, *FAT4* gene is recurrently mutated in several types of human cancers, such as melanoma (40 %), pancreatic cancer (8 %), HNSCC (6 %), and gastric cancer (5 %) (Nikolaev et al. 2011).

9.2.7 Signaling of Cadherins

In contrast to integrins, evidence for cadherin-induced outside–in signaling came into focus only slowly. Over the last 10 years, a number of studies have appeared to agree that signaling cascades emanating from cadherins play an important role in confluency-dependent growth arrest, migration, invasion, and differentiation. Changes in expression or function of cell adhesion molecules can therefore contribute to tumor progression both by altering the adhesion status and by affecting cell signaling. To date, no enzymatic activity has been attributed to the cytoplasmic tails of adhesion molecules like E-cadherin or N-cadherin. The signaling capability emanates from intracellularly bound kinases and phosphatases that link to the cytoplasmic tail of adhesion receptors (Fig. 9.3).

9.2.7.1 Signaling Cascades of E-Cadherin

Four modes of E-cadherin signaling are known:

1. Modulation of receptor tyrosinase signaling (RTK) (see also Chap. 7)
2. Inhibition of the Wnt signaling pathway (see also Chap. 7)
3. Regulation of cytoplasmic β-catenin signaling
4. Regulation of signaling through Rho GTPases

One way by which E-cadherin transmits growth-inhibiting outside–in signals appears to follow a strikingly similar scheme to that of the integrins. By using an immortalized nontumorigenic keratinocyte cell line, HaCaT, as a model system, Pece and Gutkind (2000) provide evidence that the assembly of calcium-dependent adherens junctions leads to a rapid and remarkable increase in the state of activation of MAPK and that this event is mediated by E-cadherin. Furthermore, it was found in these studies about HaCaTs that E-cadherin stimulates the MAPK pathway through ligand-independent activation of receptor tyrosine kinases, in particular EGF-receptors (Pece and Gutkind 2000). They speculated that upon adherens junction formation, signals emanating as a result of the E-cadherin-EGFR interaction might be involved in maintaining the functional and structural integrity of quiescent epithelia and, as a function of the adhesion status of the cells, possibly in promoting epithelial cell differentiation rather than proliferation. In contrast, another group detected signaling

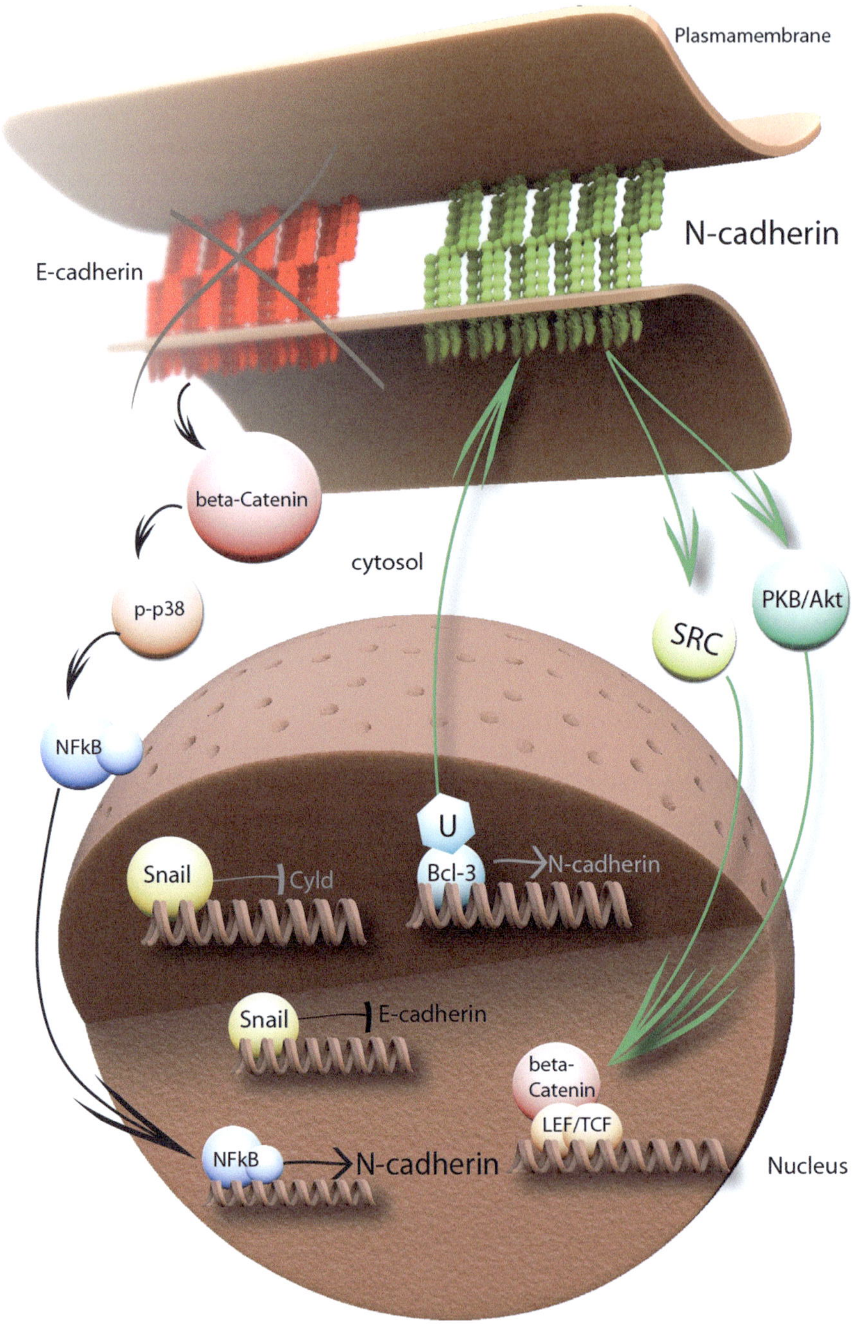

Fig. 9.3 Schematic depiction of cadherin signaling in melanoma. The transcriptional repressor Snail inactivates E-cadherin expression in melanoma. With the loss of E-cadherin cytosolic beta-catenin activates the MAP kinase p38, which stimulates the transcriptional activity of NFkappaB. NFkappaB has N-cadherin as target gene. Additionally, Snail represses the expression of the tumor suppressor Cyld, which in turn leads to ubiquitination of Bcl-3 which also has N-cadherin as target gene. The overexpression of N-cadherin activates signaling cascades of SRC and PKB/Akt which leads to tumor progression (Illustration R.J. Bauer)

cascade inhibition through EGF-receptor/E-cadherin complex formation in melanoma and breast cancer cells (Qian et al. 2004). Unfortunately, most of the literature on E-cadherin signaling does not cover melanoma. Studies on keratinocytes and other cancer cell types revealed that the E-cadherin complex associates and cooperates with an EGF-receptor family member to activate the PI3K/Akt pathway in a Src-family kinase-dependent manner (Muller et al. 2008; Perrais et al. 2007) (see also Chap. 7).

Some studies showed that homophilic ligation of E-cadherin signals directly through Rho GTPase activity (Braga 2000; Braga et al. 1997). Loss of E-cadherin in melanoma may involve changes in the organization of the cytoskeleton which is exerted by members of the Rho family. They control not only the cytoskeletal organization but also cell motility, migration, and tumor progression to malignancy at the same time. As example, E-cadherin suppresses RhoA activity in melanoma by activating p190RhoGAP (Molina-Ortiz et al. 2009). E-cadherin overexpression led to association of p190RhoGAP and p120^{ctn} on the plasma membrane where E-cadherin bounds p120^{ctn}. Recently, it was shown that E-cadherin also regulates RhoC GTPase. Here, loss of E-cadherin activates the expression of the RhoC in melanoma through upregulation of the transcription factor ETS-1, which results in increased c-Jun protein stabilization and activation (Spangler et al. 2012).

In addition to its role in adhesion, nuclear β-catenin is involved in Wnt signal transduction, and it interacts with transcription factors of the leukocyte enhancer factor (LEF)/T-cell factor (TCF) family to regulate transcription of target genes implicated in cell growth control such as cyclin D1 and c-myc (van Noort and Clevers 2002). By sequestering β-catenin at the cell surface, E-cadherin has been shown to antagonize nuclear β-catenin signaling pathways and to induce growth inhibition (Gottardi et al. 2001; Shtutman et al. 1999). Furthermore, β-catenin bound to E-cadherin inhibits phosphorylation of p38 and prevents activation of NFkappaB. Unbound cytoplasmic β-catenin activates the signaling pathway ending at transcriptional activation of N-cadherin expression in melanoma cells (Kuphal et al. 2004). In general, it was shown by Onder et al. (2008) that loss of E-cadherin promotes metastasis via multiple downstream transcriptional pathways. The publication presents ~84 of 617 genes differentially expressed in shE-cadherin human breast epithelial cells (HMLE). They presented, e.g., *twist* and *TCF-8* among other 19 transcription factors as upregulated after loss of E-cadherin.

9.2.7.2 Signaling Cascades of N-Cadherin

N-cadherin-mediated intercellular interactions promote survival and migration of melanoma cells through activation of cytoplasmic signaling cascades. The Src family kinases are involved in the regulation of N-cadherin-mediated cell adhesion and signaling during, e.g., melanoma cell transendothelial migration. Src is localized at the heterotypic contacts of N-cadherin and becomes activated when melanoma cells are transmigrating across the endothelium. Activated Src has the Tyrosine-860 at the cytoplasmic domain of N-cadherin as target site for phosphorylation. The phosphorylation leads to disruption of β-catenin binding followed by nuclear translocation of this molecule to activate gene transcription of genes responsible for proliferation (Qi et al. 2006). N-cadherin mediates cell adhesion-activated antiapoptotic protein Akt/PKB and subsequently increases β-catenin and inactivates proapoptotic factor Bad (Li et al. 2001).

9.2.8 Desmosomes/Hemidesmosomes

Desmosomes, composed of desmogleins and desmocollins, are localized spot-like adhesions randomly arranged on the lateral sides of plasma membranes and are also members of the cadherin family. The extracellular domain of the desmosome is called the extracellular core domain (ECD) or the Desmoglea, and is bisected by an electron-dense midline where the desmoglein and desmocollin proteins bind to each other. On the cytoplasmic side of the plasma membrane, there are two dense structures called the outer dense plaque (ODP) and the inner dense plaque (IDP). In the ODP, the cytoplasmic domains of the cadherins desmoglein and desmocollin attach to desmoplakin via plakoglobin and plakophilin, while in the IDP, desmoplakin attaches to the intermediate filaments such as keratine filaments.

A number of melanoma cell lines synthesize, in the absence of desmosomes, the desmosomal cadherin desmoglein 2 (Dsg2) as a frequent plasma membrane glycoprotein that is not assembled into any junction but is dispersed over large parts of the cell surface. Indeed, in tissue microarrays, Dsg2 has been demonstrated in a sizable subset of nevi and primary melanomas (Rickelt et al. 2008). In contrast, Dsg1, Dsg3, and desmocollins 1–3, were absent in the analyzed melanoma cell lines but plakoglobin and plakophilin3 were also expressed in several melanoma cell lines (Schmitt et al. 2007). Future studies will have to clarify the diagnostic and prognostic significance of these different adhesion protein subtypes.

9.3 Integrins

Integrins are transmembrane adhesion receptors localized at cell–matrix contact sites where they link ECM (extracellular matrix) components, e.g., vitronectin, fibronectin, laminin, osteopontin, or collagen, to the actin cytoskeleton and interact with multiple structural and signaling molecules including talin, kindlin, paxillin, vinculin, α-actinin, FAK (focal adhesion kinase), ILK (integrin-linked kinase), Rho GTPases, and SHC (Berrier and Yamada 2007; Papusheva and Heisenberg 2010). The latter are important mediators downstream of integrins by which they interact either directly or indirectly to effect adhesion-dependent responses (Playford and Schaller 2004). The metastatic transformation of melanocytes is associated with altered expression of integrins, which transduce signals upon ligation to ECM proteins that regulate tumor growth and metastasis, apoptosis, differentiation as well as tumor angiogenesis. Integrin receptors are functional dimers of α- and β-integrin subunits, which each have a large ectodomain, a single transmembrane domain, and a generally short cytoplasmic tail (except for β4 integrin). The combination of different α- and β-subunits determines the substrate specificity of the dimer (Danen and Sonnenberg 2003). There are at least 18 known α-chains and 8 β-chains, allowing for at least 24 unique heterodimers.

The pattern of integrins on the cell surface is usually very specific, which makes the cell fit perfectly into its surrounding environment. Importantly, integrin expression patterns differ considerably in vitro versus in vivo. Thus, in vitro studies may not translate into the in vivo situation.

Several publications have shown that the expression levels mainly of αvβ3, α2β1, α3β1, α4β1, and α5β1 appear to increase from primary melanomas to metastatic melanoma tissue sections, whereas there was a significant decrease in α1β1, α2β1, and α6β1 expression levels in metastatic melanoma compared to primary melanoma (Friedl et al. 1998; Natali et al. 1993; Schadendorf et al. 1993). Although many integrins have been implicated in mediating melanoma growth and metastasis, perhaps none have been studied as much as the vitronectin receptor, αvβ3 (Danen et al. 1995; Mortarini and Anichini 1993; Seftor et al. 1999). αvβ3 integrin adheres to vitronectin, fibronectin, laminin, collagen, and osteopontin. Binding fibronectin and vitronectin induces the expression of MMP-2, which is able to degrade the collagen of the basement membrane (Felding-Habermann et al. 2002). Furthermore, osteopontin's RGD-sequence (Arg–Gly–Asp) has high binding affinity and specificity to αvβ3. As the aggressiveness of melanoma has been associated with high osteopontin expression (Sieg et al. 2000), this interaction of αvβ3 and osteopontin is important for melanoma progression. Interaction between αvβ3 and extracellular matrix molecules serves to promote cell attachment, spreading, and migration. αvβ3 integrin also undergoes heterophilic binding with two members of the immunoglobulin superfamily of cell adhesion molecules, PECAM-1 and L1. The αv subunit is widely expressed on melanomas regardless of disease stage. This stands in contrast to the β3 subunit, which is predominantly expressed on melanoma cells in the vertical growth phase. The onset of β3 integrin expression is one of the most specific markers of the transition from radial growth phase to vertical growth phase of melanoma (Albelda et al. 1990; Danen et al. 1995; Natali et al. 1997). Although many studies on human melanoma cell lines have correlated αvβ3 integrin expression with progression and metastasis, in vivo studies are less clear.

9.3.1 Integrin Signaling in Melanoma

Apart from being involved in the attachment of cells to the ECM, integrins are also responsible for signaling between the cells and the environment. Signaling works bidirectionally: "outside–in signaling" can control behavior, proliferation, cell polarity, cell growth, and migration. "Inside–out signaling," on the other hand, changes the integrins from a passive, weak binding state into an active, adhesive state and alters the interaction of the receptors with the extracellular environment. Integrins are receptors for cell movement in response to binding to ECM of the basement membrane or connective tissue or plasma membrane receptors expressed on endothelial cell surfaces. Additionally, integrins bind cytoplasmic adaptor proteins of the actin-myosin filaments and create a plasticity that allows the cell to move. In summary, integrins are bivalent linker proteins, binding simultaneously to extracellular ligands as well as cytoplasmic proteins including intracellular signaling molecules. They influence, for example, tyrosine kinases, serine/threonine kinases, phosphoinositides, and signaling cascades which determine the fate of a cell, letting it grow, proliferate, or die whenever it is necessary in the context of the whole organism. This paragraph introduces some of the most important and best studied proteins which are known to interact with integrins in melanoma.

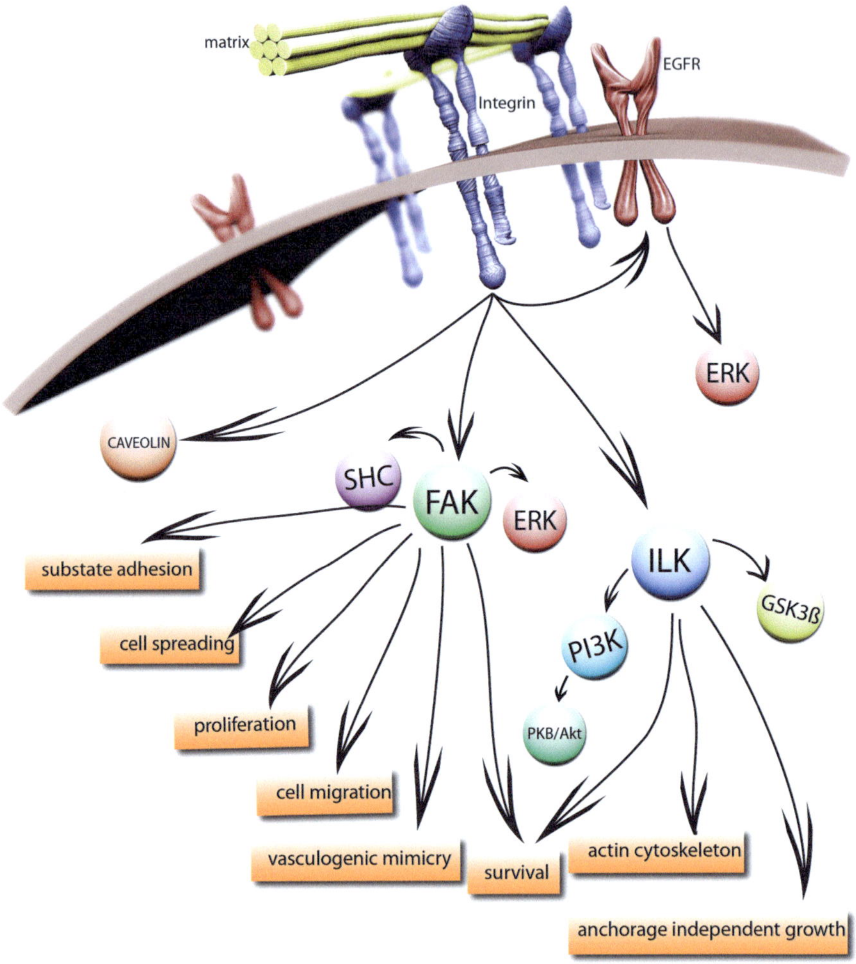

Fig. 9.4 Schematic depiction of the signaling pathways leading from integrins to focal adhesion kinase (*FAK*) and integrin-linked kinase (*ILK*), respectively, and further reactions of the cell (Illustration R.J. Bauer)

There is the non-receptor protein tyrosinase kinase FAK (focal adhesion kinase) (Fig. 9.4) that co-localizes with integrins in focal adhesions. FAK becomes phosphorylated and then controls processes like cell spreading, proliferation, motility, vasculogenic mimicry, and survival (Schaller 2001). Proteins like c-SRC, SHC, CSK, PI3K, and GRB2 are known to interact with FAK to transfer the signaling into the cytoplasm and to link FAK signaling also to MAP kinases (Chakraborty et al. 2002) (see also Chap. 7). FAK expression seems to be required in melanoma cells for substrate adhesion. It has been shown that in melanoma FAK is constitutively active and that it is essential for maintaining adhesiveness in melanoma cells (Hamamura et al. 2008; Kahana et al. 2002).

Furthermore, the integrin-linked kinase (ILK), a serine/threonine kinase, is implicated in connecting cell–extracellular matrix interaction and growth factor signaling to cell survival, cell migration, invasion, anchorage-independent growth, angiogenesis, and epithelial–mesenchymal transition. It has been shown that strong ILK expression was significantly associated with melanoma thickness, migration, and invasion (Wong et al. 2007). Increased expression of integrin-linked kinase is correlated with melanoma progression and poor patient survival (Dai et al. 2003). ILK directly phosphorylates PKB/Akt and glycogen synthase kinase-3 (GSK-3beta), which is inactivated upon phosphorylation (Delcommenne et al. 1998; Troussard et al. 1999). SHC is another protein which is implicated in integrin signaling. It is an adaptor protein capable of binding phosphotyrosine-containing sequences. So far, studies have demonstrated that SHC signaling is involved in pathways, which play a role in the development of malignancies like c-Myc activation (Gotoh et al. 1997), survival signaling (Friedmann et al. 1996; Sakai et al. 2000), cytoskeletal organization, and mitogenic signaling through RAS. It has been proposed that SHC is a substrate for FAK.

Also, the ERK/MAP kinase cascade is a pathway in which integrin-mediated adhesion is involved. In the ERK pathway, various stimuli of many important integrin signaling molecules like FAK or SHC converge and are able to influence nearly every profound cellular activity (Meier et al. 2005).

Epidermal growth factor receptor (EGFR) is also activated by integrins to generate cellular responses such as adhesion-dependent cell survival and proliferation in response to ECM. Subsequently, integrin-mediated EGFR activation induces ERK/MAP kinase signaling (Howe et al. 2002; Jost et al. 2001). Furthermore, Caveolin-1 (CAV1) is the main structural component of caveolae, which are plasma membrane invaginations that participate in vesicular trafficking and signal transduction events. Following integrin activation, B16F10 cells expressing CAV1 display reduced expression levels and activity of FAK and Src proteins. Furthermore, CAV1 expression markedly reduces the expression of integrin β3 in B16F10 melanoma cells. These findings provide experimental evidence that CAV1 may function as an antimetastatic gene in malignant melanoma (Trimmer et al. 2010).

9.4 Immunoglobulin Gene Superfamily of Cell Adhesion Molecules (CAMs)

Whereas normal melanocytes express few cell–cell adhesion receptors of the immunoglobulin gene superfamily of cell adhesion molecules (CAMs), melanoma cells show an increase in expression of melanoma cell adhesion molecule (MCAM, Mel-CAM, MUC18, CD146), L1 cell adhesion molecule (L1-CAM, CD171), activated leukocyte cell adhesion molecule (ALCAM, CD166), vascular cell adhesion molecule 1 (VCAM-1, CD106), intercellular cell adhesion molecule 1 (ICAM-1, CD54), and carcinoembryonic antigen-related cell adhesion molecule 1 (CEACAM-1, CD66a) (reviewed in Haass et al. 2005).

9.4.1 Melanoma Cell Adhesion Molecule (MCAM, Mel-CAM, MUC18, CD146)

Mel-CAM mediates homologous and heterologous interactions between melanoma cells and endothelial cells, respectively, via a heterophilic Ca^{2+}-independent adhesion to its ligand (Shih et al. 1997a, b; Johnson et al. 1997). Recently, Laminin-411 ($\alpha4\beta1\gamma1$ integrin) and Galectin-1 have been identified as Mel-CAM ligands (Flanagan et al. 2012; Jouve et al. 2013; Yazawa et al. 2015). In melanocytic cells, expression of Mel-CAM is first found in nevi, when the cells have separated from the epidermal keratinocytes and have migrated into the dermis (Shih et al. 1994; Kraus et al. 1997). With progression to malignancy, Mel-CAM expression gradually increases and is highest in metastatic melanoma cells (Xie et al. 1997; Johnson et al. 1996; Shih et al. 1994; Lehmann et al. 1987, 1989). In vitro and in vivo data supporting an important role of Mel-CAM in melanoma progression was demonstrated in several experimental studies (reviewed in Haass et al. 2005; Lei et al. 2015). Recently, the zinc finger transcription factor ZBTB7A was found to repress melanoma metastasis by directly binding to the promoter and transcriptionally repressing Mel-CAM (Liu et al. 2015).

An evaluation of tissue arrays of primary and metastatic melanomas revealed that in patients meeting the current criteria for sentinel lymph node dissection, both Mel-CAM expression positivity and intensity were independently predictive of survival and development of lymph node disease in primary melanoma over and above established markers of prognosis, such as Breslow thickness. Mel-CAM-negative patients had a 5-year survival of 92 % compared with 40 % for Mel-CAM-positive patients (Pearl et al. 2008). Recently, a study on 175 patients revealed that sequential molecular detection of Mel-CAM mRNA in the peripheral blood correlated with poor prognosis. The authors suggested to utilize Mel-CAM expression as a "molecular warning of progression" even in early stage patients in otherwise disease-free conditions (Rapanotti et al. 2014). However, larger trials to confirm this finding as a biomarker are still pending.

9.4.2 L1-Cell Adhesion Molecule (L1-CAM, CD171)

L1-CAM, originally described as a neuronal cell adhesion molecule, has also been detected in a number of other non-neuroendocrine tissues and in several malignant tumors, including melanoma (Nolte et al. 1999; Thies et al. 2002b). L1-CAM mediates adhesion both via homophilic (L1-CAM-L1-CAM) and heterophilic (L1-CAM-$\alpha_v\beta_3$ integrin) mechanisms (Hortsch 1996). In melanoma/melanoma cell and in melanoma/endothelial cell interactions, L1-CAM binds to $\alpha_v\beta_3$ integrin (Montgomery et al. 1996). The interaction of L1-CAM and $\alpha_v\beta_3$ integrin plays an important role in transendothelial migration of melanoma cells (Voura et al. 2001) whereas overexpression of L1-CAM promotes conversion from radial to vertical growth phase melanoma without upregulation of $\alpha_v\beta_3$ integrin expression (Meier et al. 2006). There is an increase in L1-CAM immunoreactivity in melanomas and metastases of melanoma compared to acquired melanocytic nevi (Fogel et al. 2003). A study that systematically identified novel melanoma-specific genes confirmed that L1-CAM is not expressed in normal skin and melanocytic nevi, but is highly and differentially expressed in primary melanoma tissues and melanoma lymph node metastases (Talantov et al. 2005). Evaluation of specimens of nevi, primary melanomas, sentinel lymph nodes, and distant metastases showed that L1-CAM can serve as a highly sensitive and specific diagnostic marker for melanoma (Thies et al. 2007). A 10-year retrospective biomarker study, evaluating 100 melanoma specimens, showed that the expression of L1-CAM in human primary cutaneous melanoma is significantly associated with metastatic spread and that L1-CAM expression is an independent predictor for the risk of metastasis (Thies et al. 2002b). A recent study revealed that the CE7 epitope of L1-CAM on a variety of tumors (however, melanoma was not included in the study) may be amenable to targeting by CE7R+ T cells, making it a promising target for adoptive immunotherapy (Hong et al. 2014).

9.4.3 Activated Leukocyte Cell Adhesion Molecule (ALCAM, CD166)

ALCAM is involved in homophilic (ALCAM-ALCAM) (Degen et al. 1998) and heterophilic (ALCAM-CD6) (Patel et al. 1995) cell–cell adhesion interactions. ALCAM is expressed in metastatic human melanoma cells, whereas it is absent in non-metastatic cells (Degen et al. 1998). Immunohistochemistry on a series of common nevi, primary melanomas, and melanoma metastases revealed that ALCAM expression correlates with melanoma progression (van Kempen et al. 2000). ALCAM is therefore proposed to be a molecular melanoma progression marker. Intact cell adhesion function of ALCAM favored primary tumor growth and represented a rate-limiting step for tissue invasion, which supported the view that dynamic control of ALCAM plays an important role in progression (van Kempen et al. 2004). An immunohistochemical biomarker study, evaluating tissue microarrays showed that a significantly greater percentage of melanomas (combined primary and metastatic) than nevi contained cells that expressed ALCAM (Klein et al. 2007). Interestingly, a recent study evaluating ALCAM expression and long-term survival in melanoma patients suggested that, in primary melanomas, high ALCAM expression was a marker of negative outcome, but in regional lymph node melanoma metastases low expression of ALCAM was a feature associated with unfavorable prognosis (Donizy et al. 2015). ALCAM upregulation in metastatic melanoma cells is driven by miR-214 and depends on transcriptional mechanisms mediated by TFAP2 and posttranscriptional mechanisms mediated by miR-148b, which itself is controlled by TFAP2. Therefore, miR-214 and miR-148b have opposite effects on melanoma cell dissemination and are part of a regulatory loop (Penna et al. 2013).

9.4.4 Intercellular Adhesion Molecule-1 (ICAM-1, CD54)

ICAM-1 can be induced in a cell-specific manner by several cytokines, e.g., TNF-α (tumor necrosis factor-alpha), IL-1 (interleukin-1), and IFN-γ (interferon-gamma). The ligands of ICAM-1 are $\alpha_L\beta_2$ (lymphocyte function-associated antigen 1, LFA-1) and Mac1 on lymphocytes (van de Stolpe and van der Saag 1996). ICAM-1 correlates with melanoma progression and increased risk of metastasis (Johnson et al. 1989). Its expression in melanoma is stronger than in common nevi and increases with the Breslow index in primary melanomas (Natali et al. 1990, 1997; Schadendorf et al. 1993, 1995). The observation that stage I patients with ICAM-1-positive melanomas had a significantly shorter disease-free interval and overall survival than those with ICAM-1-negative tumors (Natali et al. 1997) and that the suppression of ICAM-1 in an animal model reduced the metastatic capacity (Miele et al. 1994), supported the role of ICAM-1 in melanoma progression and metastasis. However, the specific role of ICAM-1 in melanoma progression remains to be determined. Expression of ICAM-1 may promote aggregate formation with leucocytes, which can enhance survival in the vascular system and encourage extravasation (Aeed et al. 1988). On the other hand, ICAM-1 is shed from melanoma cells (Giavazzi et al. 1992) – possibly in a form that inhibits lymphocyte–tumor cell interaction and thus contributes to tumor survival (Becker et al. 1993). A recent study has unraveled a mechanism by which shear flow-regulated melanoma cell adhesion to the endothelium can upregulate endothelial ICAM-1 expression (Zhang et al. 2014). Elevated ICAM-1 levels may serve as receptors to recruit neutrophils and bind fibrin, which assists melanoma cell adhesion and migration. An increase of ICAM-1 expression on endothelial cells could be a result of direct ligation of tumor CD44 and endothelial E-selectin, through the PKCα-p38-SP-1 pathway. This suggests a new mechano-signaling cascade triggered by stretching E-selectin to induce ICAM-1 expression (Zhang et al. 2014).

9.4.5 Carcinoembryonic Antigen-Related Cell Adhesion Molecule 1 (CEACAM-1, CD66a)

CEACAM1 is involved in intercellular adhesion and subsequent signal transduction events in a number of epithelia. In epithelial cells, CEACAM1 is believed to act as a growth suppressor, since its expression was shown to be lost or significantly down- or dysregulated in carcinomas of liver, prostate, endometrium, breast, and colon (reviewed in Haass et al. 2005). On the other hand, CEACAM1 is upregulated in non-small cell lung cancer (Sienel et al. 2003). CEACAM1 interacts with the β_3 integrin subunit via the CEACAM1 cytoplasmic domain. CEACAM1 and the β_3 integrin subunit co-localize at the tumor–stroma interface of invading melanoma masses, suggesting that CEACAM1–integrin β_3 interaction plays a role in melanoma cell migration and invasion (Brummer et al. 2001). The expression of CEACAM1 in primary melanomas is associated with the subsequent development of metastatic disease (Thies et al. 2002a). Furthermore, the overexpression of CEACAM1 in CEACAM1-negative melanocytic cells and melanoma cell lines increases the migratory and invasive growth potentials in vitro (Ebrahimnejad et al. 2004) supporting the role of CEACAM1 in melanoma progression and metastasis. Evaluation of specimens of nevi, primary melanomas, sentinel lymph nodes, and distant metastases showed that CEACAM1 can serve as a highly sensitive and specific diagnostic marker for melanoma (Thies et al. 2007). Indeed, CEACAM1 was shown to be one of the seven plasma markers best able to identify metastatic melanoma patients (Kluger et al. 2011).

9.5 Gap Junctions/Connexins

Connexins belong to a family of transmembrane proteins that form gap junctions (GJs), cell–cell junctions that are essential for intercellular communication. Gap junctional intercellular communication (GJIC) in the skin is involved in maintenance of homeostasis, regulation of proliferation, differentiation, barrier function, and recruitment of inflammatory cells. GJIC is thus a critical factor in the life and death balance of cells (Djalilian et al. 2006; Langlois et al. 2007; Maass et al. 2004; Man et al. 2007) (reviewed in Kretz et al. 2004; Mese et al. 2007). Furthermore, GJIC is critical in keratinocyte–melanocyte interaction (Hsu et al. 2000; Satyamoorthy et al. 2001). Alternatively, connexins can form hemichannels, which allow release (e.g., ATP, NAD^+) or putative uptake of molecules and ions to and from the cellular environment (Barr et al. 2013; Chandrasekhar and Bera 2012). Finally, connexins, especially Cx43, interact with structural and signaling molecules, which may add further functions to these molecules (Herve et al. 2007).

GJs form channels between adjacent cells allowing the intercellular transport of small metabolites, second messengers, and ions (Loewenstein 1981; Spray 1994). In addition to molecular weight and size, the ability of a solute to transverse these channels depends on its net charge, shape, and interactions with specific connexins that constitute gap junctions in particular cells (Goldberg et al. 2004). Each GJ channel consists of two hemichannels called connexons, each formed by six connexins (reviewed in Richard 2000). Twenty-one connexins have been identified, 11 of which are in the skin (Di et al. 2001; Willecke et al. 2002; Zucker et al. 2013). GJs can be homotypic, heterotypic, homomeric, and heteromeric (reviewed in Richard 2000). A connexon is homomeric if it is composed of six identical connexin subunits (e.g., Cx32 only), or heteromeric if it is composed of more than one connexin species (e.g., Cx32 and Cx43 and/or others). Channels are homotypic if both connexons are homomeric of the same type, heterotypic if homomeric connexons are of different types, and heteromeric if both connexons are heteromeric. Not all connexins are equally compatible at forming a connexon – even though they may co-exist in the same cell (reviewed in Haass et al. 2004). The type of connexin-forming GJ channels influences their selectivity and thereby controls the specificity of GJIC. For example, channels formed by Cx26 prefer cations, while those formed by Cx32 prefer anions (Brissette et al. 1994; Elfgang et al. 1995; Veenstra 1996). Thus, the up- or downregulation of a certain connexin in a tissue may change its GJIC considerably. In addition, connexins can also form hemichannels, which have been shown to be able to exchange molecules with the extracellular microenvironment. These hemichannels are relevant for signal propagation and especially for calcium homeostasis (reviewed in Evans et al. 2006).

9.5.1 Connexins Are Conditional Tumor Suppressors

Loss of gap junctional activity and/or downregulation of connexins have been reported both in cell lines as well as in tissues of many tumor types, such as hepatocellular carcinoma, gastric carcinoma, prostate cancer, lung cancer, glioma, mammary carcinoma, basal cell carcinoma, squamous cell carcinoma, and melanoma. This phenomenon was first observed half a century ago (Loewenstein and Kanno 1966) and summarized in a number of review articles (Cronier et al. 2009; Mesnil et al. 2005; Naus and Laird 2010). The type of connexins lost during tumor progression varies according to tumor type. In the 1980s and 1990s, a series of studies were published showing that reagents and/or oncogenes that promote tumor onset or progression frequently inhibit GJIC or downregulate connexin expression (Lampe 1994; Trosko et al. 1990; Atkinson et al. 1981). The role of connexins as potential tumor suppressors was also shown in gene knockdown studies (Shao et al. 2005). Correspondingly, ectopic expression of connexins in tumors restored functional communication and reduced tumor proliferation and growth both in vitro and in vivo (reviewed in Naus and Laird 2010). Importantly, ectopic expression of connexins partially differentiated transformed cells (Zhu et al. 1991; McLachlan et al. 2006; Hellmann et al. 1999; Hirschi et al. 1996). Moreover, functional abrogation of connexins, using antisense or dominant-negative mutant approaches, have demonstrated an enhancement of the malignant phenotype in several tumor types, such as Cx26 in HeLa cells (Duflot-Dancer et al. 1997), Cx32 in hepatocellular carcinoma (Dagli et al. 2004), Cx43 in lung cancer (Avanzo et al. 2004), Cx43 in glioma (Omori and Yamasaki 1998), and Cx43 in bladder carcinoma (Krutovskikh et al. 1998). Finally, Cx32 knock-out mice have an increased incidence of tumor onset when challenged with carcinogens (Temme et al. 1997; King and Lampe 2004a, b; Moennikes et al. 2000).

This may lead to the assumption that connexins are general tumor suppressors, but it appears that this is only the case in the earlier steps of cancerogenesis. In fact, the role of connexins in invasion and metastasis is very complex, and connexins might facilitate invasion, intravasation, extravasation, and metastasis (Krutovskikh et al. 1994; el-Sabban and Pauli 1991, 1994; Ito et al. 2000; Saunders et al. 2001; Lin et al. 2002; Miekus et al. 2005; Pollmann et al. 2005; Kanczuga-Koda et al. 2006; Bates et al. 2007; Li et al. 2007; Dobrowolski et al. 2008; Cotrina et al. 2008; Elzarrad et al. 2008; Ezumi et al. 2008). The following model supports both the tumor suppressor and the tumor driver theories (Cronier et al. 2009): for the step from primary to invasive tumors, there is a need for disruption of intercellular junctions including GJs, consistent with the model that connexins are tumor suppressors. In contrast, for the tumor cell dissemination and metastasis steps, increased cell contacts and communication are needed in order to enable interaction with the tumor stroma – especially between cancer cells and endothelial cells. Therefore, connexins might be better classified as conditional tumor suppressors that modulate cell proliferation as well as adhesion and migration (Naus and Laird 2010).

9.5.2 Cx43 in Cancer

Cx43 is decreased in prostate cancer (Tsai et al. 1996), mammary cancer (Hirschi et al. 1996), glioma (Huang et al. 1999), lung cancer (Jinn et al. 1998; Zhang et al. 1998), bladder carcinoma (Krutovskikh et al. 2000), cervical carcinoma (King et al. 2000), and various skin cancers including melanoma (Haass et al. 2006; Tada and Hashimoto 1997; Wilgenbus et al. 1992). Electron microscopy investigations have shown that basal and squamous cell carcinomas do not have fully developed GJs, and that Cx43 is not restricted to these poorly developed GJs but is present in the cytoplasm (Tada and Hashimoto 1997). In several cancers, Cx43 acts as a tumor suppressor gene with loss of Cx43 contributing to metastasis (Czyz 2008; Gershon et al. 2008; Shen et al. 2007). Functional abrogation of Cx43 enhances the malignant phenotype in lung cancer (Avanzo et al. 2004), glioma (Omori and Yamasaki 1998), and bladder carcinoma (Krutovskikh et al. 1998).

In contrast to other cancers, hepatocellular carcinoma is associated with an induction of Cx43, which is, however, localized in the cytoplasm, and thus is not involved in GJIC (Krutovskikh et al. 1994). The loss of GJIC might help the tumor cells to survive, as GJIC has been shown to spread cell-killing signals, most likely Ca^{2+} ions (Krutovskikh et al. 2002). In addition, downregulation of Cx43 expression or function resulted in increased proliferation and migration in primary keratinocytes, implying a contribution of Cx43 to controlling early stages of tumorigenesis (Mori et al. 2006; Wright et al. 2009; Pollok et al. 2011). Finally, increased opening of hemichannels formed by connexins resulted in cell death in cochlear supporting cells of the ear and in keratinocytes of the epidermis (Xu and Nicholson 2013).

Conversely, expression of Cx43 has also been shown to increase tumor metastasis in breast cancer, glioma as well as in melanoma through increased attachment and communication with the vascular endothelium (Bates et al. 2007; Kanczuga-Koda et al. 2006; Cotrina et al. 2008; Lin et al. 2002; el-Sabban and Pauli 1991, 1994; Pollmann et al. 2005; Elzarrad et al. 2008).

9.5.3 Cx32 in Cancer

Cx32 is downregulated in gastric carcinoma (Uchida et al. 1995), lung cancer (Jinn et al. 1998), and hepatocellular carcinoma (Eghbali et al. 1991; Loewenstein and Rose 1992; Krutovskikh et al. 1994; Yamaoka et al. 1995). In the latter case, the remaining Cx32 is localized in the cytoplasm or in the plasma membrane free from contact with other cells. In addition, it was found that there was no mutation in the coding sequence of Cx32 in hepatocellular carcinoma; instead, it appears that the aberrant localization of Cx32 is a consequence of the disruption of Cx32 gap junction plaque formation (Krutovskikh et al. 1994). Functional abrogation of Cx32 enhances the malignant phenotype in hepatocellular carcinoma (Dagli et al. 2004). Cx32 knock-out mice have an increased incidence of tumor onset when challenged with carcinogens (Temme et al. 1997; King and Lampe 2004a, b; Moennikes et al. 2000). In contrast to most other tumors, Cx32 is upregulated in some breast cancer cells (Saunders et al. 2001).

9.5.4 Cx26 in Cancer

Whereas in mammary carcinoma cells, there is a downregulation of both Cx43 and Cx26 (Hirschi et al. 1996); in human basal cell carcinoma, Cx43 is downregulated but there is an induction of Cx26 (Haass et al. 2006; Wilgenbus et al. 1992). Cx26 is also highly expressed in HeLa cells, where its functional abrogation enhances the malignant phenotype (Duflot-Dancer et al. 1997).

9.5.5 Connexins in Melanoma

Reflecting the situation in many other cancer types as discussed above, the role of connexins and GJIC is still highly controversial also in melanoma and its tumor microenvironment.

Cx43 is the most-studied connexin in melanoma. Western blotting revealed Cx43 protein expression in foreskin-derived melanocytes and several melanoma cell lines (Hsu et al. 2000). This was confirmed by immunofluorescence detecting Cx43 expression in human melanoma cell lines (Lin et al. 2010). While neither study quantified the Cx43 protein expression levels, a qRT-PCR and immunofluorescence study demonstrated lower Cx43 expression levels in human melanoma cell lines compared to human melanocytes (Schiffner et al. 2011). Also, a microarray study revealed that Cx43 was expressed at low levels in human melanoma cell lines and, importantly, that its overexpression suppressed anchorage-independent growth in colony-forming efficiency assays, suggesting a tumor-suppressor role of Cx43 in melanoma (Su et al. 2000). By qRT-PCR, no expression for Cx26, Cx30, Cx31.1, Cx36, and Cx37; low expression for Cx30.3 and Cx31; and higher expression levels for Cx32, Cx40, Cx43, and Cx45 were detected in human melanoma cell lines (Zucker et al. 2013). Surprisingly, Western blotting showed much higher Cx43 expression levels in migrating than in non-migrating cells (Zucker et al. 2013). Consistently, high levels of Cx43 protein expression were found in human metastatic melanoma cell lines (Villares et al. 2009). Loss of protease-activated receptor-1 (PAR-1) expression resulted in the loss of Cx43 and, correspondingly, overexpression of PAR-1 contributed to melanoma metastasis via upregulation of Cx43 (Villares et al. 2009, 2011). Interestingly, while initial levels of Cx43 were low in B16 mouse melanoma cells, Cx43 protein levels increased after infection with bacteria or treatment with interferon-γ (Saccheri et al. 2010). This was followed by the transfer of preprocessed antigenic peptides from melanoma cells to dendritic cells, which then presented those peptides on their surface and activated cytotoxic T cells against the tumor antigen. Correspondingly, melanoma cells in which Cx43 had been silenced, failed to elicit a cytotoxic antitumor response after infection with bacteria (Saccheri et al. 2010).

In addition to the discussed in vitro data, there are also a number of studies on human melanoma tissue. Using immunofluorescence on human tissue samples, we did not detect Cx43 (nor Cx26 and Cx30) in nevi, primary melanomas, or cutaneous melanoma metastases, while the internal controls (adjacent epidermis) were positive in the expected layers (Haass et al. 2006, 2010). In contrast, using immunohistochemistry, other groups reported Cx43 expression in human melanoma tissue, higher than in human nevi (Rezze et al. 2011; Sargen et al. 2013). However, neither of these studies provided high magnification images to confirm the subcellular localization nor did they show appropriate positive and negative controls. Indeed, in both studies, Cx43 expression in melanoma cells appeared to be cytoplasmic and hence would argue for a cell–cell or cell–matrix communication-independent role of these connexins. This would not support the mechanism for melanoma survival in brain metastasis proposed by Lin and colleagues, who showed that reactive astrocytes protect metastatic melanoma cells in the brain from chemotherapy by sequestering intracellular calcium through direct cell–cell communication (Lin et al. 2010). Moreover, in the Rezze and Sargen studies, the expression pattern of Cx43 in nevi and different melanoma stages appeared very variable and the typical Cx43 staining in the epidermis was missing (Rezze et al. 2011; Sargen et al. 2013). An Oncomine analysis of human tissue showed that increased Cx43 (and Cx26) gene expression in primary lesions correlated with metastasis and poor patient survival (Stoletov et al. 2013).

Cx26 and Cx30 are much less studied. Cx26 was found to be upregulated in the highly aggressive BL6 sub-line of B16 mouse melanoma cells compared to the less aggressive F10 sub-line (Ito et al. 2000). F10 cells transfected with wild-type Cx26 exhibited similar metastatic behavior to the BL6 cells. Correspondingly, BL6 cells transfected with a dominant-negative Cx26 mutant showed the less aggressive behavior characteristic of F10 cells. Cx26 was not found to be expressed in human melanoma in situ but was upregulated in invasive melanomas (Ito et al. 2000). However, in this study, Cx26 staining in both melanoma cells and epidermal keratinocytes was cytoplasmic. Moreover, the study did not distinguish between Cx26 and Cx30. In contrast, we showed in immunofluorescence studies on human melanoma tissue samples, that all areas of melanocytic nevi, primary melanomas, and cutaneous melanoma metastases lacked Cx26 and Cx30 expression (Haass et al. 2006, 2010) – similar to our findings in Merkel cell carcinoma (Haass et al. 2003a). This was confirmed by other groups who did not detect Cx26 in melanoma using immunohistochemistry on human tissue samples (Sargen et al. 2013) or did not find Cx26 and Cx30 expression in human melanoma cell lines using qRT-PCR (Zucker et al. 2013). Contrastingly, a positive correlation between Cx26 expression and metastatic potential was reported using Cx26 shRNA in B16 mouse melanoma cells (Stoletov et al. 2013). This was supported by an Oncomine analysis of human tissue, which showed that increased Cx26 expression in primary lesions correlated with metastasis and poor patient survival (Stoletov et al. 2013).

Interestingly, loss of Pannexin 1, a channel-forming glycoprotein remotely related to connexins, attenuated melanoma progression by reversion to a melanocyte-like phenotype (Penuela et al. 2013).

The Oncomine data (Stoletov et al. 2013) do not seem to match the data on primary melanomas in other studies; however, it would be interesting to re-analyze these data more in detail. As there appears to be a correlation to tumor thickness, is there no or little expression on thin tumors and a differential expression pattern in different areas of thick melanomas?

The discrepancies between the different studies in Cx43, Cx26, and Cx30 in melanoma may be due to the following reasons:

1. Several studies investigated the molecules on mRNA level only. The presence of mRNA does not necessarily mean that the respective protein is present.
2. In tissues, it is difficult to separate between connexins present in melanoma cells and those present in epidermal, mesenchymal, or endothelial tissues enclosed by the tumor.
3. Immunohistochemistry is often dependent on staining conditions and can result in false-positive and false-negative results. Appropriate positive and negative controls showing the sensitivity and specificity of the antibody are indispensable for the interpretation of these results. For example, the Cx26 antibody used in some of the discussed studies shows cross-reactivity with Cx30.

Importantly, most of the apparent discrepancies in this paragraph can be explained by a model, which implies that connexins are tumor suppressors during early melanomagenesis but tumor drivers during metastasis (Cronier et al. 2009). During early melanomagenesis, the respective connexins are typically located in the cell membranes indicating that they are functioning through GJIC. In contrast, in advanced stages, connexins are typically located in the cytoplasm indicating a different function – possibly through interaction with signaling molecules.

9.5.6 Connexins in the Epidermal Tumor Environment of Melanoma

Keratinocytes communicate with melanocytes but not with melanoma cells via GJIC; instead, melanoma cells communicate among themselves and with fibroblasts and endothelial cells (Hsu et al. 2000). This switch in communication partners coincides with the E- to N-cadherin switch, suggesting that the gain of N-cadherin with the concurrent loss of E-cadherin facilitates GJ formation with fibroblasts and endothelial cells (Hsu et al. 2000). Additionally, GJ formation in human melanoma cell lines appears to require MCAM (Satyamoorthy et al. 2001). This switch will allow melanoma cells to de-couple from the epidermal microenvironment and to communicate with cell types important for their metastatic spread. Several studies have suggested that connexins may promote metastasis in melanoma and other tumors by forming intercellular connections between cancer cells and vascular endothelium that are able to initiate tumor cell diapedesis (Hsu et al. 2000; Villares et al. 2009; el-Sabban and Pauli 1991, 1994; Saito-Katsuragi et al. 2007; Pollmann et al. 2005). Melanoma cells expressing higher levels of Cx43 show increased coupling to vascular endothelial cells (el-Sabban and Pauli 1991) and the ability of tumor cells to metastasize appears to correlate with the ability of tumor cells to communicate with endothelial cells (Pollmann et al. 2005). Also, Cx26 may contribute to the metastasis of melanoma by facilitating communication between melanoma cells and their surrounding endothelial cells (Saito-Katsuragi et al. 2007).

Cx26 expression is associated with lymphatic vessel invasion and poor prognosis in human breast cancer (Naoi et al. 2007).

Melanoma brain metastases are surrounded and infiltrated by astrocytes, and these astrocytes can play a role similar to their established ability to protect neurons from apoptosis (Lin et al. 2010). In co-culture experiments, astrocytes reduced apoptosis in human melanoma cells treated with various chemotherapeutic drugs. This chemoprotective effect was dependent on physical contact and GJIC between astrocytes, which express high levels of Cx43, and tumor cells. Moreover, the protective effect of astrocytes resulted from their sequestering calcium from the cytoplasm of tumor cells. These data suggest that brain metastases can harness the neuroprotective effects of reactive astrocytes for their own survival (Lin et al. 2010). In a chick embryo model, B16 mouse melanoma cells, which express Cx26 but not Cx43, colonized the chicken brain forming numerous microtumors invading along the preexisting vasculature (Stoletov et al. 2013). In contrast, Cx26 knockdown B16 cells formed significantly fewer and less invasive tumors, suggesting that in metastatic melanoma cells Cx26 expression enhances microtumor formation in the brain in association with the existing vasculature (Stoletov et al. 2013).

While these studies demonstrate the interaction of melanoma cells with the stroma and the role of connexins and/or GJIC in the early and late steps of melanomagenesis, interactions between melanoma and the epidermal tumor microenvironment (ETM) – the multilayered epithelium of the skin – are poorly understood. In this regard, we have demonstrated the induction of Cx26 and Cx30 in the epidermis adjacent to malignant tumors (e.g., melanoma and Merkel cell carcinoma), but not in the epidermis adjacent to benign tumors (e.g., melanocytic nevi and angiomas) (Haass et al. 2003a, 2006). Subsequently, we found correlation between (a) tumor thickness (Breslow index) and vertical Cx26 and Cx30 expression in the ETM, (b) tumor thickness and horizontal Cx26 dissemination in the ETM, (c) metastasis and horizontal Cx26 expression in the ETM, and (d) vertical epidermal expression patterns of Cx26 and Cx30 and the proliferative index in the ETM. We thus provided evidence for the association of ETM alteration with tumor malignancy and progression (Haass et al. 2010). The results of this study, which included dysplastic nevi as well as thin melanomas which are often difficult to distinguish (reviewed in Haass and Smalley 2009), suggest that membrane expression of Cx26 and Cx30 in the epidermal tumor microenvironment may be a useful diagnostic aid for the distinction of melanomas and melanocytic nevi (Haass et al. 2010). As neither Cx26 nor Cx30 are expressed in the melanoma itself, but both are induced in its tumor microenvironment, they may be useful complementary melanoma markers.

Cx26 and Cx30 upregulation in the epidermal tumor microenvironment did not correlate with the proliferative index of the melanoma cells, but correlated significantly with the proliferative index in the epidermis. In transgenic mice expressing Cx26 ectopically, proliferation was increased in the epidermis (Djalilian et al. 2006), suggesting that Cx26 influences keratinocyte proliferation and not vice versa. Interestingly, Cx26 overexpressing mice showed a delay in wound healing, which needs to be explored with regards to ulceration, a biomarker associated with very poor prognosis for melanoma patients (Balch et al. 2001). In our study, all melanomas with ulceration showed Cx26 (and Cx30) expression in all layers of the epidermal tumor microenvironment (Haass et al. 2010). Induction of angiogenesis by the hyperplastic epithelium could stimulate growth and progression of melanoma (McCarty et al. 2003). This suggests a positive feedback mechanism: tumor cells induce alterations in keratinocytes, which results in the production of growth factors which, in turn, stimulate tumor survival via endothelial cells. The induction of Cx26 and Cx30 in the epidermis adjacent to melanoma putatively leading to GJIC or signaling via hemichannels may play a role in this feedback mechanism by inducing proliferation and other functions. An interruption of this vicious circle may provide a novel therapeutic approach.

9.6 Tight Junctions

In simple epithelia and endothelia, tight junctions (TJs) are responsible for the formation and maintenance of the tissue barrier between distinct compartments by controlling the paracellular pathway ("barrier function") (reviewed in Stevenson and Keon 1998; Tsukita et al. 2001). Subsequently, the involvement of TJs in the barrier function of a complex epithelium, the epidermis, was shown (Pummi et al. 2001; Brandner et al. 2002, 2003; Furuse et al. 2002; Langbein et al. 2002). In addition, TJs prevent the diffusion of membrane proteins and lipids from the apical to the basolateral side of an epithelial cell sheet, helping to maintain cell polarity ("fence function") (reviewed in Mitic and Anderson 1998; Tsukita et al. 2001). Therefore, TJs are crucial for the epithelium to generate chemical and electrical gradients that is necessary for vectorial transport processes such as absorption and secretion (reviewed in Martin and Jiang 2009). Moreover, TJ molecules act as intermediates and transducers in cell signaling, thus playing a role in the processes of polarity, cell differentiation, cell growth, and differentiation. Finally, TJs act as cell–cell adhesion molecules and as a barrier to cell migration (reviewed in Martin and Jiang 2009).

TJs are composed of integral transmembrane proteins (claudin 1–24, occludin, and junctional adhesion molecules A-C, 4 (JAMs)), peripheral plaque proteins (zonula occludens (ZO) proteins 1–3, MAGI 1–3, MUPP-1, PAR-3, PAR-6, AF-6, CASK, and CAROM), and associated proteins (symplekin, ZONAB, cingulin, Rab-13, Rab-3B, c-src, α-catenin, PKA, ZAK, and Rho GTPases). The molecular composition of TJs is highly complex and varies according to the cell type and degree of differentiation. TJ molecules from neighboring cells associate and form paired strands which seal the paracellular pathway and which contain aqueous pores or paracellular channels, explaining the ion and size selectivity for passaging molecules of TJ (Tsukita and Furuse 2000).

In cancer, disruption of TJs should occur in three critical steps: (1) detachment of the tumor cell from the primary tumor, (2) intravasation of the tumor through the endothelium, and (3) extravastion of the circulating tumor cell (reviewed in Martin and Jiang 2009). Early studies have shown a correlation between lack of TJs and tumor differentiation and there is evidence that TJs need to be overcome by cancer cells in order to metastasize (reviewed in Martin and Jiang 2001, 2009). Cancer cells frequently exhibit deficiencies in TJ function, as well as decreased differentiation and cell polarity (Weinstein et al. 1976; Soler et al. 1999). Loss of TJ integrity may be particularly important in allowing the diffusion of nutrients and other factors necessary for the survival and growth of the tumor cells (Mullin et al. 1997). In addition, decreased polarity and differentiation may be important for the metastatic phenotype, where individual cells must leave the primary site and enter the blood vessels to reach distant sites (Ren et al. 1990).

Electron microscopy studies in human thyroid tumors showed that TJs decrease in number and are attenuated during carcinogenesis, which is associated with loss of tumor differentiation (Kerjaschki et al. 1979). Expression of TJ proteins is decreased in some cancer types, e.g., ZO-1 and occludin in gastrointestinal adenocarcinoma (Kimura et al. 1997), occludin in epithelial-derived tumors (Li and Mrsny 2000), claudin 3 in glioblastoma multiforme (Wolburg et al. 2003), claudin 1 in sporadic and hereditary breast cancer (Kramer et al. 2000), and claudin 7 in ductal carcinoma of the breast (Kominsky et al. 2003). On the other hand, some TJ molecules appear to be upregulated in some cancers. We found protein expression of claudins 3, 4, and 5, occludin, and ZO-1 in Merkel cell carcinoma cells (Haass et al. 2003b). Strikingly, expression of some claudin family members is highly elevated in various human cancers, e.g., claudin 7 in two breast cancer cell lines (Nacht et al. 1999), claudin 1 in colorectal cancer (Miwa et al. 2000), and claudins 3 and 4 in ovarian (Hough et al. 2001; Rangel et al. 2003) and prostate cancer (Long et al. 2001).

The expression of TJ proteins in melanoma tissues and cultured melanoma cells was described on RNA and on protein level (Cohn et al. 2005; Smalley et al. 2005; Leotlela et al. 2007; Schmitt et al. 2007; Morita et al. 2008). In a tissue array study, Claudin-1 was found to be significantly reduced in metastatic melanoma (Cohn et al. 2005). These data were, however, directly contradicted by another study (Leotlela et al. 2007). In this study Claudin-1 appeared to contribute to melanoma cell invasion, as transient transfection of melanoma cells with Claudin-1 increased metalloproteinase 2 (MMP-2) secretion and activation, and subsequently, motility of melanoma cells as demonstrated by wound-healing assays. Conversely, knockdown of CLDN1 by siRNA resulted in the inhibition of motility, as well as decreases in MMP-2 secretion and activation (Leotlela et al. 2007).

In contrast to most cancers, where levels of ZO-1 are typically downregulated, leading to increased motility, we found that ZO-1 expression is upregulated in melanoma cells and is located at adherens junctions between melanoma cells and fibroblasts (Smalley et al. 2005). Immunofluorescence and co-immunoprecipitation studies showed co-localization of ZO-1 with N-cadherin. Downregulation of ZO-1 in melanoma cells through RNA interference produced marked changes in cell morphology – leading to a less dendritic, more rounded phenotype. Consistent with a role in N-cadherin-based adhesion, RNAi-treated melanoma cells were less adherent and invasive when grown in a collagen gel. These data provided the first evidence that increased ZO-1 expression in melanoma contributes to the oncogenic behavior of this tumor and further illustrated that protein products of genes, such as

ZO-1, can function in either a pro- or anti-oncogenic manner when expressed in different cellular contexts (Smalley et al. 2005).

In summary, while it appears that functional TJs may be tumor suppressors, the upregulation of certain TJ proteins can contribute to oncogenic behavior. The relationship between TJ protein overexpression and cancer initiation or progression is thus unclear at present, but may be explained by the lack of functional TJs and that the upregulated TJ proteins therefore likely function through TJ-independent mechanisms.

Acknowledgment NKH is a Cameron Fellow of the Melanoma and Skin Cancer Research Institute, Australia, and a Sydney Medical School Foundation Fellow. NKH also thanks the German Research Foundation (DFG, HA26801), Cancer Council NSW (RG 09–08, RG 13–06), Cancer Australia/Cure Cancer Australia Foundation (570778), Cancer Institute New South Wales (08/RFG/1-27), and the National Health and Medical Research Council Australia (1003637, 1084893) for contributing grant support.

References

Aeed PA, Nakajima M, Welch DR (1988) The role of polymorphonuclear leukocytes (PMN) on the growth and metastatic potential of 13762NF mammary adenocarcinoma cells. Int J Cancer 42(5):748–759

Albelda SM, Mette SA, Elder DE, Stewart R, Damjanovich L, Herlyn M, Buck CA (1990) Integrin distribution in malignant melanoma: association of the beta 3 subunit with tumor progression. Cancer Res 50:6757–6764

Alexaki VI, Javelaud D, Van Kempen LC, Mohammad KS, Dennler S, Luciani F, Hoek KS, Juarez P, Goydos JS, Fournier PJ, Sibon C, Bertolotto C, Verrecchia F, Saule S, Delmas V, Ballotti R, Larue L, Saiag P, Guise TA, Mauviel A (2010) GLI2-mediated melanoma invasion and metastasis. J Natl Cancer Inst 102:1148–1159

Atkinson MM, Menko AS, Johnson RG, Sheppard JR, Sheridan JD (1981) Rapid and reversible reduction of junctional permeability in cells infected with a temperature-sensitive mutant of avian sarcoma virus. J Cell Biol 91(2 Pt 1):573–578

Avanzo JL, Mesnil M, Hernandez-Blazquez FJ, Mackowiak II, Mori CM, da Silva TC, Oloris SC, Garate AP, Massironi SM, Yamasaki H, Dagli ML (2004) Increased susceptibility to urethane-induced lung tumors in mice with decreased expression of connexin43. Carcinogenesis 25(10):1973–1982. doi:10.1093/carcin/bgh193bgh193 [pii]

Bachmann IM, Straume O, Puntervoll HE, Kalvenes MB, Akslen LA (2005) Importance of P-cadherin, beta-catenin, and Wnt5a/frizzled for progression of melanocytic tumors and prognosis in cutaneous melanoma. Clin Cancer Res 11:8606–8614

Balch CM, Soong SJ, Gershenwald JE, Thompson JF, Reintgen DS, Cascinelli N, Urist M, McMasters KM, Ross MI, Kirkwood JM, Atkins MB, Thompson JA, Coit DG, Byrd D, Desmond R, Zhang Y, Liu PY, Lyman GH, Morabito A (2001) Prognostic factors analysis of 17,600 melanoma patients: validation of the American Joint Committee on Cancer melanoma staging system. J Clin Oncol 19(16):3622–3634

Barr TP, Albrecht PJ, Hou Q, Mongin AA, Strichartz GR, Rice FL (2013) Air-stimulated ATP release from keratinocytes occurs through connexin hemichannels. PLoS One 8(2):e56744. doi:10.1371/journal.pone.0056744

Bates DC, Sin WC, Aftab Q, Naus CC (2007) Connexin43 enhances glioma invasion by a mechanism involving the carboxy terminus. Glia 55(15):1554–1564. doi:10.1002/glia.20569

Batlle E, Sancho E, Francí C, Domínguez D, Monfar M, Baulida J, García De Herreros A (2000) The transcription factor snail is a repressor of E-cadherin gene expression in epithelial tumour cells. Nat Cell Biol 2(2):84–89

Bauer R, Bosserhoff AK (2006) Functional implication of truncated P-cadherin expression in malignant melanoma. Exp Mol Pathol 81:224–230
Bauer R, Hein R, Bosserhoff AK (2005) A secreted form of P-cadherin is expressed in malignant melanoma. Exp Cell Res 305:418–426
Bauer R, Wild PJ, Meyer S, Bataille F, Pauer A, Klinkhammer-Schalke M, Hofstaedter F, Bosserhoff AK (2006) Prognostic relevance of P-cadherin expression in melanocytic skin tumours analysed by high-throughput tissue microarrays. J Clin Pathol 59:699–705
Becker JC, Termeer C, Schmidt RE, Brocker EB (1993) Soluble intercellular adhesion molecule-1 inhibits MHC-restricted specific T cell/tumor interaction. J Immunol 151(12):7224–7232
Berrier AL, Yamada KM (2007) Cell-matrix adhesion. J Cell Physiol 213:565–573
Bissell MJ, Radisky D (2001) Putting tumours in context. Nat Rev Cancer 1(1):46–54
Billion K, Ibrahim H, Mauch C, Niessen CM (2006) Increased soluble E-cadherin in melanoma patients. Skin Pharmacol Physiol 19:65–70
Bolós V, Peinado H, Pérez-Moreno MA, Fraga MF, Esteller M, Cano A (2003) The transcription factor Slug represses E-cadherin expression and induces epithelial to mesenchymal transitions: a comparison with Snail and E47 repressors. J Cell Sci 116(Pt 3):499–511
Boveri T (1914) Zur frage der entstehung maligner tumoren. Gustav Fischer Verlag, Jena
Brandner JM, Haass NK (2013) Melanoma's connections to the tumour microenvironment. Pathology 45(5):443–452. doi:10.1097/PAT.0b013e328363b3bd
Brandner JM, Kief S, Grund C, Rendl M, Houdek P, Kuhn C, Tschachler E, Franke WW, Moll I (2002) Organization and formation of the tight junction system in human epidermis and cultured keratinocytes. Eur J Cell Biol 81(5):253–263
Brandner JM, McIntyre M, Kief S, Wladykowski E, Moll I (2003) Expression and localization of tight junction-associated proteins in human hair follicles. Arch Dermatol Res 295(5):211–221
Braga V (2000) Epithelial cell shape: cadherins and small GTPases. Exp Cell Res 261:83–90
Braga VM, Machesky LM, Hall A, Hotchin NA (1997) The small GTPases Rho and Rac are required for the establishment of cadherin-dependent cell-cell contacts. J Cell Biol 137:1421–1431
Brissette JL, Kumar NM, Gilula NB, Hall JE, Dotto GP (1994) Switch in gap junction protein expression is associated with selective changes in junctional permeability during keratinocyte differentiation. Proc Natl Acad Sci U S A 91(14):6453–6457
Brummer J, Ebrahimnejad A, Flayeh R, Schumacher U, Loning T, Bamberger AM, Wagener C (2001) cis Interaction of the cell adhesion molecule CEACAM1 with integrin beta(3). Am J Pathol 159(2):537–546
Caramel J, Papadogeorgakis E, Hill L, Browne GJ, Richard G, Wierinckx A, Saldanha G, Osborne J, Hutchinson P, Tse G, Lachuer J, Puisieux A, Pringle JH, Ansieau S, Tulchinsky E (2013) A switch in the expression of embryonic EMT-inducers drives the development of malignant melanoma. Cancer Cell 24:466–480
Chandrasekhar A, Bera AK (2012) Hemichannels: permeants and their effect on development, physiology and death. Cell Biochem Funct 30(2):89–100. doi:10.1002/cbf.2794
Chakraborty C, Gleeson LM, McKinnon T, Lala PK (2002) Regulation of human trophoblast migration and invasiveness. Can J Physiol Pharmacol 80:116–124
Cohn ML, Goncharuk VN, Diwan AH, Zhang PS, Shen SS, Prieto VG (2005) Loss of claudin-1 expression in tumor-associated vessels correlates with acquisition of metastatic phenotype in melanocytic neoplasms. J Cutan Pathol 32(8):533–536, CUP324 [pii] 10.1111/j.0303-6987.2005.00324.x
Comijn J, Berx G, Vermassen P, Verschueren K, van Grunsven L, Bruyneel E, Mareel M, Huylebroeck D, van Roy F (2001) The two-handed E box binding zinc fingerprotein SIP1 downregulates E-cadherin and induces invasion. Mol Cell 7(6):1267–1278
Cotrina ML, Lin JH, Nedergaard M (2008) Adhesive properties of connexin hemichannels. Glia 56(16):1791–1798. doi:10.1002/glia.20728
Cronier L, Crespin S, Strale PO, Defamie N, Mesnil M (2009) Gap junctions and cancer: new functions for an old story. Antioxid Redox Signal 11(2):323–338. doi:10.1089/ars.2008.2153
Czyz J (2008) The stage-specific function of gap junctions during tumourigenesis. Cell Mol Biol Lett 13(1):92–102. doi:10.2478/s11658-007-0039-5

Dai DL, Makretsov N, Campos EI, Huang C, Zhou Y, Huntsman D, Martinka M, Li G (2003) Increased expression of integrin-linked kinase is correlated with melanoma progression and poor patient survival. Clin Cancer Res 9:4409–4414
Danen EH, Sonnenberg A (2003) Integrins in regulation of tissue development and function. J Pathol 201:632–641
Danen EH, Jansen KF, Van Kraats AA, Cornelissen IM, Ruiter DJ, van Muijen GN (1995) Alpha v-integrins in human melanoma: gain of alpha v beta 3 and loss of alpha v beta 5 are related to tumor progression in situ but not to metastatic capacity of cell lines in nude mice. Int J Cancer 61:491–496
Danen EH, de Vries TJ, Morandini R, Ghanem GG, Ruiter DJ, van Muijen GN (1996) E-cadherin expression in human melanoma. Melanoma Res 6:127–131
Dagli ML, Yamasaki H, Krutovskikh V, Omori Y (2004) Delayed liver regeneration and increased susceptibility to chemical hepatocarcinogenesis in transgenic mice expressing a dominant-negative mutant of connexin32 only in the liver. Carcinogenesis 25(4):483–492. doi:10.1093/carcin/bgh050bgh050 [pii]
Delcommenne M, Tan C, Gray V, Rue L, Woodgett J, Dedhar S (1998) Phosphoinositide-3-OH kinase-dependent regulation of glycogen synthase kinase 3 and protein kinase B/AKT by the integrin-linked kinase. Proc Natl Acad Sci U S A 95:11211–11216
Degen WG, van Kempen LC, Gijzen EG, van Groningen JJ, van Kooyk Y, Bloemers HP, Swart GW (1998) MEMD, a new cell adhesion molecule in metastasizing human melanoma cell lines, is identical to ALCAM (activated leukocyte cell adhesion molecule). Am J Pathol 152(3):805–813
Di WL, Rugg EL, Leigh IM, Kelsell DP (2001) Multiple epidermal connexins are expressed in different keratinocyte subpopulations including connexin 31. J Invest Dermatol 117(4):958–964
Djalilian AR, McGaughey D, Patel S, Seo EY, Yang C, Cheng J, Tomic M, Sinha S, Ishida-Yamamoto A, Segre JA (2006) Connexin 26 regulates epidermal barrier and wound remodeling and promotes psoriasiform response. J Clin Invest 116(5):1243–1253
Dobrowolski R, Sasse P, Schrickel JW, Watkins M, Kim JS, Rackauskas M, Troatz C, Ghanem A, Tiemann K, Degen J, Bukauskas FF, Civitelli R, Lewalter T, Fleischmann BK, Willecke K (2008) The conditional connexin43G138R mouse mutant represents a new model of hereditary oculodentodigital dysplasia in humans. Hum Mol Genet 17(4):539–554. doi:10.1093/hmg/ddm329
Donizy P, Zietek M, Halon A, Leskiewicz M, Kozyra C, Matkowski R (2015) Prognostic significance of ALCAM (CD166/MEMD) expression in cutaneous melanoma patients. Diagn Pathol 10:86. doi:10.1186/s13000-015-0331-z
Duflot-Dancer A, Mesnil M, Yamasaki H (1997) Dominant-negative abrogation of connexin-mediated cell growth control by mutant connexin genes. Oncogene 15(18):2151–2158. doi:10.1038/sj.onc.1201393
Ebrahimnejad A, Streichert T, Nollau P, Horst AK, Wagener C, Bamberger AM, Brummer J (2004) CEACAM1 enhances invasion and migration of melanocytic and melanoma cells. Am J Pathol 165(5):1781–1787
Eger A, Aigner K, Sonderegger S, Dampier B, Oehler S, Schreiber M, Berx G, Cano A, Beug H, Foisner R (2005) DeltaEF1 is a transcriptional repressor of E-cadherin and regulates epithelial plasticity in breast cancer cells. Oncogene 24(14):2375–2385
Eghbali B, Kessler JA, Reid LM, Roy C, Spray DC (1991) Involvement of gap junctions in tumorigenesis: transfection of tumor cells with connexin 32 cDNA retards growth in vivo. Proc Natl Acad Sci U S A 88(23):10701–10705
el-Sabban ME, Pauli BU (1991) Cytoplasmic dye transfer between metastatic tumor cells and vascular endothelium. J Cell Biol 115(5):1375–1382
el-Sabban ME, Pauli BU (1994) Adhesion-mediated gap junctional communication between lung-metastatatic cancer cells and endothelium. Invasion Metastasis 14(1–6):164–176
Elfgang C, Eckert R, Lichtenberg-Frate H, Butterweck A, Traub O, Klein RA, Hulser DF, Willecke K (1995) Specific permeability and selective formation of gap junction channels in connexin-transfected HeLa cells. J Cell Biol 129(3):805–817

Elzarrad MK, Haroon A, Willecke K, Dobrowolski R, Gillespie MN, Al-Mehdi AB (2008) Connexin-43 upregulation in micrometastases and tumor vasculature and its role in tumor cell attachment to pulmonary endothelium. BMC Med 6:20. doi:10.1186/1741-7015-6-20, 1741-7015-6-20 [pii]

Evans WH, De Vuyst E, Leybaert L (2006) The gap junction cellular internet: connexin hemichannels enter the signalling limelight. Biochem J 397(1):1–14

Ezumi K, Yamamoto H, Murata K, Higashiyama M, Damdinsuren B, Nakamura Y, Kyo N, Okami J, Ngan CY, Takemasa I, Ikeda M, Sekimoto M, Matsuura N, Nojima H, Monden M (2008) Aberrant expression of connexin 26 is associated with lung metastasis of colorectal cancer. Clin Cancer Res 14(3):677–684. doi:10.1158/1078-0432.CCR-07-1184

Felding-Habermann B, Fransvea E, O'Toole TE, Manzuk L, Faha B, Hensler M (2002) Involvement of tumor cell integrin alpha v beta 3 in hematogenous metastasis of human melanoma cells. Clin Exp Metastasis 19:427–436

Fidler IJ (2003) The pathogenesis of cancer metastasis: the 'seed and soil' hypothesis revisited. Nat Rev Cancer 3(6):453–458. doi:10.1038/nrc1098

Fitzpatrick TB, Breathnach AS (1963) The epidermal melanin unit system. Dermatol Wochenschr 147:481–489

Fitzpatrick TB, Szabo G, Seiji M, Quevedo WC Jr (1979) Biology of the melanin pigmentary system. In: Fitzpatrick TB, Eisen A, Wolff K, Freedberg I, Austen K (eds) Dermatology in general medicine. McGraw-Hill, New York, pp 131–145

Flanagan K, Fitzgerald K, Baker J, Regnstrom K, Gardai S, Bard F, Mocci S, Seto P, You M, Larochelle C, Prat A, Chow S, Li L, Vandevert C, Zago W, Lorenzana C, Nishioka C, Hoffman J, Botelho R, Willits C, Tanaka K, Johnston J, Yednock T (2012) Laminin-411 is a vascular ligand for MCAM and facilitates TH17 cell entry into the CNS. PLoS One 7(7):e40443. doi:10.1371/journal.pone.0040443

Fogel M, Mechtersheimer S, Huszar M, Smirnov A, Abu-Dahi A, Tilgen W, Reichrath J, Georg T, Altevogt P, Gutwein P (2003) L1 adhesion molecule (CD 171) in development and progression of human malignant melanoma. Cancer Lett 189(2):237–247

Franke WW (2009) Discovering the molecular components of intercellular junctions – a historical view. Cold Spring Harb Perspect Biol 1:a003061

Friedl P, Zanker KS, Brocker EB (1998) Cell migration strategies in 3-D extracellular matrix: differences in morphology, cell matrix interactions, and integrin function. Microsc Res Tech 43:369–378

Friedmann MC, Migone TS, Russell SM, Leonard WJ (1996) Different interleukin 2 receptor beta-chain tyrosines couple to at least two signaling pathways and synergistically mediate interleukin 2-induced proliferation. Proc Natl Acad Sci U S A 93:2077–2082

Furuse M, Hata M, Furuse K, Yoshida Y, Haratake A, Sugitani Y, Noda T, Kubo A, Tsukita S (2002) Claudin-based tight junctions are crucial for the mammalian epidermal barrier: a lesson from claudin-1-deficient mice. J Cell Biol 156(6):1099–1111

Furukawa F, Fujii K, Horiguchi Y, Matsuyoshi N, Fujita M, Toda K, Imamura S, Wakita H, Shirahama S, Takigawa M (1997) Roles of E- and P-cadherin in the human skin. Microsc Res Tech 38:343–352

Gershon E, Plaks V, Dekel N (2008) Gap junctions in the ovary: expression, localization and function. Mol Cell Endocrinol 282(1–2):18–25. doi:10.1016/j.mce.2007.11.001, S0303-7207(07)00411-X [pii]

Giavazzi R, Chirivi RG, Garofalo A, Rambaldi A, Hemingway I, Pigott R, Gearing AJ (1992) Soluble intercellular adhesion molecule 1 is released by human melanoma cells and is associated with tumor growth in nude mice. Cancer Res 52(9):2628–2630

Goldberg GS, Valiunas V, Brink PR (2004) Selective permeability of gap junction channels. Biochim Biophys Acta 1662(1–2):96–101. doi:10.1016/j.bbamem.2003.11.022

Gottardi CJ, Wong E, Gumbiner BM (2001) E-cadherin suppresses cellular transformation by inhibiting beta-catenin signaling in an adhesion-independent manner. J Cell Biol 153:1049–1060

Gotoh N, Toyoda M, Shibuya M (1997) Tyrosine phosphorylation sites at amino acids 239 and 240 of Shc are involved in epidermal growth factor-induced mitogenic signaling that is distinct from Ras/mitogen-activated protein kinase activation. Mol Cell Biol 17:1824–1831

Graff JR, Greenberg VE, Herman JG, Westra WH, Boghaert ER, Ain KB, Saji M, Zeiger MA, Zimmer SG, Baylin SB (1998) Distinct patterns of E-cadherin CpG island methylation in papillary, follicular, Hurthle's cell, and poorly differentiated human thyroid carcinoma. Cancer Res 58:2063–2066

Gregory PA, Bert AG, Paterson EL, Barry SC, Tsykin A, Farshid G, Vadas MA, Khew-Goodall Y, Goodall GJ (2008) The miR-200 family and miR-205 regulate epithelial to mesenchymal transition by targeting ZEB1 and SIP1. Nat Cell Biol 10:593–601

Groebe K, Mueller-Klieser W (1991) Distributions of oxygen, nutrient, and metabolic waste concentrations in multicellular spheroids and their dependence on spheroid parameters. Eur Biophys J 19(4):169–181

Haass NK (2015) Dynamic tumor heterogeneity in melanoma therapy: how do we address this in a novel model system? Melanoma Manag 2(2):93–95

Haass NK, Beaumont KA, Hill DS, Anfosso A, Mrass P, Munoz MA, Kinjyo I, Weninger W (2014) Real-time cell cycle imaging during melanoma growth, invasion, and drug response. Pigment Cell Melanoma Res 27(5):764–776. doi:10.1111/pcmr.12274

Haass NK, Herlyn M (2005) Normal human melanocyte homeostasis as a paradigm for understanding melanoma. J Investig Dermatol Symp Proc 10(2):153–163

Haass NK, Houdek P, Brandner JM, Moll I (2003a) Expression patterns of connexins in Merkel cell carcinoma and adjacent epidermis. In: Baumann KI, Moll I, Halata Z (eds) The Merkel cell – structure – development – function – and cancerogenesis. Springer, Berlin/Heidelberg/New York/Tokyo, pp 219–222

Haass NK, Houdek P, Wladykowski E, Moll I, Brandner JM (2003b) Expression patterns of tight junction proteins in Merkel cell carcinoma. In: Baumann KI, Moll I, Halata Z (eds) The Merkel cell – structure – development – function – and cancerogenesis. Springer, Berlin/Heidelberg/New York/Tokyo, pp 223–226

Haass NK, Ripperger D, Wladykowski E, Dawson P, Gimotty PA, Blome C, Fischer F, Schmage P, Moll I, Brandner JM (2010) Melanoma progression exhibits a significant impact on connexin expression patterns in the epidermal tumor microenvironment. Histochem Cell Biol 133(1):113–124. doi:10.1007/s00418-009-0654-5

Haass NK, Smalley KS (2009) Melanoma biomarkers: current status and utility in diagnosis, prognosis, and response to therapy. Mol Diagn Ther 13(5):283–296. doi:10.2165/11317270-000000000-00000, 2 [pii]

Haass NK, Smalley KS, Herlyn M (2004) The role of altered cell-cell communication in melanoma progression. J Mol Histol 35(3):309–318

Haass NK, Smalley KS, Li L, Herlyn M (2005) Adhesion, migration and communication in melanocytes and melanoma. Pigment Cell Res 18(3):150–159

Haass NK, Wladykowski E, Kief S, Moll I, Brandner JM (2006) Differential induction of connexins 26 and 30 in skin tumors and their adjacent epidermis. J Histochem Cytochem 54(2):171–182

Hanahan D, Weinberg RA (2000) The hallmarks of cancer. Cell 100(1):57–70

Hanahan D, Weinberg RA (2011) Hallmarks of cancer: the next generation. Cell 144(5):646–674

Hamamura K, Tsuji M, Ohkawa Y, Nakashima H, Miyazaki S, Urano T, Yamamoto N, Ueda M, Furukawa K, Furukawa K (2008) Focal adhesion kinase as well as p130Cas and paxillin is crucially involved in the enhanced malignant properties under expression of ganglioside GD3 in melanoma cells. Biochim Biophys Acta 1780:513–519

Hajra KM, Chen DY, Fearon ER (2002) The SLUG zinc-finger protein represses E-cadherin in breast cancer. Cancer Res 62(6):1613–1618

Hendrix MJ, Seftor EA, Meltzer PS, Gardner LM, Hess AR, Kirschmann DA, Schatteman GC, Seftor RE (2001) Expression and functional significance of VE-cadherin in aggressive human melanoma cells: role in vasculogenic mimicry. Proc Natl Acad Sci U S A 98:8018–8023

Hendrix MJ, Seftor EA, Hess AR, Seftor RE (2003) Molecular plasticity of human melanoma cells. Oncogene 22:3070–3075

Hellmann P, Grummer R, Schirrmacher K, Rook M, Traub O, Winterhager E (1999) Transfection with different connexin genes alters growth and differentiation of human choriocarcinoma cells. Exp Cell Res 246(2):480–490. doi:10.1006/excr.1998.4332, S0014-4827(98)94332-4 [pii]

Herve JC, Bourmeyster N, Sarrouilhe D, Duffy HS (2007) Gap junctional complexes: from partners to functions. Prog Biophys Mol Biol 94(1–2):29–65. doi:10.1016/j.pbiomolbio.2007.03.010
Hirschi KK, Xu CE, Tsukamoto T, Sager R (1996) Gap junction genes Cx26 and Cx43 individually suppress the cancer phenotype of human mammary carcinoma cells and restore differentiation potential. Cell Growth Differ 7(7):861–870
Hong H, Stastny M, Brown C, Chang WC, Ostberg JR, Forman SJ, Jensen MC (2014) Diverse solid tumors expressing a restricted epitope of L1-CAM can be targeted by chimeric antigen receptor redirected T lymphocytes. J Immunother 37(2):93–104. doi:10.1097/CJI.0000000000000018
Hortsch M (1996) The L1 family of neural cell adhesion molecules: old proteins performing new tricks. Neuron 17(4):587–593
Hough CD, Cho KR, Zonderman AB, Schwartz DR, Morin PJ (2001) Coordinately up-regulated genes in ovarian cancer. Cancer Res 61(10):3869–3876
Howe AK, Aplin AE, Juliano RL (2002) Anchorage-dependent ERK signaling – mechanisms and consequences. Curr Opin Genet Dev 12:30–35
Hsu MY, Wheelock MJ, Johnson KR, Herlyn M (1996) Shifts in cadherin profiles between human normal melanocytes and melanomas. J Investig Dermatol Symp Proc 1:188–194
Hsu M, Andl T, Li G, Meinkoth JL, Herlyn M (2000) Cadherin repertoire determines partner-specific gap junctional communication during melanoma progression. J Cell Sci 113(Pt 9):1535–1542
Huang RP, Hossain MZ, Sehgal A, Boynton AL (1999) Reduced connexin43 expression in high-grade human brain glioma cells. J Surg Oncol 70(1):21–24. doi:10.1002/(SICI)1096-9098(199901)70:1<21::AID-JSO4>3.0.CO;2–0, [pii]#
Hurteau GJ, Carlson JA, Spivack SD, Brock GJ (2007) Overexpression of the microRNA hsa-miR-200c leads to reduced expression of transcription factor 8 and increased expression of E-cadherin. Cancer Res 67:7972–7976
Ito A, Katoh F, Kataoka TR, Okada M, Tsubota N, Asada H, Yoshikawa K, Maeda S, Kitamura Y, Yamasaki H, Nojima H (2000) A role for heterologous gap junctions between melanoma and endothelial cells in metastasis. J Clin Invest 105(9):1189–1197
Jacobs K, Feys L, Vanhoecke B, Van Marck V, Bracke M (2011) P-cadherin expression reduces melanoma growth, invasion, and responsiveness to growth factors in nude mice. Eur J Cancer Prev 20(3):207–216
Jimbow K, Quevedo WC Jr, Fitzpatrick TB, Szabo G (1976) Some aspects of melanin biology: 1950–1975. J Invest Dermatol 67(1):72–89
Jinn Y, Ichioka M, Marumo F (1998) Expression of connexin32 and connexin43 gap junction proteins and E-cadherin in human lung cancer. Cancer Lett 127(1–2):161–169
Johnson JP, Bar-Eli M, Jansen B, Markhof E (1997) Melanoma progression-associated glycoprotein MUC18/MCAM mediates homotypic cell adhesion through interaction with a heterophilic ligand. Int J Cancer 73(5):769–774
Johnson JP, Rummel MM, Rothbacher U, Sers C (1996) MUC18: a cell adhesion molecule with a potential role in tumor growth and tumor cell dissemination. Curr Top Microbiol Immunol 213(Pt 1):95–105
Johnson JP, Stade BG, Holzmann B, Schwable W, Riethmuller G (1989) De novo expression of intercellular-adhesion molecule 1 in melanoma correlates with increased risk of metastasis. Proc Natl Acad Sci U S A 86(2):641–644
Joshi MB, Ivanov D, Philippova M, Kyriakakis E, Erne P, Resink TJ (2008) A requirement for thioredoxin in redox-sensitive modulation of T-cadherin expression in endothelial cells. Biochem J 416:271–280
Jost M, Huggett TM, Kari C, Boise LH, Rodeck U (2001) Epidermal growth factor receptor-dependent control of keratinocyte survival and Bcl-xL expression through a MEK-dependent pathway. J Biol Chem 276:6320–6326
Jouve N, Despoix N, Espeli M, Gauthier L, Cypowyj S, Fallague K, Schiff C, Dignat-George F, Vely F, Leroyer AS (2013) The involvement of CD146 and its novel ligand Galectin-1 in apoptotic regulation of endothelial cells. J Biol Chem 288(4):2571–2579. doi:10.1074/jbc.M112.418848

Kanai Y, Ushijima S, Hui AM, Ochiai A, Tsuda H, Sakamoto M, Hirohashi S (1997) The E-cadherin gene is silenced by CpG methylation in human hepatocellular carcinomas. Int J Cancer 71:355–359

Kanczuga-Koda L, Sulkowski S, Lenczewski A, Koda M, Wincewicz A, Baltaziak M, Sulkowska M (2006) Increased expression of connexins 26 and 43 in lymph node metastases of breast cancer. J Clin Pathol 59(4):429–433. doi:10.1136/jcp.2005.029272, 59/4/429 [pii]

Kahana O, Micksche M, Witz IP, Yron I (2002) The focal adhesion kinase (P125FAK) is constitutively active in human malignant melanoma. Oncogene 21:3969–3977

Kerjaschki D, Krisch K, Sleyter UB, Umrath W, Jakesz R, Depisch D, Kokoschka R, Horandner H (1979) The structure of tight junctions in human thyroid tumors. A systematic freeze-fracture study. Am J Pathol 96(1):207–225

Khanna P, Yunkunis T, Muddana HS, Peng HH, August A, Dong C (2010) p38 MAP kinase is necessary for melanoma-mediated regulation of VE-cadherin disassembly. Am J Physiol Cell Physiol 298:C1140–C1150

Kimura Y, Shiozaki H, Hirao M, Maeno Y, Doki Y, Inoue M, Monden T, Ando-Akatsuka Y, Furuse M, Tsukita S, Monden M (1997) Expression of occludin, tight-junction-associated protein, in human digestive tract. Am J Pathol 151(1):45–54

King TJ, Fukushima LH, Hieber AD, Shimabukuro KA, Sakr WA, Bertram JS (2000) Reduced levels of connexin43 in cervical dysplasia: inducible expression in a cervical carcinoma cell line decreases neoplastic potential with implications for tumor progression. Carcinogenesis 21(6):1097–1109

King TJ, Lampe PD (2004a) The gap junction protein connexin32 is a mouse lung tumor suppressor. Cancer Res 64(20):7191–7196. doi:10.1158/0008-5472.CAN-04-0624, 64/20/7191 [pii]

King TJ, Lampe PD (2004b) Mice deficient for the gap junction protein Connexin32 exhibit increased radiation-induced tumorigenesis associated with elevated mitogen-activated protein kinase (p44/Erk1, p42/Erk2) activation. Carcinogenesis 25(5):669–680. doi:10.1093/carcin/bgh071bgh071 [pii]

Klein WM, Wu BP, Zhao S, Wu H, Klein-Szanto AJ, Tahan SR (2007) Increased expression of stem cell markers in malignant melanoma. Mod Pathol 20(1):102–107

Kluger HM, Hoyt K, Bacchiocchi A, Mayer T, Kirsch J, Kluger Y, Sznol M, Ariyan S, Molinaro A, Halaban R (2011) Plasma markers for identifying patients with metastatic melanoma. Clin Cancer Res 17(8):2417–2425. doi:10.1158/1078-0432.CCR-10-2402

Kominsky SL, Argani P, Korz D, Evron E, Raman V, Garrett E, Rein A, Sauter G, Kallioniemi OP, Sukumar S (2003) Loss of the tight junction protein claudin-7 correlates with histological grade in both ductal carcinoma in situ and invasive ductal carcinoma of the breast. Oncogene 22(13):2021–2033

Kramer F, White K, Kubbies M, Swisshelm K, Weber BH (2000) Genomic organization of claudin-1 and its assessment in hereditary and sporadic breast cancer. Hum Genet 107(3):249–256

Kraus A, Masat L, Johnson JP (1997) Analysis of the expression of intercellular adhesion molecule-1 and MUC18 on benign and malignant melanocytic lesions using monoclonal antibodies directed against distinct epitopes and recognizing denatured, non-glycosylated antigen. Melanoma Res 7(Suppl 2):S75–S81

Kretz M, Maass K, Willecke K (2004) Expression and function of connexins in the epidermis, analyzed with transgenic mouse mutants. Eur J Cell Biol 83(11–12):647–654

Krutovskikh V, Mazzoleni G, Mironov N, Omori Y, Aguelon AM, Mesnil M, Berger F, Partensky C, Yamasaki H (1994) Altered homologous and heterologous gap-junctional intercellular communication in primary human liver tumors associated with aberrant protein localization but not gene mutation of connexin 32. Int J Cancer 56(1):87–94

Krutovskikh VA, Piccoli C, Yamasaki H (2002) Gap junction intercellular communication propagates cell death in cancerous cells. Oncogene 21(13):1989–1999. doi:10.1038/sj.onc.1205187

Krutovskikh VA, Troyanovsky SM, Piccoli C, Tsuda H, Asamoto M, Yamasaki H (2000) Differential effect of subcellular localization of communication impairing gap junction protein connexin43 on tumor cell growth in vivo. Oncogene 19(4):505–513. doi:10.1038/sj.onc.1203340

Krutovskikh VA, Yamasaki H, Tsuda H, Asamoto M (1998) Inhibition of intrinsic gap-junction intercellular communication and enhancement of tumorigenicity of the rat bladder carcinoma cell line BC31 by a dominant-negative connexin 43 mutant. Mol Carcinog 23(4):254–261. doi:10.1002/(SICI)1098-2744(199812)23:4<254::AID-MC9>3.0.CO;2-4 [pii]

Kuphal S, Poser I, Jobin C, Hellerbrand C, Bosserhoff AK (2004) Loss of E-cadherin leads to upregulation of NFkappaB activity in malignant melanoma. Oncogene 23:8509–8519

Kuphal S, Martyn AC, Pedley J, Crowther LM, Bonazzi VF, Parsons PG, Bosserhoff AK, Hayward NK, Boyle GM (2009) H-cadherin expression reduces invasion of malignant melanoma. Pigment Cell Melanoma Res 22:296–306

Bosserhoff AK, Ellmann L, Quast AS, Eberle J, Boyle GM, Kuphal S (2014) Loss of T-cadherin (CDH-13) regulates AKT signaling and desensitizes cells to apoptosis in melanoma. Mol Carcinog 53(8):635–647

Kuphal S, Haass NK (2011) Cell–cell and cell–matrix contacts in melanoma and the tumor microenvironment. In: Bosserhoff AK (ed) Melanoma development – molecular biology, genetics and clinical application. Springer, Wien, pp 181–215

Lampe PD (1994) Analyzing phorbol ester effects on gap junctional communication: a dramatic inhibition of assembly. J Cell Biol 127(6 Pt 2):1895–1905

Langbein L, Grund C, Kuhn C, Praetzel S, Kartenbeck J, Brandner JM, Moll I, Franke WW (2002) Tight junctions and compositionally related junctional structures in mammalian stratified epithelia and cell cultures derived therefrom. Eur J Cell Biol 81(8):419–435

Langlois S, Maher AC, Manias JL, Shao Q, Kidder GM, Laird DW (2007) Connexin levels regulate keratinocyte differentiation in the epidermis. J Biol Chem 282(41):30171–30180

Larue L, Ohsugi M, Hirchenhain J, Kemler R (1994) E-cadherin null mutant embryos fail to form a trophectoderm epithelium. Proc Natl Acad Sci U S A 91:8263–8267

Lehmann JM, Holzmann B, Breitbart EW, Schmiegelow P, Riethmuller G, Johnson JP (1987) Discrimination between benign and malignant cells of melanocytic lineage by two novel antigens, a glycoprotein with a molecular weight of 113,000 and a protein with a molecular weight of 76,000. Cancer Res 47(3):841–845

Lehmann JM, Riethmuller G, Johnson JP (1989) MUC18, a marker of tumor progression in human melanoma, shows sequence similarity to the neural cell adhesion molecules of the immunoglobulin superfamily. Proc Natl Acad Sci U S A 86(24):9891–9895

Lei X, Guan CW, Song Y, Wang H (2015) The multifaceted role of CD146/MCAM in the promotion of melanoma progression. Cancer Cell Int 15(1):3. doi:10.1186/s12935-014-0147-z

Leotlela PD, Wade MS, Duray PH, Rhode MJ, Brown HF, Rosenthal DT, Dissanayake SK, Earley R, Indig FE, Nickoloff BJ, Taub DD, Kallioniemi OP, Meltzer P, Morin PJ, Weeraratna AT (2007) Claudin-1 overexpression in melanoma is regulated by PKC and contributes to melanoma cell motility. Oncogene 26(26):3846–3856. doi:10.1038/sj.onc.1210155, 1210155 [pii]

Li D, Mrsny RJ (2000) Oncogenic Raf-1 disrupts epithelial tight junctions via downregulation of occludin. J Cell Biol 148(4):791–800

Li G, Satyamoorthy K, Herlyn M (2001) N-cadherin-mediated intercellular interactions promote survival and migration of melanoma cells. Cancer Res 61:3819–3825

Li Q, Omori Y, Nishikawa Y, Yoshioka T, Yamamoto Y, Enomoto K (2007) Cytoplasmic accumulation of connexin32 protein enhances motility and metastatic ability of human hepatoma cells in vitro and in vivo. Int J Cancer 121(3):536–546. doi:10.1002/ijc.22696

Liu S, Kumar SM, Lu H, Liu A, Yang R, Pushparajan A, Guo W, Xu X (2012) MicroRNA-9 up-regulates E-cadherin through inhibition of NF-kB1-Snail1 pathway in melanoma. J Pathol 226:61–72

Lin JH, Takano T, Cotrina ML, Arcuino G, Kang J, Liu S, Gao Q, Jiang L, Li F, Lichtenberg-Frate H, Haubrich S, Willecke K, Goldman SA, Nedergaard M (2002) Connexin 43 enhances the adhesivity and mediates the invasion of malignant glioma cells. J Neurosci 22(11):4302–4311, 2002645022/11/4302 [pii]

Lin Q, Balasubramanian K, Fan D, Kim SJ, Guo L, Wang H, Bar-Eli M, Aldape KD, Fidler IJ (2010) Reactive astrocytes protect melanoma cells from chemotherapy by sequestering intracellular calcium through gap junction communication channels. Neoplasia 12(9):748–754

Liu XS, Genet MD, Haines JE, Mehanna EK, Wu S, Chen HI, Chen Y, Qureshi AA, Han J, Chen X, Fisher DE, Pandolfi PP, Yuan ZM (2015) ZBTB7A suppresses melanoma metastasis by transcriptionally repressing MCAM. Mol Cancer Res 13(8):1206–1217. doi:10.1158/1541-7786.MCR-15-0169

Loewenstein WR (1981) Junctional intercellular communication: the cell-to-cell membrane channel. Physiol Rev 61(4):829–913

Loewenstein WR, Kanno Y (1966) Intercellular communication and the control of tissue growth: lack of communication between cancer cells. Nature 209(5029):1248–1249

Loewenstein WR, Rose B (1992) The cell-cell channel in the control of growth. Semin Cell Biol 3(1):59–79

Long H, Crean CD, Lee WH, Cummings OW, Gabig TG (2001) Expression of Clostridium perfringens enterotoxin receptors claudin-3 and claudin-4 in prostate cancer epithelium. Cancer Res 61(21):7878–7881

Maass K, Ghanem A, Kim JS, Saathoff M, Urschel S, Kirfel G, Grummer R, Kretz M, Lewalter T, Tiemann K, Winterhager E, Herzog V, Willecke K (2004) Defective epidermal barrier in neonatal mice lacking the C-terminal region of connexin43. Mol Biol Cell 15(10):4597–4608

Man YK, Trolove C, Tattersall D, Thomas AC, Papakonstantinopoulou A, Patel D, Scott C, Chong J, Jagger DJ, O'Toole EA, Navsaria H, Curtis MA, Kelsell DP (2007) A deafness-associated mutant human connexin 26 improves the epithelial barrier in vitro. J Membr Biol 218(1–3):29–37

Martin TA, Jiang WG (2001) Tight junctions and their role in cancer metastasis. Histol Histopathol 16(4):1183–1195

Martin TA, Jiang WG (2009) Loss of tight junction barrier function and its role in cancer metastasis. Biochim Biophys Acta 1788(4):872–891. doi:10.1016/j.bbamem.2008.11.005, S0005-2736(08)00373-8 [pii]

Massoumi R, Kuphal S, Hellerbrand C, Haas B, Wild P, Spruss T, Pfeifer A, Fassler R, Bosserhoff AK (2009) Down-regulation of CYLD expression by snail promotes tumor progression in malignant melanoma. J Exp Med 206:221–232

McCarty MF, Bielenberg DR, Nilsson MB, Gershenwald JE, Barnhill RL, Ahearne P, Bucana CD, Fidler IJ (2003) Epidermal hyperplasia overlying human melanoma correlates with tumour depth and angiogenesis. Melanoma Res 13(4):379–387

McLachlan E, Shao Q, Wang HL, Langlois S, Laird DW (2006) Connexins act as tumor suppressors in three-dimensional mammary cell organoids by regulating differentiation and angiogenesis. Cancer Res 66(20):9886–9894. doi:10.1158/0008-5472.CAN-05-4302, 66/20/9886 [pii]

Meier F, Busch S, Gast D, Goppert A, Altevogt P, Maczey E, Riedle S, Garbe C, Schittek B (2006) The adhesion molecule L1 (CD171) promotes melanoma progression. Int J Cancer 119(3):549–555

Meier F, Schittek B, Busch S, Garbe C, Smalley K, Satyamoorthy K, Li G, Herlyn M (2005) The RAS/RAF/MEK/ERK and PI3K/AKT signaling pathways present molecular targets for the effective treatment of advanced melanoma. Front Biosci 10(2986–3001):2986–3001

Mese G, Richard G, White TW (2007) Gap junctions: basic structure and function. J Invest Dermatol 127(11):2516–2524

Mesnil M, Crespin S, Avanzo JL, Zaidan-Dagli ML (2005) Defective gap junctional intercellular communication in the carcinogenic process. Biochim Biophys Acta 1719(1–2):125–145. doi:10.1016/j.bbamem.2005.11.004, S0005-2736(05)00361-5 [pii]

Miekus K, Czernik M, Sroka J, Czyz J, Madeja Z (2005) Contact stimulation of prostate cancer cell migration: the role of gap junctional coupling and migration stimulated by heterotypic cell-to-cell contacts in determination of the metastatic phenotype of dunning rat prostate cancer cells. Biol Cell 97(12):893–903. doi:10.1042/BC20040129

Miele ME, Bennett CF, Miller BE, Welch DR (1994) Enhanced metastatic ability of TNF-alpha-treated malignant melanoma cells is reduced by intercellular adhesion molecule-1 (ICAM-1, CD54) antisense oligonucleotides. Exp Cell Res 214(1):231–241

Minchinton AI, Tannock IF (2006) Drug penetration in solid tumours. Nat Rev Cancer 6(8):583–592

Mitic LL, Anderson JM (1998) Molecular architecture of tight junctions. Annu Rev Physiol 60:121–142

Miwa N, Furuse M, Tsukita S, Niikawa N, Nakamura Y, Furukawa Y (2000) Involvement of claudin-1 in the beta-catenin/Tcf signaling pathway and its frequent upregulation in human colorectal cancers. Oncol Res 12(11–12):469–476

Moennikes O, Buchmann A, Willecke K, Traub O, Schwarz M (2000) Hepatocarcinogenesis in female mice with mosaic expression of connexin32. Hepatology 32(3):501–506. doi:10.1053/jhep.2000.16598, S0270913900790100

Molina-Ortiz I, Bartolome RA, Hernandez-Varas P, Colo GP, Teixido J (2009) Overexpression of E-cadherin on melanoma cells inhibits chemokine-promoted invasion involving p190RhoGAP/p120ctn-dependent inactivation of RhoA. J Biol Chem 284:15147–15157

Montgomery AM, Becker JC, Siu CH, Lemmon VP, Cheresh DA, Pancook JD, Zhao X, Reisfeld RA (1996) Human neural cell adhesion molecule L1 and rat homologue NILE are ligands for integrin alpha v beta 3. J Cell Biol 132(3):475–485

Mori R, Power KT, Wang CM, Martin P, Becker DL (2006) Acute downregulation of connexin43 at wound sites leads to a reduced inflammatory response, enhanced keratinocyte proliferation and wound fibroblast migration. J Cell Sci 119(Pt 24):5193–5203

Morita K, Morita NI, Nemoto K, Nakamura Y, Miyachi Y, Muto M (2008) Expression of claudin in melanoma cells. J Dermatol 35(1):36–38. doi:10.1111/j.1346-8138.2007.00409.x, JDE409 [pii]

Mortarini R, Anichini A (1993) From adhesion to signalling: roles of integrins in the biology of human melanoma. Melanoma Res 3:87–97

Mullin JM, Kampherstein JA, Laughlin KV, Saladik DT, Soler AP (1997) Transepithelial paracellular leakiness induced by chronic phorbol ester exposure correlates with polyp-like foci and redistribution of protein kinase C-alpha. Carcinogenesis 18(12):2339–2345

Muller EJ, Williamson L, Kolly C, Suter MM (2008) Outside-in signaling through integrins and cadherins: a central mechanism to control epidermal growth and differentiation? J Invest Dermatol 128:501–516

Nacht M, Ferguson AT, Zhang W, Petroziello JM, Cook BP, Gao YH, Maguire S, Riley D, Coppola G, Landes GM, Madden SL, Sukumar S (1999) Combining serial analysis of gene expression and array technologies to identify genes differentially expressed in breast cancer. Cancer Res 59(21):5464–5470

Naoi Y, Miyoshi Y, Taguchi T, Kim SJ, Arai T, Tamaki Y, Noguchi S (2007) Connexin26 expression is associated with lymphatic vessel invasion and poor prognosis in human breast cancer. Breast Cancer Res Treat 106(1):11–17. doi:10.1007/s10549-006-9465-8

Natali P, Nicotra MR, Cavaliere R, Bigotti A, Romano G, Temponi M, Ferrone S (1990) Differential expression of intercellular adhesion molecule 1 in primary and metastatic melanoma lesions. Cancer Res 50(4):1271–1278

Natali PG, Hamby CV, Felding-Habermann B, Liang B, Nicotra MR, Di Filippo F, Giannarelli D, Temponi M, Ferrone S (1997) Clinical significance of alpha(v)beta3 integrin and intercellular adhesion molecule-1 expression in cutaneous malignant melanoma lesions. Cancer Res 57(8):1554–1560

Natali PG, Nicotra MR, Bartolazzi A, Cavaliere R, Bigotti A (1993) Integrin expression in cutaneous malignant melanoma: association of the alpha 3/beta 1 heterodimer with tumor progression. Int J Cancer 54:68–72

Naus CC, Laird DW (2010) Implications and challenges of connexin connections to cancer. Nat Rev Cancer 10(6):435–441. doi:10.1038/nrc2841, nrc2841 [pii]

Nikolaev SI, Rimoldi D, Iseli C, Valsesia A, Robyr D, Gehrig C, Harshman K, Guipponi M, Bukach O, Zoete V, Michielin O, Muehlethaler K, Speiser D, Beckmann JS, Xenarios I, Halazonetis TD, Jongeneel CV, Stevenson BJ, Antonarakis SE (2011) Exome sequencing identifies recurrent somatic *MAP2K1* and *MAP2K2* mutations in melanoma. Nat Genet 44:133–139

Nishimura EK, Yoshida H, Kunisada T, Nishikawa SI (1999) Regulation of E- and P-cadherin expression correlated with melanocyte migration and diversification. Dev Biol 215:155–166

Nolte C, Moos M, Schachner M (1999) Immunolocalization of the neural cell adhesion molecule L1 in epithelia of rodents. Cell Tissue Res 298(2):261–273

Omori Y, Yamasaki H (1998) Mutated connexin43 proteins inhibit rat glioma cell growth suppression mediated by wild-type connexin43 in a dominant-negative manner. Int J Cancer 78(4):446–453. doi:10.1002/(SICI)1097-0215(19981109)78:4<446::AID-IJC10>3.0.CO;2-4 [pii]

Onder TT, Gupta PB, Mani SA, Yang J, Lander ES, Weinberg RA (2008) Loss of E-cadherin promotes metastasis via multiple downstream transcriptional pathways. Cancer Res 68:3645–3654

Overduin M, Harvey TS, Bagby S, Tong KI, Yau P, Takeichi M, Ikura M (1995) Solution structure of the epithelial cadherin domain responsible for selective cell adhesion. Science 267:386–389

Papusheva E, Heisenberg CP (2010) Spatial organization of adhesion: force-dependent regulation and function in tissue morphogenesis. EMBO J 29:2753–2768

Park CC, Bissell MJ, Barcellos-Hoff MH (2000) The influence of the microenvironment on the malignant phenotype. Mol Med Today 6(8):324–329

Patel DD, Wee SF, Whichard LP, Bowen MA, Pesando JM, Aruffo A, Haynes BF (1995) Identification and characterization of a 100-kD ligand for CD6 on human thymic epithelial cells. J Exp Med 181(4):1563–1568

Pearl RA, Pacifico MD, Richman PI, Wilson GD, Grover R (2008) Stratification of patients by melanoma cell adhesion molecule (MCAM) expression on the basis of risk: implications for sentinel lymph node biopsy. J Plast Reconstr Aesthet Surg 61(3):265–271

Pece S, Gutkind JS (2000) Signaling from E-cadherins to the MAPK pathway by the recruitment and activation of epidermal growth factor receptors upon cell-cell contact formation. J Biol Chem 275:41227–41233

Penna E, Orso F, Cimino D, Vercellino I, Grassi E, Quaglino E, Turco E, Taverna D (2013) miR-214 coordinates melanoma progression by upregulating ALCAM through TFAP2 and miR-148b downmodulation. Cancer Res 73(13):4098–4111. doi:10.1158/0008-5472.CAN-12-3686

Penuela S, Gehi R, Laird DW (2013) The biochemistry and function of pannexin channels. Biochim Biophys Acta 1828(1):15–22. doi:10.1016/j.bbamem.2012.01.017

Perrais M, Chen X, Perez-Moreno M, Gumbiner BM (2007) E-cadherin homophilic ligation inhibits cell growth and epidermal growth factor receptor signaling independently of other cell interactions. Mol Biol Cell 18:2013–2025

Perez-Moreno MA, Locascio A, Rodrigo I, Dhondt G, Portillo F, Nieto MA, Cano A (2001) A new role for E12/E47 in the repression of E-cadherin expression and epithelial-mesenchymal transitions. J Biol Chem 276(29):27424–27431

Pollmann MA, Shao Q, Laird DW, Sandig M (2005) Connexin 43 mediated gap junctional communication enhances breast tumor cell diapedesis in culture. Breast Cancer Res 7(4):R522–R534. doi:10.1186/bcr1042, bcr1042 [pii]

Pollok S, Pfeiffer AC, Lobmann R, Wright CS, Moll I, Martin PE, Brandner JM (2011) Connexin 43 mimetic peptide Gap27 reveals potential differences in the role of Cx43 in wound repair between diabetic and non-diabetic cells. J Cell Mol Med 15(4):861–873. doi:10.1111/j.1582-4934.2010.01057.x

Poser I, Dominguez D, de Herreros AG, Varnai A, Buettner R, Bosserhoff AK (2001) Loss of E-cadherin expression in melanoma cells involves up-regulation of the transcriptional repressor Snail. J Biol Chem 276:24661–24666

Place RF, Li LC, Pookot D, Noonan EJ, Dahiya R (2008) MicroRNA-373 induces expression of genes with complementary promoter sequences. Proc Natl Acad Sci U S A 105:1608–1613

Playford MP, Schaller MD (2004) The interplay between Src and integrins in normal and tumor biology. Oncogene 23:7928–7946

Pummi K, Malminen M, Aho H, Karvonen SL, Peltonen J, Peltonen S (2001) Epidermal tight junctions: ZO-1 and occludin are expressed in mature, developing, and affected skin and in vitro differentiating keratinocytes. J Invest Dermatol 117(5):1050–1058

Qi J, Wang J, Romanyuk O, Siu CH (2006) Involvement of Src family kinases in N-cadherin phosphorylation and beta-catenin dissociation during transendothelial migration of melanoma cells. Mol Biol Cell 17:1261–1272

Qian X, Karpova T, Sheppard AM, McNally J, Lowy DR (2004) E-cadherin-mediated adhesion inhibits ligand-dependent activation of diverse receptor tyrosine kinases. EMBO J 23:1739–1748

Rangel LB, Agarwal R, D'Souza T, Pizer ES, Alo PL, Lancaster WD, Gregoire L, Schwartz DR, Cho KR, Morin PJ (2003) Tight junction proteins claudin-3 and claudin-4 are frequently overexpressed in ovarian cancer but not in ovarian cystadenomas. Clin Cancer Res 9(7):2567–2575

Rapanotti MC, Suarez Viguria TM, Costanza G, Ricozzi I, Pierantozzi A, Di Stefani A, Campione E, Bernardini S, Chimenti S, Orlandi A, Bianchi L (2014) Sequential molecular analysis of circulating MCAM/MUC18 expression: a promising disease biomarker related to clinical outcome in melanoma. Arch Dermatol Res 306(6):527–537. doi:10.1007/s00403-014-1473-7

Ren J, Hamada J, Takeichi N, Fujikawa S, Kobayashi H (1990) Ultrastructural differences in junctional intercellular communication between highly and weakly metastatic clones derived from rat mammary carcinoma. Cancer Res 50(2):358–362

Rezze GG, Fregnani JH, Duprat J, Landman G (2011) Cell adhesion and communication proteins are differentially expressed in melanoma progression model. Hum Pathol 42(3):409–418. doi:10.1016/j.humpath.2010.09.004

Richard G (2000) Connexins: a connection with the skin. Exp Dermatol 9(2):77–96

Rickelt S, Franke WW, Doerflinger Y, Goerdt S, Brandner JM, Peitsch WK (2008) Subtypes of melanocytes and melanoma cells distinguished by their intercellular contacts: heterotypic adherens junctions, adhesive associations, and dispersed desmoglein 2 glycoproteins. Cell Tissue Res 334:401–422

Rodriguez M, Aladowicz E, Lanfrancone L, Goding CR (2008) Tbx3 represses E-cadherin expression and enhances melanoma invasiveness. Cancer Res 68(19):7872–7881

Rubina KA, Yurlova EI, Sysoeva VY, Semina EV, Kalinina NI, Poliakov AA, Mikhaylova IN, Andronova NV, Treshalina HM (2013) T-cadherin stimulates melanoma cell proliferation and mesenchymal stromal cell recruitment, but inhibits angiogenesis in a mouse melanoma model. In: Jianyuan Chai (ed) Cardiology and Cardiovascular Medicine. "Research Directions in Tumor Angiogenesis", pp 143–174

Sadeqzadeh E, de Bock CE, Zhang XD, Shipman KL, Scott NM, Song C, Yeadon T, Oliveira CS, Jin B, Hersey P, Boyd AW, Burns GF, Thorne RF (2011) Dual processing of FAT1 cadherin protein by human melanoma cells generates distinct protein products. J Biol Chem 286:28181–28191

Saccheri F, Pozzi C, Avogadri F, Barozzi S, Faretta M, Fusi P, Rescigno M (2010) Bacteria-induced gap junctions in tumors favor antigen cross-presentation and antitumor immunity. Sci Transl Med 2(44):44ra57. doi:10.1126/scitranslmed.3000739

Saito-Katsuragi M, Asada H, Niizeki H, Katoh F, Masuzawa M, Tsutsumi M, Kuniyasu H, Ito A, Nojima H, Miyagawa S (2007) Role for connexin 26 in metastasis of human malignant melanoma: communication between melanoma and endothelial cells via connexin 26. Cancer 110(5):1162–1172

Saito Y, Takazawa H, Uzawa K, Tanzawa H, Sato K (1998) Reduced expression of E-cadherin in oral squamous cell carcinoma: relationship with DNA methylation of 5' CpG island. Int J Oncol 12:293–298

Sakai R, Henderson JT, O'Bryan JP, Elia AJ, Saxton TM, Pawson T (2000) The mammalian ShcB and ShcC phosphotyrosine docking proteins function in the maturation of sensory and sympathetic neurons. Neuron 28:819–833

Sanders DS, Blessing K, Hassan GA, Bruton R, Marsden JR, Jankowski J (1999) Alterations in cadherin and catenin expression during the biological progression of melanocytic tumours. Mol Pathol 52:151–157

Santiago-Walker A, Li L, Haass NK, Herlyn M (2009) Melanocytes: from morphology to application. Skin Pharmacol Physiol 22(2):114–121

Sargen MR, Gormley RH, Pasha TL, Yum S, Acs G, Xu X, Zhang PJ (2013) Melanocytic tumors express connexin 43 but not 26: immunohistochemical analysis with potential significance in melanocytic oncogenesis. Am J Dermatopathol 35(8):813–7. doi:10.1097/DAD.0b013e318278d401

Satyamoorthy K, Muyrers J, Meier F, Patel D, Herlyn M (2001) Mel-CAM-specific genetic suppressor elements inhibit melanoma growth and invasion through loss of gap junctional communication. Oncogene 20(34):4676–4684

Saunders MM, Seraj MJ, Li Z, Zhou Z, Winter CR, Welch DR, Donahue HJ (2001) Breast cancer metastatic potential correlates with a breakdown in homospecific and heterospecific gap junctional intercellular communication. Cancer Res 61(5):1765–1767

Schadendorf D, Gawlik C, Haney U, Ostmeier H, Suter L, Czarnetzki BM (1993) Tumour progression and metastatic behaviour in vivo correlates with integrin expression on melanocytic tumours. J Pathol 170(4):429–434

Schadendorf D, Heidel J, Gawlik C, Suter L, Czarnetzki BM (1995) Association with clinical outcome of expression of VLA-4 in primary cutaneous malignant melanoma as well as P-selectin and E-selectin on intratumoral vessels. J Natl Cancer Inst 87(5):366–371

Schaller MD (2001) Biochemical signals and biological responses elicited by the focal adhesion kinase. Biochim Biophys Acta 1540:1–21

Schiffner S, Zimara N, Schmid R, Bosserhoff AK (2011) p54nrb is a new regulator of progression of malignant melanoma. Carcinogenesis 32(8):1176–1182. doi:10.1093/carcin/bgr103

Schmitt CJ, Franke WW, Goerdt S, Falkowska-Hansen B, Rickelt S, Peitsch WK (2007) Homo- and heterotypic cell contacts in malignant melanoma cells and desmoglein 2 as a novel solitary surface glycoprotein. J Invest Dermatol 127(9):2191–2206. doi:10.1038/sj.jid.5700849, 5700849 [pii]

Seftor RE, Seftor EA, Hendrix MJ (1999) Molecular role(s) for integrins in human melanoma invasion. Cancer Metastasis Rev 18:359–375

Shao Q, Wang H, McLachlan E, Veitch GI, Laird DW (2005) Down-regulation of Cx43 by retroviral delivery of small interfering RNA promotes an aggressive breast cancer cell phenotype. Cancer Res 65(7):2705–2711. doi:10.1158/0008-5472.CAN-04-2367, 65/7/2705 [pii]

Shen Y, Khusial PR, Li X, Ichikawa H, Moreno AP, Goldberg GS (2007) SRC utilizes Cas to block gap junctional communication mediated by connexin43. J Biol Chem 282(26):18914–18921. doi:10.1074/jbc.M608980200, M608980200 [pii]

Shih IM, Elder DE, Speicher D, Johnson JP, Herlyn M (1994) Isolation and functional characterization of the A32 melanoma-associated antigen. Cancer Res 54(9):2514–2520

Shih IM, Speicher D, Hsu MY, Levine E, Herlyn M (1997a) Melanoma cell-cell interactions are mediated through heterophilic Mel-CAM/ligand adhesion. Cancer Res 57(17):3835–3840

Shih LM, Hsu MY, Palazzo JP, Herlyn M (1997b) The cell-cell adhesion receptor Mel-CAM acts as a tumor suppressor in breast carcinoma. Am J Pathol 151(3):745–751

Shtutman M, Zhurinsky J, Simcha I, Albanese C, D'Amico M, Pestell R, Ben Ze'ev A (1999) The cyclin D1 gene is a target of the beta-catenin/LEF-1 pathway. Proc Natl Acad Sci U S A 96:5522–5527

Sieg DJ, Hauck CR, Ilic D, Klingbeil CK, Schaefer E, Damsky CH, Schlaepfer DD (2000) FAK integrates growth-factor and integrin signals to promote cell migration. Nat Cell Biol 2:249–256

Sienel W, Dango S, Woelfle U, Morresi-Hauf A, Wagener C, Brummer J, Mutschler W, Passlick B, Pantel K (2003) Elevated expression of carcinoembryonic antigen-related cell adhesion molecule 1 promotes progression of non-small cell lung cancer. Clin Cancer Res 9(6):2260–2266

Silye R, Karayiannakis AJ, Syrigos KN, Poole S, van Noorden S, Batchelor W, Regele H, Sega W, Boesmueller H, Krausz T, Pignatelli M (1998) E-cadherin/catenin complex in benign and malignant melanocytic lesions. J Pathol 186:350–355

Smalley KS, Brafford P, Haass NK, Brandner JM, Brown E, Herlyn M (2005) Up-regulated expression of zonula occludens protein-1 in human melanoma associates with N-cadherin and contributes to invasion and adhesion. Am J Pathol 166(5):1541–1554

Soler AP, Marano CW, Bryans M, Miller RD, Garulacan LA, Mauldin SK, Stamato TD, Mullin JM (1999) Activation of NF-kappaB is necessary for the restoration of the barrier function of an epithelium undergoing TNF-alpha-induced apoptosis. Eur J Cell Biol 78(1):56–66

Spangler B, Kappelmann M, Schittek B, Meierjohann S, Vardimon L, Bosserhoff AK, Kuphal S (2012) ETS1/RhoC signaling regulates the transcription factor c-Jun in melanoma. Int J Cancer 130:2801–2811

Spray DC (1994) Physiological and pharmacological regulation of gap junction channels. In: Citi S (ed) Molecular mechanisms of epithelial cell junctions: from development to disease. R. G. Landes Company, Austin, pp 195–215

Stevenson BR, Keon BH (1998) The tight junction: morphology to molecules. Annu Rev Cell Dev Biol 14:89–109

Stoletov K, Strnadel J, Zardouzian E, Momiyama M, Park FD, Kelber JA, Pizzo DP, Hoffman R, Vandenberg SR, Klemke RL (2013) Role of connexins in metastatic breast cancer and melanoma brain colonization. J Cell Sci 126(Pt 4):904–913. doi:10.1242/jcs.112748

Strathdee G (2002) Epigenetic versus genetic alterations in the inactivation of E-cadherin. Semin Cancer Biol 12:373–379

Su YA, Bittner ML, Chen Y, Tao L, Jiang Y, Zhang Y, Stephan DA, Trent JM (2000) Identification of tumor-suppressor genes using human melanoma cell lines UACC903, UACC903(+6), and SRS3 by comparison of expression profiles. Mol Carcinog 28(2):119–127

Tada J, Hashimoto K (1997) Ultrastructural localization of gap junction protein connexin 43 in normal human skin, basal cell carcinoma, and squamous cell carcinoma. J Cutan Pathol 24(10):628–635

Talantov D, Mazumder A, Yu JX, Briggs T, Jiang Y, Backus J, Atkins D, Wang Y (2005) Novel genes associated with malignant melanoma but not benign melanocytic lesions. Clin Cancer Res 11(20):7234–7242

Tang A, Eller MS, Hara M, Yaar M, Hirohashi S, Gilchrest BA (1994) E-cadherin is the major mediator of human melanocyte adhesion to keratinocytes in vitro. J Cell Sci 107:983–992

Temme A, Buchmann A, Gabriel HD, Nelles E, Schwarz M, Willecke K (1997) High incidence of spontaneous and chemically induced liver tumors in mice deficient for connexin32. Curr Biol 7(9):713–716

Thies A, Berlin A, Brunner G, Schulze HJ, Moll I, Pfuller U, Wagener C, Schachner M, Altevogt P, Schumacher U (2007) Glycoconjugate profiling of primary melanoma and its sentinel node and distant metastases: implications for diagnosis and pathophysiology of metastases. Cancer Lett 248(1):68–80

Thies A, Moll I, Berger J, Wagener C, Brummer J, Schulze HJ, Brunner G, Schumacher U (2002a) CEACAM1 expression in cutaneous malignant melanoma predicts the development of metastatic disease. J Clin Oncol 20(10):2530–2536

Thies A, Schachner M, Moll I, Berger J, Schulze HJ, Brunner G, Schumacher U (2002b) Overexpression of the cell adhesion molecule L1 is associated with metastasis in cutaneous malignant melanoma. Eur J Cancer 38(13):1708–1716

Trimmer C, Whitaker-Menezes D, Bonuccelli G, Milliman JN, Daumer KM, Aplin AE, Pestell RG, Sotgia F, Lisanti MP, Capozza F (2010) CAV1 inhibits metastatic potential in melanomas through suppression of the integrin/Src/FAK signaling pathway. Cancer Res 70:7489–7499

Trosko JE, Chang CC, Madhukar BV, Klaunig JE (1990) Chemical, oncogene and growth factor inhibition gap junctional intercellular communication: an integrative hypothesis of carcinogenesis. Pathobiology 58(5):265–278

Troussard AA, Tan C, Yoganathan TN, Dedhar S (1999) Cell-extracellular matrix interactions stimulate the AP-1 transcription factor in an integrin-linked kinase- and glycogen synthase kinase 3-dependent manner. Mol Cell Biol 19:7420–7427

Tsai H, Werber J, Davia MO, Edelman M, Tanaka KE, Melman A, Christ GJ, Geliebter J (1996) Reduced connexin 43 expression in high grade, human prostatic adenocarcinoma cells. Biochem Biophys Res Commun 227(1):64–69

Tsukita S, Furuse M (2000) Pores in the wall: claudins constitute tight junction strands containing aqueous pores. J Cell Biol 149(1):13–16
Tsukita S, Furuse M, Itoh M (2001) Multifunctional strands in tight junctions. Nat Rev Mol Cell Biol 2(4):285–293
Uchida Y, Matsuda K, Sasahara K, Kawabata H, Nishioka M (1995) Immunohistochemistry of gap junctions in normal and diseased gastric mucosa of humans. Gastroenterology 109(5):1492–1496
van Marck V, Stove C, Van Den Bossche K, Stove V, Paredes J, Vander Haeghen Y (2005) P-cadherin promotes cell-cell adhesion and counteracts invasion in human melanoma. Cancer Res 65(19):8774–8783
van de Stolpe A, van der Saag PT (1996) Intercellular adhesion molecule-1. J Mol Med 74(1):13–33
van Kempen LC, Meier F, Egeblad M, Kersten-Niessen MJ, Garbe C, Weidle UH, Van Muijen GN, Herlyn M, Bloemers HP, Swart GW (2004) Truncation of activated leukocyte cell adhesion molecule: a gateway to melanoma metastasis. J Invest Dermatol 122(5):1293–1301
van Kempen LC, van den Oord JJ, van Muijen GN, Weidle UH, Bloemers HP, Swart GW (2000) Activated leukocyte cell adhesion molecule/CD166, a marker of tumor progression in primary malignant melanoma of the skin. Am J Pathol 156(3):769–774
van Noort M, Clevers H (2002) TCF transcription factors, mediators of Wnt-signaling in development and cancer. Dev Biol 244:1–8
Veenstra RD (1996) Size and selectivity of gap junction channels formed from different connexins. J Bioenerg Biomembr 28(4):327–337
Villanueva J, Herlyn M (2008) Melanoma and the tumor microenvironment. Curr Oncol Rep 10(5):439–446
Villares GJ, Dobroff AS, Wang H, Zigler M, Melnikova VO, Huang L, Bar-Eli M (2009) Overexpression of protease-activated receptor-1 contributes to melanoma metastasis via regulation of connexin 43. Cancer Res 69(16):6730–6737. doi:10.1158/0008-5472.CAN-09-0300, 69/16/6730 [pii]
Villares GJ, Zigler M, Bar-Eli M (2011) The emerging role of the thrombin receptor (PAR-1) in melanoma metastasis – a possible therapeutic target. Oncotarget 2(1–2):8–17
Voura EB, Ramjeesingh RA, Montgomery AM, Siu CH (2001) Involvement of integrin alpha(v) beta(3) and cell adhesion molecule L1 in transendothelial migration of melanoma cells. Mol Biol Cell 12(9):2699–2710
Watson-Hurst K, Becker D (2006) The role of N-cadherin, MCAM and beta3 integrin in melanoma progression, proliferation, migration and invasion. Cancer Biol Ther 5:1375–1382
Weinstein RS, Merk FB, Alroy J (1976) The structure and function of intercellular junctions in cancer. Adv Cancer Res 23:23–89
Wilgenbus KK, Kirkpatrick CJ, Knuechel R, Willecke K, Traub O (1992) Expression of Cx26, Cx32 and Cx43 gap junction proteins in normal and neoplastic human tissues. Int J Cancer 51(4):522–529
Wiklund ED, Bramsen JB, Hulf T, Dyrskjot L, Ramanathan R, Hansen TB, Villadsen SB, Gao S, Ostenfeld MS, Borre M, Peter ME, Orntoft TF, Kjems J, Clark SJ (2011) Coordinated epigenetic repression of the miR-200 family and miR-205 in invasive bladder cancer. Int J Cancer 128:1327–1334
Willecke K, Eiberger J, Degen J, Eckardt D, Romualdi A, Guldenagel M, Deutsch U, Sohl G (2002) Structural and functional diversity of connexin genes in the mouse and human genome. Biol Chem 383(5):725–737
Wolburg H, Wolburg-Buchholz K, Kraus J, Rascher-Eggstein G, Liebner S, Hamm S, Duffner F, Grote EH, Risau W, Engelhardt B (2003) Localization of claudin-3 in tight junctions of the blood–brain barrier is selectively lost during experimental autoimmune encephalomyelitis and human glioblastoma multiforme. Acta Neuropathol (Berl) 105(6):586–592
Wong RP, Ng P, Dedhar S, Li G (2007) The role of integrin-linked kinase in melanoma cell migration, invasion, and tumor growth. Mol Cancer Ther 6:1692–1700

Wright CS, van Steensel MA, Hodgins MB, Martin PE (2009) Connexin mimetic peptides improve cell migration rates of human epidermal keratinocytes and dermal fibroblasts in vitro. Wound Repair Regen 17(2):240–249. doi:10.1111/j.1524-475X.2009.00471.x

Xie S, Luca M, Huang S, Gutman M, Reich R, Johnson JP, Bar-Eli M (1997) Expression of MCAM/MUC18 by human melanoma cells leads to increased tumor growth and metastasis. Cancer Res 57(11):2295–2303

Xu J, Nicholson BJ (2013) The role of connexins in ear and skin physiology – functional insights from disease-associated mutations. Biochim Biophys Acta 1828(1):167–178. doi:10.1016/j.bbamem.2012.06.024

Yamaoka K, Nouchi T, Tazawa J, Hiranuma S, Marumo F, Sato C (1995) Expression of gap junction protein connexin 32 and E-cadherin in human hepatocellular carcinoma. J Hepatol 22(5):536–539, 0168-8278(95)80447-1 [pii]

Yang J, Mani SA, Donaher JL, Ramaswamy S, Itzykson RA, Come C, Savagner P, Gitelman I, Richardson A, Weinberg RA (2004) Twist, a master regulator of morphogenesis, plays an essential role in tumor metastasis. Cell 117(7):927–939

Yazawa EM, Geddes-Sweeney JE, Cedeno-Laurent F, Walley KC, Barthel SR, Opperman MJ, Liang J, Lin JY, Schatton T, Laga AC, Mihm MC, Qureshi AA, Widlund HR, Murphy GF, Dimitroff CJ (2015) Melanoma cell galectin-1 ligands functionally correlate with malignant potential. J Invest Dermatol 135(7):1849–1862. doi:10.1038/jid.2015.95

Zhang P, Goodrich C, Fu C, Dong C (2014) Melanoma upregulates ICAM-1 expression on endothelial cells through engagement of tumor CD44 with endothelial E-selectin and activation of a PKCalpha-p38-SP-1 pathway. FASEB J 28(11):4591–4609. doi:10.1096/fj.11-202747

Zhang ZQ, Zhang W, Wang NQ, Bani-Yaghoub M, Lin ZX, Naus CC (1998) Suppression of tumorigenicity of human lung carcinoma cells after transfection with connexin43. Carcinogenesis 19(11):1889–1894

Zhu D, Caveney S, Kidder GM, Naus CC (1991) Transfection of C6 glioma cells with connexin 43 cDNA: analysis of expression, intercellular coupling, and cell proliferation. Proc Natl Acad Sci U S A 88(5):1883–1887

Zigler M, Kamiya T, Brantley EC, Villares GJ, Bar-Eli M (2011) PAR-1 and thrombin: the ties that bind the microenvironment to melanoma metastasis. Cancer Res 71(21):6561–6566. doi:10.1158/0008-5472.CAN-11-1432

Zucker SN, Bancroft TA, Place DE, Des Soye B, Bagati A, Berezney R (2013) A dominant negative Cx43 mutant differentially affects tumorigenic and invasive properties in human metastatic melanoma cells. J Cell Physiol 228(4):853–859. doi:10.1002/jcp.24235

Regulation of Apoptosis in Melanoma Cells: Critical Targets for Therapeutic Strategies

10

Jürgen Eberle and Lothar F. Fecker

10.1 Introduction: Critical Roles of Apoptosis Deficiency for Melanoma

While the incidence of most solid tumors has decreased or stabilized in the last decades, melanoma incidence continued to rise with approximately 3 % per year (Siegel et al. 2014). The until recently almost unbroken high mortality resulted from an early dissemination associated with pronounced chemotherapy resistance. In the past, neither chemotherapy regimens nor biotherapy (IL-2 and IFN-α) or vaccination protocols could significantly improve the fatal situation of metastasized melanoma patients (Fang et al. 2008; Garbe et al. 2012). This has changed recently with the development of selective BRAF inhibitors and targeted immune modulators such as anti-CTLA4 and anti-PD1, which for the first time could significantly improve the overall survival (Menzies and Long 2014; Hughes et al. 2015). Nevertheless, after initial tumor reduction and clinical improvement, tumor relapse and therapy resistance often follow within only a few months (Chen and Davies 2014), thus challenging for combination therapies that may further improve the clinical outcome.

Although different cellular mechanisms may contribute to therapy resistance in cancer, apoptosis deficiency appears as a major cause. This is explained by the fact that the final elimination of cancer cells by proapoptotic programs represents a

J. Eberle (✉)
Department of Dermatology and Allergy, Skin Cancer Center Charité, Charité – Universitätsmedizin Berlin, Charité Campus Mitte, Charitéplatz 1, Berlin 10117, Germany
e-mail: juergen.eberle@charite.de

L.F. Fecker
Department of Dermatology and Allergy, Skin Cancer Center Charité, Charité – Universitätsmedizin Berlin, Charité Campus Mitte, Charitéplatz 1, Berlin 10117, Germany
e-mail: l-fecker@web.de

A. Bosserhoff (ed.), *Melanoma Development*,
DOI 10.1007/978-3-319-41319-8_10

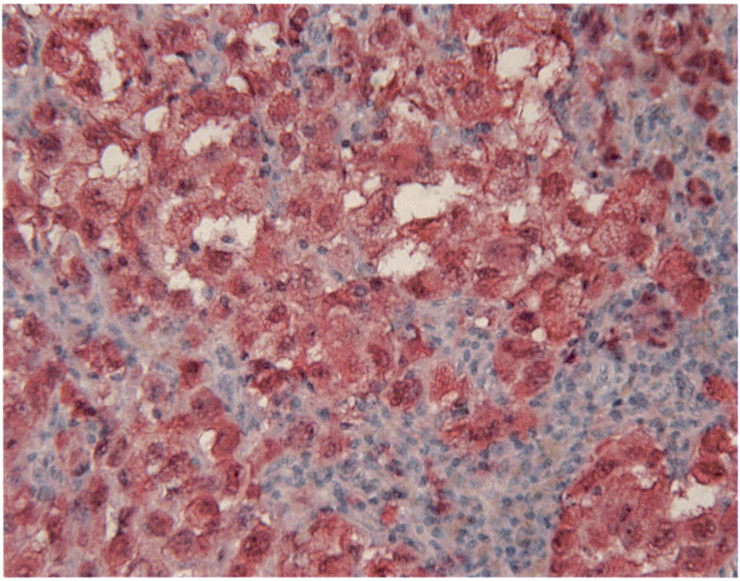

Fig. 10.1 Immunogenicity of melanoma. Massive lymphocytic tumor infiltrates are seen in a section of a primary melanoma. Lymphocytes: *gray* with small nuclei. Melanoma cells: *stained red* by S100 antibody

common final path of most anticancer therapies. For example, different chemotherapeutic drugs cause cellular or DNA damage, which induces cell-intrinsic proapoptotic pathways, and also, BRAF inhibitors have been related to an induction of apoptosis or sensitization for proapoptotic programs (Eberle et al. 2007b; Beck et al. 2013; Berger et al. 2014). Furthermore, immune stimulation results in cytotoxic T-lymphocytes, which express death ligands to trigger extrinsic proapoptotic pathways in target cancer cells (Martinez-Lostao et al. 2015).

Proapoptotic pathways serve as essential safeguard mechanisms preventing the growth of abnormal tumor cells in multicellular organisms (Eberle et al. 2007a). Thus, intrinsic proapoptotic pathways are activated by different kinds of cellular stress situations and dysfunction, also including typical characteristics of cancer cells as oncogene activation. Furthermore, the elimination of cancer cells in an immune response is based on the extrinsic induction of apoptosis. Thus, resistance to apoptosis appears as a prerequisite of early cancer growth, and in the second run, it may enable tumor cells to survive anticancer therapy (Hanahan and Weinberg 2011).

Melanoma is a particular example for pronounced chemotherapy resistance and large resistance to immune cells. The latter is suggested by the frequently high immunoreactivity in initial tumor stages and high numbers of tumor-infiltrating lymphocytes (Fig. 10.1). Nevertheless, the tumor grows and may finally form metastases. Thus, the sensitization of melanoma cells for apoptosis may support the therapeutic effects both of BRAF inhibitors (intrinsic proapoptotic pathways) and of immunotherapy due to a strengthening of extrinsic proapoptotic pathways (Fig. 10.2).

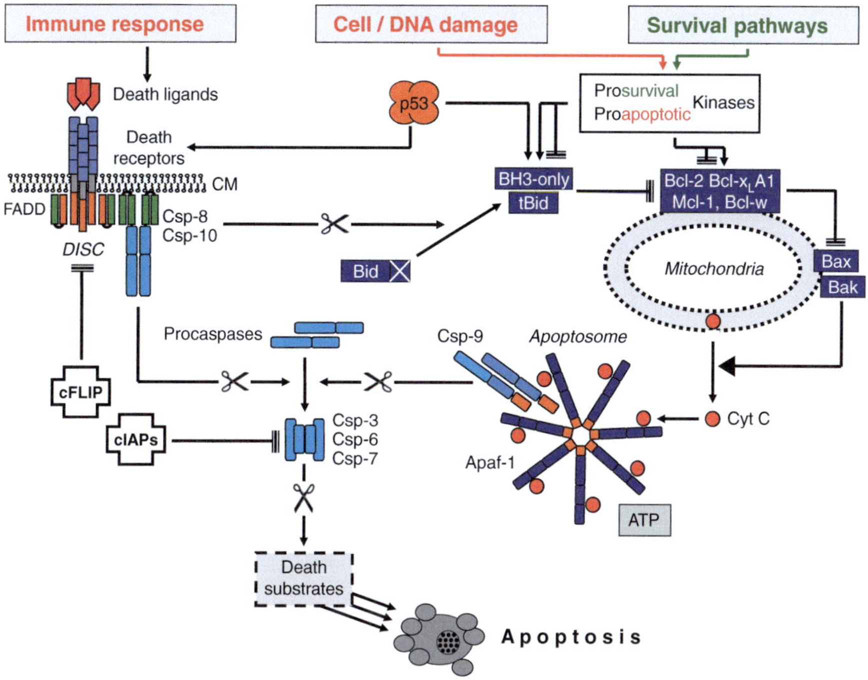

Fig. 10.2 Signaling pathways for regulation of apoptosis. Extrinsic proapoptotic pathways (*left*) are triggered by death ligands released from immune cells in an immune response, whereas intrinsic proapoptotic pathways (*right side*) are initiated upon cellular damage via p53 activation or via proapoptotic kinases. Kinases are affected in the opposite way by survival pathways, e.g., the BRAF-initiated MAP kinase pathway. Prosurvival and proapoptotic kinases in particular control the activity of antiapoptotic Bcl-2 proteins (Bcl-2, Bcl-x_L, A1, Mcl-1, and Bcl-w) as well as the proapoptotic BH3-only proteins. Two multiprotein complexes, the death-inducing signaling complex (DISC) and the apoptosome are employed for caspase activation. Caspase 8/10 binding to the DISC is mediated by the adaptor protein FADD and the interaction of death domains (*orange*) and death effector domains (*green*), while binding of caspase-9 to the apoptosome is mediated by the caspase recruitment domains (*orange*). The caspase-8/-10 homolog cFLIP inhibits activation of the initiator caspases at the DISC, while cIAPs block effector caspases (-3, -6, -7). *FADD*, Fas-associated death domain; *Csp*, caspase; *tBid*, truncated Bid; *APAF-1*, apoptotic protease-activating factor-1; *ATP*, adenosine triphosphate; *Cyt C*, cytochrome C; *BH3-only*, BH3-only proteins. *c-FLIP* cellular homolog of FLICE-inhibitory protein, *c-IAPs* cellular inhibitor of apoptosis proteins, *CM* cytoplasmic membrane. Scissors indicate protease activity

Apoptosis deficiency is based on an inactivation of proapoptotic factors or the activation of antiapoptotic factors. Both options are linked to activated survival pathways. In normal tissues, homeostasis is maintained by a well-balanced equilibrium of cell proliferation and cell death. In this way, programmed cell death (apoptosis) represents an active cellular process, whose physiological endpoint is phagocytosis by macrophages or neighboring cells (Kerr et al. 1972). Due to this key function, apoptosis pathways are tightly regulated. Various cellular options for counter-regulation, necessary for the survival of normal cells, abet tumor cells to escape from apoptosis control.

10.2 Intrinsic Apoptosis Pathways

Intrinsic proapoptotic pathways can be induced by different kinds of cellular stress situations as by DNA damage, hypoxia, oncogene activation, or other intrinsic problems. They can be mediated by the tumor suppressor and transcription factor p53 or by proapoptotic kinases (Fig. 10.2). P53 is negatively regulated by ubiquitin ligation through HDM-2 resulting in its early degradation. In response to cellular stress situations, it is stabilized by different kinds of protein modifications as by phosphorylation. Apoptosis by p53 is related to transcriptional upregulation of death receptors and proapoptotic Bcl-2 proteins as Bax, Noxa, Puma, Bik/Nbk, and Bid (Zuckerman et al. 2009).

The large family of pro- and antiapoptotic Bcl-2 proteins control mitochondria-mediated apoptosis pathways. Bcl-2 proteins are characterized by up to four conserved Bcl-2 homology domains (BH1–BH4) (Fig. 10.3). Whereas most antiapoptotic proteins as Bcl-2 share all four domains, proapoptotic proteins subdivide in multidomain proteins as Bax, Bak, and Bok which enclose BH1, BH2, and BH3 as well as the large subfamily of BH3-only proteins (Chipuk et al. 2010). Other proteins reveal further domain combinations. Thus, Bcl-x_S (BH3, BH4) and Bcl-x_{AK} (BH2, BH4), which derive from the *Bcl-x* gene by alternative splicing, showed characteristic proapoptotic functions in melanoma cells by activating the Bak or the Bax and Bak pathway, respectively (Plötz et al. 2012a, b).

Multidomain proapoptotic proteins as Bax and Bak are believed to induce pores in mitochondrial membranes for release of mitochondrial factors, such as cytochrome C. They are negatively controlled by antiapoptotic Bcl-2 family members,

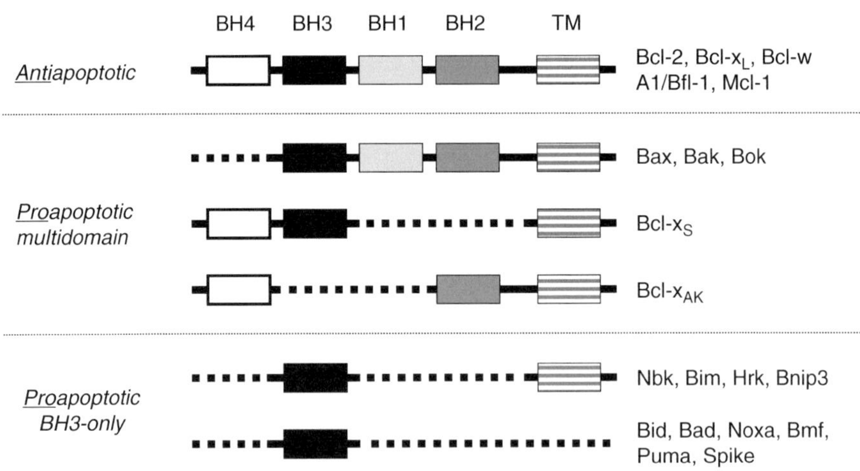

Fig. 10.3 Structure of pro- and antiapoptotic Bcl-2 proteins. A schematic view is given of the principle structures of Bcl-2 proteins. The presence of up to four Bcl-2 homology domains (*BH*) is indicated. Unlike the schematic view, Bcl-2 proteins have variable lengths. Besides the main groups of multidomain antiapoptotic, multidomain proapoptotic (Bax/Bak group), and BH3-only proteins, two proapoptotic splice variants of Bcl-x with an unusual domain structure are shown. BH3-only proteins may have a transmembrane domain (*TM*) or not

which neutralize proapoptotic Bcl-2 proteins through heterodimerization, thus protecting the mitochondrial membrane integrity. Finally, BH3-only proteins function as sensors in apoptosis control. When activated by cellular stress signals, they bind to antiapoptotic Bcl-2 proteins thus to free Bax and Bak. Some were even reported to activate Bax in a direct way as Bid and Bim (Chipuk et al. 2010).

Bax and Bak are mutually exchangeable, seen in mice deficient for either one of the two. These mice are viable, whereas the double knockout strongly impairs developmental apoptosis, resulting in perinatal death. Also cultured cells deficient for both proteins are largely apoptosis-resistant (Lindsten et al. 2000). Deficiency of Bcl-x_L is also lethal, whereas Bcl-2 knockout mice are viable, but reveal developmental defects particularly concerning increased apoptosis in melanocyte precursors, thus underlining the particular role of Bcl-2 for the melanocytic lineage (Korsmeyer 1999).

The balance between pro- and antiapoptotic Bcl-2 proteins controls the permeability of the outer mitochondrial membrane. Once a certain threshold is reached, a rapid release of mitochondrial intermembrane factors is induced, which exert specific proapoptotic functions in the cytoplasm, as reported for cytochrome C, endonuclease G, AIF (apoptosis-inducing factor), Smac/DIABLO, and HtrA2/Omi. Thus, cytochrome C released into the cytosol induces formation of the apoptosome, a protein complex consisting of Apaf-1, ATP, cytochrome C, and the initiator caspase-9 (Chipuk et al. 2010). Here, caspase-9 is activated by induced proximity, which initiates a subsequent caspase signaling cascade. Caspases (aspartate-specific cysteine proteases) represent hallmarks in apoptosis. They are synthesized as inactive zymogens and activate each other by proteolytic processing. Proapoptotic caspases separate in initiator caspases (2, 8, 9, and 10) and effector caspases (3, 6, and 7), which have a large number of cellular target proteins (Pop and Salvesen 2009) (Fig. 10.2).

10.3 Extrinsic Apoptotic Pathways

Cytotoxic T-lymphocytes and natural killer cells employ death ligands as tumor necrosis factor (TNF-α), CD95L/FasL, and TNF-related apoptosis-inducing ligand (TRAIL), which trigger extrinsic apoptosis in target cells (Fig. 10.2) (Chan and Housseau 2008). They bind to four death receptors (TNF-R1, CD95, TRAIL-R1/DR4, and TRAIL-R2/DR5), whereas decoy receptors (DcR 1–3 and OPG) do not forward the proapoptotic signal (Fig. 10.4). Characteristic for the proapoptotic program is receptor oligomerization upon ligand binding and formation of membrane-bound, death-inducing signaling complexes (DISC). Here, attached initiator caspases (8 and 10) become activated due to induced proximity and/or autocatalytic proteolysis. Besides their proapoptotic function, death receptors may also activate NF-kB and MAPK-related pathways, and NF-kB is also activated by TNF-R2, which does not trigger caspases (Guicciardi and Gores 2009) (Fig. 10.4). The NF-kB-mediated transcriptional activation of antiapoptotic proteins as c-FLIP, Bcl-x_L, and c-IAPs may enable a balanced response to death signals (Karin 2006).

Thus, both extrinsic and intrinsic pathways result in the activation of initiator caspases, which in turn promote a caspase cascade leading to active effector

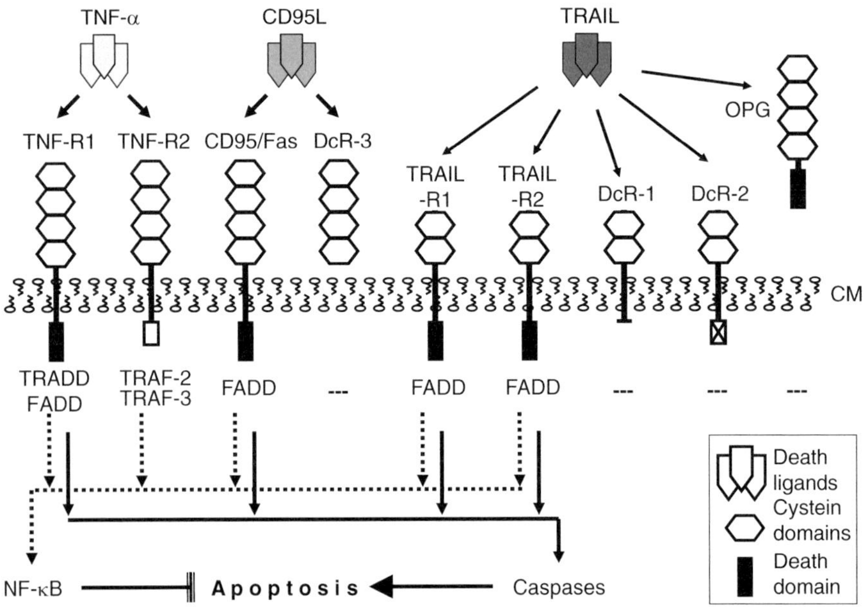

Fig. 10.4 Death receptors and death ligands. Receptors of TNF-α, CD95L/FasL, and TRAIL are shown. They enclose four death receptors, characterized by the death domain (black), four decoy receptors (DcR, OPG), and TNF-R2. While the death domain is lacking or not functional in DcR-1 and DcR-2, respectively, DcR-3 and OPG lack a functional transmembrane domain. Finally, the cytoplasma domain of TNF-R2 does not trigger DISC formation but a complex to activate NF-kB. The four death receptors can activate both pathways (caspases and NF-kB). *FADD*, Fas-associated death domain; *TRADD*, TNF receptor-associated death domain; *TRAF*, TNF receptor-associated factor; *CM*, cytoplasma membrane. Outside the cytoplasma membrane, the receptors have 2–4 cysteine-rich domains (hexagons)

caspases. These cleave a large subset of cellular proteins (death substrates) including enzymes for DNA repair and modification as well as signaling and structural proteins, in this way reprogramming the cell for apoptosis (Fischer et al. 2003). Crosstalk between the pathways may lead to mutual enhancements, e.g., transactivation of death receptors by p53 or cleavage and activation of the proapoptotic Bcl-2 protein Bid by caspase-8. Truncated Bid is a BH3-only protein and involved in activation of the mitochondrial pathway (Fig. 10.2).

10.4 Less Obvious Roles of p53 in Melanoma

The tumor suppressor gene p53 is mutated in around 50 % of human cancer cases but only in 10–20 % of human melanoma (Mar et al. 2013). Nevertheless, the tumor-suppressive function of p53 in melanoma cells is largely lost. The important role of p53 for suppression of melanoma growth is suggested by the rapid proliferation of BRAFV600E-mutated melanocytes on loss of p53 function (Yu et al. 2009). Inactivation of the p53 pathway may also result from overexpression/amplification of its antagonists MDM2 and MDM4 as well as from mutation/deletion of CDKN4, which encodes the cell cycle inhibitor p16 as well as the MDM2 inhibitor $p14^{ARF}$ (Lu et al. 2014).

In addition, p53 transcriptional activity may be modulated. Thus, p53 frequently found accumulated in the nucleus of melanoma cells seems to exhibit only little transcriptional activity, likely indicative for a post-translational inactivation. Accordingly, melanoma cell lines with wild-type p53 did not respond to exogeneous p53 overexpression, whereas apoptosis was induced in p53-mutated melanoma cells by overexpression of a functional p53 (Satyamoorthy et al. 2000). Transcriptional activity of p53 is critically modulated by the evolutionarily conserved ASPP family of proteins. Thus, phosphorylated nuclear iASPP was found in 90 % of wild-type p53-expressing melanoma cell lines. Compared to unphosphorylated cytoplasmic iASPP, phosphorylated nuclear iASPP binds p53 better and is more potent in inhibiting p53's apoptotic function. Furthermore, high levels of phosphorylated nuclear iASPP are associated with poor survival in melanoma patients (Lu et al. 2013).

10.5 Role of Caspase Downregulation and Inhibitor of Apoptosis Proteins

The initiator caspases 8 and 10, which are essential for death ligand-induced apoptosis (Fig. 10.2), are frequently downregulated in tumors, which may result from gene silencing by DNA methylation. In melanoma cell lines, both caspases are highly expressed but are downregulated in cells selected for TRAIL resistance (Kurbanov et al. 2007).

Many proapoptotic pathways merge at the level of effector caspases, which are suppressed by cIAPs (Nachmias et al. 2004). In melanoma, expression of survivin, livin/ML-IAP, and X-linked IAP (XIAP) correlated with drug resistance, progression, and survival, and their downregulation increased melanoma cell chemosensitivity in vitro and in xenotransplants (Yan et al. 2006). The antiapoptotic function of XIAP in melanoma cells, which is antagonized by Smac release, is suggested by an incomplete processing of caspase-3 upon TRAIL treatment. The role of the Smac/XIAP rheostat in TRAIL-induced apoptosis was proven by XIAP overexpression and/or by Smac knockdown, which both protected melanoma cells from TRAIL-induced apoptosis (Hornle et al. 2011; Quast et al. 2012; Berger et al. 2013). High XIAP activities thus appear as one of the major barriers for efficient apoptosis induction in melanoma (Quast et al. 2014).

10.6 The Role of Bcl-2 Proteins in Melanoma Apoptosis Resistance

The mitochondrial, proapoptotic pathway is critically controlled by three groups of Bcl-2 proteins (Figs. 10.2 and 10.3). The expression of both antiapoptotic proteins as Bcl-2, Bcl-x_L, and Mcl-1 as well as many proapoptotic proteins as Bax, Bak, Bid,

Bad, PUMA, and Noxa was reported in melanoma cells. A high Bcl-2/Bax ratio correlated to apoptosis resistance, and exogeneous Bcl-2 overexpression almost abrogated melanoma cell sensitivity for many strategies as CD95L, TRAIL, ceramide and kinase inhibitors (Eberle et al. 2007b; Quast et al. 2014). Expression and activity of antiapoptotic Bcl-2 proteins is controlled by different survival pathways (Fig. 10.2), e.g., Bcl-2 is controlled by microphthalmia-associated transcription factor (MITF) or Bcl-x_L is controlled by NF-kB (Eberle et al. 2007b; Karin 2006).

Despite the significant role of Bcl-2 in melanocyte cell survival, its contribution to chemoresistance of metastasized melanoma remains unclear because Bcl-2 levels did not correlate with prognosis in primary melanoma and even reduced expression was found in metastases, whereas Bcl-x_L and Mcl-1 were upregulated (Zhuang et al. 2007). On the other hand, several proapoptotic Bcl-2 proteins may be upregulated in course of chemotherapy or kinase inhibition. Thus, taurolidine-induced apoptosis in melanoma cells correlated with enhanced Bax and reduced Bcl-2 expression (Sun et al. 2007), or Puma and Bim were upregulated by BRAF inhibition (Beck et al. 2013; Berger et al. 2014). Particularly, the expression of proapoptotic Bcl-2 proteins as Bax and Bak appears of prognostic value, as their downregulation in primary melanomas was correlated with unfavorable prognosis (Fecker et al. 2006), and inactivation of Bax appeared as a critical step in TRAIL resistance of melanoma cells (Quast et al. 2014).

Thus, high expression of antiapoptotic Bcl-2 proteins in melanoma and/or low activity of proapoptotic family members may elevate the threshold for an activation of the mitochondrial pathway and may thus critically contribute to chemoresistance. In agreement, significant induction of apoptosis was enabled by overexpression of different proapoptotic Bcl-2 proteins in melanoma (Eberle et al. 2007b; Plötz et al. 2012a, b; Plötz et al. 2013).

10.7 Blockage of Death Receptor–Mediated Pathways in Melanoma

Despite a high immunoreactivity, proliferating melanomas withstand apoptosis induction by immune cells (Fig. 10.1). Expression of TNF-α, CD95L, and TRAIL was proven for melanoma-infiltrating lymphocytes (Thomas and Hersey 1998). This indicates a high selective pressure for melanomas to acquire death ligand resistance. Accordingly, molecular changes in the death receptor-mediated pathways are frequently seen. Thus, melanoma cell lines often reveal resistance to CD95 activation, and cultures of metastases were more resistant than those of primary tumors. Loss of CD95 expression and missense mutations in the death domain as well as high Bcl-2 or Mcl-1 expression have been related to resistance to CD95 (Chetoui et al. 2008; Eberle et al. 2007b).

Also, resistance to TNF-α and loss of TNF-R1 have been reported for melanoma cells, which may be correlated to promoter hypermethylation (Kaminski et al. 2004). In contrast, neither mutations of TRAIL death receptors nor involvement of decoy receptors (DcR-1, DcR-2) have been identified in melanoma cells so far. However, expression of TRAIL-R1, which mediates high TRAIL sensitivity in melanoma cells when expressed, was frequently lost. In contrast, TRAIL-R2 is constitutively expressed, but the downstream pathways may be inactive as shown in melanoma cell lines (Kurbanov et al. 2005). Inactivation of TRAIL-R2 may result from its decreased glycosylation or from high c-FLIP expression (Wagner et al. 2007; Geserick et al. 2008).

Whereas no clear correlation was found to the expression of antiapoptotic factors, TRAIL resistance in TRAIL-selected melanoma cells clearly correlated with downregulation of proapoptotic regulators as initiator caspases, DR4 and BH3-only proteins (Kurbanov et al. 2007). Furthermore, melanoma resistance to TRAIL was explained by three major steps, namely, high levels of antiapoptotic Bcl-2 proteins, high levels of inhibitor of apoptosis proteins (cIAPs), and suppressed Bax activity (Quast et al. 2014).

10.8 Roles of MAP Kinase Pathways in Apoptosis Resistance

Central signaling pathways downstream of growth factor receptors as of MAPKs, PI3K/Akt, and NF-kB are not only critically implicated in enhanced proliferation of cancer cells but also in their apoptosis resistance (see also Chap. 13). As seen by BRAF mutations, these survival pathways are activated in melanoma. They contribute to the control of a number of apoptosis regulators either by affecting the transcriptional level through regulation of respective transcription factors or by regulating the activity of apoptosis factors directly through phosphorylation (Eberle et al. 2007b).

High activity of the canonical MAPK pathway via RAF, MEK, and ERK in melanoma is mainly attributed to the activating mutations in *B-Raf* and *N-Ras* (Davies et al. 2002). Downstream are a multitude of transcription factors that also control the expression of many apoptosis regulators. For example, the transcription factor MITF plays a particular role in apoptosis resistance of melanoma cells due to its upregulation of Bcl-2 as well as the cIAP Livin (Dynek et al. 2008). Further transcription factors involved in apoptosis resistance have been identified within the Ets and CREB/ATF families, which may contribute to upregulation of also Bcl-2 or of Bcl-x_L downstream of MAPK activation (Eberle et al. 2007b) (see also Chap. 7). An example for the direct regulation of apoptosis factors by kinases is the inactivation of the BH3-only proteins, Bad, Bim, and Puma, through phosphorylation by MAPKs (Inamdar et al. 2010; Beck et al. 2013; Berger et al. 2014). Thus, selective BRAF inhibitors induced apoptosis and/or sensitized for proapoptotic strategies, e.g., for TRAIL (Beck et al. 2013; Berger et al. 2014). Similarly, targeting of the MAPK pathway downstream of BRAF as by MEK inhibitors induced apoptosis, sensitized melanoma cells for TRAIL, and reduced the growth of lung metastases in mice (Inamdar et al. 2010; Berger et al. 2014). These effects have been related to upregulation or activation of the BH3-only proteins Puma, Bim, and Bmf, downregulation of Mcl-1, as well as activation of Bax (VanBrocklin et al. 2009; Wang et al. 2007;

Quast et al. 2014). Thus, clinical efficiency of MAPK inhibitors appears as strongly related to enhanced apoptosis sensitivity, which may be further improved by combination therapies.

10.9 Targeting of the PI3K/Akt/mTOR Pathway

A central role in cell survival has been ascribed to the phosphoinositide 3-kinase (PI3K)/AKT pathway, which is related to increased chemoresistance in many tumors (see also Chap. 16). Akt may directly phosphorylate and inactivate several proapoptotic proteins such as Bax, Bad, and caspase-9, and may further inactivate proapoptotic transcription factors such as FoxO and p53. In addition, AKT is linked to the survival pathway of mTOR (mammalian target of rapamycin), which inhibits cell death pathways as apoptosis and autophagy (Stiles 2009). Melanomas reveal high immunoreactivity for activated, phosphorylated AKT, which may partly be related to mutations of its inhibitor phosphatase and tensin homolog on chromosome 10 (PTEN). Antiapoptotic activities of AKT have been described for melanoma cells, such as inactivation of Bad and activation of IKK (I-kB kinase) leading to a cross-activation of the NF-kB pathway. The critical role of the AKT survival pathway in melanoma was demonstrated by expression of a dominant negative AKT mutant, by its siRNA downregulation as well as by overexpression of PTEN, which all triggered apoptosis (Robertson 2005).

By using small molecule approaches, inhibition of PI3K-reduced melanoma growth in mice, particularly in combination with inhibition of MEK (Inamdar et al. 2010), and both AKT and mTOR inhibition consistently enhanced apoptosis and chemosensitivity of melanoma cells (Sinnberg et al. 2009). Also, the farnesyl transferase inhibitor lonafarnib, which inhibits mTOR signaling, enhanced sorafenib-induced apoptosis in melanoma cells, which was related to induction of ER stress and downregulation of Mcl-1 (Niessner et al. 2011). However, inhibitors of AKT as well as of mTOR did not result in significant clinical responses in metastatic melanoma patients, when used as monotherapy (Eberle et al. 2007b). But PI3K and AKT inhibitors showed synergistic enhancement of apoptosis in combination with TRAIL, which was explained by a novel so far not well described pathway that is based on the generation of reactive oxygen species (ROS) (Quast et al. 2013). Thus although inhibition of this pathway may not be sufficient by itself, combination strategies may be an option.

10.10 New Proapoptotic Strategies by BH3 Mimetics

To further improve the clinical efficiency of melanoma therapy, combinations of survival pathway inhibitors with proapoptotic strategies appear as highly promising. Frequently, chemotherapeutics were used in combinations, which cause cellular stress situations as DNA damage to trigger apoptosis via intrinsic pathways. A selective induction of apoptosis in cancer cells may, however, be more efficient and better tolerated.

When considering the important role of mitochondrial proapoptotic pathways in melanoma, approaches that target the Bcl-2 protein family appear of particular interest. Thus Bcl-2 antisense strategies have been applied, which revealed in vitro and in mouse models significant apoptosis induction and sensitization for chemotherapy. However, in clinical trials in melanoma, the combination of Bcl-2 antisense with chemotherapy did not prove as effective enough (Bedikian et al. 2006). This may be related to the finding that Bcl-2 may be even downregulated in metastatic melanoma and may be substituted by other antiapoptotic Bcl-2 proteins (Zhuang et al. 2007). Thus, the simultaneous targeting of several antiapoptotic Bcl-2 proteins may be necessary. Alternatively, proapoptotic Bcl-2 proteins may be overexpressed to trigger the rheostat of pro- and antiapoptotic Bcl-2 proteins from the other side. The efficiency of such strategies has been demonstrated by plasmid or adenovirus-mediated overexpression of Bax, Bik/NBK, Bcl-x_S, Bcl-x_{AK}, and Bim (Eberle et al. 2007b; Plötz et al. 2012a, b, 2013).

Of particular interest are effectors that mimic the BH3 domain of proapoptotic Bcl-2 proteins. BH3 is required for the interaction between proapoptotic Bcl-2 proteins and the hydrophobic pocket of antiapoptotic Bcl-2 proteins formed by BH1, BH2, and BH3. These are peptides or small molecules structurally related to BH3 domains of different proteins and may have the potential to block different antiapoptotic Bcl-2 proteins (Adams and Cory 2007; Plötz and Eberle 2014).

There are several preclinical reports on the effects of BH3 mimetics in melanoma. Thus, the natural BH3 mimetic gossypol, a compound of cotton seeds, induced cell death in melanoma cells with even higher efficacy than some chemotherapeutics (Shelley et al. 1999). Apoptosis resistance due to high levels of antiapoptotic Bcl-2 proteins was overcome by the BH3 mimetic TW-37 when used in combination with the MEK inhibitor U0126 (Verhaegen et al. 2006). A synergistic induction of mitochondrial apoptosis has been reported in melanoma cells by combination of the BH3 mimetic ABT-737 and the proteasome inhibitor MG-132, which resulted in simultaneous upregulation of Noxa (Miller et al. 2009). Efficient induction of apoptosis has also been described for the combination of ABT-737 and a Mcl-1 knockdown (Keuling et al. 2009). A combination of obatoclax, a BH3 mimetic with inhibitory activity against Mcl-1, with an ER stress-inducing compound resulted in marked induction of apoptosis in melanoma cells, which was dependent on Mcl-1 inhibition and again induction of Noxa (Jiang et al. 2009).

New BH3 mimetics designed by computer-based modeling are presently developed and more effective ones, preferentially targeting several antiapoptotic Bcl-2 proteins, may be expected in the future. Considering the high dependency of apoptosis induction in melanoma cells on the mitochondrial pathway, BH3 mimetics provide hope for an efficient targeting of melanoma (Plötz and Eberle 2014; Liu et al. 2015). The complex mutual regulation of Bcl-2 proteins, however, needs further clarification in melanoma to optimize these approaches.

10.11 TRAIL as a Combination Partner

As suggested by the high immunoreactivity of melanoma (Fig. 10.1) and by its frequent resistance to death ligands (Kurbanov et al. 2007), strategies for enhancing death ligand sensitivity and for overcoming resistance appear as also highly promising. In contrast to chemotherapy, death ligands trigger apoptosis independently of p53 and thus may overcome drug resistance related to p53 inactivation. Although CD95 agonistic antibodies and TNF-α have shown efficiency in mouse xenotransplants, their application in patients is largely prevented due to systemic inflammation (TNF-α) or liver toxicity (CD95L) (Kelley and Ashkenazi 2004; Trauth et al. 1989). Their selective expression in gene therapeutic approaches, however, remains an alternative strategy. Thus, expression of CD95L prevented growth of melanoma xenotransplants in mice (Eberle et al. 2003), and its selective expression via melanoma-selective replication-competent adenoviral vectors appeared as an efficient approach for targeting melanoma cells (Fecker et al. 2010).

As compared to TNF-α and CD95L, systemic application of TRAIL is much better tolerated. Induction of apoptosis and eradication of xenotransplants were demonstrated in a variety of tumor models, whereas toxicity for normal cells remained at a low level. Both TRAIL receptors (DR4 and DR5) may be targeted by recombinant TRAIL or by selective agonistic antibodies, which showed efficiency and synergistic effects with chemotherapy in preclinical studies. TRAIL also demonstrated antitumor activities in clinical trials; it appeared, however, not as efficient enough when used as monotherapy, as shown in a phase III trial with agonistic DR4 antibodies for therapy of patients with refractory colorectal cancer (Newsom-Davis et al. 2009; Trarbach et al. 2010).

All melanoma cell lines express TRAIL-R1/DR5, which may or may not mediate TRAIL sensitivity. However, all melanoma cell lines that have TRAIL-R1/DR4 in addition revealed pronounced sensitivity to TRAIL. Importantly, the majority of primary melanomas are DR4-positive, as proven by immunohistochemistry, thus suggesting principle TRAIL sensitivity (Kurbanov et al. 2005). However, DR4-positive melanoma cells respond to TRAIL treatment with an inducible TRAIL resistance that was correlated to downregulation of DR4 and initiator caspases as well as to an inactivation of Bax (Kurbanov et al. 2007; Quast et al. 2014). Chemotherapy, which may upregulate death receptors (Singh et al. 2003), proteasome inhibitors, which may prevent death receptor degradation (Kurbanov et al. 2007) or IFN-γ, which may upregulate initiator caspases (Fulda and Debatin 2006), may thus be helpful in countering TRAIL resistance. Furthermore, several signal pathway inhibitors showed high efficiency in combination with TRAIL as they mediated Bax activation (Quast et al. 2014).

Indeed, melanoma cells could be sensitized for TRAIL by multiple different strategies, e.g., resveratrol (Ivanov et al. 2008), chemotherapeutics (Fecker et al. 2011), the multi-kinase inhibitor indirubin (Berger et al. 2011), the ion channel inhibitor TRAM-34 (Quast et al. 2012), IKK inhibition (Berger et al. 2013), PI3K or AKT inhibition (Quast et al. 2013) as well as BRAF and MEK inhibition (Berger et al. 2014). A common principle of TRAIL sensitization appeared to be the inhibition of the cell cycle by different inhibitors and the activation of Bax (Quast et al. 2015). Due to the multiple strategies that could sensitize melanoma cells for TRAIL, this ligand appears as an ideal combination partner for melanoma therapy.

References

Adams JM, Cory S (2007) The Bcl-2 apoptotic switch in cancer development and therapy. Oncogene 26:1324–1337

Bedikian AY, Millward M, Pehamberger H, Conry R, Gore M, Trefzer U, Pavlick AC, DeConti R, Hersh EM, Hersey P, Kirkwood JM, Haluska FG (2006) Bcl-2 antisense (oblimersen sodium) plus dacarbazine in patients with advanced melanoma: the oblimersen melanoma study group. J Clin Oncol 24:4738–4745

Beck D, Niessner H, Smalley KS, Flaherty K, Paraiso KH, Busch C, Sinnberg T, Vasseur S, Iovanna JL, Drießen S, Stork B, Wesselborg S, Schaller M, Biedermann T, Bauer J, Lasithiotakis K, Weide B, Eberle J, Schittek B, Schadendorf D, Garbe C, Kulms D, Meier F (2013) Vemurafenib potently induces endoplasmic reticulum stress-mediated apoptosis in BRAFV600E melanoma cells. Sci Signal 6:ra7

Berger A, Quast SA, Plotz M, Hein M, Kunz M, Langer P, Eberle J (2011) Sensitization of melanoma cells for death ligand-induced apoptosis by an indirubin derivative – enhancement of both extrinsic and intrinsic apoptosis pathways. Biochem Pharmacol 81:71–81

Berger A, Quast SA, Plötz M, Kammermeier A, Eberle J (2013) Sensitization of melanoma cells for TRAIL-induced apoptosis by BMS-345541 correlates with altered phosphorylation and activation of Bax. Cell Death Dis 4, e477

Berger A, Quast SA, Plötz M, Kuhn NF, Trefzer U, Eberle J (2014) RAF inhibition overcomes resistance to TRAIL-induced apoptosis in melanoma cells. J Invest Dermatol 134:430–440

Chan CW, Housseau F (2008) The 'kiss of death' by dendritic cells to cancer cells. Cell Death Differ 15:58–69

Chen G, Davies MA (2014) Targeted therapy resistance mechanisms and therapeutic implications in melanoma. Hematol Oncol Clin North Am 28:523–536

Chetoui N, Sylla K, Gagnon-Houde JV, Alcaide-Loridan C, Charron D, Al Daccak R, Aoudjit F (2008) Down-regulation of mcl-1 by small interfering RNA sensitizes resistant melanoma cells to fas-mediated apoptosis. Mol Cancer Res 6:42–52

Chipuk JE, Moldoveanu T, Llambi F, Parsons MJ, Green DR (2010) The BCL-2 family reunion. Mol Cell 37:299–310

Davies H, Bignell GR, Cox C, Stephens P, Edkins S, Clegg S, Teague J, Woffendin H, Garnett MJ, Bottomley W, Davis N, Dicks E, Ewing R, Floyd Y, Gray K, Hall S, Hawes R, Hughes J, Kosmidou V, Menzies A, Mould C, Parker A, Stevens C, Watt S, Hooper S, Wilson R, Jayatilake H, Gusterson BA, Cooper C, Shipley J, Hargrave D, Pritchard-Jones K, Maitland N, Chenevix-Trench G, Riggins GJ, Bigner DD, Palmieri G, Cossu A, Flanagan A, Nicholson A, Ho JW, Leung SY, Yuen ST, Weber BL, Seigler HF, Darrow TL, Paterson H, Marais R, Marshall CJ, Wooster R, Stratton MR, Futreal PA (2002) Mutations of the BRAF gene in human cancer. Nature 417:949–954

Dynek JN, Chan SM, Liu J, Zha J, Fairbrother WJ, Vucic D (2008) Microphthalmia-associated transcription factor is a critical transcriptional regulator of melanoma inhibitor of apoptosis in melanomas. Cancer Res 68:3124–3132

Eberle J, Fecker LF, Hossini AM, Wieder T, Daniel PT, Orfanos CE, Geilen CC (2003) CD95/Fas signaling in human melanoma cells: conditional expression of CD95L/FasL overcomes the intrinsic apoptosis resistance of malignant melanoma and inhibits growth and progression of human melanoma xenotransplants. Oncogene 22:9131–9141

Eberle J, Fecker LF, Forschner T, Ulrich C, Röwert-Huber J, Stockfleth E (2007a) Apoptosis pathways as promising targets for skin cancer therapy. Br J Dermatol 156(S3):18–24

Eberle J, Kurbanov BM, Hossini AM, Trefter U, Fecker LF (2007b) Overcoming apoptosis deficiency of melanoma – hope for new therapeutic approaches. Drug Resist Updat 10:218–234
Fang L, Lonsdorf AS, Hwang ST (2008) Immunotherapy for advanced melanoma. J Invest Dermatol 128:2596–2605
Fecker LF, Geilen CC, Tchernev G, Trefzer U, Assaf C, Kurbanov BM, Schwarz C, Daniel PT, Eberle J (2006) Loss of proapoptotic Bcl-2-related multidomain proteins in primary melanomas is associated with poor prognosis. J Invest Dermatol 126:1366–1371
Fecker LF, Ruckert S, Kurbanov BM, Schmude M, Stockfleth E, Fechner H, Eberle J (2011) Efficient melanoma cell killing and reduced melanoma growth in mice by a selective replicating adenovirus armed with TNF-related apoptosis inducing ligand. Hum Gene Ther 22, PMID 20977303
Fecker LF, Schmude M, Jost S, Hossini AM, Pico AH, Wang X, Schwarz C, Fechner H, Eberle J (2010) Efficient and selective tumor cell lysis and induction of apoptosis in melanoma cells by a conditional replication-competent CD95L adenovirus. Exp Dermatol 19:e56–e66
Fischer U, Janicke RU, Schulze-Osthoff K (2003) Many cuts to ruin: a comprehensive update of caspase substrates. Cell Death Differ 10:76–100
Fulda S, Debatin KM (2006) 5-Aza-2′-deoxycytidine and IFN-gamma cooperate to sensitize for TRAIL-induced apoptosis by upregulating caspase-8. Oncogene 25:5125–5133
Garbe C, Peris K, Hauschild A, Saiag P, Middleton M, Spatz A, Grob JJ, Malvehy J, Newton-Bishop J, Stratigos A, Pehamberger H, Eggermont AM, European Dermatology Forum, European Association of Dermato-Oncology, European Organization of Research and Treatment of Cancer (2012) Diagnosis and treatment of melanoma. European consensus-based interdisciplinary guideline - update. Eur J Cancer 48:2375–2390
Geserick P, Drewniok C, Hupe M, Haas TL, Diessenbacher P, Sprick MR, Schon MP, Henkler F, Gollnick H, Walczak H, Leverkus M (2008) Suppression of cFLIP is sufficient to sensitize human melanoma cells to TRAIL- and CD95L-mediated apoptosis. Oncogene 27:3211–3220
Guicciardi ME, Gores GJ (2009) Life and death by death receptors. FASEB J 23:1625–1637
Hanahan D, Weinberg RA (2011) Hallmarks of cancer: the next generation. Cell 144:646–674
Hornle M, Peters N, Thayaparasingham B, Vorsmann H, Kashkar H, Kulms D (2011) Caspase-3 cleaves XIAP in a positive feedback loop to sensitize melanoma cells to TRAIL-induced apoptosis. Oncogene 30:575–587
Hughes T, Klairmont M, Sharfman WH, Kaufman HL (2015) Interleukin-2, ipilimumab, and anti-PD-1: clinical management and the evolving role of immunotherapy for the treatment of patients with metastatic melanoma. Cancer Biol Ther 29, Epub ahead of print
Inamdar GS, Madhunapantula SV, Robertson GP (2010) Targeting the MAPK pathway in melanoma: why some approaches succeed and other fail. Biochem Pharmacol 80:624–637
Ivanov VN, Partridge MA, Johnson GE, Huang SX, Zhou H, Hei TK (2008) Resveratrol sensitizes melanomas to TRAIL through modulation of antiapoptotic gene expression. Exp Cell Res 314:1163–1176
Jiang CC, Wroblewski D, Yang F, Hersey P, Zhang XD (2009) Human melanoma cells under endoplasmic reticulum stress are more susceptible to apoptosis induced by the BH3 mimetic obatoclax. Neoplasia 11:945–955
Kaminski R, Kozar K, Niderla J, Grzela T, Wilczynski G, Skierski JS, Koronkiewicz M, Jakobisiak M, Golab J (2004) Demethylating agent 5-aza-2′-deoxycytidine enhances expression of TNFRI and promotes TNF-mediated apoptosis in vitro and in vivo. Oncol Rep 12:509–516
Karin M (2006) Nuclear factor-kappaB in cancer development and progression. Nature 441:431–436
Kelley SK, Ashkenazi A (2004) Targeting death receptors in cancer with Apo2L/TRAIL. Curr Opin Pharmacol 4:333–339
Kerr JF, Wyllie AH, Currie AR (1972) Apoptosis: a basic biological phenomenon with wide-ranging implications in tissue kinetics. Br J Cancer 26:239–257
Keuling AM, Felton KE, Parker AA, Akbari M, Andrew SE, Tron VA (2009) RNA silencing of Mcl-1 enhances ABT-737-mediated apoptosis in melanoma: role for a caspase-8-dependent pathway. PLoS One 4, e6651

Korsmeyer SJ (1999) BCL-2 gene family and the regulation of programmed cell death. Cancer Res 59:1693s–1700s

Kurbanov BM, Fecker LF, Geilen CC, Sterry W, Eberle J (2007) Resistance of melanoma cells to TRAIL does not result from upregulation of antiapoptotic proteins by NF-kappaB but is related to downregulation of initiator caspases and DR4. Oncogene 26:3364–3377

Kurbanov BM, Geilen CC, Fecker LF, Orfanos CE, Eberle J (2005) Efficient TRAIL-R1/DR4-mediated apoptosis in melanoma cells by tumor necrosis factor-related apoptosis-inducing ligand (TRAIL). J Invest Dermatol 125:1010–1019

Lindsten T, Ross AJ, King A, Zong WX, Rathmell JC, Shiels HA, Ulrich E, Waymire KG, Mahar P, Frauwirth K, Chen Y, Wei M, Eng VM, Adelman DM, Simon MC, Ma A, Golden JA, Evan G, Korsmeyer SJ, MacGregor GR, Thompson CB (2000) The combined functions of proapoptotic Bcl-2 family members bak and bax are essential for normal development of multiple tissues. Mol Cell 6:1389–1399

Liu Y, Xie M, Song T, Sheng H, Yu X, Zhang Z (2015) A novel BH3 mimetic efficiently induces apoptosis in melanoma cells through direct binding to anti-apoptotic Bcl-2 family proteins, including phosphorylated Mcl-1. Pigment Cell Melanoma Res 28:161–170

Lu M, Miller P, Lu X (2014) Restoring the tumour suppressive function of p53 as a parallel strategy in melanoma therapy. FEBS Lett 588:2616–2621

Lu M, Breyssens H, Salter V, Zhong S, Hu Y, Baer C, Ratnayaka I, Sullivan A, Brown NR, Endicott J, Knapp S, Kessler BM, Middleton MR, Siebold C, Jones EY, Sviderskaya EV, Cebon J, John T, Caballero OL, Goding CR, Lu X (2013) Restoring p53 function in human melanoma cells by inhibiting MDM2 and cyclin B1/CDK1-phosphorylated nuclear iASPP. Cancer Cell 23:618–633

Mar VJ, Wong SQ, Li J, Scolyer RA, McLean C, Papenfuss AT, Tothill RW, Kakavand H, Mann GJ, Thompson JF, Behren A, Cebon JS, Wolfe R, Kelly JW, Dobrovic A, McArthur GA (2013) BRAF/NRAS wild-type melanomas have a high mutation load correlating with histologic and molecular signatures of UV damage. Clin Cancer Res 19:4589–4598

Martinez-Lostao L, de Miguel D, Al-Wasaby S, Gallego-Lleyda A, Anel A (2015) Death ligands and granulysin: mechanisms of tumor cell death induction and therapeutic opportunities. Immunotherapy 7:883–892

Menzies AM, Long GV (2014) Systemic treatment for BRAF-mutant melanoma: where do we go next? Lancet Oncol 15:e371–e381

Miller LA, Goldstein NB, Johannes WU, Walton CH, Fujita M, Norris DA, Shellman YG (2009) BH3 mimetic ABT-737 and a proteasome inhibitor synergistically kill melanomas through noxa-dependent apoptosis. J Invest Dermatol 129:964–971

Nachmias B, Ashhab Y, Ben Yehuda D (2004) The inhibitor of apoptosis protein family (IAPs): an emerging therapeutic target in cancer. Semin Cancer Biol 14:231–243

Newsom-Davis T, Prieske S, Walczak H (2009) Is TRAIL the holy grail of cancer therapy? Apoptosis 14:607–623

Niessner H, Beck D, Sinnberg T, Lasithiotakis K, Maczey E, Gogel J, Venturelli S, Berger A, Mauthe M, Toulany M, Flaherty K, Schaller M, Schadendorf D, Proikas-Cezanne T, Schittek B, Garbe C, Kulms D, Meier F (2011) The farnesyl transferase inhibitor lonafarnib inhibits mTOR signaling and enforces sorafenib-induced apoptosis in melanoma cells. J Invest Dermatol 131:468–479

Plötz M, Gillissen B, Hossini AM, Daniel PT, Eberle J (2012a) Disruption of the VDAC2-Bak interaction by Bcl-x(S) mediates efficient induction of apoptosis in melanoma cells. Cell Death Differ 19:1928–1938

Plötz M, Hossini AM, Gillissen B, Daniel PT, Stockfleth E, Eberle J (2012b) Mutual regulation of Bcl-2 proteins independent of the BH3 domain as shown by the BH3-lacking protein Bcl-x(AK). PLoS One 7, e34549

Plötz M, Gillissen B, Quast SA, Berger A, Daniel PT, Eberle J (2013) The BH3-only protein Bim(L) overrides Bcl-2-mediated apoptosis resistance in melanoma cells. Cancer Lett 335:100–108

Plötz M, Eberle J (2014) BH3-only proteins: possible proapoptotic triggers for melanoma therapy. Exp Dermatol 23:375–378

Pop C, Salvesen GS (2009) Human caspases: activation, specificity, and regulation. J Biol Chem 284:21777–21781
Quast SA, Berger A, Buttstädt N, Friebel K, Schönherr R, Eberle J (2012) General Sensitization of melanoma cells for TRAIL-induced apoptosis by the potassium channel inhibitor TRAM-34 depends on release of SMAC. PLoS One 7, e39290
Quast SA, Berger A, Eberle J (2013) ROS-dependent phosphorylation of Bax by wortmannin sensitizes melanoma cells for TRAIL-induced apoptosis. Cell Death Dis 4, e839
Quast SA, Berger A, Plötz M, Eberle J (2014) Sensitization of melanoma cells for TRAIL-induced apoptosis by activation of mitochondrial pathways via Bax. Eur J Cell Biol 93:42–48
Quast SA, Steinhorst K, Plötz M, Eberle J (2015) Sensitization of melanoma cells for death ligand TRAIL is based on cell cycle arrest, ROS production, and activation of proapoptotic Bcl-2 proteins. J Invest Dermatol 135:2794–2804
Robertson GP (2005) Functional and therapeutic significance of Akt deregulation in malignant melanoma. Cancer Metastasis Rev 24:273–285
Satyamoorthy K, Chehab NH, Waterman MJ, Lien MC, El Deiry WS, Herlyn M, Halazonetis TD (2000) Aberrant regulation and function of wild-type p53 in radioresistant melanoma cells. Cell Growth Differ 11:467–474
Shelley MD, Hartley L, Fish RG, Groundwater P, Morgan JJG, Mort D, Mason M, Evans A (1999) Stereo-specific cytotoxic effects of gossypol enantiomers and gossypolone in tumour cell lines. Cancer Lett 135:171–180
Siegel R, Ma J, Zou Z, Jemal A (2014) Cancer statistics 2014. CA Cancer J Clin 64:9–29
Singh TR, Shankar S, Chen X, Asim M, Srivastava RK (2003) Synergistic interactions of chemotherapeutic drugs and tumor necrosis factor-related apoptosis-inducing ligand/Apo-2 ligand on apoptosis and on regression of breast carcinoma in vivo. Cancer Res 63:5390–5400
Sinnberg T, Lasithiotakis K, Niessner H, Schittek B, Flaherty KT, Kulms D, Maczey E, Campos M, Gogel J, Garbe C, Meier F (2009) Inhibition of PI3K-AKT-mTOR signaling sensitizes melanoma cells to cisplatin and temozolomide. J Invest Dermatol 129:1500–1515
Stiles BL (2009) PI-3-K and AKT: onto the mitochondria. Adv Drug Deliv Rev 61:1276–1282
Sun BS, Wang JH, Liu LL, Gong SL, Redmond HP (2007) Taurolidine induces apoptosis of murine melanoma cells in vitro and in vivo by modulation of the Bcl-2 family proteins. J Surg Oncol 96(3):241–248
Thomas WD, Hersey P (1998) TNF-related apoptosis-inducing ligand (TRAIL) induces apoptosis in Fas ligand-resistant melanoma cells and mediates CD4 T cell killing of target cells. J Immunol 161:2195–2200
Trarbach T, Moehler M, Heinemann V, Kohne CH, Przyborek M, Schulz C, Sneller V, Gallant G, Kanzler S (2010) Phase II trial of mapatumumab, a fully human agonistic monoclonal antibody that targets and activates the tumour necrosis factor apoptosis-inducing ligand receptor-1 (TRAIL-R1), in patients with refractory colorectal cancer. Br J Cancer 102:506–512
Trauth BC, Klas C, Peters AM, Matzku S, Moller P, Falk W, Debatin KM, Krammer PH (1989) Monoclonal antibody-mediated tumor regression by induction of apoptosis. Science 245:301–305
VanBrocklin MW, Verhaegen M, Soengas MS, Holmen SL (2009) Mitogen-activated protein kinase inhibition induces translocation of Bmf to promote apoptosis in melanoma. Cancer Res 69:1985–1994
Verhaegen M, Bauer JA, de la Vega CM, Wang G, Wolter KG, Brenner JC, Nikolovska-Coleska Z, Bengtson A, Nair R, Elder JT, Van BM, Carey TE, Bradford CR, Wang S, Soengas MS (2006) A novel BH3 mimetic reveals a mitogen-activated protein kinase-dependent mechanism of melanoma cell death controlled by p53 and reactive oxygen species. Cancer Res 66:11348–11359
Wagner KW, Punnoose EA, Januario T, Lawrence DA, Pitti RM, Lancaster K, Lee D, von Goetz M, Yee SF, Totpal K, Huw L, Katta V, Cavet G, Hymowitz SG, Amler L, Ashkenazi A (2007) Death-receptor O-glycosylation controls tumor-cell sensitivity to the proapoptotic ligand Apo2L/TRAIL. Nat Med 13:1070–1077

Wang YF, Jiang CF, Kiejda KF, Gillespie SF, Zhang XF, Hersey P (2007) Apoptosis induction in human melanoma cells by inhibition of MEK is caspase-independent and mediated by the Bcl-2 family members PUMA, Bim, and Mcl-1. Clin Cancer Res 13:4934–4942

Yan H, Thomas J, Liu T, Raj D, London N, Tandeski T, Leachman SA, Lee RM, Grossman D (2006) Induction of melanoma cell apoptosis and inhibition of tumor growth using a cell-permeable survivin antagonist. Oncogene 25:6968–6974

Yu H, McDaid R, Lee J, Possik P, Li L, Kumar SM, Elder DE, Van Belle P, Gimotty P, Guerra M, Hammond R, Nathanson KL, Dalla Palma M, Herlyn M, Xu X (2009) The role of BRAF mutation and p53 inactivation during transformation of a subpopulation of primary human melanocytes. Am J Pathol 174:2367–2377

Zhuang L, Lee CS, Scolyer RA, McCarthy SW, Zhang XD, Thompson JF, Hersey P (2007) Mcl-1, Bcl-XL and Stat3 expression are associated with progression of melanoma whereas Bcl-2, AP-2 and MITF levels decrease during progression of melanoma. Mod Pathol 20:416–426

Zuckerman V, Wolyniec K, Sionov RV, Haupt S, Haupt Y (2009) Tumour suppression by p53: the importance of apoptosis and cellular senescence. J Pathol 219:3–15

Senescence 11

Helen Rizos, Sebastian Haferkamp, and Lyndee L. Scurr

11.1 Introduction

Cellular senescence is regarded as an intrinsic stress response mechanism that limits the proliferative lifespan of cells. Senescence is induced by various signals, including telomere attrition (a response often referred to as replicative senescence), activated oncogenes (a process known as oncogene-induced senescence), DNA damage, oxidative lesions, and suboptimal culture conditions (reviewed in Collado and Serrano 2006). Irrespective of the initiating trigger, the hallmark of cellular senescence is permanent proliferative arrest, and whereas quiescent cells can be stimulated to resume proliferation, senescence cells cease to respond to mitogenic stimuli.

The limited proliferative capacity of normal human cells was recognised by Hayflick and Moorehead more than five decades ago (Hayflick and Moorhead 1961). They reported that primary human fibroblasts ceased proliferating after serial cultivation in vitro and although these arrested fibroblasts remained metabolically active for many weeks, they did not initiate DNA replication despite adequate culture conditions. Replicative senescence has since been described in many normal somatic human cells, including epidermal keratinocytes and melanocytes as well as

H. Rizos (✉)
Department of Biomedical Sciences, Macquarie University,
Sydney, NSW 2109, Australia
e-mail: helen.rizos@mq.edu.au

S. Haferkamp
Department of Dermatology, University Hospital Regensburg,
Franz-Josef-Strauss-Allee 11
D-93053, Regensburg, Germany

L.L. Haferkamp
Department of Medicine, Westmead Institute, University of Sydney,
Westmead, NSW 2145, Australia

A. Bosserhoff (ed.), *Melanoma Development*,
DOI 10.1007/978-3-319-41319-8_11

in cells derived from rodents, birds, and several other species (Campisi 2001; Kim et al. 2002). The Hayflick limit is often used to refer to the maximum number of population doublings for any given cell population.

11.2 Characteristics of Senescent Cells

Senescent cells have been identified both in vitro and in vivo using a series of phenotypic features and markers that are not exclusive to the senescent state but act as powerful predictors of senescence when used in combination (reviewed in Collado and Serrano 2006; Campisi and d'Adda di Fagagna 2007). Increased activity of acidic ß-galactosidase, termed senescence-associated ß-galactosidase (SA-ß-gal) is the most widely accepted marker of senescent cells (Dimri et al. 1995). The expression of this

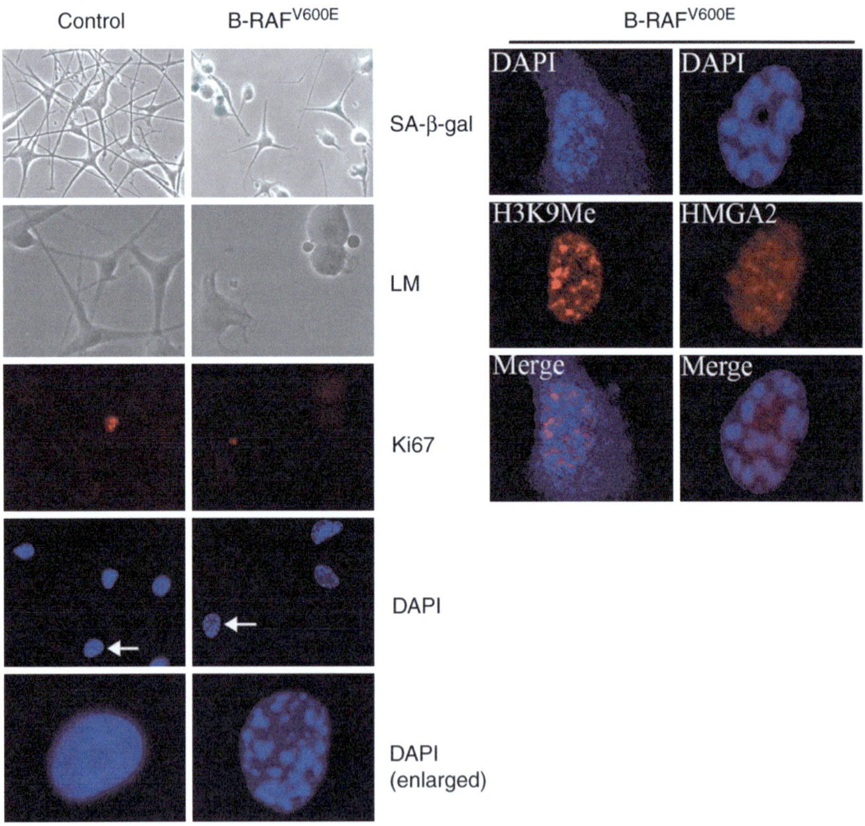

Fig. 11.1 Senescence is associated with positive SA-ß-gal activity and appearance of condensed chromatin. B-RAF^{V600E}-induced senescence in human melanocytes is characterised by rapid cell cycle arrest (reduced Ki67), appearance of SAHF (DAPI foci), and increased SA-ß-gal activity (*left panel*). Cells enlarged to show DAPI-stained SAHF foci are indicated with arrows. SAHF are enriched for markers of heterochromatin, including H3K9Me and HMGA2 (*right panels*)

enzyme correlates strongly with the senescence state (Fig. 11.1), although it can also be induced by cellular stresses such as serum withdrawal and prolonged cell culture (Severino et al. 2000). SA-ß-gal activity derives from residual lysosomal ß-galactosidase activity at the suboptimal pH 6.0 (pH 4.5 is optimal) and reflects the increased lysosomal content of senescent cells (Kurz et al. 2000; Lee et al. 2006). The appearance of DAPI-stained heterochromatic regions, known as senescence-associated heterochromatic foci (SAHF) (Fig. 11.1), which promote the stable repression of certain E2F target genes involved in proliferation, is also associated with senescence (Narita et al. 2003). SAHF occur preferentially with oncogene-induced DNA replication stress, and although global heterochromatin marks can co-exist with cellular proliferation, the accumulation of repressive chromatin marks at the promoters of E2F-target genes is a marker of oncogene-induced senescence (Di Micco et al. 2011). Each SAHF contains portions of a single condensed chromosome, which is enriched for common markers of heterochromatin, including heterochromatin protein 1γ, histone H3 methylated at lysine 9 (H3K9Me), and the non-histone chromatin protein, HMGA2 (Fig. 11.1) (Narita et al. 2003; reviewed in Adams 2007).

Several other markers of senescence have also been described and validated, including accumulation of the cyclin-dependent kinase (CDK) inhibitors $p16^{INK4a}$, $p15^{INK4b}$, an anti-apoptotic bcl-2 member Mcl-1, and the transcription factor Dec1 (Collado and Serrano 2005). Levels of the p53 transcription target and CDK inhibitor $p21^{Waf1}$, the plasminogen activator inhibitor-1 (PAI-1) protein and miR-34 family of microRNAs are also elevated in senescent cells (Goldstein et al. 1994; Wong and Riabowol 1996; He et al. 2007). Finally, morphological changes such as cell enlargement with a concomitant increase in nuclear size, vacuolisation, and cell flattening are typical of senescent cells in vitro (reviewed in Sharpless and Sherr 2015).

11.3 Senescent Cells In Vivo

The existence of senescence cells in vivo has important implications for multicellular organisms; the onset of stress-induced premature senescence may prevent the development of malignant cancer, but the accumulation of damaged senescent cells may eventually compromise tissue integrity and prove detrimental.

11.3.1 Cellular Senescence and Cancer

The observation that aberrant activity of many oncogenes, including RAS, c-MYC, and B-RAF, triggers senescence in vitro (reviewed in Gorgoulis and Halazonetis 2010) suggested that oncogene-induced senescence may act as a barrier to tumourigenesis. Compelling evidence for the tumour suppressor role of oncogene-induced senescence stems from studies in mouse cancer models and human tumours. For instance, pre-malignant lesions in the lung (which developed in a conditional knock-in mouse model expressing oncogenic $K\text{-}RAS^{G12D}$) contained many cells expressing markers of oncogene-induced senescence including $p16^{INK4a}$, $p15^{INK4b}$, SAHF, and

SA-ß-gal, whereas lung adenocarcinomas were almost completely devoid of cells positive for these markers (Collado and Serrano 2005). Similarly, constitutively active N-RAS^{G12D} prevented lymphomagenesis by triggering potent senescence in murine lymphocytes (Braig et al. 2005) and H-RAS^{G12V} triggered a dose-dependent senescence response in mammary epithelia (Sarkisian et al. 2007). Further, inactivation of the PTEN tumour suppressor, which acts as a phosphoinositide 3-kinase (PI3K) pathway inhibitor, in mouse prostate triggered an acute senescence response that suppressed the development of invasive adenocarcinoma (Chen et al. 2005). Finally, consistent with tumour suppression, oncogene-induced senescent cells exhibit a metabolic shift favouring mitochondrial oxidative phosphorylation, rather than the abnormal glycolytic metabolism common to cancer (Kaplon et al. 2013; Li et al. 2013).

Senescence markers are also abundant in human pre-malignant lesions of the skin, colon, prostate, and nervous system, whereas they are almost completely absent in malignant tumours (Chen et al. 2005; Michaloglou et al. 2005; Bartkova et al. 2006; Courtois-Cox et al. 2006; Kuilman et al. 2008). Perhaps the most compelling data come from studies with human naevi (moles), which are small benign tumours of melanocytes that frequently harbour oncogenic mutations in the B-RAF kinase (Pollock et al. 2003). Naevi remain growth arrested for decades and rarely become melanomas (Kuwata et al. 1993; Maldonado et al. 2004), presumably because aberrant B-RAF signalling induces potent senescence (Michaloglou et al. 2005; Gray-Schopfer et al. 2006; Dankort et al. 2009; Dhomen et al. 2009; Goel et al. 2009). Human naevi display some features of oncogene-induced senescence, including intact telomeres (the repetitive sequences at the ends of each chromosome), increased p16^{INK4a} expression, and positive SA-ß-gal activity (Miracco et al. 2002; Michaloglou et al. 2005; Mooi and Peeper 2006), although the expression of senescence-associated features, including SA-ß-gal, that should distinguish human naevus cells from primary and transformed melanocytes remains controversial (Cotter et al. 2007, 2008; Michaloglou et al. 2008; Tran et al. 2012). There is also some discord regarding the clonality of B-RAF^{V600E} mutations in melanocytic naevi, although recent data using sensitive droplet digital PCR in combination with immunohistochemistry support the notion that oncogenic B-RAF initiates melanocytic hyperplasia (Ichii-Nakato et al. 2006; Lin et al. 2009; Yeh et al. 2013).

11.3.2 Cellular Senescence and Aging

Evidence that replicative (telomere-associated) senescence reflects organismal aging and may contribute to age-related decrements in tissue structure and function is more contentious. Certainly, telomeres progressively shorten with each cell division and DNA damage foci marking telomere dysfunction increase with age to approximately 20 % in very old primates (Herbig et al. 2006). Further, cells with a senescent phenotype are prevalent at sites of age-related diseases, such as osteoarthritis and atherosclerosis (Chang and Harley 1995; Price et al. 2002) and mice lacking the mitotic regulator BubR1 or the p53 homologue, p63, developed age-related pathologies that were associated with cellular senescence (Baker et al. 2004; Keyes et al. 2005).

SAHF-positive senescent fibroblasts also increase with age in primate skin (Herbig et al. 2006) and SA-ß-gal-positive senescent cells were found to accumulate in the skin of elderly people (Dimri et al. 1995; Dekker et al. 2009) although this latter result was not reproduced (Severino et al. 2000). Conversely, in some 13 studies involving 79 patients with accelerated aging disorders, such as Werner and Hutchinson–Gilford syndromes, the replicative capacity of fibroblasts was consistently lower than fibroblasts derived from age-matched controls (reviewed in Davis et al. 2007; Maier and Westendorp 2009). Early reports described a weak inverse relationship between replicative lifespan of fibroblasts in vitro and the chronological age of the donor, although there was large variability in the data and recent studies using larger cohorts have found no significant association between age and replicative lifespan (Cristofalo et al. 1998; reviewed in Maier and Westendorp 2009). It is worth considering that the majority of these studies utilise mass cell cultures, so that the Hayflick limit, which is comparable in young and older individuals, reflects the cells with the longest proliferative capacity. This does not preclude the possibility that overall replicative capacity declines with age, in fact the replicative lifespan of individual human fibroblast clones were related to donor age (McCarron et al. 1987).

The accumulation of senescent cells may contribute to the aging process by depleting the regenerative potential of stem cells or by altering tissue structure and function. Many studies suggest that the expression of p16^{INK4a}, which increases during senescence and with age in many rodent, baboon, and human tissues (Zindy et al. 1997; Melk et al. 2003; Krishnamurthy et al. 2004; Herbig et al. 2006; Edwards et al. 2007; Liu et al. 2009), limits the proliferative capacity of self-renewing stem cells and thus impairs tissue regeneration. Mice lacking p16^{INK4a} retain stem cell division and tissue regeneration with advancing age (Janzen et al. 2006; Krishnamurthy et al. 2006; Molofsky et al. 2006; Signer et al. 2008). In contrast, p16^{INK4a} inhibits the reprogramming of differentiated human cells into induced pluripotent stem cells. Reprogramming can be likened to a rejuvenation process and there is an age-related decline in reprogramming efficiency that can be reversed by inactivation of the *p16INK4a* gene (Banito et al. 2009; Li et al. 2009).

In spite of the substantial evidence linking p16^{INK4a} expression with senescence and molecular aging in humans, a recent study suggested that p16^{INK4a}, and its homologue p15^{INK4b}, may have anti-aging functions. This work was based on a mouse model genetically engineered to carry two copies of the *INK4a/ARF* locus, which encodes the p16^{INK4a}, p19ARF, and p15^{INK4b} tumour suppressor proteins. These mice were less susceptible to cancer, showed increased median longevity and a lower incidence of aging-associated kidney lesions and DNA damage response (Matheu et al. 2009). Although, the additional p15^{INK4b} and p19ARF genes complicate interpretation of these data, it is conceivable that the role of p16^{INK4a} in aging reflects its expression. The progressive upregulation of p16^{INK4a} may delay aging by reducing cell proliferation and maintaining stem cell reserves. In contrast, the acute, mitogen-driven upregulation of p16^{INK4a} may promote aging by initiating senescence and permanently preventing stem cell proliferation and tissue regeneration.

Senescent cells may also contribute to aging by altering tissue structure and function; senescent cells secrete many extracellular matrix associated factors and inflammatory proteins. Many of these secreted factors, including TGFß, IL-6, and PAI1, accumulate with aging. Some, including PAI1 and matrix metalloproteinases, may damage or alter tissue integrity (reviewed in Campisi and d'Adda di Fagagna 2007; Kuilman and Peeper 2009).

Taken together, these findings suggest that irreversibly growth-arrested senescent cells can act as a barrier against tumour formation in young organisms, but their net accumulation may reach a point that compromises tissue function and stem cell renewal leading to the development of deleterious phenotypes with age (Campisi and d'Adda di Fagagna 2007).

11.4 Critical Pathways in Cellular Senescence

Although diverse stimuli can induce a senescence response, they appear to converge on two pathways that initiate and maintain this programme. These pathways are regulated by the tumour suppressor proteins p53 and the retinoblastoma protein (pRb), both of which are frequently lost in human cancer cells (Sherr 1996). Importantly, although cancer cells have partially lost the capacity to initiate senescence, the senescence response can be re-engaged by restoring the p53 and pRb pathways, and tumour regression through senescence may be achieved. It has been shown, for instance, that re-instating $p16^{INK4a}$ in human tumour cells resulted in the establishment and maintenance of a senescence response (Sugrue et al. 1997; Haferkamp et al. 2008).

The senescent states induced by the p53 and pRb pathways may be distinct and whether cells engage one or the other pathway appears to reflect the type of stress signal, the tissue and species of origin. Recent data also reveal senescence-inducing pathways that appear to be independent of the p53- and pRb-pathways. For instance, neither p53 nor $p16^{INK4a}$ were required for H-RAS-induced senescence in melanocytes and senescence induced by $B\text{-}RAF^{V600E}$ or $N\text{-}RAS^{Q61R}$ did not depend on $p16^{INK4a}$ or p53 (Denoyelle et al. 2006; Zhuang et al. 2008; Haferkamp et al. 2009a, b).

11.4.1 The p53 Pathway and Senescence

p53 engages a formidable proliferative arrest by transactivating genes, such as $p21^{Waf1}$ and the miR-34 class of microRNAs (Smith et al. 1996; Brown et al. 1997; He et al. 2007) primarily in response to DNA-damage checkpoint signals triggered by telomere dysfunction and activated oncogenes (Ramirez et al. 2001; Herbig et al. 2004; Bartkova et al. 2006; Di Micco et al. 2006). Shortened dysfunctional telomeres are recognised as DNA double-strand breaks and lead to the activation of the DNA damage checkpoint (d'Adda di Fagagna et al. 2003). Aberrant oncogenic activity also triggers DNA replication stress and a DNA damage response, possibly via the suppression of RRM2, a key rate-limiting regulatory unit in dNTP synthesis (Bartkova et al. 2006; Aird et al. 2013). Thus, senescent cells are characterised by persistent DNA damage foci, termed DNA segments with chromatin alterations reinforcing senescence (DNA-SCARS). DNA-SCARS are associated with promyelocytic leukaemia protein nuclear bodies and the accumulation of activated DNA damage response mediators, including ataxia telangiectasia mutated (ATM) and checkpoint-2 (Chk2) kinases (Rodier et al. 2011).

Dampening the DNA damage checkpoint via the inactivation of p53-regulators (including ATM and Chk2) or p53 itself can overcome oncogene-induced and telomere-dependent senescence in human fibroblasts (d'Adda di Fagagna et al. 2003; Di Micco et al. 2006). Similarly, inactivation of the upstream p53 activator, ARF, overcame oncogene-induced senescence in mouse embryo fibroblasts (MEFs) (Serrano et al. 1996; Kamijo et al. 1997), while the loss of $p21^{Waf1}$ caused cells to bypass telomere-dependent replicative- and oncogene-induced senescence in normal human fibroblasts and MEFs, respectively (Brown et al. 1997; Pantoja and Serrano 1999; Wei and Sedivy 1999).

Despite the substantial evidence that p53 promotes senescence, recent data indicate that physiological p53 signalling promotes longevity and favours quiescence over senescence (Matheu et al. 2007, 2008; Demidenko et al. 2010). Mice engineered to express mildly elevated levels of wild-type p53 display strong resistance to tumourigenesis, normal longevity but decreased levels of aging-associated damage (Garcia-Cao et al. 2002, 2006). In contrast, mice expressing constitutively activate forms of p53 showed accelerated aging and an increase in the proportion of senescent cells in vivo (Dumble et al. 2004; Hinkal et al. 2009). It is likely that the cellular context of the p53 response dictates whether quiescence or senescence is triggered. For instance, inhibition of the growth-promoting mTOR pathway by p53 favours quiescence, whereas the simultaneous activation of p53 signalling along with mTOR (i.e., via oncogenic RAS, loss of PTEN) promotes senescence (Fig. 11.2) (Alimonti et al. 2010; Galluzzi et al. 2010; Korotchkina et al. 2010).

11.4.2 The $p16^{INK4a}$/pRb Pathway

Although inactivation of the p53 pathway can reverse the senescence arrest in some cells, there is an emerging consensus that this reversal is blocked in cells with an activated $p16^{INK4a}$/pRb pathway (Sakamoto et al. 1993; Beausejour et al. 2003; Herbig et al. 2004). Active, hypophosphorylated pRb interacts with E2F transcription factors and facilitates chromosome condensation at E2F target promoters. The reorganisation of chromatin leads to the formation of SAHF and the stable repression of proliferation-promoting genes, resulting in the irreversible growth arrest associated with senescence (Narita et al. 2003).

$p16^{INK4a}$ is a positive regulator of pRb and is crucial in generating SAHFs (Narita et al. 2003). Not surprisingly, $p16^{INK4a}$ also acts as a tumour suppressor and is frequently inactivated in established human tumours and inactivating melanoma-associated mutations in $p16^{INK4a}$ are inherited in melanoma-dense kindreds (Goldstein et al. 2006). In fact, $p16^{INK4a}$-deficient human melanocytes, derived from melanoma affected individuals, show an extended lifespan and can be immortalised by ectopic expression of telomerase reverse transcriptase, whereas normal melanocytes display neither of these features (Bennett 2003; Sviderskaya et al. 2003).

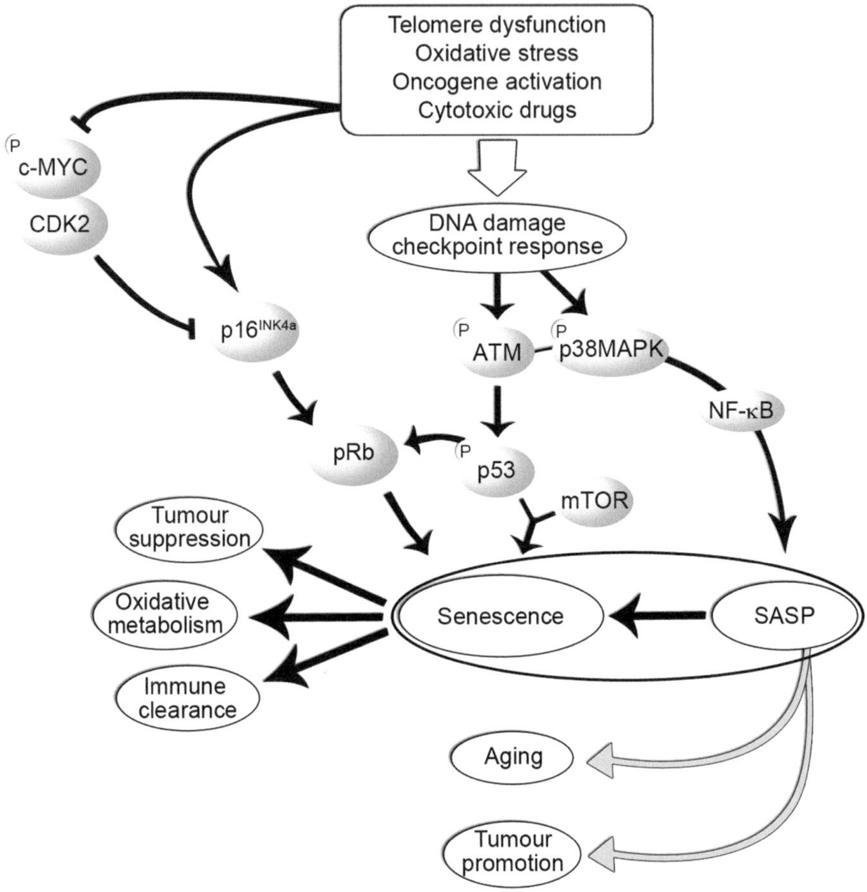

Fig. 11.2 Diverse stress stimuli activate cellular senescence via the DNA damage checkpoint response. Persistent DNA damage leads to the activation of the p53-signalling cascade, which favours senescence when the mTOR growth-promoting pathway is switched on. p53 also signals through the pRb tumour suppressor pathway via the transcriptional induction of the CDK inhibitor $p21^{Waf1}$ (not shown). pRb activation is reinforced by the CDK inhibitor, $p16^{INK4a}$, which is induced by oncogenic signalling, in part by inhibition of c-MYC-CDK2 transcription activity. Sustained damage to DNA also promotes the secretion of a large number of proteins, a phenomenon known as the senescence-associated secretory phenotype (*SASP*), via ATM and p38MAPK-mediated activation of NF-kB. SASP can have different effects on cancer and aging; it can suppress cancer by reinforcing the senescent state and inhibiting mitogenic signals, it can activate the innate immune response leading to improved clearance of tumour cells, it can impair the function of stem cells and promote aging, and it can stimulate the proliferation of neighbouring tumour cells

Furthermore, replicative- and oncogene-induced senescence are accompanied by accumulation of $p16^{INK4a}$ in primary human cells (Alcorta et al. 1996; Hara et al. 1996; Serrano et al. 1997), while ectopically expressed $p16^{INK4a}$ initiates a senescence programme characterised by cell cycle arrest, senescence-associated changes in cell morphology, increased SA-ß-gal activity, and the appearance of SAHF (Dai and Enders 2000; Haferkamp et al. 2008).

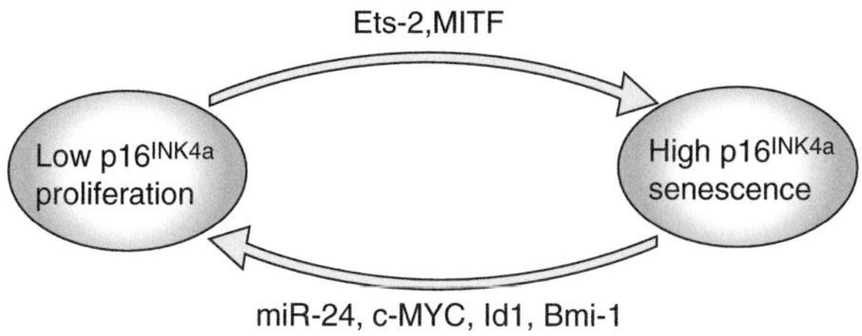

Fig. 11.3 Acute activation of the CDK inhibitor p16^{INK4a} favours senescence. Aberrant oncogenic activity promotes p16^{INK4a} accumulation by suppressing the MYC, Id1, and Bmi-1 transcription factors, while inducing the accumulation of the Ets-2 and MITF transcription regulators. As cells near replicative senescence the p16^{INK4a}-inhibitory microRNA, miR24, is depleted and p16^{INK4a} translation is restored

p16^{INK4a} expression is maintained at low levels prior to senescence by miR-24, a negative-regulator microRNA that suppresses p16^{INK4a} translation. As cells near senescence, miR-24 expression diminishes and p16^{INK4a} protein accumulates (Lal et al. 2008). Oncogenic signalling also induces p16^{INK4a} expression by reducing the levels of the p16^{INK4a} transcriptional repressors Bmi-1 and Id1 (Jacobs et al. 1999a; Ohtani et al. 2001) and increasing the activity of the p16^{INK4a} transcription enhancers, Ets-2 and MITF (Fig. 11.3) (Ohtani et al. 2001; Loercher et al. 2005). Importantly, Bmi-1 is a direct transcription target of c-MYC, and reduced c-MYC signalling is associated with oncogenic N-RAS and B-RAF activity in melanocytes (Zhuang et al. 2008). Thus, decreased c-MYC activity leads to senescence by regulating Bmi-1 and p16^{INK4a} (Jacobs et al. 1999b; Guney et al. 2006). Further, Bmi-1 deficiency inhibits stem cell renewal via p16^{INK4a} induction in mice and Bmi-1 downregulation was associated with increased p16^{INK4a} expression in human keratinocytes derived from older individuals (Molofsky et al. 2003, 2005; Park et al. 2003; Cordisco et al. 2010).

11.4.3 The Senescence-Associated Secretory Network

Senescent cells secrete a complex range of chemokines, interleukins, proteases, and growth factors that are associated with inflammation and malignancy. Collectively, these senescence-associated soluble factors have been termed the senescence-associated secretory phenotype (SASP) and the senescence-messaging secretome (SMS) (Coppe et al. 2008; Kuilman and Peeper 2009; Gorgoulis and Halazonetis 2010). Detailed lists of SASP factors have been provided in several recent articles and are briefly summarised in Table 11.1 (Kuilman and Peeper 2009; Coppe et al. 2010; Gorgoulis and Halazonetis 2010, reviewed in Lasry and Ben-Neriah 2015). This review will focus on the role of SASP in senescence and its relationship with DNA damage response, p53 and pRb pathways.

SASP is not triggered by senescence but is induced in response to persistent DNA damage signalling and via activation of the stress-inducible kinase p38MAPK,

Table 11.1 The senescence-associated secretory phenotype

Soluble signalling factors	
Interleukins	IL-6, −7, −1a, −1b, −13, −15
Chemokines	IL-8; GROa, −ß; MCP-2, −4; HCC-4; cotaxin-3; MIP-3a, −1a; IGFBP-2, −3, −4, −5, −6, −7; G-CSF; GM-CSF
Growth factors	EGF; bFGF; HGF; IGF, SCF; TGFß, NGF; VEGF
Non-protein factors	Nitric oxide, reactive oxygen species
Serine proteases	
	MMP-1, −3, −10, −12, −13, −14; TIMP-1, −2; PAI-1, −2
Secreted insoluble factors	
	Fibronectin, collagen, laminin

A subset of factors significantly altered during senescence

both of which lead to the phosphorylation and activation of the transcription factor target, NF-kB. DNA-damaged induced ATM and p38MAPK synergistically phosphorylated and activated the NF-kB transcription factor, which induced the majority of SASP factors in senescent human fibroblasts (Freund et al. 2011). SASP relies on upstream elements of the DNA damage response cascade, including NBS1 (a sensor of DNA damage), ATM kinase and its target Chk2, but does not require the downstream DNA damage signalling target p53. Thus, cells induced to senescence in response to $p16^{INK4a}$, in the absence of DNA damage, do not initiate SASP. Similarly, oncogenic RAS promotes senescence with limited SASP in ATM-deficient cells (Rodier et al. 2009). Although SASP is not restricted to the senescence programme, it can reinforce senescence growth arrest. For instance, human fibroblasts depleted for IL-6 bypassed $B\text{-}RAF^{V600E}$-induced senescence and showed a strong suppression of other inflammatory regulators including IL-8, IL-1α, and IL-1β (Kuilman et al. 2008). Similarly, the disruption of SASP via inhibition of NF-kB confirmed the importance of SASP in stabilising cell cycle arrest and promoting immune clearance (Chien et al. 2011). SASP molecules IL-8 and the chemokine receptor 2 (CXCR2) ligands support senescence by boosting the DNA damage response, while IGFBP7, IL-6, and PAI-1 contribute to senescence by inhibiting proliferative and mitogenic pathways (Kortlever et al. 2006; Acosta et al. 2008; Kuilman et al. 2008; Wajapeyee et al. 2008; Acosta and Gil 2009). Thus, the onset of a protracted DNA damage response controls senescence by initiating a rapid p53- and/or pRb-dependent proliferative arrest, followed by induction of a DNA damage responsive cytokine secretory response (Fig. 11.2).

The secretion of soluble factors into the extracellular environment can also have pro-tumourigenic effects. This probably reflects a complex combination of cellular and genetic context along with the level of SASP activity. SASP factors such as IL-6 and IL-8 can promote cancer progression by stimulating proliferation, angiogenesis, invasiveness, and inducing epithelial–mesenchymal transition (Ancrile et al. 2007; Coppe et al. 2008; Kuilman et al. 2008; Rodier et al. 2009). Others, such as matrix metalloproteinases, promote breast tumourigenesis by altering the differentiation of epithelial tumour cells and increasing tumour cell migration by weakening tissue integrity (Liu and Hornsby 2007; Acosta and Gil 2009). The combined loss of p53 with the aberrant activation of RAS amplifies and accelerates the development of SASP and this coincides with the potent stimulation of growth, invasiveness, and epithelial–mesenchymal transition of nonaggressive human cancer cells (Coppe et al. 2008). In vivo cytokine secretion is a feature of preneoplastic lesions of the colon and breast, which display markers of DNA damage and senescence, while IL-6 expression correlates with ATM (DNA damage sensor) kinase activity in invasive ductal breast carcinomas (Kuilman et al. 2008; Rodier et al. 2009). Conversely, the selective suppression of SASP factors with the mTORC1 inhibitor rapamycin, which also inhibited IL1A-NF-kB signalling, diminished the ability of senescent fibroblasts to stimulate prostate tumour growth in mice (Laberge et al. 2015).

Finally, the innate immune system can be activated by SASP inflammatory cytokines and can effectively restrict oncogenic SASP activity by clearing damaged and senescent cells (Xue et al. 2007). The accumulation of inflammatory cytokines is associated with several age-associated diseases, and it is not surprising that accumulation of SASP factors such as IL-6, TGFß, PAI, and fibronectin also correlate with aging (Goldstein et al. 1994; Rasoamanantena et al. 1994; Ershler and Keller 2000; Carrieri et al. 2004; Herbig et al. 2006; Rossi et al. 2007). Although the precise impact of the SASP in vivo remains unresolved, these data indicate that damaged senescent cells mount a complex cytokine response that communicates with neighbouring cells, modifies the tissue microenvironment, and leads to multiple pathologies. In particular, cytokines may reinforce senescence in surrounding non-malignant cells (Acosta et al. 2013), generate a potent immune response to clear damaged cells, affect the function of stem cells, or even promote tumourigenesis of high-grade pre-malignant and malignant cells in a paracrine manner (Fig. 11.2).

11.4.4 p53- and p16^{INK4a}-Independent Oncogene-Induced Senescence in Melanocytes

Recent reports have shown that pro-oncogenic forms of the H- and N-RAS GTPases, and their downstream kinase B-RAF, are not functionally equivalent and each may induce senescence via distinct programmes that do not require pRb or p53. Certainly, the inactivation of p16^{INK4a}, pRb, or p53 did not prevent cell cycle arrest, DNA damage signalling, or SA-ß-gal activity in human melanocytes transduced to express these oncogenes (Michaloglou et al. 2005; Denoyelle et al. 2006; Zhuang et al. 2008; Haferkamp et al. 2009a, b). One alternative pathway appears to involve the endoplasmic reticulum-associated unfolded protein response (UPR). Ectopic expression of H-RAS^{G12V} in human melanocytes induced the UPR and inhibition of this response (by silencing expression of several UPR proteins) suppressed H-RAS-induced senescence (Denoyelle et al. 2006). The RAS-mediated activation of the PI3K pathway was required for UPR induction and this was most potently achieved by oncogenic H-RAS, as UPR was poorly induced by N-RAS and not activated by B-RAF. Consistent with these data, Spitz naevi expressing mutated H-RAS showed a significantly greater expansion of the endoplasmic reticulum and activation of the

UPR compared to benign naevi expressing mutated B-RAF or N-RAS (Denoyelle et al. 2006). It has been suggested that UPR-induced senescence may account for the bias against H-RAS mutations in melanoma (Denoyelle et al. 2006), although it should be noted that the efficiency of UPR signalling declines during aging (Naidoo 2009a, b) and melanomas seem to have adapted to the presence of extreme endoplasmic reticulum stress (Jiang et al. 2007; Hersey and Zhang 2008).

Another alternative senescence pathway has been proposed for oncogenic B-RAF in human melanocytes. Ectopic expression of the oncogenic transcription factor c-MYC was found to partially rescue B-RAF^{V600E}-induced senescence, and more weakly, N-RAS^{Q61R}-induced senescence of human melanocytes. c-MYC did not influence the UPR pathway and this may account for the inability of c-MYC to overcome N-RAS-induced senescence (Zhuang et al. 2008). Suppression of c-MYC has been shown to induce senescence in several mouse tumour models, including lymphoma, osteosarcoma, and hepatocellular carcinoma (Wu et al. 2007), and in human melanoma cells expressing B-RAF^{V600E} or N-RAS^{Q61R} (Zhuang et al. 2008). The requirement for p16^{INK4a} or p53 in senescence caused by c-MYC depletion remains controversial; intact p16^{INK4a}, pRb, and p53 were required in mouse tumours for the initiation of senescence by c-MYC inactivation (Wu et al. 2007), whereas c-MYC depletion led to senescence of p16^{INK4a}-null and p53-null human melanoma cells (Zhuang et al. 2008). The impact of p16^{INK4a} and p53 expression on c-MYC activity in human melanocytes remains to be investigated. Importantly, c-MYC is frequently upregulated in human tumours and is up to sevenfold higher in metastatic melanomas compared to benign naevi (Zhuang et al. 2008).

The anti-senescence function of c-MYC requires phosphorylation of MYC at Ser-62 by cyclin E/CDK2. CDK2 acts as a c-MYC transcription co-factor altering the MYC-dependent regulation of genes, such as Bmi-1, p16^{INK4a}, and p21^{Waf1}, all of which participate in senescence control. Inhibition of CDK2 leads to the upregulation of p16^{INK4a} and p21^{Waf1} and the repression of Bmi-1. Thus, MYC can induce senescence in MEFs lacking CDK2, but not in wild-type MEFs (Hydbring et al. 2010; Hydbring and Larsson 2010). This has important implications, as the inhibition of CDK2 (via pharmacological inhibition or induction of the CDK2 inhibitor p27^{Kip1}) can drive MYC-transformed cells into senescence and prevents c-MYC from bypassing RAS-induced senescence (reviewed in Hydbring and Larsson 2010). Accordingly, depletion of CDK2 delayed MYC-induced B-cell lymphomas, −neuroblastoma cells, −breast cancers, and -melanoma cell lines (Du et al. 2004; Deans et al. 2006; Molenaar et al. 2009; Campaner et al. 2010) and deletion of Skp2 (an oncogenic E3 ligase that targets p27^{Kip1} and MYC for degradation) suppressed tumourigenesis through senescence (Lin et al. 2010).

11.5 Re-establishing Senescence Mechanisms

The concept of re-instating senescence as a cancer therapy is being approached with caution because the retention of damaged senescent cancer cells that are metabolically active and capable of secreting cytokines and growth factors could be harmful. It is important to consider, however, that many current cancer treatments cause senescence as a result of acute DNA damage (te Poele et al. 2002; Roberson et al. 2005), and the presence of senescent cells in colon carcinomas contributed to improved overall outcome to therapy (Haugstetter et al. 2010). The existence of sporadic senescent cells in tumours may indicate a retained susceptibility to senescence induction and this may translate to sensitivity to senescence-inducing therapies.

Senescence can be triggered by reactivating tumour suppressor molecules or targeting oncogenes. For instance, reactivation of p53 induces a potent senescence response in sarcomas and liver carcinomas that were subsequently cleared by the innate immune system (Ventura et al. 2007; Xue et al. 2007). Presumably, SASP molecules were responsible for the activation of the immune cells. Targeting the oncogenic E3-ubiquitin ligase, Skp2, triggered senescence in H-RAS^{G12V} expressing or PTEN-deficient prostate cancer cells (Lin et al. 2010). Likewise, deleting CDK2 induced senescence in c-MYC expressing MEFs (Campaner et al. 2010). Importantly, senescence was also triggered in these oncogenic model systems with small molecule inhibitors of Skp2 and CDK2 function (Lin et al. 2010). Similarly, the selective inhibition of B-RAF and MEK triggered senescence in B-RAF^{V600E}-mutant human melanoma cells and inhibition of MEK sensitised melanoma cells to radiotherapy (Haferkamp et al. 2013; Schick et al. 2015). Intriguingly, melanoma resistance to B-RAF inhibition commonly involves the hyperactivation of MAPK signalling, often via mutational activation of NRAS, MEK, or *B-RAF* amplification, and this appears to confer a fitness deficit to tumour cells by promoting senescence (Das Thakur et al. 2013). These data coincide with genetic evidence that RAS and B-RAF mutations are mutually exclusive in cancer, and recent evidence confirming that co-expression of mutant KRAS and B-RAF resulted in elevated MAPK activity, increased p16^{INK4a} production, and promoted SA-ß-gal in MEFs (Cisowski et al. 2016).

The pharmacological induction of senescence has been shown to suppress the in vivo growth of prostate cancer cells (Alimonti et al. 2010; Lin et al. 2010), and therapy-induced senescence is detectable in tumour biopsies after neoadjuvant chemotherapy (Roberson et al. 2005). Mouse models of chemotherapy have also shown that MYC-initiated lymphomas responded to cycloheximide by inducing tumour cell senescence, which contributed to better prognosis (Schmitt et al. 2002). This suggests that delivery of chemotherapy to cells undergoing senescence could be used to augment senescence or to transform cell cycle arrest into cell death.

Heterochromatin may also prove a useful target in oncogene-expressing senescent and proliferating tumour cells. The condensation of chromatin hinders access of DNA damage response proteins to DNA lesions and this diminishes DNA damage response signalling (Di Micco et al. 2011). Perturbation of heterochromatin, using histone deacetylase (HDAC) inhibitors, augmented DNA damage response activity, induced apoptosis and tumour regression in a K-RAS-driven colorectal cancer xenograft model (Di Micco et al. 2011). HDAC inhibitors have shown encouraging anti-tumour activity with manageable toxicities in clinical trials, and several have been granted approval by the US Food and Drug Administration for cancer treatment (West and Johnstone 2014).

Despite the contribution of senescence to tumour suppression, the possibility that drug-induced senescent cancer cells may accumulate and contribute to drug resistance and tumour recurrence must be considered. As described above, the secretion of inflammatory factors can stimulate tumour cell proliferation and angiogenesis, and escape from drug-induced senescence in breast cancer cells resulted in the generation of aggressive tumour clones with stem cell-like properties (Achuthan et al. 2011).

Conclusions

Together, these data confirm that senescence plays an important role in suppressing tumourigenesis and possibly predicting treatment outcome. The long-term impact of senescent tumour cells in vivo remains largely unknown and much more work is needed to resolve the complex regulation of the pro- and anti-tumourigenic activities of senescent cells. The finding that the senescent phenotype can be uncoupled from cell cycle arrest suggests that it may be possible to minimise the detrimental aspects of senescence (Dulic et al. 2000; Wang et al. 2004; Rodier et al. 2009). For instance, p53 activity and the miR-146 class of microRNAs suppress excessive SASP activity (Coppe et al. 2008; Bhaumik et al. 2009) and ectopic expression of CDK inhibitors, including $p16^{INK4a}$ and $p21^{Waf1}$, can induce senescence without SASP (Coppe et al. 2011). Disrupting SASP, however, weakened the proliferative arrest and diminished the immune recognition and clearance of senescent Eμ-MYC lymphoma cells in vivo (Chien et al. 2011). Thus, in order to maximise the therapeutic potential of senescence, we may need to establish a new equilibrium that favours immune-mediated clearance of permanently arrested preneoplastic cells, while limiting the deleterious paracrine effects that disrupt tissue homeostasis.

Acknowledgements Our work is supported by the National Health and Medical Research Council of Australia (NHMRC), the Cancer Council of New South Wales. HR is a NHMRC Research Fellow.

References

Achuthan S, Santhoshkumar TR, Prabhakar J, Nair SA, Pillai MR (2011) Drug-induced senescence generates chemoresistant stemlike cells with low reactive oxygen species. J Biol Chem 286:37813–37829

Acosta JC, Gil J (2009) A role for CXCR2 in senescence, but what about in cancer? Cancer Res 69:2167–2170

Acosta JC, O'Loghlen A, Banito A, Guijarro MV, Augert A, Raguz S, Fumagalli M, Da Costa M, Brown C, Popov N, Takatsu Y, Melamed J, d'Adda di Fagagna F, Bernard D, Hernando E, Gil J (2008) Chemokine signaling via the CXCR2 receptor reinforces senescence. Cell 133:1006–1101

Acosta JC, Banito A, Wuestefeld T, Georgilis A, Janich P, Morton JP, Athineos D, Kang TW, Lasitschka F, Andrulis M, Pascual G, Morris KJ, Khan S, Jin H, Dharmalingam G, Snijders AP, Carroll T, Capper D, Pritchard C, Inman GJ, Longerich T, Sansom OJ, Benitah SA, Zender L, Gil J (2013) A complex secretory program orchestrated by the inflammasome controls paracrine senescence. Nat Cell Biol 15:978–990

Adams PD (2007) Remodeling of chromatin structure in senescent cells and its potential impact on tumor suppression and aging. Gene 397:84–93
Aird KM, Zhang G, Li H, Tu Z, Bitler BG, Garipov A, Wu H, Wei Z, Wagner SN, Herlyn M, Zhang R (2013) Suppression of nucleotide metabolism underlies the establishment and maintenance of oncogene-induced senescence. Cell Rep 3:1252–1265
Alcorta DA, Xiong Y, Phelps D, Hannon G, Beach D, Barrett JC (1996) Involvement of the cyclin-dependent kinase inhibitor p16 (INK4a) in replicative senescence of normal human fibroblasts. Proc Natl Acad Sci U S A 93:13742–13747
Alimonti A, Nardella C, Chen Z, Clohessy JG, Carracedo A, Trotman LC, Cheng K, Varmeh S, Kozma SC, Thomas G, Rosivatz E, Wosholski R, Cognetti F, Scher HI, Pandolfi PP (2010) A novel type of cellular senescence that can be enhanced in mouse models and human tumor xenografts to suppress prostate tumorigenesis. J Clin Invest 120(3):681–693
Ancrile B, Lim KH, Counter CM (2007) Oncogenic Ras-induced secretion of IL6 is required for tumorigenesis. Genes Dev 21:1714–1719
Baker DJ, Jeganathan KB, Cameron JD, Thompson M, Juneja S, Kopecka A, Kumar R, Jenkins RB, de Groen PC, Roche P, van Deursen JM (2004) BubR1 insufficiency causes early onset of aging-associated phenotypes and infertility in mice. Nat Genet 36:744–749
Banito A, Rashid ST, Acosta JC, Li S, Pereira CF, Geti I, Pinho S, Silva JC, Azuara V, Walsh M, Vallier L, Gil J (2009) Senescence impairs successful reprogramming to pluripotent stem cells. Genes Dev 23:2134–2139
Bartkova J, Rezaei N, Liontos M, Karakaidos P, Kletsas D, Issaeva N, Vassiliou LV, Kolettas E, Niforou K, Zoumpourlis VC, Takaoka M, Nakagawa H, Tort F, Fugger K, Johansson F, Sehested M, Andersen CL, Dyrskjot L, Orntoft T, Lukas J, Kittas C, Helleday T, Halazonetis TD, Bartek J, Gorgoulis VG (2006) Oncogene-induced senescence is part of the tumorigenesis barrier imposed by DNA damage checkpoints. Nature 444:633–637
Beausejour CM, Krtolica A, Galimi F, Narita M, Lowe SW, Yaswen P, Campisi J (2003) Reversal of human cellular senescence: roles of the p53 and p16 pathways. EMBO J 22:4212–4222
Bennett DC (2003) Human melanocyte senescence and melanoma susceptibility genes. Oncogene 22:3063–3069
Bhaumik D, Scott GK, Schokrpur S, Patil CK, Orjalo AV, Rodier F, Lithgow GJ, Campisi J (2009) MicroRNAs miR-146a/b negatively modulate the senescence-associated inflammatory mediators IL-6 and IL-8. Aging (Albany NY) 1:402–411
Braig M, Lee S, Loddenkemper C, Rudolph C, Peters AH, Schlegelberger B, Stein H, Dorken B, Jenuwein T, Schmitt CA (2005) Oncogene-induced senescence as an initial barrier in lymphoma development. Nature 436:660–665
Brown JP, Wei W, Sedivy JM (1997) Bypass of senescence after disruption of p21CIP1/WAF1 gene in normal diploid human fibroblasts. Science 277:831–834
Campaner S, Doni M, Hydbring P, Verrecchia A, Bianchi L, Sardella D, Schleker T, Perna D, Tronnersjo S, Murga M, Fernandez-Capetillo O, Barbacid M, Larsson LG, Amati B (2010) Cdk2 suppresses cellular senescence induced by the c-myc oncogene. Nat Cell Biol 12:54–59; sup pp 51–14
Campisi J (2001) From cells to organisms: can we learn about aging from cells in culture? Exp Gerontol 36:607–618
Campisi J, d'Adda di Fagagna F (2007) Cellular senescence: when bad things happen to good cells. Nat Rev Mol Cell Biol 8:729–740
Carrieri G, Marzi E, Olivieri F, Marchegiani F, Cavallone L, Cardelli M, Giovagnetti S, Stecconi R, Molendini C, Trapassi C, De Benedictis G, Kletsas D, Franceschi C (2004) The G/C915 polymorphism of transforming growth factor beta1 is associated with human longevity: a study in Italian centenarians. Aging Cell 3:443–448
Chang E, Harley CB (1995) Telomere length and replicative aging in human vascular tissues. Proc Natl Acad Sci U S A 92:11190–11194
Chen Z, Trotman LC, Shaffer D, Lin HK, Dotan ZA, Niki M, Koutcher JA, Scher HI, Ludwig T, Gerald W, Cordon-Cardo C, Pandolfi PP (2005) Crucial role of p53-dependent cellular senescence in suppression of Pten-deficient tumorigenesis. Nature 436:725–730

Chien Y, Scuoppo C, Wang X, Fang X, Balgley B, Bolden JE, Premsrirut P, Luo W, Chicas A, Lee CS, Kogan SC, Lowe SW (2011) Control of the senescence-associated secretory phenotype by NF-kappaB promotes senescence and enhances chemosensitivity. Genes Dev 25:2125–2136

Cisowski J, Sayin VI, Liu M, Karlsson C, Bergo MO (2016) Oncogene-induced senescence underlies the mutual exclusive nature of oncogenic KRAS and B-RAF. Oncogene 35:1328-33

Collado M, Serrano M (2005) The senescent side of tumor suppression. Cell Cycle 4:1722–1724

Collado M, Serrano M (2006) The power and the promise of oncogene-induced senescence markers. Nat Rev Cancer 6:472–476

Coppe JP, Patil CK, Rodier F, Sun Y, Munoz DP, Goldstein J, Nelson PS, Desprez PY, Campisi J (2008) Senescence-associated secretory phenotypes reveal cell-nonautonomous functions of oncogenic RAS and the p53 tumor suppressor. PLoS Biol 6:2853–2868

Coppe JP, Desprez PY, Krtolica A, Campisi J (2010) The senescence-associated secretory phenotype: the dark side of tumor suppression. Annu Rev Pathol 5:99–118

Coppe JP, Rodier F, Patil CK, Freund A, Desprez PY, Campisi J (2011) Tumor suppressor and aging biomarker p16(INK4a) induces cellular senescence without the associated inflammatory secretory phenotype. J Biol Chem 286:36396–36403

Cordisco S, Maurelli R, Bondanza S, Stefanini M, Zambruno G, Guerra L, Dellambra E (2010) Bmi-1 reduction plays a key role in physiological and premature aging of primary human keratinocytes. J Invest Dermatol 130:1048–1062

Cotter MA, Florell SR, Leachman SA, Grossman D (2007) Absence of senescence-associated beta-galactosidase activity in human melanocytic nevi in vivo. J Invest Dermatol 127:2469–2471

Cotter MA, Florell SR, Leachman SA, Grossman D (2008) Response to Gray-Schopfer et al. and Michaloglou et al. J Invest Dermatol 128:1583–1584

Courtois-Cox S, Genther Williams SM, Reczek EE, Johnson BW, McGillicuddy LT, Johannessen CM, Hollstein PE, MacCollin M, Cichowski K (2006) A negative feedback signaling network underlies oncogene-induced senescence. Cancer Cell 10:459–472

Cristofalo VJ, Allen RG, Pignolo RJ, Martin BG, Beck JC (1998) Relationship between donor age and the replicative lifespan of human cells in culture: a reevaluation. Proc Natl Acad Sci U S A 95:10614–10619

d'Adda di Fagagna F, Reaper PM, Clay-Farrace L, Fiegler H, Carr P, Von Zglinicki T, Saretzki G, Carter NP, Jackson SP (2003) A DNA damage checkpoint response in telomere-initiated senescence. Nature 426:194–198

Dai CY, Enders GH (2000) p16 INK4a can initiate an autonomous senescence program. Oncogene 19:1613–1622

Dankort D, Curley DP, Cartlidge RA, Nelson B, Karnezis AN, Damsky WE Jr, You MJ, Depinho RA, McMahon M, Bosenberg M (2009) B-RAF(V600E) cooperates with Pten loss to induce metastatic melanoma. Nat Genet 12:12

Das Thakur M, Salangsang F, Landman AS, Sellers WR, Pryer NK, Levesque MP, Dummer R, McMahon M, Stuart DD (2013) Modelling vemurafenib resistance in melanoma reveals a strategy to forestall drug resistance. Nature 474:251–255

Davis T, Wyllie FS, Rokicki MJ, Bagley MC, Kipling D (2007) The role of cellular senescence in Werner syndrome: toward therapeutic intervention in human premature aging. Ann N Y Acad Sci 1100:455–469

Deans AJ, Khanna KK, McNees CJ, Mercurio C, Heierhorst J, McArthur GA (2006) Cyclin-dependent kinase 2 functions in normal DNA repair and is a therapeutic target in BRCA1-deficient cancers. Cancer Res 66:8219–8226

Dekker P, Maier AB, van Heemst D, de Koning-Treurniet C, Blom J, Dirks RW, Tanke HJ, Westendorp RG (2009) Stress-induced responses of human skin fibroblasts in vitro reflect human longevity. Aging Cell 8:595–603

Demidenko ZN, Korotchkina LG, Gudkov AV, Blagosklonny MV (2010) Paradoxical suppression of cellular senescence by p53. Proc Natl Acad Sci U S A 107:9660–9664

Denoyelle C, Abou-Rjaily G, Bezrookove V, Verhaegen M, Johnson TM, Fullen DR, Pointer JN, Gruber SB, Su LD, Nikiforov MA, Kaufman RJ, Bastian BC, Soengas MS (2006)

Anti-oncogenic role of the endoplasmic reticulum differentially activated by mutations in the MAPK pathway. Nat Cell Biol 8:1053–1063

Dhomen N, Reis-Filho JS, da Rocha DS, Hayward R, Savage K, Delmas V, Larue L, Pritchard C, Marais R (2009) Oncogenic B-RAF induces melanocyte senescence and melanoma in mice. Cancer Cell 15:294–303

Di Micco R, Fumagalli M, Cicalese A, Piccinin S, Gasparini P, Luise C, Schurra C, Garre M, Nuciforo PG, Bensimon A, Maestro R, Pelicci PG, d'Adda di Fagagna F (2006) Oncogene-induced senescence is a DNA damage response triggered by DNA hyper-replication. Nature 444:638–642

Di Micco R, Sulli G, Dobreva M, Liontos M, Botrugno OA, Gargiulo G, Dal Zuffo R, Matti V, d'Ario G, Montani E, Mercurio C, Hahn WC, Gorgoulis V, Minucci S, d'Adda di Fagagna F (2011) Interplay between oncogene-induced DNA damage response and heterochromatin in senescence and cancer. Nat Cell Biol 13:292–302

Dimri GP, Lee X, Basile G, Acosta M, Scott G, Roskelley C, Medrano EE, Linskens M, Rubelj I, Pereira-Smith O, Peacocke M, Campisi J (1995) A biomarker that identifies senescent human cells in culture and in aging skin in vivo. Proc Natl Acad Sci U S A 92:9363–9367

Du J, Widlund HR, Horstmann MA, Ramaswamy S, Ross K, Huber WE, Nishimura EK, Golub TR, Fisher DE (2004) Critical role of CDK2 for melanoma growth linked to its melanocyte-specific transcriptional regulation by MITF. Cancer Cell 6:565–576

Dulic V, Beney GE, Frebourg G, Drullinger LF, Stein GH (2000) Uncoupling between phenotypic senescence and cell cycle arrest in aging p21-deficient fibroblasts. Mol Cell Biol 20:6741–6754

Dumble M, Gatza C, Tyner S, Venkatachalam S, Donehower LA (2004) Insights into aging obtained from p53 mutant mouse models. Ann N Y Acad Sci 1019:171–177

Edwards MG, Anderson RM, Yuan M, Kendziorski CM, Weindruch R, Prolla TA (2007) Gene expression profiling of aging reveals activation of a p53-mediated transcriptional program. BMC Genomics 8:80

Ershler WB, Keller ET (2000) Age-associated increased interleukin-6 gene expression, late-life diseases, and frailty. Annu Rev Med 51:245–270

Freund A, Patil CK, Campisi J (2011) p38MAPK is a novel DNA damage response-independent regulator of the senescence-associated secretory phenotype. MBO J 30:1536–1548

Galluzzi L, Kepp O, Kroemer G (2010) TP53 and MTOR crosstalk to regulate cellular senescence. Aging 18:18

Garcia-Cao I, Garcia-Cao M, Martin-Caballero J, Criado LM, Klatt P, Flores JM, Weill JC, Blasco MA, Serrano M (2002) "Super p53" mice exhibit enhanced DNA damage response, are tumor resistant and age normally. EMBO J 21:6225–6235

Garcia-Cao I, Garcia-Cao M, Tomas-Loba A, Martin-Caballero J, Flores JM, Klatt P, Blasco MA, Serrano M (2006) Increased p53 activity does not accelerate telomere-driven ageing. EMBO Rep 7:546–552

Goel VK, Ibrahim N, Jiang G, Singhal M, Fee S, Flotte T, Westmoreland S, Haluska FS, Hinds PW, Haluska FG (2009) Melanocytic nevus-like hyperplasia and melanoma in transgenic BRAFV600E mice. Oncogene 28:2289–2298

Goldstein S, Moerman EJ, Fujii S, Sobel BE (1994) Overexpression of plasminogen activator inhibitor type-1 in senescent fibroblasts from normal subjects and those with Werner syndrome. J Cell Physiol 161:571–579

Goldstein AM, Chan M, Harland M, Gillanders EM, Hayward NK, Avril MF, Azizi E, Bianchi-Scarra G, Bishop DT, Bressac-de Paillerets B, Bruno W, Calista D, Cannon Albright LA, Demenais F, Elder DE, Ghiorzo P, Gruis NA, Hansson J, Hogg D, Holland EA, Kanetsky PA, Kefford RF, Landi MT, Lang J, Leachman SA, Mackie RM, Magnusson V, Mann GJ, Niendorf K, Newton Bishop J, Palmer JM, Puig S, Puig-Butille JA, de Snoo FA, Stark M, Tsao H, Tucker MA, Whitaker L, Yakobson E (2006) High-risk melanoma susceptibility genes and pancreatic cancer, neural system tumors, and uveal melanoma across GenoMEL. Cancer Res 66:9818–9828

Gorgoulis VG, Halazonetis TD (2010) Oncogene-induced senescence: the bright and dark side of the response. Curr Opin Cell Biol 29:29

Gray-Schopfer VC, Cheong SC, Chong H, Chow J, Moss T, Abdel-Malek ZA, Marais R, Wynford-Thomas D, Bennett DC (2006) Cellular senescence in naevi and immortalisation in melanoma: a role for p16? Br J Cancer 95:496–505

Guney I, Wu S, Sedivy JM (2006) Reduced c-Myc signaling triggers telomere-independent senescence by regulating Bmi-1 and p16(INK4a). Proc Natl Acad Sci U S A 103:3645–3650

Haferkamp S, Becker TM, Scurr LL, Kefford RF, Rizos H (2008) p16INK4a-induced senescence is disabled by melanoma-associated mutations. Aging Cell 7:733–745

Haferkamp S, Scurr LL, Becker TM, Frausto M, Kefford RF, Rizos H (2009a) Oncogene-induced senescence does not require the p16(INK4a) or p14ARF melanoma tumor suppressors. J Invest Dermatol 129:1983–1991

Haferkamp S, Tran SL, Becker TM, Scurr LL, Kefford RF, Rizos H (2009b) The relative contributions of the p53 and pRb pathways in oncogene-induced melanocyte senescence. Aging 1:542–556

Haferkamp S, Borst A, Adam C, Becker TM, Motschenbacher S, Windhovel S, Hufnagel AL, Houben R, Meierjohann S (2013) Vemurafenib induces senescence features in melanoma cells. J Invest Dermatol 15:6

Hara E, Smith R, Parry D, Tahara H, Steven S, Peters G (1996) Regulation of p16(CDKN2) expression and its implications for cell immortalization and senescence. Mol Cell Biol 16:859–867

Haugstetter AM, Loddenkemper C, Lenze D, Grone J, Standfuss C, Petersen I, Dorken B, Schmitt CA (2010) Cellular senescence predicts treatment outcome in metastasised colorectal cancer. Br J Cancer 103:505–509

Hayflick L, Moorhead PS (1961) The serial cultivation of human diploid cell strains. Exp Cell Res 25:585–621

He L, He X, Lim LP, de Stanchina E, Xuan Z, Liang Y, Xue W, Zender L, Magnus J, Ridzon D, Jackson AL, Linsley PS, Chen C, Lowe SW, Cleary MA, Hannon GJ (2007) A microRNA component of the p53 tumour suppressor network. Nature 447:1130–1134

Herbig U, Jobling WA, Chen BP, Chen DJ, Sedivy JM (2004) Telomere shortening triggers senescence of human cells through a pathway involving ATM, p53, and p21(CIP1), but not p16(INK4a). Mol Cell 14:501–513

Herbig U, Ferreira M, Condel L, Carey D, Sedivy JM (2006) Cellular senescence in aging primates. Science 311:1257

Hersey P, Zhang XD (2008) Adaptation to ER stress as a driver of malignancy and resistance to therapy in human melanoma. Pigment Cell Melanoma Res 21:358–367

Hinkal GW, Gatza CE, Parikh N, Donehower LA (2009) Altered senescence, apoptosis, and DNA damage response in a mutant p53 model of accelerated aging. Mech Ageing Dev 130:262–271

Hydbring P, Larsson LG (2010) Tipping the balance: Cdk2 enables Myc to suppress senescence. Cancer Res 70:6687–6691

Hydbring P, Bahram F, Su Y, Tronnersjo S, Hogstrand K, von der Lehr N, Sharifi HR, Lilischkis R, Hein N, Wu S, Vervoorts J, Henriksson M, Grandien A, Luscher B, Larsson LG (2010) Phosphorylation by Cdk2 is required for Myc to repress Ras-induced senescence in cotransformation. Proc Natl Acad Sci U S A 107:58–63

Ichii-Nakato N, Takata M, Takayanagi S, Takashima S, Lin J, Murata H, Fujimoto A, Hatta N, Saida T (2006) High frequency of B-RAFV600E mutation in acquired nevi and small congenital nevi, but low frequency of mutation in medium-sized congenital nevi. J Invest Dermatol 126:2111–2118

Jacobs JJ, Kieboom K, Marino S, DePinho RA, van Lohuizen M (1999a) The oncogene and Polycomb-group gene bmi-1 regulates cell proliferation and senescence through the ink4a locus. Nature 397:164–168

Jacobs JJ, Scheijen B, Voncken JW, Kieboom K, Berns A, van Lohuizen M (1999b) Bmi-1 collaborates with c-Myc in tumorigenesis by inhibiting c-Myc- induced apoptosis via INK4a/ARF. Genes Dev 13:2678–2690

Janzen V, Forkert R, Fleming HE, Saito Y, Waring MT, Dombkowski DM, Cheng T, DePinho RA, Sharpless NE, Scadden DT (2006) Stem-cell ageing modified by the cyclin-dependent kinase inhibitor p16INK4a. Nature 443:421–426

Jiang CC, Chen LH, Gillespie S, Kiejda KA, Mhaidat N, Wang YF, Thorne R, Zhang XD, Hersey P (2007) Tunicamycin sensitizes human melanoma cells to tumor necrosis factor-related apoptosis-inducing ligand-induced apoptosis by up-regulation of TRAIL-R2 via the unfolded protein response. Cancer Res 67:5880–5888

Kamijo T, Zindy F, Roussel MF, Quelle DE, Downing JR, Ashmun RA, Grosveld G, Sherr CJ (1997) Tumor suppression at the mouse INK4a locus mediated by the alternative reading frame product $p19^{ARF}$. Cell 91:649–659

Kaplon J, Zheng L, Meissl K, Chaneton B, Selivanov VA, Mackay G, van der Burg SH, Verdegaal EM, Cascante M, Shlomi T, Gottlieb E, Peeper DS (2013) A key role for mitochondrial gatekeeper pyruvate dehydrogenase in oncogene-induced senescence. Nature 498:109–112

Keyes WM, Wu Y, Vogel H, Guo X, Lowe SW, Mills AA (2005) p63 deficiency activates a program of cellular senescence and leads to accelerated aging. Genes Dev 19:1986–1999

Kim H, You S, Farris J, Kong BW, Christman SA, Foster LK, Foster DN (2002) Expression profiles of p53-, p16(INK4a)-, and telomere-regulating genes in replicative senescent primary human, mouse, and chicken fibroblast cells. Exp Cell Res 272:199–208

Korotchkina LG, Leontieva OV, Bukreeva EI, Demidenko ZN, Gudkov AV, Blagosklonny MV (2010) The choice between p53-induced senescence and quiescence is determined in part by the mTOR pathway. Aging (Albany NY) 2:344–352

Kortlever RM, Higgins PJ, Bernards R (2006) Plasminogen activator inhibitor-1 is a critical downstream target of p53 in the induction of replicative senescence. Nat Cell Biol 8:877–884

Krishnamurthy J, Torrice C, Ramsey MR, Kovalev GI, Al-Regaiey K, Su L, Sharpless NE (2004) Ink4a/Arf expression is a biomarker of aging. J Clin Invest 114:1299–1307

Krishnamurthy J, Ramsey MR, Ligon KL, Torrice C, Koh A, Bonner-Weir S, Sharpless NE (2006) p16INK4a induces an age-dependent decline in islet regenerative potential. Nature 443:453–457

Kuilman T, Peeper DS (2009) Senescence-messaging secretome: SMS-ing cellular stress. Nat Rev Cancer 9:81–94

Kuilman T, Michaloglou C, Vredeveld LC, Douma S, van Doorn R, Desmet CJ, Aarden LA, Mooi WJ, Peeper DS (2008) Oncogene-induced senescence relayed by an interleukin-dependent inflammatory network. Cell 133:1019–1031

Kurz DJ, Decary S, Hong Y, Erusalimsky JD (2000) Senescence-associated (beta)-galactosidase reflects an increase in lysosomal mass during replicative ageing of human endothelial cells. J Cell Sci 113(Pt 20):3613–3622

Kuwata T, Kitagawa M, Kasuga T (1993) Proliferative activity of primary cutaneous melanocytic tumours. Virchows Arch A Pathol Anat Histopathol 423:359–364

Laberge RM, Sun Y, Orjalo AV, Patil CK, Freund A, Zhou L, Curran SC, Davalos AR, Wilson-Edell KA, Liu S, Limbad C, Demaria M, Li P, Hubbard GB, Ikeno Y, Javors M, Desprez PY, Benz CC, Kapahi P, Nelson PS, Campisi J (2015) MTOR regulates the pro-tumorigenic senescence-associated secretory phenotype by promoting IL1A translation. Nat Cell Biol 17:1049–1061

Lal A, Kim HH, Abdelmohsen K, Kuwano Y, Pullmann R Jr, Srikantan S, Subrahmanyam R, Martindale JL, Yang X, Ahmed F, Navarro F, Dykxhoorn D, Lieberman J, Gorospe M (2008) p16(INK4a) translation suppressed by miR-24. PLoS One 3:e1864

Lasry A, Ben-Neriah Y (2015) Senescence-associated inflammatory responses: aging and cancer perspectives. Trends Immunol 36:217–228. doi:10.1016/j.it.2015.1002.1009, Epub 2015 Mar 1021

Lee BY, Han JA, Im JS, Morrone A, Johung K, Goodwin EC, Kleijer WJ, DiMaio D, Hwang ES (2006) Senescence-associated beta-galactosidase is lysosomal beta-galactosidase. Aging Cell 5:187–195

Li H, Collado M, Villasante A, Strati K, Ortega S, Canamero M, Blasco MA, Serrano M (2009) The Ink4/Arf locus is a barrier for iPS cell reprogramming. Nature 460:1136–1139

Li M, Durbin KR, Sweet SM, Tipton JD, Zheng Y, Kelleher NL (2013) Oncogene-induced cellular senescence elicits an anti-Warburg effect. Proteomics 13:2585–2596

Lin J, Takata M, Murata H, Goto Y, Kido K, Ferrone S, Saida T (2009) Polyclonality of BRAF mutations in acquired melanocytic nevi. J Natl Cancer Inst 101:1423–1427

Lin HK, Chen Z, Wang G, Nardella C, Lee SW, Chan CH, Yang WL, Wang J, Egia A, Nakayama KI, Cordon-Cardo C, Teruya-Feldstein J, Pandolfi PP (2010) Skp2 targeting suppresses tumorigenesis by Arf-p53-independent cellular senescence. Nature 464:374–379

Liu D, Hornsby PJ (2007) Senescent human fibroblasts increase the early growth of xenograft tumors via matrix metalloproteinase secretion. Cancer Res 67:3117–3126

Liu Y, Sanoff HK, Cho H, Burd CE, Torrice C, Ibrahim JG, Thomas NE, Sharpless NE (2009) Expression of p16(INK4a) in peripheral blood T-cells is a biomarker of human aging. Aging Cell 8:439–448

Loercher AE, Tank EMH, Delston RB, Harbour JW (2005) MITF links differentiation with cell cycle arrest in melanocytes by transcriptional activation of INK4A. J Cell Biol 168:35–40

Maier AB, Westendorp RG (2009) Relation between replicative senescence of human fibroblasts and life history characteristics. Ageing Res Rev 8:237–243

Maldonado JL, Timmerman L, Fridlyand J, Bastian BC (2004) Mechanisms of cell-cycle arrest in Spitz nevi with constitutive activation of the MAP-kinase pathway. Am J Pathol 164:1783–1787

Matheu A, Maraver A, Klatt P, Flores I, Garcia-Cao I, Borras C, Flores JM, Vina J, Blasco MA, Serrano M (2007) Delayed ageing through damage protection by the Arf/p53 pathway. Nature 448:375–379

Matheu A, Maraver A, Serrano M (2008) The Arf/p53 pathway in cancer and aging. Cancer Res 68:6031–6034

Matheu A, Maraver A, Collado M, Garcia-Cao I, Canamero M, Borras C, Flores JM, Klatt P, Vina J, Serrano M (2009) Anti-aging activity of the Ink4/Arf locus. Aging Cell 8:152–161

McCarron M, Osborne Y, Story CJ, Dempsey JL, Turner DR, Morley AA (1987) Effect of age on lymphocyte proliferation. Mech Ageing Dev 41:211–218

Melk A, Kittikowit W, Sandhu I, Halloran KM, Grimm P, Schmidt BM, Halloran PF (2003) Cell senescence in rat kidneys in vivo increases with growth and age despite lack of telomere shortening. Kidney Int 63:2134–2143

Michaloglou C, Vredeveld LC, Soengas MS, Denoyelle C, Kuilman T, van der Horst CM, Majoor DM, Shay JW, Mooi WJ, Peeper DS (2005) BRAFE600-associated senescence-like cell cycle arrest of human naevi. Nature 436:720–724

Michaloglou C, Soengas MS, Mooi WJ, Peeper DS (2008) Comment on "Absence of senescence-associated beta-galactosidase activity in human melanocytic nevi in vivo". J Invest Dermatol 128:1582–1583; author reply 1583–1584

Miracco C, Margherita De Santi M, Schurfeld K, Santopietro R, Lalinga AV, Fimiani M, Biagioli M, Brogi M, De Felice C, Luzi P, Andreassi L (2002) Quantitative in situ evaluation of telomeres in fluorescence in situ hybridization-processed sections of cutaneous melanocytic lesions and correlation with telomerase activity. Br J Dermatol 146:399–408

Molenaar JJ, Ebus ME, Geerts D, Koster J, Lamers F, Valentijn LJ, Westerhout EM, Versteeg R, Caron HN (2009) Inactivation of CDK2 is synthetically lethal to MYCN over-expressing cancer cells. Proc Natl Acad Sci U S A 106:12968–12973

Molofsky AV, Pardal R, Iwashita T, Park IK, Clarke MF, Morrison SJ (2003) Bmi-1 dependence distinguishes neural stem cell self-renewal from progenitor proliferation. Nature 425:962–967

Molofsky AV, He S, Bydon M, Morrison SJ, Pardal R (2005) Bmi-1 promotes neural stem cell self-renewal and neural development but not mouse growth and survival by repressing the p16Ink4a and p19Arf senescence pathways. Genes Dev 19:1432–1437

Molofsky AV, Slutsky SG, Joseph NM, He S, Pardal R, Krishnamurthy J, Sharpless NE, Morrison SJ (2006) Increasing p16INK4a expression decreases forebrain progenitors and neurogenesis during ageing. Nature 443:448–452

Mooi WJ, Peeper DS (2006) Oncogene-induced cell senescence--halting on the road to cancer. N Engl J Med 355:1037–1046

Naidoo N (2009a) The endoplasmic reticulum stress response and aging. Rev Neurosci 20:23–37

Naidoo N (2009b) ER and aging-Protein folding and the ER stress response. Ageing Res Rev 8:150–159

Narita M, Nunez S, Heard E, Lin AW, Hearn SA, Spector DL, Hannon GJ, Lowe SW (2003) Rb-mediated heterochromatin formation and silencing of E2F target genes during cellular senescence. Cell 113:703–716

Ohtani N, Zebedee Z, Huot TJ, Stinson JA, Sugimoto M, Ohashi Y, Sharrocks AD, Peters G, Hara E (2001) Opposing effects of Ets and Id proteins on p16INK4a expression during cellular senescence. Nature 409:1067–1070

Pantoja C, Serrano M (1999) Murine fibroblasts lacking p21 undergo senescence and are resistant to transformation by oncogenic Ras. Oncogene 18:4974–4982

Park IK, Qian D, Kiel M, Becker MW, Pihalja M, Weissman IL, Morrison SJ, Clarke MF (2003) Bmi-1 is required for maintenance of adult self-renewing haematopoietic stem cells. Nature 423:302–305

Pollock PM, Harper UL, Hansen KS, Yudt LM, Stark M, Robbins CM, Moses TY, Hostetter G, Wagner U, Kakareka J, Salem G, Pohida T, Heenan P, Duray P, Kallioniemi O, Hayward NK, Trent JM, Meltzer PS (2003) High frequency of BRAF mutations in nevi. Nat Genet 33:19–20

Price JS, Waters JG, Darrah C, Pennington C, Edwards DR, Donell ST, Clark IM (2002) The role of chondrocyte senescence in osteoarthritis. Aging Cell 1:57–65

Ramirez RD, Morales CP, Herbert BS, Rohde JM, Passons C, Shay JW, Wright WE (2001) Putative telomere-independent mechanisms of replicative aging reflect inadequate growth conditions. Genes Dev 15:398–403

Rasoamanantena P, Thweatt R, Labat-Robert J, Goldstein S (1994) Altered regulation of fibronectin gene expression in Werner syndrome fibroblasts. Exp Cell Res 213:121–127

Roberson RS, Kussick SJ, Vallieres E, Chen SY, Wu DY (2005) Escape from therapy-induced accelerated cellular senescence in p53-null lung cancer cells and in human lung cancers. Cancer Res 65:2795–2803

Rodier F, Coppe JP, Patil CK, Hoeijmakers WA, Munoz DP, Raza SR, Freund A, Campeau E, Davalos AR, Campisi J (2009) Persistent DNA damage signalling triggers senescence-associated inflammatory cytokine secretion. Nat Cell Biol 11:973–979

Rodier F, Munoz DP, Teachenor R, Chu V, Le O, Bhaumik D, Coppe JP, Campeau E, Beausejour CM, Kim SH, Davalos AR, Campisi J (2011) DNA-SCARS: distinct nuclear structures that sustain damage-induced senescence growth arrest and inflammatory cytokine secretion. J Cell Sci 124:68–81

Rossi DJ, Bryder D, Seita J, Nussenzweig A, Hoeijmakers J, Weissman IL (2007) Deficiencies in DNA damage repair limit the function of haematopoietic stem cells with age. Nature 447:725–729

Sakamoto K et al (1993) Relative mitogenic activities of wild-type and retinoblastoma binding deficient SV40 T antigens in serum-deprived human diploid fibroblasts. Oncogene 8:1887–1893

Sarkisian CJ, Keister BA, Stairs DB, Boxer RB, Moody SE, Chodosh LA (2007) Dose-dependent oncogene-induced senescence in vivo and its evasion during mammary tumorigenesis. Nat Cell Biol 9:493–505

Schick U, Kyula J, Barker H, Patel R, Zaidi S, Gregory C, Hafsi H, Roulstone V, Deutsch E, McLaughlin M, Harrington K (2015) Trametinib radiosensitises RAS- and BRAF-mutated melanoma by perturbing cell cycle and inducing senescence. Radiother Oncol 117(2): 364–375, 026

Schmitt CA, Fridman JS, Yang M, Lee S, Baranov E, Hoffman RM, Lowe SW (2002) A senescence program controlled by p53 and p16INK4a contributes to the outcome of cancer therapy. Cell 109:335–346

Serrano M, Lee H-W, Chin L, Cordon-Cardo C, Beach D, DePinho RA (1996) Role of the *INK4a* locus in tumor suppression and cell mortality. Cell 85:27–37

Serrano M, Lin AW, McCurrach ME, Beach D, Lowe SW (1997) Oncogenic ras provokes premature cell senescence associated with accumulation of p53 and p16INK4a. Cell 85:593–602
Severino J, Allen RG, Balin S, Balin A, Cristofalo VJ (2000) Is beta-galactosidase staining a marker of senescence in vitro and in vivo? Exp Cell Res 257:162–171
Sharpless NE, Sherr CJ (2015) Forging a signature of in vivo senescence. Nat Rev Cancer 15:397–408. doi:10.1038/nrc3960
Sherr CJ (1996) Cancer cell cycles. Science 274:1672–1677
Signer RA, Montecino-Rodriguez E, Witte ON, Dorshkind K (2008) Aging and cancer resistance in lymphoid progenitors are linked processes conferred by p16Ink4a and Arf. Genes Dev 22:3115–3120
Smith JR, Nakanishi M, Robetorye RS, Venable SF, Pereira-Smith OM (1996) Studies demonstrating the complexity of regulation and action of the growth inhibitory gene SDI1. Exp Gerontol 31:327–335
Sugrue MM, Shin DY, Lee SW, Aaronson SA (1997) Wild-type p53 triggers a rapid senescence program in human tumor cells lacking functional p53. Proc Natl Acad Sci U S A 94:9648–9653
Sviderskaya EV, Gray-Schopfer VC, Hill SP, Smit NP, Evans-Whipp TJ, Bond J, Hill L, Bataille V, Peters G, Kipling D, Wynford-Thomas D, Bennett DC (2003) p16/cyclin-dependent kinase inhibitor 2A deficiency in human melanocyte senescence, apoptosis, and immortalization: possible implications for melanoma progression. J Natl Cancer Inst 95:723–732
te Poele RH, Okorokov AL, Jardine L, Cummings J, Joel SP (2002) DNA damage is able to induce senescence in tumor cells in vitro and in vivo. Cancer Res 62:1876–1883
Tran SL, Haferkamp S, Scurr LL, Gowrishankar K, Becker TM, Desilva C, Thompson JF, Scolyer RA, Kefford RF, Rizos H (2012) Absence of distinguishing senescence traits in human melanocytic nevi. J Invest Dermatol 19:126
Ventura A, Kirsch DG, McLaughlin ME, Tuveson DA, Grimm J, Lintault L, Newman J, Reczek EE, Weissleder R, Jacks T (2007) Restoration of p53 function leads to tumour regression in vivo. Nature 445:661–665
Wajapeyee N, Serra RW, Zhu X, Mahalingam M, Green MR (2008) Oncogenic BRAF induces senescence and apoptosis through pathways mediated by the secreted protein IGFBP7. Cell 132:363–374
Wang Y, Meng A, Zhou D (2004) Inhibition of phosphatidylinostol 3-kinase uncouples H2O2-induced senescent phenotype and cell cycle arrest in normal human diploid fibroblasts. Exp Cell Res 298:188–196
Wei W, Sedivy JM (1999) Differentiation between senescence (M1) and crisis (M2) in human fibroblast cultures. Exp Cell Res 253:519–522
West AC, Johnstone RW (2014) New and emerging HDAC inhibitors for cancer treatment. J Clin Invest 124:30–39
Wong H, Riabowol K (1996) Differential CDK-inhibitor gene expression in aging human diploid fibroblasts. Exp Gerontol 31:311–325
Wu CH, van Riggelen J, Yetil A, Fan AC, Bachireddy P, Felsher DW (2007) Cellular senescence is an important mechanism of tumor regression upon c-Myc inactivation. Proc Natl Acad Sci U S A 104:13028–13033
Xue W, Zender L, Miething C, Dickins RA, Hernando E, Krizhanovsky V, Cordon-Cardo C, Lowe SW (2007) Senescence and tumour clearance is triggered by p53 restoration in murine liver carcinomas. Nature 445:656–660
Yeh I, von Deimling A, Bastian BC (2013) Clonal BRAF mutations in melanocytic nevi and initiating role of BRAF in melanocytic neoplasia. J Natl Cancer Inst 105:917–919
Zhuang D, Mannava S, Grachtchouk V, Tang WH, Patil S, Wawrzyniak JA, Berman AE, Giordano TJ, Prochownik EV, Soengas MS, Nikiforov MA (2008) C-MYC overexpression is required for continuous suppression of oncogene-induced senescence in melanoma cells. Oncogene 27:6623–6634
Zindy F, Quelle DE, Roussel MF, Sherr CJ (1997) Expression of the p16INK4a tumor suppressor versus other INK4 family members during mouse development and aging. Oncogene 15:203–211

Melanoma Stem Cells

12

Tobias F.I. Schatton and Markus H. Frank

12.1 Introduction

The hypothesis that cancers and tissue stem cells might share several biological traits is many decades old (Bruce and Van Der Gaag 1963; Hamburger and Salmon 1977; Park et al. 1971). Indeed, the defining stem cell traits of (a) self-renewal, (b) differentiation, and (c) potential to proliferate nearly indefinitely are commonly observed among cancer subpopulations (Reya et al. 2001). Moreover, interactions with stromal elements and signaling pathways that govern physiologic stem cell behavior were also found to play important roles during tumor development (Frank et al. 2010). Together, these observations have led to the cancer stem cells (CSCs) theory of tumor initiation and growth, which postulates that the tumorigenic process relies on a reservoir of self-renewing, aggressive cells that confer clinical virulence, that is, CSCs (Reya et al. 2001). Such tumorigenic minority populations or CSCs have since been characterized in a growing number of tumor entities (Schatton et al. 2009), including in human melanoma (Boiko et al. 2010; Boonyaratanakornkit et al. 2010; Schatton et al. 2008).

In this chapter, we will review the current knowledge of CSCs and their biological features with particular emphasis on human malignant melanoma and discuss controversial aspects of the CSC theory. Furthermore, we will explore the

T.F.I. Schatton, Ph.D., Pharm.D.
Assistant Professor of Dermatology, Department of Dermatology, Brigham and Women's Hospital, 77 Avenue Louis Pasteur, Boston 02115, MA, USA

M.H. Frank (✉)
Department of Dermatology, Harvard Skin Disease Research Center, Brigham and Women's Hospital, Harvard Medical School, 77 Avenue Louis Pasteur, Boston 02115, MA, USA

Transplant Research Program, Boston Children's Hospital, Harvard Medical School, 300 Longwood Avenue, Boston 02115, MA, USA
e-mail: markus.frank@childrens.harvard.edu

A. Bosserhoff (ed.), *Melanoma Development*,
DOI 10.1007/978-3-319-41319-8_12

implications of the findings of melanoma as a CSC-driven disease for the development of more effective treatment modalities for melanoma patients.

12.2 What Is a "Cancer Stem Cell"?

It has long been established that tumors comprise multiple phenotypically and functionally distinct populations of cancer cells (Hanahan and Weinberg 2000). Several theories have been put forward to account for the occurrence of such tumor heterogeneity. According to the classic view of tumorigenesis, tumor heterogeneity can be explained by both intrinsic factors (i.e., progressive accumulations of genetic alterations over time) and extrinsic stimuli (e.g., distinct cues from the tumor microenvironment, Hanahan and Weinberg 2000). The so-called stochastic theory of tumor initiation postulates that all malignant cells within a cancer, regardless of their phenotype, possess equivalent capacities to proliferate, form new tumors, and cause relapse (Nowell 1976). The CSC hypothesis, on the other hand, provides an alternative explanation for tumor heterogeneity (Reya et al. 2001): It posits that cancers, like physiologic tissues, are organized as developmentally defined hierarchies of cells with divergent differentiation features and disparate capabilities for self-renewal and neoplastic proliferation. The CSC concept thus proposes that only a subpopulation of tumor cells within a cancer, namely CSCs, bears the competence to fuel tumor growth by continuously undergoing self-renewal and differentiation, whereas the bulk of differentiated cancer components lacks the capacity for tumor initiation and unlimited proliferation (Murphy et al. 2014) (Fig. 12.1).

According to a consensus definition (Clarke et al. 2006), a CSC is a cell within a tumor that possesses the capacity to undergo both self-renewing cell divisions that expand the CSC pool, and cell divisions that result in more differentiated cancer cell progeny. Therefore, CSCs can only be defined experimentally by their ability to recapitulate the generation of a continuously growing tumor (Clarke et al. 2006).

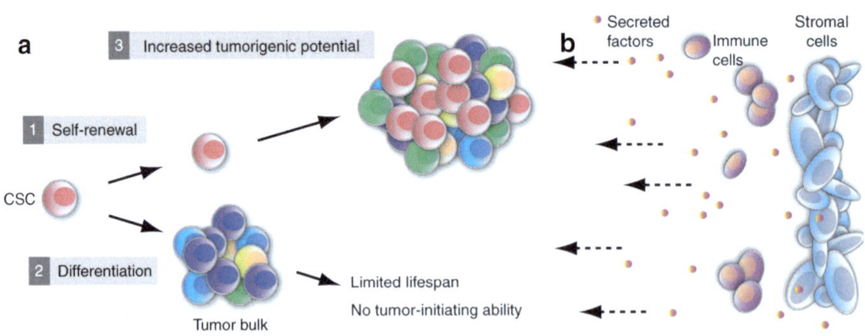

Fig. 12.1 *The cardinal features of CSCs*. Illustrated are (**a**) the defining features of CSCs, that is, (*1*) self-renewal capacity, (*2*) differentiation capacity, and (*3*) increased tumorigenic potential. (**b**) TME characteristics, that is, secreted factors, host immunity, and stromal cell interactions also regulate CSC-dependent tumor growth

Accordingly, the experimental characterization of a putative CSC population relies on the use of an in vivo model system that allows for a rigorous confirmation of the traits used to define CSCs. The gold standard assay that fulfills this criterion for identification of human CSC populations is serial xenotransplantation at limiting dilution of marker-defined clinical cancer subpopulations into an orthotopic site of immunocompromised mice (typically NOD/SCID), which although imperfect is considered the best experimental system to evaluate CSC activity (Clarke et al. 2006). Using this approach, CSCs capable of sustained self-renewal and tumor propagation were first described in cancers of the hematopoietic lineage (Bonnet and Dick 1997). These initial studies demonstrated that it is possible to isolate from a single tumor sample two distinct cancer subpopulations that differ in their cell surface antigen profile and their tumor-seeding properties: (1) a CSC-enriched subset, as defined by its exclusive ability to self-renew as well as differentiate into nontumorigenic cancer cell progeny and its competence to seed new tumors upon serial xenotransplantation, and (2) the bulk of tumor cells that lack the capacity to generate tumors in animal hosts (Bonnet and Dick 1997). Subsequent studies extended these findings to a variety of additional hematological malignancies and solid tumor entities (Al-Hajj et al. 2003; Castor et al. 2005; Chan et al. 2009; Cox et al. 2004, 2007; Dalerba et al. 2007; Hermann et al. 2007; Ishikawa et al. 2007; Li et al. 2007; O'Brien et al. 2007; Prince et al. 2007; Ricci-Vitiani et al. 2007; Singh et al. 2004; Suva et al. 2009; Yang et al. 2008; Zhang et al. 2008), including malignant melanoma (Boiko et al. 2010; Schatton et al. 2008). Hierarchical tumor organization has been confirmed in syngeneic mouse models in which only fractions of murine tumor cells possessed the fundamental CSC features of extensive self-renewal, differentiation, and enhanced tumorigenic capacity (Cho et al. 2008; Deshpande et al. 2006; Held et al. 2010; Wu et al. 2008).

Despite these advances in our understanding of functional tumor heterogeneity, the CSC model has represented a topic of considerable controversy (Hill 2006; Jordan 2009). Some of this controversy appears to arise from uncertainty regarding the term "CSC." For instance, the term CSC has been interpreted to mean that the cellular precursors of such tumorigenic subpopulations were originally physiologic stem cells, which accumulated genetic alterations resulting in cancerous transformation. While this may be the case in some malignancies (Barker et al. 2009; Zhu et al. 2009), CSCs in other cancers may originate from more differentiated cells that reacquired stem-like properties through a series of mutagenic events (Huntly et al. 2004; Jamieson et al. 2004; Krivtsov et al. 2006). Additionally, differentiation in the context of CSC biology does not refer to multipotent differentiation plasticity as it occurs during organogenesis or physiologic tissue regeneration, but rather to the ability of CSCs to give rise to cancer cells that lack tumor-initiating capacity (Clarke et al. 2006). Furthermore, in contrast to physiologic stem cells, which represent only a small cellular fraction of a particular tissue, CSCs may represent larger relative proportions of a total cancer cell population, depending on tumor type, variance of genetic alterations, and stage of disease progression (Gupta et al. 2009). In support of this notion, the frequency of leukemic CSCs varied more than hundred-fold between distinct patient specimens (Bonnet and Dick 1997). CSC representation may also vary within a single cancer specimen, in which undifferentiated regions may harbor larger numbers of CSCs compared to more differentiated tumor areas (Gupta et al. 2009). Importantly, the number of cells needed to initiate a tumor is not part of the CSC definition (Reya et al. 2001; Schatton et al. 2009). Hence, a larger relative proportion of tumorigenic cells does not contradict the CSC model of tumor initiation and growth. Given the potential confusion associated with the term "CSC," many investigators in the field refer to them as tumor-initiating or tumor-propagating cells (Clarke et al. 2006).

The determination of relative CSC frequencies is influenced by the experimental model system used to assess cancer "stemness" (Boiko et al. 2010; Bonnet and Dick 1997; Lapidot et al. 1994; O'Brien et al. 2007; Quintana et al. 2008, 2010; Ricci-Vitiani et al. 2007; Schatton et al. 2008; Shmelkov et al. 2008). In this regard, it has been established for some time that biological aspects of the tumor microenvironment, including growth factor availability, extracellular matrix (ECM) composition, or the degree of vascularization, as well as host immunocompetence can control the tumorigenic potential of cancer subpopulations (Scadden 2006) (Fig. 12.1). Given this dependence of a defining CSC feature on microenvironmental factors and the immune status of the host, it is not surprising that animal models that offer a more hospitable microenvironment for tumor growth – that is, through the exogenous addition of ECM factors (e.g., Matrigel) (Quintana et al. 2008) and/or the use of more severely immunocompromised mice (Bonnet and Dick 1997; Quintana et al. 2008) – can yield higher relative CSC counts compared to CSC frequencies assessed in the absence of cografted stromal factors in more immunocompetent mouse models (Lapidot et al. 1994; Quintana et al. 2008; Schatton et al. 2008). Based on these considerations, more permissive xenotransplantation conditions might be inadequate for the accurate assessment of CSC biology as it occurs in humans, as they could enable non-CSCs to initiate and maintain experimental tumor growth (Gupta et al. 2009; Murphy et al. 2014).

The tumor biospecimens used for the isolation and characterization of putative CSC populations also influence the assessment of CSC frequency (Gupta et al. 2009). For instance, utilizing tumor cell isolates from tumor xenografts that have been passaged in vivo for extended periods of time Quintana et al. (2008, 2010) in lieu of fresh patient-derived tumor samples likely obscures the accurate assessment of CSC frequencies and biological functions (Boiko et al. 2010). Indeed, Boiko and colleagues demonstrated that both in vitro and in vivo passaging of melanoma cells can result in the emergence of tumorigenic subclones that drive experimental tumor growth independent of their immunophenotype (Boiko et al. 2010). Similarly, tumor cell lines may have lost the hierarchical structure of the primary tumor from which they originated (Zhou et al. 2009). Variations in tumor dissociation, isolation, and/or inoculation techniques could also account for differences in calculated CSC frequencies between different laboratories (Shackleton 2010). Moreover, the use of tumor specimens from patients with more advanced disease (Quintana et al. 2008), which have been demonstrated to contain elevated CSC numbers compared to primary tumors (Schatton et al. 2008), could yield higher estimated CSC frequencies (Boiko et al. 2010).

Clearly, a considerable variability has been observed in the course of CSC identification efforts with regard to estimated frequencies of tumorigenic cells depending on the mouse model used. While the relative frequency of CSCs is not directly relevant for their identification as it is not a CSC-defining feature, it is nevertheless important to define the factors responsible for this variability because such studies could help identify additional CSC-specific functions (Schatton et al. 2009). For example, the tumor microenvironment, including that of an immunocompromised host, may govern not only the tumorigenic potential of cancer subpopulations but also additional CSC-defining traits, including differentiation and self-renewal (Postovit et al. 2006). It is thus possible that a very permissive milieu for tumor growth may not only enable non-CSCs to seed cancers but could also facilitate the "de-differentiation" of such nontumorigenic bulk populations into CSC phenotype-expressing cells (Hoek and Goding 2010). The conversion of non-CSCs into CSC-like cells may, however, not occur in more hostile cancer environments observed in patient tumors, which are typically characterized by low nutrient availability, marked levels of hypoxia, necrosis, and inflammation, and the presence of antitumor immune responses. Only a minority of tumor cells, that is, CSCs, might possess the ability to survive and fuel the tumorigenic process under these selective pressures. In support of this hypothesis, hypoxia-inducible factors (HIFs) are preferentially expressed in CSCs, and blockade of HIF2α on glioma CSCs attenuated their potential to initiate experimental tumors (Li et al. 2009b). Furthermore, viable glioma CSCs preferentially localize to perivascular niches in both clinical and experimental cancer specimens (Calabrese et al. 2007). The bulk of tumor cells within cancerous lesions that have reached a significant size, on the other hand, is often necrotic or undergoes apoptosis (Cotter 2009), indicating that their conversion into apoptosis-resistant stem-like cancer cells does not commonly occur under these conditions.

The complexity of CSC biology and its implications for the type of animal model utilized for their characterization is further highlighted by the identification of novel CSC functions (Frank et al. 2010), including their intrinsic property to evade or actively modulate antitumor immune responses (Chan et al. 2009; Di Tomaso et al. 2010; Majeti et al. 2009; Schatton and Frank 2009; Schatton et al. 2010; Todaro et al. 2009; Wei et al. 2010a, b). Such mechanisms, which may confer selective growth advantages to the CSC pool, need to be taken into consideration when designing biologically relevant assays for their characterization. These findings highlight the importance of establishing translationally relevant assays for the study of CSCs, which accurately mimic the environmental factors found in clinical cancers (e.g., presence of human stromal cells, low-nutrient levels, necrosis, hypoxia, and relatively intact antitumor immunity) rather than further deviating from the naturally occurring microenvironmental characteristics. Current xenotransplantation protocols and animal models for the study of tumorigenic subpopulations that do not accurately reflect the pathological environment of spontaneously occurring human malignancies might favor niche-independent tumor growth (Quintana et al. 2008). Similarly, the so-called tumor sphere culture assay, which favors anchorage-independent in vitro passaging of cancer cells, and which has been proposed to serve as a surrogate tool for the identification of tumor-initiating cells (Fang et al. 2005; Keshet et al. 2008; Perego et al. 2010), represents an inadequate stand-alone assay for the relevant study of CSC biology in the absence of an in vivo confirmation of CSC-defining traits of a marker-defined tumor subset (Schatton and Frank 2010).

Although much work is still required to fully characterize CSCs and to reach consensus about clinically relevant model systems for their study, efforts directed toward identifying strategies that effectively target tumorigenic minority populations could significantly enhance current treatment modalities. In the following sections, we will discuss how the study of MMICs can yield new insights into melanomagenesis that could potentially lead to the development of improved melanoma treatment strategies.

12.3 Melanoma Stem Cells: Evidence for Their Clinical Relevance

The study of CSCs in human malignant melanoma has recently elicited considerable interest. Given its marked heterogeneity, pronounced resistance to conventional anticancer therapy, and highly aggressive behavior, it has been speculated for some time that melanoma, like numerous additional solid cancers, may follow the CSC model of tumor initiation and growth (Hendrix et al. 2003a; Schatton and Frank 2008). Melanoma remains the most lethal form of skin cancer and melanoma incidence is increasing faster than any other cancer worldwide (Jemal et al. 2010). Although the survival rate of patients diagnosed with melanoma has improved over the past decades (Linos et al. 2009), and greatly accelerated to improve in recent years with the advent of novel molecular targeted therapies and checkpoint blockade immunotherapies (Ugurel et al. 2016), there continues to exist a clear need for novel strategies to eradicate the melanoma subpopulation in which clinical virulence and therapeutic resistance reside, which appear to coincide with MMICs.

Initial support for the potential existence of MMICs came from the demonstration that CSC phenotype-expressing cancer subpopulations are present in melanoma cell lines and clinical melanomas (Frank et al. 2005). Specifically, this study showed that a number of stem cell markers, including the prospective CSC determinant, *CD133* (Hermann et al. 2007; O'Brien et al. 2007; Ricci-Vitiani et al. 2007; Singh et al. 2004; Suva et al. 2009), were over-expressed by chemoresistant tumor subsets among heterogeneous malignant melanoma cultures and within clinical melanoma biospecimens (Frank et al. 2005). Subsequently, Monzani and colleagues showed that $CD133^+$ melanoma fractions had the preferential ability to initiate primary tumor formation in NOD/SCID mice compared to $CD133^-$ melanoma bulk populations (Monzani et al. 2007), demonstrating the existence of tumorigenic melanoma subpopulations. The authors of the study did not examine, however, whether $CD133^+$ melanoma subsets were capable of self-renewal and differentiation in serial xenotransplantation experiments (Monzani et al. 2007). In the absence of stringent in vivo assays aimed at dissecting these key CSC-defining features, no definitive conclusions can be made about the potential relationship of $CD133^+$ or other melanoma minority populations to MMICs. This limitation also applies to a study characterizing melanoma subpopulations based on their ability to grow in spheroid bodies in vitro (Fang et al. 2005). Melanoma cells isolated from such "melanospheres" preferentially expressed the marker of mature B cells, *CD20*, and were more tumorigenic when grafted to immunodeficient mice compared to melanoma cells grown as adherent in vitro cultures (Fang et al. 2005). While the results by Fang and colleagues (Fang et al. 2005) did not establish the existence of MMICs, they suggested, however, that melanomas might comprise functionally distinct subpopulations with divergent tumorigenic capacities.

Unequivocal evidence for the existence of melanoma CSCs, capable of long-term self-renewal and differentiation, was first provided when the chemoresistance mediator (Cheung et al. 2011; Elliott and Al-Hajj 2009; Frank et al. 2005; Fukunaga-Kalabis et al. 2010; Huang et al. 2004; Yang et al. 2010) and cell surface molecule, *ABCB5*, was established as a prospective biomarker of MMICs (Schatton et al. 2008). This study demonstrated that $ABCB5^+$ melanoma fractions, but not $ABCB5^-$ melanoma bulk populations, isolated from patient biopsies were capable of initiating primary and secondary neoplasms upon serial xenotransplantation at limiting dilution into NOD/SCID mice (Schatton et al. 2008). In addition, $ABCB5^+$ melanoma cells were capable of generating phenocopies of the original patient tumors, indicating their ability to both self-renew (i.e., to maintain the $ABCB5^+$ cell pool by generating more copies of themselves) and differentiate (i.e., to give rise to more differentiated, $ABCB5^-$ tumor cell progeny, incapable of initiating experimental tumor growth) upon serial xenotransplantation (Schatton et al. 2008). These results thus established that $ABCB5^+$ melanoma subpopulations represent MMICs (Zabierowski and Herlyn 2008) as per the CSC consensus definition (Clarke et al. 2006) outlined above.

To further confirm the selective capacity of $ABCB5^+$ MMICs for enhanced tumorigenic growth, self-renewal, and differentiation, genetic lineage tracking was performed in human melanoma to NOD/SCID mouse xenotransplantation experiments employing genetically encoded DsRed (red fluorescent protein) and EYFP (enhanced yellow–green fluorescent protein) labeling of MMICs and melanoma bulk populations, respectively (Schatton et al. 2008). Xenotransplantation of $ABCB5^+DsRed^+$ melanoma cells and $ABCB5^-EYFP^+$ tumor bulk components, reconstituted at naturally occurring ratios, resulted in markedly increased relative frequencies of $DsRed^+$ cells of $ABCB5^+$ origin in melanoma xenografts (Schatton et al. 2008), confirming the enhanced tumorigenic capacity of $ABCB5^+$ MMICs. In addition, these lineage-tracing experiments revealed a tumor hierarchy, in which $ABCB5^+$ cells had the ability to generate both $ABCB5^+$ and $ABCB5^-$ tumor progeny, whereas $ABCB5^-$ melanoma cells exclusively gave rise to more copies of themselves (Schatton et al. 2008). In more recent work, the increased tumorigenic capacity of $ABCB5^+$ vis-a-vis $ABCB5^-$ melanoma subpopulations has been independently confirmed not only in human to NOD *scid* gamma (NSG) mouse xenotransplantation experiments (Kupas et al. 2011), but also for murine melanomas in syngeneic tumor transplantation models (Zhang et al. 2016). Thus, two fundamentally different cell types with divergent tumorigenic potentials exist within melanomas, only one of which is capable of self-renewal and differentiation – that is, ABCB5⁺ MMICs. To further establish that the melanoma subpopulation marked by ABCB5 is required for efficient tumor growth, as anticipated by the MMIC model, our laboratory examined whether selective ablation of MMICs could inhibit tumor development (Schatton et al. 2008). Indeed, administration of an anti-ABCB5 monoclonal antibody into nude mice xenografted with human melanomas impaired tumor initiation and slowed tumorigenic growth via antibody-dependent cell-mediated cytotoxicity (ADCC) directed at $ABCB5^+$ MMICs (Schatton et al. 2008). These results provided proof-of-concept for the potential therapeutic utility of targeting MMICs and provided evidence that melanoma is a CSC-driven disease.

In the same study, using an established melanocytic tumor tissue microarray (Kim et al. 2006), a positive correlation between $ABCB5^+$ melanoma cell frequency and clinical melanoma progression was established (Schatton et al. 2008). Specifically, there was higher ABCB5 expression in primary melanomas versus benign nevi, and in metastatic melanomas versus primary melanomas, showing that ABCB5 correlates with neoplastic progression (Schatton et al. 2008). A role for ABCB5 in clinical melanoma initiation/progression has recently also been established by additional laboratories (Gazzaniga et al. 2010; Sharma et al. 2010), and these findings have been extended to acral melanomas (Vasquez-Moctezuma et al. 2010) and in vivo human melanoma model systems (Fukunaga-Kalabis et al. 2010; Ma et al. 2010). ABCB5 expression also correlates with neoplastic progression in additional malignancies, including hepatocellular carcinoma, where it serves as a major independent clinical biomarker of poor survival (Cheung et al. 2011). The potential importance of ABCB5 as a biomarker of metastatic melanoma progression and disseminated disease was initially further supported by an additional study from our laboratory (Ma et al. 2010): ABCB5 mRNA could be detected in peripheral blood mononuclear cell preparations from human stage IV melanoma patients but not healthy controls (Ma et al. 2010). Similarly, human ABCB5 mRNA expression could also be detected among peripheral blood mononuclear cells isolated from NOD *scid* gamma (NSG) recipients of subcutaneous human melanoma xenografts (Ma et al. 2010), indicating that circulating melanoma-initiating cells might be present in both murine models and stage IV melanoma patients. Indeed, viable circulating tumor cells (CTCs), isolated from the blood circulation of tumor-bearing hosts, were capable of primary melanoma and metastasis formation in serial xenotransplantation experiments (Ma et al. 2010). Strikingly, CTCs capable of melanoma initiation demonstrated significantly increased ABCB5 expression levels compared to primary tumor xenografts and metastatic lesions (Ma et al. 2010). These results provided initial evidence that circulating melanoma cells are tumorigenic and capable of metastasis formation, and showed that CTCs are enriched for MMICs. Indeed, subsequent clinical studies showed that ABCB5 subpopulations are also more common among CTCs than in solid tumors in melanoma patients (Gray et al. 2015) and that ABCB5 mRNA levels in the peripheral circulation of melanoma patients had significant prognostic value in inferring disease recurrence (Reid et al. 2013). Together, these results highlighted that ABCB5 identifies clinically important disseminated melanoma subpopulations that warrant future research investigations regarding their potential role as a novel diagnostic and therapeutic biomarker.

Additional support for the CSC properties of ABCB5$^+$ melanoma fractions has also come from syngeneic melanoma mouse models (Ehira et al. 2010). Specifically, a tumorigenic B16 murine melanoma cell line variant demonstrated increased Abcb5 expression upon in vivo tumor formation (Ehira et al. 2010) alongside with other markers previously shown to enrich for murine MMIC-like cells with increased clonogenic and tumorigenic potentials (Dou et al. 2007). Taken together, these findings indicate that murine Abcb5$^+$ B16 melanoma subpopulations, like human ABCB5$^+$ MMICs, represent CSC-like cells that amplify during the tumorigenic process (Ehira et al. 2010). Similarly, the ABCB5 gene was also preferentially expressed by human melanomas with high in vivo tumorigenic capacity in human to murine xenotransplantation experiments Hoek et al. (2004, 2008). Consistent with these findings, human melanoma subpopulations with enhanced in vitro clonogenic and self-renewal capacities demonstrated increased ABCB5 expression levels (Keshet et al. 2008). In a separate study, induction of terminal differentiation of human melanoma cells resulted in a significant decrease in ABCB5 expression concomitant with reduced proliferation and enhanced susceptibility to chemotherapeutic agents (Botelho et al. 2010). Thus, both in vitro and in vivo substantiation of the CSC properties of ABCB5$^+$ melanoma fractions was established in settings that are independent of the foreign host milieu given in human to mouse xenotransplantation assays (Botelho et al. 2010; Ehira et al. 2010; Keshet et al. 2008).

Recently, additional evidence that melanoma follows the CSC model of tumor initiation and growth was provided in serial human melanoma to mouse xenotransplantation experiments (Boiko et al. 2010; Boonyaratanakornkit et al. 2010; Civenni et al. 2011). Boiko et al. and Civenni et al. demonstrated that MMICs can be prospectively isolated from melanoma patient specimens based on their expression of the nerve growth factor receptor (NGFR) *CD271* (also known as p75) (Boiko et al. 2010; Civenni et al. 2011). Serial xenotransplantation of CD271$^+$ melanoma subsets into engrafted human skin or bone in severely immunocompromised, T-, B-, and natural-killer deficient Rag2$^{-/-}\gamma^{-/-}$ mice resulted in experimental tumor growth in 70 % of injected animals (Boiko et al. 2010). In contrast, only 7 % of mice inoculated with CD271$^-$ melanoma cells developed tumors (Boiko et al. 2010). In addition, CD271$^+$ melanoma subpopulations demonstrated both self-renewal and differentiation capacity through serial in vivo passaging (Boiko et al. 2010), consistent with the existence of a functional melanoma hierarchy (Dirks 2010). Importantly, CD271$^+$ melanoma cells were also capable of metastasis in vivo (Boiko et al. 2010), suggesting a critical role for MMICs not only in tumor initiation but also in neoplastic progression. Remarkably, we found the MMIC markers ABCB5 (Schatton et al. 2008) and CD271 (Boiko et al. 2010) preferentially coexpressed on the same tumor subpopulation in human melanoma specimens (Schatton et al. 2010). The preferential coexpression of both markers has also been similarly documented by others (Civenni et al. 2011), indicating significant overlap of these MMIC populations.

In a separate study, the detoxifying enzyme, aldehyde dehydogenase (ALDH), was used to select for tumorigenic melanoma cell fractions (Boonyaratanakornkit et al. 2010). Of note, ALDH expression identifies CSCs in human breast cancer (Ginestier et al. 2007) and colon cancer (Carpentino et al. 2009; Huang et al. 2009). Similarly, high ALDH activity enriched for tumorigenic cells with sustained self-renewal capacity in human malignant melanoma was determined in both NOD/SCID and NSG recipients mice (Boonyaratanakornkit et al. 2010), confirming that not all melanoma cells are equally adept at tumor initiation, including in NSG recipients. Consistently, ALDH^{+} cells were found to give rise to ALDH^{-} melanoma progeny, while the conversion of ALDH^{-} into ALDH^{+} melanoma cells was rarely observed in a separate study (Prasmickaite et al. 2010), suggesting a preferential self-renewal ability of the ALDH^{high} cell pool. However, in this study ALDH activity did not enrich for melanoma subsets with enhanced tumorigenic potential (Prasmickaite et al. 2010), pointing to potential limitations of ALDH as a universal MMIC identifier. The relationship of ALDH expression to ABCB5 and/or CD271 is currently unknown and deserves further investigation, especially given the importance of the ALDH enzyme for conferring chemoresistance to alkylating agents (Vasiliou et al. 2004).

In summary, several recent studies independently demonstrated that not all melanoma cells possess equal capacities to initiate and maintain tumor growth in immunodeficient hosts (Boiko et al. 2010; Boonyaratanakornkit et al. 2010; Schatton et al. 2008; Civenni et al. 2011). Rather, a distinct subpopulation of MMICs capable of self-renewal and differentiation exists (Boiko et al. 2010; Schatton et al. 2008). Both the ABCB5 (Schatton et al. 2008) and the CD271 (Boiko et al. 2010) surface molecules have been established as prospective biomarkers of MMICs, and important links of these unique melanoma subpopulations to neoplastic progression (Fukunaga-Kalabis et al. 2010; Gazzaniga et al. 2010; Ma et al. 2010; Schatton et al. 2008; Sharma et al. 2010; Vasquez-Moctezuma et al. 2010) and melanoma chemotherapy (Elliott and Al-Hajj 2009; Frank et al. 2005; Fukunaga-Kalabis et al. 2010; Huang et al. 2004) and immunotherapy resistance (Boiko et al. 2010; Schatton et al. 2010) have emerged. Taken together, these findings highlight the clinical relevance of MMICs and emphasize the potential importance of research investigations directed at targeting these tumorigenic melanoma subpopulations to achieve better response rates in patients with advanced stage disease.

12.4 Melanoma Stem Cell Assays

Despite increasing knowledge regarding MMICs and their established relationship to melanocytic tumor progression and therapy resistance, a range of opinions exists with regard to the most relevant assay systems for CSC identification and frequency determination. MMIC frequencies in human melanoma to NOD/SCID mouse xenotransplantation experiments have been estimated to be approximately 1 in 10^{6} cells among unfractionated melanoma populations when tumor formation was assessed 8 weeks post melanoma cell inoculation (Quintana et al. 2008; Schatton et al. 2008). Determination of experimental tumorigenicity in NOD/SCID recipients at 32 weeks post melanoma cell inoculation yielded a higher estimated frequency of tumorigenic melanoma cells of approximately 1 in 10^5 cells (Quintana et al. 2008). The use of more immunocompromised NSG hosts for assessment of tumor formation under otherwise equal experimental conditions yielded a further increase in estimated MMIC frequencies to approximately 1 in 5.5×10^3 cells among unsegregated patient-derived melanoma populations (Quintana et al. 2008). An even greater enrichment of tumorigenic cells was observed when melanoma cells were co-injected into NSG mice with matrigel (Quintana et al. 2008). Under these modified conditions, an average of 1 in 9 melanoma cells formed tumors at 8 weeks post melanoma cell inoculation (Quintana et al. 2008). While this study did not directly address CSC-defining features, such as sustained self-renewal and differentiation capacity in serial xenotransplantation experiments, the results support the view that alterations of the tumor environment can govern MMIC behavior.

Specifically, host environments characterized by absence of immune selective forces could permit tumor bulk populations, which do not normally initiate tumors and may not possess CSC-specific self-renewal and differentiation capacity to also cause experimental tumor growth. MMICs, on the other hand, might possess the preferential capacity to evade host immunosurveillance and initiate tumor growth (Schatton and Frank 2009), which would explain findings of lower estimated MMIC frequencies in more immunocompetent hosts. Indeed, several mechanisms by which MMICs evade antitumor immunity have recently been identified (Boiko et al. 2010; Schatton et al. 2010). For example, MMICs were found to express low to absent levels of immunogenic tumor-associated antigens (TAAs) (Boiko et al. 2010; Schatton et al. 2010), suggesting evasion from antitumor immune responses directed at TAAs. Furthermore, $ABCB5^+$ MMICs also preferentially blocked production of the proliferative cytokine IL-2 by cocultured lymphocytes (Schatton et al. 2010). Additional recently unraveled immunomodulatory functions of MMICs include the secretion of immunosuppressive factors and contact-dependent immunoregulatory mechanisms requiring engagement of immune-inhibitory surface molecules (Schatton et al. 2010), which will be discussed in more detail below. A relative immune privilege of CSCs was also demonstrated in alternative malignancies, including glioblastoma (Di Tomaso et al. 2010; Wei et al. 2010a, b), bladder cancer (Chan et al. 2009), colorectal carcinoma (Todaro et al. 2009), and leukemias (Majeti et al. 2009), indicating that immunomodulation might represent a common feature of CSCs (Schatton and Frank 2009). Clearly, the possibility of a CSC-driven tumor immune escape has profound implications not only for the development of improved cancer immunotherapeutic protocols but also for the design of biologically relevant assays for the study of CSC behavior. Specifically, assessment of tumor-initiating ability in the absence of antitumor immunity now appears to represent an inadequate assay system for the study of MMICs, because host immune environments incapable of immunologic tumor clearance might enable melanoma bulk populations to also initiate and sustain experimental tumor growth. Because preferential inhibition of IL-2 production is one mechanism by which MMICs evade antitumor immunity (Schatton et al. 2010), assessment of melanoma initiation in a murine model, that is, IL-2 receptor null (i.e., NSG mice) (Quintana et al. 2008) is not an appropriate environment for the accurate enumeration of MMIC frequency, because host immunity is abnormally impaired. In light of these considerations, it is not surprising that tumorigenicity experiments performed using more immunocompromised hosts with defective IL-2 receptors (i.e., NSG mice) (Quintana et al. 2008) yielded higher estimated MMIC frequencies compared to xenotransplantation assays utilizing more immunocompetent hosts (i.e., NOD/SCID mice) (Quintana et al. 2008; Schatton et al. 2008). In our view, tumor initiation in melanoma, one of the most immunogenic cancers, should be assessed in a setting that allows for host antitumor immune responses to occur. Ideally, model systems for the accurate assessment of MMIC biology might involve chimeric murine xenograft recipients that are orthotopically xenografted with human cancer cells into syngeneic human tissues of cancer origin in the presence of an adoptively transferred hematopoietic system originating from the same patient (Frank et al. 2010).

In addition to alterations of host antitumor immune response, co-injection of matrigel, a solution containing growth factors and ECM constituents (Kleinman and Martin 2005), accounted for a marked increase in tumorigenic capacity of unfractionated human melanoma cells and estimated MMIC frequencies in NSG mice (Quintana et al. 2008). In our view, these findings imply that the stage can be set for MMICs to appear more abundant by exposing them to microenvironmental stimulants such as ECM and growth factors. It is conceivable that in the absence of such growth-promoting signals, only MMICs might possess the ability to survive and as a consequence maintain the tumorigenic process. This possibility is indeed supported by findings in other CSC-driven cancers (Calabrese et al. 2007; Li et al. 2009b). The clinical cancer scenario is typically characterized by low nutrient and growth factor availability and deregulated ECM function (Hendrix et al. 2003b). It thus seems plausible that MMICs might preferentially produce both ECM and growth factors, thereby sustaining tumor maintenance. In support of this hypothesis, Duda and colleagues demonstrated that circulating cancer cells, which are coated with autologous stromal components, including ECM factors, have the preferential capacity to seed distant metastasis and promote initial tumor growth compared to those cancer cells that are not incorporated in stromal elements (Duda et al. 2010). Upon establishment of a growth-promoting environment through ECM-expressing tumor subsets at the early stage of metastatic foci, additional cancer populations can also home to secondary tumor sites and contribute to neoplastic growth and progression during later disease stages (Duda et al. 2010). Similarly, genetic lineage-tracing experiments revealed that melanoma bulk populations could furnish the growing tumor with cellular progeny in the presence of MMICs (Schatton et al. 2008). Thus, it is conceivable that the co-injection of growth-promoting factors to melanoma cell inocula may mask MMIC-specific functions and could allow most melanoma cells to initiate experimental tumor growth. Subpopulations of differentiated cancer cells that do not normally initiate tumors and do not display the ability for sustained self-renewal under clinical conditions may thus be able do so in the presence of the appropriate microenvironment. Similarly, melanoma cells can give rise to induced pluripotent stem cells (iPSCs) through exogenous reprogramming factors (Utikal et al. 2009). While these findings clearly establish the *potential* of melanoma cells to generate iPSCs, it seems, however, unlikely that such gains of cellular plasticity occur naturally in human patients. In aggregate, these findings further highlight the importance of establishing translationally relevant assays for the study of MMICs, which accurately mimic the environmental factors found in clinical cancers (e.g., low-nutrient levels, necrosis, hypoxia, and relatively intact antitumor immunity) rather than further deviating from them. Assays that are very permissive to revealing the tumorigenic potential of melanoma cells might thus vastly overestimate MMIC frequencies. A major weakness of the hypothesis that the CSC model might not apply to melanoma Quintana et al. (2008, 2010) is that MMICs must be rare. The observation that tumorigenic melanoma cells may be more common when assay conditions are modified does not imply that MMICs might not exist. Indeed, rarity is clearly not a defining criterion of CSCs according to the consensus definition (Clarke et al. 2006).

While the above outlined differences in microenvironmental cues (i.e., immune selective pressures and growth and ECM factor availability) could account for variations in estimated MMIC frequencies in NOD/SCID vis-à-vis NSG xenotransplantation experiments (Quintana et al. 2008; Schatton et al. 2008), they cannot explain apparent discrepancies in tumor-initiating ability of unfractionated melanoma cells assayed in the presence of matrigel and using identical mouse models (Boiko et al. 2010; Boonyaratanakornkit et al. 2010; Quintana et al. 2008). Specifically, the marked frequency of up to 1 in 4 unfractionated human melanoma cells with tumor-seeding ability in NSG hosts described by Quintana and colleagues (Quintana et al. 2010; Quintana et al. 2008) has not been confirmed to date. Indeed, independent laboratories have found that a minimum of 100 unfractionated patient-derived melanoma cells were required to consistently initiate tumors in NSG mice under equivalent experimental conditions (i.e., in the presence of matrigel) (Boiko et al. 2010; Boonyaratanakornkit et al. 2010), paralleling findings in additional CSC-driven malignancies, including pancreatic and head and neck cancers (Ishizawa et al. 2010). These new studies (Boiko et al. 2010; Boonyaratanakornkit et al. 2010; Ishizawa et al. 2010) alert us to the fact that MMICs might generally not be as common as suggested by Quintana et al. (2008, 2010). Thus, even experimental models that are very permissive to experimental tumor growth support the view that only a minority of melanoma cells is capable of initiating and maintaining the disease.

How can the differences of the findings by Quintana and colleagues and other studies using apparently identical model systems (Boiko et al. 2010; Boonyaratanakornkit et al. 2010) be explained? For instance, variations in enzymatic tumor dissociation, isolation, and/or inoculation techniques between different laboratories could lead to different estimated MMIC frequencies (Shackleton 2010). Specifically, the aforementioned laboratory procedures could potentially account for differences in surface marker expression and/or viability among inoculated melanoma cell suspensions (Murphy et al. 2014). Also, the use of distinct matrigel batches with varying growth and/or ECM factor compositions could result in altered melanoma growth. Alternatively, the use of tumor specimens from patients with more advanced disease (Quintana et al. 2008), which have been demonstrated to contain elevated CSC numbers compared to primary tumors (Schatton et al. 2008), might also account for higher relative proportions of melanoma cells capable of initiating experimental tumor growth. In addition, the assessment of CSC frequency, utilizing tumor cell isolates from melanoma xenografts that have been passaged in vivo for extended periods of time in lieu of directly patient-derived tumor samples, could further obscure the accurate assessment of CSC frequencies and biological functions (Boiko et al. 2010; Quintana et al. 2008). Indeed, Boiko and colleagues demonstrated that both in vitro and in vivo passaging of melanoma cells can result in the emergence of tumorigenic subclones independent of their immunophenotype (Boiko et al. 2010). Similarly, tumor cell lines may have lost the hierarchical structure of the primary tumor from which they originated (Zhou et al. 2009). A lesson to be learned from the apparently conflicting evidence regarding the frequency of tumorigenic melanoma cells in NSG mice (Boiko et al. 2010; Boonyaratanakornkit et al. 2010; Quintana et al. 2008) is that careful comparison of experimental methodologies may serve to explain differing results. Clearly, these discordant studies demonstrate that both the tumor environment and experimental procedures can govern tumor growth and underline the importance of establishing standardized assays for the study of MMIC biology that could enable the consolidation of experimental findings from different laboratories.

In summary, differences in MMIC frequency and function suggested by results obtained in alternative host immune milieus in the presence or absence of co-injected ECM and/or growth factors (Boiko et al. 2010; Quintana et al. 2008, 2010; Schatton et al. 2008, Murphy et al. 2014) strongly suggest critical interactions of MMIC with the tumor host environment. Thus, bioassays and experimental model systems for the detection of clinically relevant MMICs require further approximation of, rather than further abstraction from, the naturally occurring tumor–host interactions in human patients (Frank et al. 2010; Schatton et al. 2009; Murphy et al. 2014).

12.5 Melanoma Stem Biology: Therapeutic Opportunities

The ability to prospectively identify CSCs has permitted researchers to begin characterizing specific molecular and cellular mechanisms preferentially associated with CSCs that may contribute to tumor initiation and growth, in addition to those associated with their defining features of unlimited self-renewal and proliferative capacities (Frank et al. 2010). Among the recently uncovered CSC functions likely to influence tumor development are mechanisms of tumor immune evasion (Schatton and Frank 2009). Findings of increased tumor incidence in immunocompromised patients suggest that immunosurveillance might serve to eliminate malignant cells at early stages of tumorigenesis (Mapara and Sykes 2004). Relative immune privilege and/or selective immunomodulatory functions could thus enable CSCs to evade antitumor immune responses in favor of inexorable tumor growth (Schatton and Frank 2009). This possibility is especially relevant to melanoma development because melanoma is a particularly immunogenic cancer (Rosenberg et al. 2008). Indeed, several mechanisms by which MMICs evade antitumor immunity have recently been identified (Boiko et al. 2010; Schatton et al. 2010).

For example, MMICs can downregulate their expression of TAAs, such as MART-1, tyrosinase, ML-IAP, and the cancer testis antigens NY-ESO-1, and MAGE-A (Boiko et al. 2010; Schatton et al. 2010). Importantly, T cells reactive against TAAs are commonly observed in melanoma patients where they elicit antitumor immune responses directed at TAA-expressing melanoma cells (Lee et al. 1999; Stockert et al. 1998). Decreased expression of TAAs would thus enable MMICs to evade antitumor immune responses (Boiko et al. 2010; Schatton et al. 2010), providing for a potential explanation for the relative ineffectiveness of tumor-reactive T cells and autologous vaccination strategies in halting tumor growth (Schatton and Frank 2009). ABCB5$^+$ MMICs were also found to express decreased levels of MHC class I molecules (Schatton et al. 2010), which represent an established mechanism of tumor immune evasion and neoplastic progression (Aptsiauri et al. 2007; Khong et al. 2004), further suggesting preferential MMIC evasion from immunological clearance.

In addition to reduced expression of MHC class I molecules, ABCB5$^+$ MMICs selectively expressed the B7.2 (CD86) costimulatory ligand and the negative costimulatory receptor, PD-1 (Schatton et al. 2010). Of note, interactions of B7.2 with its receptor CTLA-4 and of PD-1 with its ligands PD-L1 and PD-L2 can downmodulate immune responses by inducing T cell anergy and/or by activating Tregs (Greenwald et al. 2005; Li et al. 2009a), suggesting that MMICs might regulate antitumor immune responses in favor of inexorable tumor growth via the involvement of negative costimulatory pathways. Indeed, selective blockade of MMIC-expressed B7.2 maintained CD4$^+$CD25$^+$FoxP3$^+$ Treg frequencies among cocultured lymphocytes and regulated their secretion of the immunosuppressive cytokine IL-10 (Schatton et al. 2010). Importantly, accumulating evidence in various cancers, including melanoma, suggests that Tregs might represent important mediators of clinical tumor immune evasion (Ahmadzadeh et al. 2008; Clark et al. 2008; Curiel et al. 2004), underlining the potential importance of MMIC-mediated Treg induction for melanoma progression.

In addition, MMICs were also found to inhibit human peripheral blood mononuclear cell proliferation more efficiently than tumor bulk populations (Schatton et al. 2010). Consistently, ABCB5$^+$ melanoma subpopulations preferentially inhibited production of the proliferative cytokine, IL-2, by both cocultured mitogen-activated lymphocytes and patient-identical peripheral blood mononuclear cells in the absence of a mitogenic stimulus (Schatton et al. 2010). Importantly, decreased IL-2 levels correlate with increased melanoma growth in animal models and human patients (Eklund and Kuzel 2004). Given its immune-activating effects, IL-2 is used as adjuvant therapy for the treatment of advanced stage melanoma (Eklund and Kuzel 2004). Thus, preferential inhibition of IL-2 signaling might not only represent an important mechanism underlying MMIC-driven tumor growth but could also provide for a novel explanation for the commonly observed inability of therapeutic regimens involving IL-2 in producing durable patient responses (Eklund and Kuzel 2004). The preferential inhibition of IL-2 production by ABCB5$^+$ MMICs might also explain observed differences in MMIC frequency in NSG (IL-2R$\gamma^{-/-}$) (Quintana et al. 2008) versus NOD/SCID (IL-2R^{WT}) hosts (Quintana et al. 2008;

Schatton et al. 2008). Specifically, assessment of tumorigenicity outcomes in the absence of functional IL-2 signaling might overestimate MMIC frequency because a host environment characterized by abnormally impaired antitumor immunity might enable melanoma bulk populations to also contribute to tumor growth.

Additional immunomodulatory functions of MMICs include the secretion of immunosuppressive factors, such as immune-inhibitory TGF-β pathway members (Schatton et al. 2010). Importantly, these soluble mediators can be produced by tumors to dampen the anticancer immune response (Gorelik and Flavell 2001; Inge et al. 1992).

In sum, numerous MMIC-specific immunological mechanisms have been unraveled that may enable them to evade and/or modulate the antitumor immune response to promote neoplastic growth and progression. Strikingly, a relative immune privilege of CSCs was also demonstrated in alternative malignancies, including glioblastoma (Di Tomaso et al. 2010; Wei et al. 2010a, b), bladder cancer (Chan et al. 2009), colorectal carcinoma (Todaro et al. 2009), and leukemias (Majeti et al. 2009), indicating that immunomodulation might represent a common feature of CSCs (Schatton and Frank 2009). Clearly, the possibility of CSC-driven tumor immune escape has profound implications for the design of biologically relevant assays for the study of CSC behavior.

Perhaps, most significant are the implications of an MMIC-driven tumor immune escape for the development of improved cancer immunotherapeutic protocols. In addition, MMIC biology could provide a highly relevant tool for the evaluation of patient responses to current immunotherapeutic regimens, including those aimed at modulating critical regulatory elements of patient immune cells to enhance their antitumor reactivity. Importantly, a number of such novel immunotherapeutics have recently entered clinical practice or ongoing trials (Kirkwood et al. 2008; Ugurel et al. 2016). These include inhibitors of costimulatory molecules or paracrine immunosuppressive cytokines, including monoclonal antibodies directed at CTLA-4, PD-1, 4-1BB, and TGF-β (Fong and Small 2008; Kirkwood et al. 2008; Lahn et al. 2005; Lynch, 2008). In contrast to current immunotherapeutic regimens, these novel agents exert inhibitory effects on both immune effector cells and Treg function (Kirkwood et al. 2008). They might thus prove more effective in inducing durable patient responses. Indeed, a phase III study demonstrated that treatment of stage III or IV melanoma patients with therapy-resistant disease with the anti-CTLA-4 antibody Ipilimumab resulted in improved overall survival compared to patients treated with a gp100 peptide vaccine (Hodi et al. 2010) and Ipilimumab was subsequently approved for clinical use. A potential additional explanation for this anti-melanoma effect of CTLA-4 inhibition arises from the fact that tumorigenic MMICs preferentially expressed the CTLA-4 ligand, B7.2, and induced Tregs in a B7.2-dependent fashion (Schatton et al. 2010). Inhibition of MMIC-specific immune escape mechanisms might thus contribute to the antitumor efficacy of Ipilimumab. Given the preferential expression of PD-1, 4-1BBL, and TGF-β pathway members by MMICs, it is further conceivable that responses observed in melanoma patients treated with clinically approved anti-PD-1 antibodies (Brahmer et al. 2010), or therapeutic agents directed at 4-1BB (Lynch 2008) or TGF-β (Kirkwood et al. 2008), might potentially also relate to the ability of these immunotherapeutics to block MMIC-specific immunomodulatory functions. The observed failure of immunotherapies directed at the bulk of tumor cells (e.g., vaccination strategies targeting differentiation antigens such as MART-1 or tyrosinase) or those that elicit nonspecific immune activation (e.g., neoadjuvant IL-2 therapy) in mediating sustained patient responses (Rosenberg et al. 2004) might, on the other hand, relate to the inability of such regimens to effectively target the MMIC compartment (Schatton and Frank 2009), given its low expression levels of TAAs (Boiko et al. 2010; Schatton et al. 2010) and its preferential ability to inhibit IL-2 production (Schatton et al. 2010). Taken together, these findings highlight the possibility that immunotherapeutic strategies aimed at enhancing the endogenous immune responses to melanoma might prove most efficient if MMIC-specific immune escape mechanisms are concurrently impaired. In light of this intriguing possibility, it might be relevant to analyze the clinical effectiveness of novel immunotherapeutic agents, including Ipilimumab or PD-1 antibodies, not only with regard to the pattern and duration of immune responses (Reuben et al. 2006) but also in the context of their impact on the MMIC subset and its immunomodulatory properties (Schatton and Frank 2009).

In addition to their preferential refractoriness to current immunotherapeutic protocols, MMICs also demonstrate enhanced resistance to several structurally unrelated chemotherapeutic agents with distinct mechanisms of action (Schatton et al. 2009), a phenomenon also termed multidrug resistance (MDR) (Dean et al. 2005). MDR can result through several different means, including impairment of tumor apoptotic pathways, alterations in cell cycle checkpoints, and decreased drug accumulation (Gottesman et al. 2002). The latter mechanism is of particular interest to MMICs because one mechanism resulting in reduced intracellular drug levels is the excretion of cytotoxic agents by energy-dependent efflux pumps, known as ATP-binding cassette (ABC) transporters (Gottesman et al. 2002). Specifically, the MMIC determinant, ABCB5 (Schatton et al. 2008), mediates resistance to multiple chemotherapeutic agents in malignant melanoma, hepatocellular carcinoma, breast cancer, and leukemias, including doxorubicin (Cheung et al. 2011; Elliott and Al-Hajj 2009; Frank et al. 2005; Fukunaga-Kalabis et al. 2010; Yang et al. 2010), camptothecin, mitoxantrone, and 5-fluorouracil (Huang et al. 2004; Lehne et al. 2009). A broader role for the ABCB5 transporter in chemotherapeutic resistance to additional agents is suggested by the observation that ABCB5 mRNA expression levels across a panel of human cancer cell lines used by the National Cancer Institute for drug screening correlated significantly with chemoresistance to 45 out of 119 anticancer agents (Frank et al. 2005). Evidence for a preferential resistance of CSCs to both chemotherapy and radiotherapy has also been generated in numerous additional CSC-driven malignancies, including leukemias, gliomas, breast carcinomas, and pancreatic cancer (reviewed in (Schatton et al. 2009)), underscoring the need to dissect further the molecular pathways responsible for CSC-specific therapy resistance. For example, Chartrain et al. showed that ABCB5-expressing melanoma cells selectively survive not only when exposed to dacarbazine, a long-standing reference treatment of metastatic melanoma, but also to vemurafenib, a recently approved inhibitor of the mutated kinase V600E BRAF and other various chemotherapeutic drugs. These results showed that anti-melanoma chemotherapy might participate in the chemoresistance acquisition by selecting tumor cell subpopulations expressing ABCB5. This is of particular importance in understanding the relapses observed after anti-melanoma treatments and reinforces the interest of ABCB5 and ABCB5-expressing cells as potential therapeutic targets in melanoma (Chartrain et al. 2012). The therapeutic promise of MMIC-directed treatment strategies, which could enhance current treatment modalities for patients with advanced stage melanoma, is further highlighted by recent findings of a relationship of MMICs to neoplastic melanoma progression (Fukunaga-Kalabis et al. 2010; Gazzaniga et al. 2010; Ma et al. 2010; Schatton et al. 2008; Sharma et al. 2010; Vasquez-Moctezuma et al. 2010; Gray et al. 2015; Reid et al. 2013) and adverse clinical outcome (Sharma et al. 2010; Reid et al. 2013). In light of the CSC concept and findings of MMIC-specific immunoregulatory properties, a number of novel therapeutic approaches can be envisioned that could potentially increase the efficacy of current forms of therapy (reviewed in Frank et al. 2010), if MMICs are indeed the major culprits of melanoma initiation and clinical virulence. For instance, MMIC ablation through prospective markers might prove useful in enhancing current anti-melanoma therapies. In support of this possibility, selective killing of MMICs via ADCC using an anti-ABCB5 monoclonal antibody halted experimental tumor growth (Schatton et al. 2008). Alternatively, targeting of MMICs via preferentially expressed surface molecules and/or MMIC-specific pathway interference might also yield improved melanoma patient responses. Such treatment strategies could include inhibition of costimulatory signaling events mediated by MMIC-expressed (Schatton et al. 2010) B7.2, PD-1, and/or 4-1BB. Disruption of surrogate MMIC-specific immune evasion pathways could also represent treatment modalities that might enhance responsiveness to current anti-melanoma regimens. Additionally, melanoma cell-intrinsic functions of PD-1 expressed on ABCB5^{+} MMIC could potentially be exploited for therapeutic benefit. Recently, we showed that melanoma cell-intrinsic PD-1 promotes tumorigenesis, even in mice lacking adaptive immunity. PD-1 inhibition on melanoma cells by RNAi, blocking antibodies, or mutagenesis of melanoma-PD-1 signaling motifs suppressed tumor growth in immunocompetent, immunocompromised, and PD-1-deficient tumor graft recipient mice. Conversely, melanoma-specific PD-1 overexpression enhanced tumorigenicity, as did engagement of melanoma-PD-1 by its ligand, PD-L1, whereas melanoma-PD-L1 inhibition or knockout of host-PD-L1 attenuated growth of PD-1-positive melanomas. Mechanistically, the melanoma-PD-1 receptor modulated downstream effectors of mTOR signaling. These results identified melanoma cell-intrinsic functions of the PD-1:PD-L1 axis in tumor growth and suggested that blocking melanoma-PD-1 might contribute to the striking clinical efficacy of anti-PD-1 therapy (Kleffel et al. 2015). In addition, driving MMICs into differentiation could lead to improved therapeutic outcomes. Consistent with this possibility, differentiation of glioblastoma CSCs via bone morphogenetic protein 4 (BMP4) exposure resulted in inhibition of experimental tumor growth concomitant with enhanced survival (Piccirillo et al. 2006). Interestingly, the BMP4 receptor, BMPR1a, is preferentially expressed by ABCB5^{+} MMICs (Schatton et al. 2008), suggesting that a similar strategy could also be promising in this malignancy. Additionally, the ABCB5 marker of MMIC itself has been shown to provide a target for melanoma differentiation therapy: In MMIC, we showed that ABCB5 controls IL1beta secretion, which serves to maintain slow cycling, chemoresistant cells through an IL1beta/IL8/CXCR1 cytokine signaling circuit. This CSC maintenance circuit involved reciprocal paracrine interactions with ABCB5-negative cancer cell populations. ABCB5 blockade-induced cellular differentiation, reversed resistance to multiple chemotherapeutic agents, and impaired tumor growth in vivo. Together, these results defined a novel function for ABCB5 in CSC maintenance and tumor growth that could be therapeutically targeted (Wilson et al. 2014). An additional MMIC-directed targeting strategy could involve the use of antiangiogenic and/or antivasculogenic regimens. This possibility is indicated by findings of a preferential induction of neovascularization by CSCs in other cancers (Bao et al. 2006b). MMICs might likewise be involved in angiogenesis and/or vasculogenesis given their preferential expression of vasculogenic differentiation markers VE-cadherin and TIE-1 (Schatton et al. 2008). For example, we showed that VEGFR-1 expressed by MMIC is required for tumor growth and that melanoma-specific shRNA-mediated knockdown of VEGFR-1 blocked the development of $ABCB5^+$ vasculogenic mimicry (VM) morphology and inhibited $ABCB5^+$ VM-associated production of the secreted melanoma mitogen laminin. Moreover, melanoma-specific VEGFR-1 knockdown markedly inhibited tumor growth, identifying VEGFR-1 as a novel MMIC therapeutic target (Frank et al. 2011) Reversal of chemoresistance and/or radioresistance mechanisms operative in MMICs might also successfully increase anti-melanoma therapeutic efficacy (Elliott and Al-Hajj 2009; Frank et al. 2005; Fukunaga-Kalabis et al. 2010; Huang et al. 2004). This is further suggested by findings in glioblastoma CSCs (Bao et al. 2006a), among other cancers (Diehn et al. 2009; Vlashi et al. 2009). Lastly, given the importance of the tumor environment in governing CSC behavior (Scadden 2006), the disruption of protumorigenic MMIC-niche interactions could also optimize anticancer therapeutic protocols. It is important to recognize that therapeutic efficacy will often depend also on a significant reduction of melanoma bulk populations, which may cause excessive tumor burden. Therefore, combination therapies that involve both MMIC-directed agents as well as debulking regimens would be predicted to prove most effective in improving clinical treatment responses and patient outcomes.

In summary, several biological functions of MMICs have recently been identified, including their preferential ability to modulate and/or evade antitumor immune responses (Boiko et al. 2010; Schatton et al. 2010). In addition to their refractoriness to current immunotherapeutic protocols, MMICs also demonstrate increased resistance to a number of chemotherapy agents (Elliott and Al-Hajj 2009; Frank et al. 2005; Fukunaga-Kalabis et al. 2010; Huang et al. 2004; Chartrain et al. 2012). Taken together with the recently established relationship of MMICs to melanocytic tumor progression (Fukunaga-Kalabis et al. 2010; Gazzaniga et al. 2010; Ma et al. 2010; Schatton et al. 2008; Sharma et al. 2010; Vasquez-Moctezuma et al. 2010; Gray et al. 2015; Reid et al. 2013), these findings underscore the potential clinical relevance of MMIC-directed targeting approaches. Importantly, proof-of-principle for the potential therapeutic utility of targeting MMICs has been established, by demonstrating that selective eradication of ABCB5$^+$ melanoma subpopulations can halt experimental tumorigenesis (Schatton et al. 2008). A number of additional targeting approaches might likewise prove useful in blocking MMIC-driven tumor development and progression, including disruption of immune-inhibitory pathways, differentiation therapy, and chemoresistance reversal. While more work is required to translate these research developments into the clinic, they point to a critical relevance of MMICs for successful melanoma therapy. Further molecular screens of purified MMIC populations employing microarrays, RNA-interference, or drug-screening libraries could allow identification of further targetable pathways leading to MMIC-tailored eradication strategies for melanoma therapy.

Conclusions

A growing body of literature supports the existence of MMICs (Boiko et al. 2010; Boonyaratanakornkit et al. 2010; Schatton et al. 2008; Civenni et al. 2011). Additionally, important links have been established between MMICs, neoplastic progression (Fukunaga-Kalabis et al. 2010; Gazzaniga et al. 2010; Ma et al. 2010; Schatton et al. 2008; Sharma et al. 2010; Vasquez-Moctezuma et al. 2010; Gray et al. 2015; Reid et al. 2013), chemoresistance (Elliott and Al-Hajj 2009; Frank et al. 2005; Fukunaga-Kalabis et al. 2010; Huang et al. 2004; Chartrain et al. 2012), and refractoriness to immunotherapy (Boiko et al. 2010; Schatton et al. 2010). Moreover, novel biological features of MMICs are currently being intensively explored. For instance, the ability of MMICs to modulate the antitumor immune response (Schatton and Frank 2009; Schatton et al. 2008) might be especially informative for the optimization and/or evaluation of targeted immunotherapies that were recently found to improve overall survival in patients with recurrent metastatic melanoma (Hodi et al. 2010; Ugurel et al. 2016). Together, these findings highlight the relevance and promise of novel MMIC-centered diagnostic and therapeutic approaches in human melanoma.

Acknowledgments This work was supported by National Cancer Institute, NIH, grants 1RO1CA113796, 1RO1CA138231, and 2P50CA093683. T. Schatton is supported by an Outrun the Sun, Inc. 2010 National Melanoma Research Scholar Award.

References

Ahmadzadeh M, Felipe-Silva A, Heemskerk B, Powell DJ Jr, Wunderlich JR, Merino MJ, Rosenberg SA (2008) FOXP3 expression accurately defines the population of intratumoral regulatory T cells that selectively accumulate in metastatic melanoma lesions. Blood 112:4953–4960

Al-Hajj M, Wicha MS, Benito-Hernandez A, Morrison SJ, Clarke MF (2003) Prospective identification of tumorigenic breast cancer cells. Proc Natl Acad Sci U S A 100:3983–3988

Aptsiauri N, Cabrera T, Mendez R, Garcia-Lora A, Ruiz-Cabello F, Garrido F (2007) Role of altered expression of HLA class I molecules in cancer progression. Adv Exp Med Biol 601:123–131

Bao S, Wu Q, McLendon RE, Hao Y, Shi Q, Hjelmeland AB, Dewhirst MW, Bigner DD, Rich JN (2006a) Glioma stem cells promote radioresistance by preferential activation of the DNA damage response. Nature 444:756–760

Bao S, Wu Q, Sathornsumetee S, Hao Y, Li Z, Hjelmeland AB, Shi Q, McLendon RE, Bigner DD, Rich JN (2006b) Stem cell-like glioma cells promote tumor angiogenesis through vascular endothelial growth factor. Cancer Res 66:7843–7848

Barker N, Ridgway RA, van Es JH, van de Wetering M, Begthel H, van den Born M, Danenberg E, Clarke AR, Sansom OJ, Clevers H (2009) Crypt stem cells as the cells-of-origin of intestinal cancer. Nature 457:608–611

Boiko AD, Razorenova OV, van de Rijn M, Swetter SM, Johnson DL, Ly DP, Butler PD, Yang GP, Joshua B, Kaplan MJ, Longaker MT, Weissman IL (2010) Human melanoma-initiating cells express neural crest nerve growth factor receptor CD271. Nature 466:133–137

Bonnet D, Dick JE (1997) Human acute myeloid leukemia is organized as a hierarchy that originates from a primitive hematopoietic cell. Nat Med 3:730–737

Boonyaratanakornkit JB, Yue L, Strachan LR, Scalapino KJ, LeBoit PE, Lu Y, Leong SP, Smith JE, Ghadially R (2010) Selection of tumorigenic melanoma cells using ALDH. J Invest Dermatol 130:2799–2808

Botelho MG, Wang X, Arndt-Jovin DJ, Becker D, Jovin TM (2010) Induction of terminal differentiation in melanoma cells on downregulation of beta-amyloid precursor protein. J Invest Dermatol 130:1400–1410

Brahmer JR, Drake CG, Wollner I, Powderly JD, Picus J, Sharfman WH, Stankevich E, Pons A, Salay TM, McMiller TL, Gilson MM, Wang C, Selby M, Taube JM, Anders R, Chen L, Korman AJ, Pardoll DM, Lowy I, Topalian SL (2010) Phase I study of single-agent anti-programmed death-1 (MDX-1106) in refractory solid tumors: safety, clinical activity, pharmacodynamics, and immunologic correlates. J Clin Oncol 28(19):3167–3175

Bruce WR, Van Der Gaag H (1963) A quantitative assay for the number of murine lymphoma cells capable of proliferation in vivo. Nature 199:79–80

Calabrese C, Poppleton H, Kocak M, Hogg TL, Fuller C, Hamner B, Oh EY, Gaber MW, Finklestein D, Allen M, Frank A, Bayazitov IT, Zakharenko SS, Gajjar A, Davidoff A, Gilbertson RJ (2007) A perivascular niche for brain tumor stem cells. Cancer Cell 11:69–82

Carpentino JE, Hynes MJ, Appelman HD, Zheng T, Steindler DA, Scott EW, Huang EH (2009) Aldehyde dehydrogenase-expressing colon stem cells contribute to tumorigenesis in the transition from colitis to cancer. Cancer Res 69:8208–8215

Castor A, Nilsson L, Astrand-Grundstrom I, Buitenhuis M, Ramirez C, Anderson K, Strombeck B, Garwicz S, Bekassy AN, Schmiegelow K, Lausen B, Hokland P, Lehmann S, Juliusson G, Johansson B, Jacobsen SE (2005) Distinct patterns of hematopoietic stem cell involvement in acute lymphoblastic leukemia. Nat Med 11:630–637

Chan KS, Espinosa I, Chao M, Wong D, Ailles L, Diehn M, Gill H, Presti J Jr, Chang HY, van de Rijn M, Shortliffe L, Weissman IL (2009) Identification, molecular characterization, clinical prognosis, and therapeutic targeting of human bladder tumor-initiating cells. Proc Natl Acad Sci U S A 106:14016–14021

Chartrain M, Riond J, Stennevin A, Vandenberghe I, Gomes B, Lamant L, Meyer N, Gairin JE, Guilbaud N, Annereau JP (2012) Melanoma chemotherapy leads to the selection of ABCB5-expressing cells. PLoS One 7(5):e36762

Cheung ST, Cheung PF, Cheng CK, Wong NC, Fan ST (2011) Granulin-epithelin precursor and ATP-dependent binding cassette (ABC)B5 regulate liver cancer cell chemoresistance. Gastroenterology 140(1):344–355

Cho RW, Wang X, Diehn M, Shedden K, Chen GY, Sherlock G, Gurney A, Lewicki J, Clarke MF (2008) Isolation and molecular characterization of cancer stem cells in MMTV-Wnt-1 murine breast tumors. Stem Cells 26:364–371

Civenni G, Walter A, Kobert N, Mihic-Probst D, Zipser M, Belloni B, Seifert B, Moch H, Dummer R, van den Broek M et al (2011) Human CD271-positive melanoma stem cells associated with metastasis establish tumor heterogeneity and long-term growth. Cancer Res 71(8):3098–3109

Clark RA, Huang SJ, Murphy GF, Mollet IG, Hijnen D, Muthukuru M, Schanbacher CF, Edwards V, Miller DM, Kim JE, Lambert J, Kupper TS (2008) Human squamous cell carcinomas evade the immune response by down-regulation of vascular E-selectin and recruitment of regulatory T cells. J Exp Med 205:2221–2234

Clarke MF, Dick JE, Dirks PB, Eaves CJ, Jamieson CH, Jones DL, Visvader J, Weissman IL, Wahl GM (2006) Cancer stem cells – perspectives on current status and future directions: AACR workshop on cancer stem cells. Cancer Res 66:9339–9344
Cotter TG (2009) Apoptosis and cancer: the genesis of a research field. Nat Rev Cancer 9:501–507
Cox CV, Evely RS, Oakhill A, Pamphilon DH, Goulden NJ, Blair A (2004) Characterization of acute lymphoblastic leukemia progenitor cells. Blood 104:2919–2925
Cox CV, Martin HM, Kearns PR, Virgo P, Evely RS, Blair A (2007) Characterization of a progenitor cell population in childhood T-cell acute lymphoblastic leukemia. Blood 109:674–682
Curiel TJ, Coukos G, Zou L, Alvarez X, Cheng P, Mottram P, Evdemon-Hogan M, Conejo-Garcia JR, Zhang L, Burow M, Zhu Y, Wei S, Kryczek I, Daniel B, Gordon A, Myers L, Lackner A, Disis ML, Knutson KL, Chen L, Zou W (2004) Specific recruitment of regulatory T cells in ovarian carcinoma fosters immune privilege and predicts reduced survival. Nat Med 10:942–949
Dalerba P, Dylla SJ, Park IK, Liu R, Wang X, Cho RW, Hoey T, Gurney A, Huang EH, Simeone DM, Shelton AA, Parmiani G, Castelli C, Clarke MF (2007) Phenotypic characterization of human colorectal cancer stem cells. Proc Natl Acad Sci U S A 104:10158–10163
Dean M, Fojo T, Bates S (2005) Tumour stem cells and drug resistance. Nat Rev Cancer 5:275–284
Deshpande AJ, Cusan M, Rawat VP, Reuter H, Krause A, Pott C, Quintanilla-Martinez L, Kakadia P, Kuchenbauer F, Ahmed F, Delabesse E, Hahn M, Lichter P, Kneba M, Hiddemann W, Macintyre E, Mecucci C, Ludwig WD, Humphries RK, Bohlander SK, Feuring-Buske M, Buske C (2006) Acute myeloid leukemia is propagated by a leukemic stem cell with lymphoid characteristics in a mouse model of CALM/AF10-positive leukemia. Cancer Cell 10:363–374
Di Tomaso T, Mazzoleni S, Wang E, Sovena G, Clavenna D, Franzin A, Mortini P, Ferrone S, Doglioni C, Marincola FM, Galli R, Parmiani G, Maccalli C (2010) Immunobiological characterization of cancer stem cells isolated from glioblastoma patients. Clin Cancer Res 16:800–813
Diehn M, Cho RW, Lobo NA, Kalisky T, Dorie MJ, Kulp AN, Qian D, Lam JS, Ailles LE, Wong M, Joshua B, Kaplan MJ, Wapnir I, Dirbas FM, Somlo G, Garberoglio C, Paz B, Shen J, Lau SK, Quake SR, Brown JM, Weissman IL, Clarke MF (2009) Association of reactive oxygen species levels and radioresistance in cancer stem cells. Nature 458:780–783
Dirks P (2010) Cancer stem cells: invitation to a second round. Nature 466:40–41
Dou J, Pan M, Wen P, Li Y, Tang Q, Chu L, Zhao F, Jiang C, Hu W, Hu K, Gu N (2007) Isolation and identification of cancer stem-like cells from murine melanoma cell lines. Cell Mol Immunol 4:467–472
Duda DG, Duyverman AM, Kohno M, Snuderl M, Steller EJ, Fukumura D, Jain RK (2010) Malignant cells facilitate lung metastasis by bringing their own soil. Proc Natl Acad Sci U S A 107(50):21677–21682
Ehira N, Oshiumi H, Matsumoto M, Kondo T, Asaka M, Seya T (2010) An embryo-specific expressing TGF-beta family protein, growth-differentiation factor 3 (GDF3), augments progression of B16 melanoma. J Exp Clin Cancer Res 29:135
Eklund JW, Kuzel TM (2004) A review of recent findings involving interleukin-2-based cancer therapy. Curr Opin Oncol 16:542–546
Elliott AM, Al-Hajj MA (2009) ABCB8 mediates doxorubicin resistance in melanoma cells by protecting the mitochondrial genome. Mol Cancer Res 7:79–87
Fang D, Nguyen TK, Leishear K, Finko R, Kulp AN, Hotz S, Van Belle PA, Xu X, Elder DE, Herlyn M (2005) A tumorigenic subpopulation with stem cell properties in melanomas. Cancer Res 65:9328–9337
Fong L, Small EJ (2008) Anti-cytotoxic T-lymphocyte antigen-4 antibody: the first in an emerging class of immunomodulatory antibodies for cancer treatment. J Clin Oncol 26:5275–5283
Frank NY, Margaryan A, Huang Y, Schatton T, Waaga-Gasser AM, Gasser M, Sayegh MH, Sadee W, Frank MH (2005) ABCB5-mediated doxorubicin transport and chemoresistance in human malignant melanoma. Cancer Res 65:4320–4333

Frank NY, Schatton T, Frank MH (2010) The therapeutic promise of the cancer stem cell concept. J Clin Invest 120:41–50
Frank NY, Schatton T, Kim S, Zhan Q, Wilson BJ, Ma J, Saab KR, Osherov V, Widlund HR, Gasser M et al (2011) VEGFR-1 expressed by malignant melanoma-initiating cells is required for tumor growth. Cancer Res 71(4):1474–1485
Fukunaga-Kalabis M, Martinez G, Nguyen TK, Kim D, Santiago-Walker A, Roesch A, Herlyn M (2010) Tenascin-C promotes melanoma progression by maintaining the ABCB5-positive side population. Oncogene 29:6115–6124
Gazzaniga P, Cigna E, Panasiti V, Devirgiliis V, Bottoni U, Vincenzi B, Nicolazzo C, Petracca A, Gradilone A (2010) CD133 and ABCB5 as stem cell markers on sentinel lymph node from melanoma patients. Eur J Surg Oncol 36:1211–1214
Ginestier C, Hur MH, Charafe-Jauffret E, Monville F, Dutcher J, Brown M, Jacquemier J, Viens P, Kleer CG, Liu S, Schott A, Hayes D, Birnbaum D, Wicha MS, Dontu G (2007) ALDH1 is a marker of normal and malignant human mammary stem cells and a predictor of poor clinical outcome. Cell Stem Cell 1:555–567
Gorelik L, Flavell RA (2001) Immune-mediated eradication of tumors through the blockade of transforming growth factor-beta signaling in T cells. Nat Med 7:1118–1122
Gottesman MM, Fojo T, Bates SE (2002) Multidrug resistance in cancer: role of ATP-dependent transporters. Nat Rev Cancer 2:48–58
Gray ES, Reid AL, Bowyer S, Calapre L, Siew K, Pearce R, Cowell L, Frank MH, Millward M, Ziman M (2015) Circulating melanoma cell subpopulations: their heterogeneity and differential responses to treatment. J Invest Dermatol 135(8):2040–2048
Greenwald RJ, Freeman GJ, Sharpe AH (2005) The B7 family revisited. Annu Rev Immunol 23:515–548
Gupta PB, Chaffer CL, Weinberg RA (2009) Cancer stem cells: mirage or reality? Nat Med 15:1010–1012
Hamburger AW, Salmon SE (1977) Primary bioassay of human tumor stem cells. Science 197:461–463
Hanahan D, Weinberg RA (2000) The hallmarks of cancer. Cell 100:57–70
Held MA, Curley DP, Dankort D, McMahon M, Muthusamy V, Bosenberg MW (2010) Characterization of melanoma cells capable of propagating tumors from a single cell. Cancer Res 70:388–397
Hendrix MJ, Seftor EA, Hess AR, Seftor RE (2003a) Molecular plasticity of human melanoma cells. Oncogene 22:3070–3075
Hendrix MJ, Seftor EA, Hess AR, Seftor RE (2003b) Vasculogenic mimicry and tumour-cell plasticity: lessons from melanoma. Nat Rev Cancer 3:411–421
Hermann PC, Huber SL, Herrler T, Aicher A, Ellwart JW, Guba M, Bruns CJ, Heeschen C (2007) Distinct populations of cancer stem cells determine tumor growth and metastatic activity in human pancreatic cancer. Cell Stem Cell 1:313–323
Hill RP (2006) Identifying cancer stem cells in solid tumors: case not proven. Cancer Res 66:1891–1895; discussion 1890
Hodi FS, O'Day SJ, McDermott DF, Weber RW, Sosman JA, Haanen JB, Gonzalez R, Robert C, Schadendorf D, Hassel JC, Akerley W, van den Eertwegh AJ, Lutzky J, Lorigan P, Vaubel JM, Linette GP, Hogg D, Ottensmeier CH, Lebbe C, Peschel C, Quirt I, Clark JI, Wolchok JD, Weber JS, Tian J, Yellin MJ, Nichol GM, Hoos A, Urba WJ (2010) Improved survival with ipilimumab in patients with metastatic melanoma. N Engl J Med 363(8):711–723
Hoek K, Rimm DL, Williams KR, Zhao H, Ariyan S, Lin A, Kluger HM, Berger AJ, Cheng E, Trombetta ES, Wu T, Niinobe M, Yoshikawa K, Hannigan GE, Halaban R (2004) Expression profiling reveals novel pathways in the transformation of melanocytes to melanomas. Cancer Res 64:5270–5282
Hoek KS, Eichhoff OM, Schlegel NC, Dobbeling U, Kobert N, Schaerer L, Hemmi S, Dummer R (2008) In vivo switching of human melanoma cells between proliferative and invasive states. Cancer Res 68:650–656

Hoek KS, Goding CR (2010) Cancer stem cells versus phenotype-switching in melanoma. Pigment Cell Melanoma Res 23:746–759

Huang EH, Hynes MJ, Zhang T, Ginestier C, Dontu G, Appelman H, Fields JZ, Wicha MS, Boman BM (2009) Aldehyde dehydrogenase 1 is a marker for normal and malignant human colonic stem cells (SC) and tracks SC overpopulation during colon tumorigenesis. Cancer Res 69:3382–3389

Huang Y, Anderle P, Bussey KJ, Barbacioru C, Shankavaram U, Dai Z, Reinhold WC, Papp A, Weinstein JN, Sadee W (2004) Membrane transporters and channels: role of the transportome in cancer chemosensitivity and chemoresistance. Cancer Res 64:4294–4301

Huntly BJ, Shigematsu H, Deguchi K, Lee BH, Mizuno S, Duclos N, Rowan R, Amaral S, Curley D, Williams IR, Akashi K, Gilliland DG (2004) MOZ-TIF2, but not BCR-ABL, confers properties of leukemic stem cells to committed murine hematopoietic progenitors. Cancer Cell 6:587–596

Inge TH, Hoover SK, Susskind BM, Barrett SK, Bear HD (1992) Inhibition of tumor-specific cytotoxic T-lymphocyte responses by transforming growth factor beta 1. Cancer Res 52:1386–1392

Ishikawa F, Yoshida S, Saito Y, Hijikata A, Kitamura H, Tanaka S, Nakamura R, Tanaka T, Tomiyama H, Saito N, Fukata M, Miyamoto T, Lyons B, Ohshima K, Uchida N, Taniguchi S, Ohara O, Akashi K, Harada M, Shultz LD (2007) Chemotherapy-resistant human AML stem cells home to and engraft within the bone-marrow endosteal region. Nat Biotechnol 25:1315–1321

Ishizawa K, Rasheed ZA, Karisch R, Wang Q, Kowalski J, Susky E, Pereira K, Karamboulas C, Moghal N, Rajeshkumar NV, Hidalgo M, Tsao M, Ailles L, Waddell TK, Maitra A, Neel BG, Matsui W (2010) Tumor-initiating cells are rare in many human tumors. Cell Stem Cell 7:279–282

Jamieson CH, Ailles LE, Dylla SJ, Muijtjens M, Jones C, Zehnder JL, Gotlib J, Li K, Manz MG, Keating A, Sawyers CL, Weissman IL (2004) Granulocyte-macrophage progenitors as candidate leukemic stem cells in blast-crisis CML. N Engl J Med 351:657–667

Jemal A, Siegel R, Xu J, Ward E (2010) Cancer statistics, 2010. CA Cancer J Clin 60:277–300

Jordan CT (2009) Cancer stem cells: controversial or just misunderstood? Cell Stem Cell 4:203–205

Keshet GI, Goldstein I, Itzhaki O, Cesarkas K, Shenhav L, Yakirevitch A, Treves AJ, Schachter J, Amariglio N, Rechavi G (2008) MDR1 expression identifies human melanoma stem cells. Biochem Biophys Res Commun 368:930–936

Khong HT, Wang QJ, Rosenberg SA (2004) Identification of multiple antigens recognized by tumor-infiltrating lymphocytes from a single patient: tumor escape by antigen loss and loss of MHC expression. J Immunother 27:184–190

Kim M, Gans JD, Nogueira C, Wang A, Paik JH, Feng B, Brennan C, Hahn WC, Cordon-Cardo C, Wagner SN, Flotte TJ, Duncan LM, Granter SR, Chin L (2006) Comparative oncogenomics identifies NEDD9 as a melanoma metastasis gene. Cell 125:1269–1281

Kirkwood JM, Tarhini AA, Panelli MC, Moschos SJ, Zarour HM, Butterfield LH, Gogas HJ (2008) Next generation of immunotherapy for melanoma. J Clin Oncol 26:3445–3455

Kleffel S, Posch C, Barthel SR, Mueller H, Schlapbach C, Guenova E, Elco CP, Lee N, Juneja VR, Zhan Q et al (2015) Melanoma cell-intrinsic PD-1 receptor functions promote tumor growth. Cell 162(6):1242–1256

Kleinman HK, Martin GR (2005) Matrigel: basement membrane matrix with biological activity. Semin Cancer Biol 15:378–386

Krivtsov AV, Twomey D, Feng Z, Stubbs MC, Wang Y, Faber J, Levine JE, Wang J, Hahn WC, Gilliland DG, Golub TR, Armstrong SA (2006) Transformation from committed progenitor to leukaemia stem cell initiated by MLL-AF9. Nature 442:818–822

Kupas V, Weishaupt C, Siepmann D, Kaserer ML, Eickelmann M, Metze D, Luger TA, Beissert S, Loser K (2011) RANK is expressed in metastatic melanoma and highly upregulated on melanoma-initiating cells. J Invest Dermatol 131(4):944–955

Lahn M, Kloeker S, Berry BS (2005) TGF-beta inhibitors for the treatment of cancer. Expert Opin Investig Drugs 14:629–643

Lapidot T, Sirard C, Vormoor J, Murdoch B, Hoang T, Caceres-Cortes J, Minden M, Paterson B, Caligiuri MA, Dick JE (1994) A cell initiating human acute myeloid leukaemia after transplantation into SCID mice. Nature 367:645–648

Lee PP, Yee C, Savage PA, Fong L, Brockstedt D, Weber JS, Johnson D, Swetter S, Thompson J, Greenberg PD, Roederer M, Davis MM (1999) Characterization of circulating T cells specific for tumor-associated antigens in melanoma patients. Nat Med 5:677–685

Lehne G, Grasmo-Wendler UH, Berner JM, Meza-Zepeda LA, Adamsen BL, Flack A, Reiner A, Clausen OP, Hovig E, Myklebost O (2009) Upregulation of stem cell genes in multidrug resistant K562 leukemia cells. Leuk Res 33:1379–1385

Li C, Heidt DG, Dalerba P, Burant CF, Zhang L, Adsay V, Wicha M, Clarke MF, Simeone DM (2007) Identification of pancreatic cancer stem cells. Cancer Res 67:1030–1037

Li XC, Rothstein DM, Sayegh MH (2009a) Costimulatory pathways in transplantation: challenges and new developments. Immunol Rev 229:271–293

Li Z, Bao S, Wu Q, Wang H, Eyler C, Sathornsumetee S, Shi Q, Cao Y, Lathia J, McLendon RE, Hjelmeland AB, Rich JN (2009b) Hypoxia-inducible factors regulate tumorigenic capacity of glioma stem cells. Cancer Cell 15:501–513

Linos E, Swetter SM, Cockburn MG, Colditz GA, Clarke CA (2009) Increasing burden of melanoma in the United States. J Invest Dermatol 129:1666–1674

Lynch DH (2008) The promise of 4-1BB (CD137)-mediated immunomodulation and the immunotherapy of cancer. Immunol Rev 222:277–286

Ma J, Lin JY, Alloo A, Wilson BJ, Schatton T, Zhan Q, Murphy GF, Waaga-Gasser AM, Gasser M, Stephen Hodi F, Frank NY, Frank MH (2010) Isolation of tumorigenic circulating melanoma cells. Biochem Biophys Res Commun 402:711–717

Majeti R, Chao MP, Alizadeh AA, Pang WW, Jaiswal S, Gibbs KD Jr, van Rooijen N, Weissman IL (2009) CD47 is an adverse prognostic factor and therapeutic antibody target on human acute myeloid leukemia stem cells. Cell 138:286–299

Mapara MY, Sykes M (2004) Tolerance and cancer: mechanisms of tumor evasion and strategies for breaking tolerance. J Clin Oncol 22:1136–1151

Monzani E, Facchetti F, Galmozzi E, Corsini E, Benetti A, Cavazzin C, Gritti A, Piccinini A, Porro D, Santinami M, Invernici G, Parati E, Alessandri G, La Porta CA (2007) Melanoma contains CD133 and ABCG2 positive cells with enhanced tumourigenic potential. Eur J Cancer 43:935–946

Murphy GF, Wilson BJ, Girouard SD, Frank NY, Frank MH (2014) Stem cells and targeted approaches to melanoma cure. Mol Aspects Med 39:33–49

Nowell PC (1976) The clonal evolution of tumor cell populations. Science 194:23–28

O'Brien CA, Pollett A, Gallinger S, Dick JE (2007) A human colon cancer cell capable of initiating tumour growth in immunodeficient mice. Nature 445:106–110

Park CH, Bergsagel DE, McCulloch EA (1971) Mouse myeloma tumor stem cells: a primary cell culture assay. J Natl Cancer Inst 46:411–422

Perego M, Tortoreto M, Tragni G, Mariani L, Deho P, Carbone A, Santinami M, Patuzzo R, Mina PD, Villa A, Pratesi G, Cossa G, Perego P, Daidone MG, Alison MR, Parmiani G, Rivoltini L, Castelli C (2010) Heterogeneous phenotype of human melanoma cells with in vitro and in vivo features of tumor-initiating cells. J Invest Dermatol 130:1877–1886

Piccirillo SG, Reynolds BA, Zanetti N, Lamorte G, Binda E, Broggi G, Brem H, Olivi A, Dimeco F, Vescovi AL (2006) Bone morphogenetic proteins inhibit the tumorigenic potential of human brain tumour-initiating cells. Nature 444:761–765

Postovit LM, Seftor EA, Seftor RE, Hendrix MJ (2006) Influence of the microenvironment on melanoma cell fate determination and phenotype. Cancer Res 66:7833–7836

Prasmickaite L, Engesaeter BO, Skrbo N, Hellenes T, Kristian A, Oliver NK, Suo Z, Maelandsmo GM (2010) Aldehyde dehydrogenase (ALDH) activity does not select for cells with enhanced aggressive properties in malignant melanoma. PLoS One 5:e10731

Prince ME, Sivanandan R, Kaczorowski A, Wolf GT, Kaplan MJ, Dalerba P, Weissman IL, Clarke MF, Ailles LE (2007) Identification of a subpopulation of cells with cancer stem cell properties in head and neck squamous cell carcinoma. Proc Natl Acad Sci U S A 104:973–978

Quintana E, Shackleton M, Foster HR, Fullen DR, Sabel MS, Johnson TM, Morrison SJ (2010) Phenotypic heterogeneity among tumorigenic melanoma cells from patients that is reversible and not hierarchically organized. Cancer Cell 18:510–523

Quintana E, Shackleton M, Sabel MS, Fullen DR, Johnson TM, Morrison SJ (2008) Efficient tumour formation by single human melanoma cells. Nature 456:593–598

Reid AL, Millward M, Pearce R, Lee M, Frank MH, Ireland A, Monshizadeh L, Rai T, Heenan P, Medic S et al (2013) Markers of circulating tumour cells in the peripheral blood of patients with melanoma correlate with disease recurrence and progression. Br J Dermatol 168(1):85–92

Reuben JM, Lee BN, Li C, Gomez-Navarro J, Bozon VA, Parker CA, Hernandez IM, Gutierrez C, Lopez-Berestein G, Camacho LH (2006) Biologic and immunomodulatory events after CTLA-4 blockade with ticilimumab in patients with advanced malignant melanoma. Cancer 106:2437–2444

Reya T, Morrison SJ, Clarke MF, Weissman IL (2001) Stem cells, cancer, and cancer stem cells. Nature 414:105–111

Ricci-Vitiani L, Lombardi DG, Pilozzi E, Biffoni M, Todaro M, Peschle C, De Maria R (2007) Identification and expansion of human colon-cancer-initiating cells. Nature 445:111–115

Rosenberg SA, Restifo NP, Yang JC, Morgan RA, Dudley ME (2008) Adoptive cell transfer: a clinical path to effective cancer immunotherapy. Nat Rev Cancer 8:299–308

Rosenberg SA, Yang JC, Restifo NP (2004) Cancer immunotherapy: moving beyond current vaccines. Nat Med 10:909–915

Scadden DT (2006) The stem-cell niche as an entity of action. Nature 441:1075–1079

Schatton T, Frank MH (2008) Cancer stem cells and human malignant melanoma. Pigment Cell Melanoma Res 21:39–55

Schatton T, Frank MH (2009) Antitumor immunity and cancer stem cells. Ann N Y Acad Sci 1176:154–169

Schatton T, Frank MH (2010) The in vitro spheroid melanoma cell culture assay: cues on tumor initiation? J Invest Dermatol 130:1769–1771

Schatton T, Frank NY, Frank MH (2009) Identification and targeting of cancer stem cells. Bioessays 31:1038–1049

Schatton T, Murphy GF, Frank NY, Yamaura K, Waaga-Gasser AM, Gasser M, Zhan Q, Jordan S, Duncan LM, Weishaupt C, Fuhlbrigge RC, Kupper TS, Sayegh MH, Frank MH (2008) Identification of cells initiating human melanomas. Nature 451:345–349

Schatton T, Schutte U, Frank NY, Zhan Q, Hoerning A, Robles SC, Zhou J, Hodi FS, Spagnoli GC, Murphy GF, Frank MH (2010) Modulation of T-cell activation by malignant melanoma initiating cells. Cancer Res 70:697–708

Shackleton M (2010) Melanoma stem cells – are there devils in the detail? Pigment Cell Melanoma Res 23:693–694

Sharma BK, Manglik V, Elias EG (2010) Immuno-expression of human melanoma stem cell markers in tissues at different stages of the disease. J Surg Res 163:e11–e15

Shmelkov SV, Butler JM, Hooper AT, Hormigo A, Kushner J, Milde T, St Clair R, Baljevic M, White I, Jin DK, Chadburn A, Murphy AJ, Valenzuela DM, Gale NW, Thurston G, Yancopoulos GD, D'Angelica M, Kemeny N, Lyden D, Rafii S (2008) CD133 expression is not restricted to stem cells, and both $CD133^+$ and $CD133^-$ metastatic colon cancer cells initiate tumors. J Clin Invest 118:2111–2120

Singh SK, Hawkins C, Clarke ID, Squire JA, Bayani J, Hide T, Henkelman RM, Cusimano MD, Dirks PB (2004) Identification of human brain tumour initiating cells. Nature 432:396–401

Stockert E, Jager E, Chen YT, Scanlan MJ, Gout I, Karbach J, Arand M, Knuth A, Old LJ (1998) A survey of the humoral immune response of cancer patients to a panel of human tumor antigens. J Exp Med 187:1349–1354

Suva ML, Riggi N, Stehle JC, Baumer K, Tercier S, Joseph JM, Suva D, Clement V, Provero P, Cironi L, Osterheld MC, Guillou L, Stamenkovic I (2009) Identification of cancer stem cells in Ewing's sarcoma. Cancer Res 69:1776–1781

Todaro M, D'Asaro M, Caccamo N, Iovino F, Francipane MG, Meraviglia S, Orlando V, La Mendola C, Gulotta G, Salerno A, Dieli F, Stassi G (2009) Efficient killing of human colon cancer stem cells by gammadelta T lymphocytes. J Immunol 182:7287–7296

Ugurel S, Rohmel J, Ascierto PA, Flaherty KT, Grob JJ, Hauschild A, Larkin J, Long GV, Lorigan P, McArthur GA (2016) Survival of patients with advanced metastatic melanoma: the impact of novel therapies. Eur J Cancer 53:125–134

Utikal J, Maherali N, Kulalert W, Hochedlinger K (2009) Sox2 is dispensable for the reprogramming of melanocytes and melanoma cells into induced pluripotent stem cells. J Cell Sci 122:3502–3510

Vasiliou V, Pappa A, Estey T (2004) Role of human aldehyde dehydrogenases in endobiotic and xenobiotic metabolism. Drug Metab Rev 36:279–299

Vasquez-Moctezuma I, Meraz-Rios MA, Villanueva-Lopez CG, Magana M, Martinez-Macias R, Sanchez-Gonzalez DJ, Garcia-Sierra F, Herrera-Gonzalez NE (2010) ATP-binding cassette transporter ABCB5 gene is expressed with variability in malignant melanoma. Actas Dermosifiliogr 101:341–348

Vlashi E, McBride WH, Pajonk F (2009) Radiation responses of cancer stem cells. J Cell Biochem 108:339–342

Wei J, Barr J, Kong LY, Wang Y, Wu A, Sharma AK, Gumin J, Henry V, Colman H, Priebe W, Sawaya R, Lang FF, Heimberger AB (2010a) Glioblastoma cancer-initiating cells inhibit T-cell proliferation and effector responses by the signal transducers and activators of transcription 3 pathway. Mol Cancer Ther 9:67–78

Wei J, Barr J, Kong LY, Wang Y, Wu A, Sharma AK, Gumin J, Henry V, Colman H, Sawaya R, Lang FF, Heimberger AB (2010b) Glioma-associated cancer-initiating cells induce immunosuppression. Clin Cancer Res 16:461–473

Wilson BJ, Saab KR, Ma J, Schatton T, Putz P, Zhan Q, Murphy GF, Gasser M, Waaga-Gasser AM, Frank NY et al (2014) ABCB5 maintains melanoma-initiating cells through a proinflammatory cytokine signaling circuit. Cancer Res 74(15):4196–4207

Wu A, Oh S, Wiesner SM, Ericson K, Chen L, Hall WA, Champoux PE, Low WC, Ohlfest JR (2008) Persistence of CD133+ cells in human and mouse glioma cell lines: detailed characterization of GL261 glioma cells with cancer stem cell-like properties. Stem Cells Dev 17:173–184

Yang JY, Ha SA, Yang YS, Kim JW (2010) p-Glycoprotein ABCB5 and YB-1 expression plays a role in increased heterogeneity of breast cancer cells: correlations with cell fusion and doxorubicin resistance. BMC Cancer 10:388

Yang ZF, Ho DW, Ng MN, Lau CK, Yu WC, Ngai P, Chu PW, Lam CT, Poon RT, Fan ST (2008) Significance of CD90(+) cancer stem cells in human liver cancer. Cancer Cell 13:153–166

Zabierowski SE, Herlyn M (2008) Learning the ABCs of melanoma-initiating cells. Cancer Cell 13:185–187

Zhang S, Balch C, Chan MW, Lai HC, Matei D, Schilder JM, Yan PS, Huang TH, Nephew KP (2008) Identification and characterization of ovarian cancer-initiating cells from primary human tumors. Cancer Res 68:4311–4320

Zhang X, Cheng X, Lai Y, Zhou Y, Cao W, Hua ZC (2016) Salmonella VNP20009-mediated RNA interference of ABCB5 moderated chemoresistance of melanoma stem cell and suppressed tumor growth more potently. Oncotarget 7(12):14940–14950

Zhou BB, Zhang H, Damelin M, Geles KG, Grindley JC, Dirks PB (2009) Tumour-initiating cells: challenges and opportunities for anticancer drug discovery. Nat Rev Drug Discov 8:806–823

Zhu L, Gibson P, Currle DS, Tong Y, Richardson RJ, Bayazitov IT, Poppleton H, Zakharenko S, Ellison DW, Gilbertson RJ (2009) Prominin 1 marks intestinal stem cells that are susceptible to neoplastic transformation. Nature 457:603–607

The Birth of Malignancy: Embryogenesis and Melanoma

13

Alec Gramann, William Tyler Frantz, and Craig J. Ceol

13.1 Introduction

Embryonic development involves high levels of proliferation, migration, and differentiation to form all the tissues and organs of an organism. Under normal circumstances, cell–cell signaling in an embryo is coordinated both temporally and spatially to allow development to occur without error. Embryogenesis is a once-in-a-lifetime event, and many developmental signaling pathways and processes are not physiologically active in adult tissues, with notable exceptions in the maintenance of certain stem cell populations (Goldstein and Horsley 2012). However, in disease states such as cancer, malignant cells adopt similar characteristics to those seen in embryonic cells – proliferation, migration, and lack of differentiation. Over recent decades, investigation into various stages of melanocyte development has given great insight into specific characteristics of melanoma, leading to a deeper understanding of melanomagenesis. In this chapter, we review key literature describing connections between embryonic development and melanoma, including aspects of embryonic patterning and melanocyte lineage specification that are co-opted to promote melanoma progression.

Alec Gramann and William Tyler Frantz contributed equally with all other contributors.

A. Gramann • W.T. Frantz • C.J. Ceol (✉)
Program in Molecular Medicine, Department of Molecular, Cell and Cancer Biology, University of Massachusetts Medical School, Worcester, MA 01655, USA
e-mail: craig.ceol@umassmed.edu

A. Bosserhoff (ed.), *Melanoma Development*,
DOI 10.1007/978-3-319-41319-8_13

13.2 Role of Embryonic Patterning Factors in Melanoma

During early embryonic development, a complex signaling program directs the fates of pluripotent cells and their descendants (Sadler and Langman 2010). This process of embryonic patterning involves a balance of signals. It directs apoptosis or proliferation, fate specification or maintenance of an undifferentiated state, and varying levels of migratory capacity. Each of these properties is important in the initiation and progression of many tumor types, including melanoma (Postovit et al. 2008). Of the many signaling molecules and pathways active in early embryonic development, Nodal and Notch signaling have crucial roles in patterning and have been linked to melanoma progression.

13.2.1 Nodal

Nodal, a member of the TGF-β superfamily, is a secreted protein that binds its receptor and, acting through SMAD signaling, activates transcription of target genes to direct embryonic development (Conlon et al. 1994). While Nodal is known to have multiple roles during embryogenesis, those of most interest in the context of cancer are maintenance of pluripotency and regulation of migration during gastrulation (James et al. 2005; Quail et al. 2013). Early embryonic development relies on maintaining cells in a self-renewing, pluripotent state before cell-fate specification and differentiation. Maintenance of pluripotency is critical in mesendoderm and neurectoderm, and in these tissues, Nodal signaling is essential. Loss of Nodal causes the loss of expression of stem cell factors and leads to expression of differentiation markers of neuroectoderm (James et al. 2005; Vallier et al. 2009). During gastrulation, Nodal is required to maintain both the primitive node and the primitive streak (Conlon et al. 1994). Loss of Nodal causes disruption of the formation of the streak and node, which causes defects in the migration of mesoderm between the hypoblast and epiblast layers of the embryo. In addition, markers of mesodermal migration, such as Twist-1 and Mox-1, are absent when Nodal is lost. Interestingly, Twist affects epithelial-to-mesenchymal transition (EMT, discussed in detail below), which is implicated in metastasis of many tumor types. Nodal signaling is also crucial in defining left–right asymmetry. Nodal secreted by the primitive node acts on the left side of the embryo and is prevented from acting on the right by active cilia. The cilia sweep Nodal to the left and allow distinct signaling on the right by Lefty1 and Cerberus (Levin et al. 1995; Zhu et al. 1999). Nodal signaling in embryogenesis directs many processes crucial to normal development, but when ectopically activated, these processes contribute to the malignant phenotypes observed in cancer.

The role of Nodal in melanoma was initially proposed by Hendrix and colleagues after a screen to investigate interactions between melanoma cells and embryonic stem cells (Topczewska et al. 2006). They injected fluorescently labeled human melanoma cells, which were previously characterized for gene expression, invasiveness, and metastatic potential, into embryonic zebrafish and monitored changes in development. Those melanoma cells categorized as more aggressive induced changes in the structure of endogenous tissue, while less aggressive cell lines did not. Morphologic abnormalities observed included additional outgrowths and secondary body axes, which led to the hypothesis that melanoma cells were able to stimulate the same patterning pathways as embryonic cells. Given the nature of the morphologic abnormalities, Nodal was investigated as a candidate morphogen secreted by melanoma cells. Through evaluation of patient samples, they showed that Nodal expression is almost exclusively limited to those melanomas with more aggressive pathologic characteristics, such as an early vertical growth phase, local tissue invasion, earlier and more metastases, and lack of differentiation. Additional studies have shown that melanomas expressing Nodal have pathologic and clinical characteristics associated with a poorer prognosis than do other melanomas (Topczewska et al. 2006).

The characteristics of Nodal-expressing melanomas bear a relationship to Nodal-regulated processes in embryogenesis. For example, Nodal has been shown to activate EMT factors in melanoma, such as Snail family proteins, which, like Twist, promote embryonic mesodermal migration (Fang et al. 2013). Additionally, when melanoma cells were treated with exogenous Nodal in vitro, they became less adhesive and express increased matrix remodeling proteins. These characteristics are associated with EMT in both cancer and embryogenesis (Fang et al. 2013). Nodal has also been shown to drive dedifferentiation of melanoma cells toward a stem-cell-like state, resulting in expression of earlier melanocyte lineage markers as well as loss of pigmentation (Topczewska et al. 2006). Conversely, when Nodal is knocked down, the cells become more adherent and differentiated. Additionally, Nodal knockdown abrogates overall tumor growth in xenotransplant models (Hardy et al. 2010; Postovit et al. 2008).

The role of Nodal in aggressive melanomas has stimulated interest in it as a drug target. Nodal is expressed in few adult tissues (Hendrix et al. 2007), so an anti-Nodal therapy would be relatively tumor-specific, and off-target effects would be limited. Recently, anti-Nodal antibodies have been evaluated in vitro with dacarbazine for effects on melanoma cells (Hardy et al. 2015). Previous studies have shown Nodal-positive cell subpopulations in heterogeneous tumors are resistant to dacarbazine therapy. The combination treatment of anti-Nodal antibodies with dacarbazine decreased proliferation and increased apoptosis of melanoma cells when compared with treatments of each single agent alone. Follow-up evaluation of the combination therapy in xenografts showed a similar decrease in tumor growth rate. Anti-Nodal antibodies have been compared to $BRAF^{V600E}$ inhibitor therapy in vitro and in vivo (Strizzi et al. 2015). Notably, a greater decrease in tumor volume in xenografts treated with anti-Nodal antibodies was observed when compared to controls treated with IgG antibodies or $BRAF^{V600E}$ inhibitor. While direct targeting of Nodal for melanoma therapy shows promise in these initial evaluations, it is not yet known whether anti-Nodal therapies can improve patient clinical outcomes.

13.2.2 Notch

Notch is a highly conserved transmembrane protein that controls gene expression to regulate cell-fate determination, survival, development, and neurogenesis. There are four Notch receptors in humans, designated Notch 1–4. Five Notch ligands, designated Delta Like Ligand 1/3/4 and Jagged 1/2, activate Notch receptors. Notch ligand–receptor interactions stimulate juxtamembrane signaling, resulting in a series of proteolytic cleavage steps mediated by TNFa-converting enzyme and the γ-secretase protease complex. Following cleavage, the Notch intracellular domain (NICD) is released into the cytosol (Brou et al. 2000; Edbauer et al. 2003; Hartmann et al. 2002). NICD then translocates to the nucleus where it binds to mastermind, CBF1, and p300 and regulates transcription of genes, including the Hes and Hey gene families (Fryer et al. 2002; Nam et al. 2003; Wu et al. 2000). Notch signaling is an important part of normal embryogenesis, regulating asymmetric cell divisions that are crucial to neurogenesis, somite compartmentalization, and other developmental processes (Feller et al. 2008; Matsuzaki 2000). By regulating cell-fate specification and cell function, Notch activity contributes to a broad spectrum of biological processes, including stem cell maintenance, hematopoietic fate decisions, and intestinal epithelium renewal (Bedogni 2014; Montagne and Gonzalez-Gaitan 2014; Pinnix and Herlyn 2007). Notch targets CyclinD1, p21, and SKP2 suggesting a role in cell cycle regulation (Pinnix and Herlyn 2007). Taken together, these and many additional studies show Notch regulates cell function during embryogenesis and other contexts.

Notch signaling is required for the maintenance of melanoblasts and melanocyte stem cells (MSCs). Mice that are depleted of Notch activity in the melanocyte lineage exhibit severe coat color dilution caused by inappropriate apoptosis of melanoblasts during embryogenesis (Moriyama et al. 2006). Notch1 and Notch2 receptors are critical for melanoblast survival (Schouwey et al. 2007). Furthermore, Notch activity is required for MSC survival, as these cells are lost during successive hair cycles in Notch-depleted animals. Death within the melanocyte lineage may result from a failure to maintain melanoblasts and MSCs in a de-differentiated state. In support of this notion, gain-of-function studies by the Herlyn group found that expression of constitutively active NICD was sufficient to convert differentiated melanocytes into multipotent neural crest stem-like cells (Zabierowski et al. 2011). Notch signaling is indeed important for development of the neural crest, where it is involved in initial specification of neural crest cells and simultaneously prevents their premature differentiation (Cornell and Eisen 2002; Endo et al. 2002; Glavic et al. 2004). In cultured neural crest stem-like cells, Notch signaling is required for cell survival and is inhibited during ultraviolet-light-induced differentiation of these cells into melanocytes (Fukunaga-Kalabis et al. 2015). Overall, Notch signaling acts in cells of the melanocyte lineage, either neural crest, melanoblasts, or MSCs, to promote cell survival and prevent terminal differentiation.

Notch signaling is active in melanomas where it regulates key aspects of tumor progression (Hendrix et al. 2002). The microRNA miR-146a acts through Notch to promote melanoma cell survival and progression (Forloni et al. 2014). miR-146a is upregulated by oncogenic BRAF or NRAS signaling, and a key miR-146a target is

NUMB. Repression by miR-146a downregulates NUMB, relieving its inhibition of Notch signaling. Notch interacts with additional microRNAs to promote melanoma metastasis. Notch activation in melanoma cells through contact with neighboring keratinocytes leads to disruption of microphthalmia-associated transcription factor (MITF)/Recombination signal binding protein for immunoglobulin kappa J region (RBPJK)-mediated repression of miR-222/221 (Golan et al. 2015). This keratinocyte-induced Notch signaling results in miR-222/221 expression, which promotes melanoma invasion and metastasis. Lastly, Notch signaling is implicated in melanoma progression through an association with Nodal (Hardy et al. 2010). In aggressive melanoma cell lines, Nodal expression is correlated with and depends on Notch4 expression and activity, respectively. Inhibition of Notch4 blunts aggressive features of these cells including anchorage-independent growth. These activities of Notch in melanoma cells are consistent with its role in the melanocyte lineage of promoting a less differentiated and more proliferative state.

13.3 Adopting Melanocyte Lineage Characteristics in Promoting Melanoma

There are specific aspects of neoplasia that hold true for nearly every type of cancer – an ability to bypass cell cycle checkpoints, to suppress growth arrest and apoptotic signaling being a few commonalities. But between cancers arising from various cell types, and even between subtypes of the same cancer, there is a wide range of behaviors that are observed. Some develop more indolent characteristics, such as a slow growth rate or minimal invasion from the primary site. Others are known to be much more malignant, spreading and growing quickly, sometimes before a primary tumor is clinically apparent. While there is much variability within cancers that arise from same cell type, some malignancies are prognostically inherently worse or better than others. Some of these differences can be explained by the propensity for specific oncogenic mutations, unique environmental exposures to carcinogens, or particular viral infections. But there is also an underlying component of development that predisposes cancers to behave in specific ways.

Melanoma is often more aggressive and prone to metastasis than other cancers (Gupta et al. 2005a). While this propensity for aggressive behavior is likely related to the function of mutations in specific oncogenes and tumor suppressors, the underlying biology of melanocytes plays a role in the phenotypes observed in melanoma. In an experiment evaluating characteristics of different precursor cells with the same oncogenic mutation profile, multiple cell types were immortalized using simian virus-40-expressing LT and ST proteins and were then transformed with oncogenic Ras (Gupta et al. 2005a). The resulting transformed cells were evaluated for various malignant characteristics, such as invasive and metastatic capacity. The majority of transformed cells showed the ability to form tumors but were unable to invade or metastasize. However, transformed melanocytes were very invasive under the same transformation conditions. These results suggest that there is an inherent predisposition of melanocytes to metastasize when compared with other cell types. This predisposition is due, in part, to epigenetic differences between melanocytes and other cell types (Gupta et al. 2005a). In a more recent study, Kaufman et al. showed that in zebrafish, a marker expressed only in the neural crest during embryogenesis, *crestin*, is re-expressed during the formation of melanomas (Kaufman et al. 2016). This further supports the notion that the embryonic lineage from which a cell is derived plays a role during malignant transformation. One of the major embryonic programs operating in these precursor cells is the epithelial-to-mesenchymal transition (EMT).

As previously discussed, the first major EMT event is the migration of mesoderm during gastrulation (Conlon et al. 1994). The second major EMT event involves the migration of neural crest cells from the neural crest to multiple locations around the developing embryo (Sadler and Langman 2010). In most cases involving EMT, there are key steps that allow cells to make the transition and to begin to migrate. These steps are delineated by the expression of markers known to be associated with EMT, such as Snail1, Snail2 (previously Slug), Twist1, Zeb1, and Zeb2 (Cano et al. 2000; Comijn et al. 2001; Grooteclaes and Frisch 2000; Yang et al. 2004). The first key step is alteration of adherence molecules on the cell surface. In pre-migratory melanocytes, the major adherence molecule involved in maintaining cell–cell and cell–matrix connections is E-cadherin (reviewed in Kerosuo and Bronner-Fraser 2012). During EMT, E-cadherin expression is replaced by expression of N-cadherin, driven by the neural crest transcription factor Snail2 (Cano et al. 2000). By downregulating E-cadherin, cells are able to free themselves from neighboring cells to begin migrating. Another key step is the upregulation of metalloproteinases and other matrix remodeling proteins. Key proteins such as ADAM10, ADAM13, and MMP-2 have increased expression that correlates with the timing of delamination of the neural crest cells from the neural tube (Kuriyama and Mayor 2008). By downregulating adhesion and upregulating remodeling proteins, neural crest cells are able to migrate to their final destinations. While promoting migratory characteristics of neural crest cells and melanocyte precursors, EMT also maintains a de-differentiated and minimally proliferative state in cells during migration (Vega et al. 2004).

Many aspects of the epithelial-to-mesenchymal transition during migration of the neural crest are similar to those that are characteristic of melanoma. In support of this similarity, many factors involved in physiologic EMT during development are also active in melanoma. In particular, Twist1, Zeb1, Zeb2, and Snail family proteins have been implicated in melanoma metastasis. These EMT factors are activated through MAP kinase signaling and promote a de-differentiated and migratory state in melanoma (Caramel et al. 2013). Additionally, the proliferation rate of cells with active EMT markers is significantly decreased, making them more resistant to many cytotoxic therapies that target rapidly proliferating tumor cells.

In the context of melanoma, EMT is associated with aggressive, therapy-resistant tumor types. Thus, better understanding the role of EMT during embryogenesis and tumorigenesis offers potential clinical value. EMT factors are expressed almost exclusively during embryogenesis and are not expressed in normal adult tissues (Gupta et al. 2005b). This affords the possibility of diagnostic techniques focused on these factors as biomarkers for the presence of malignancy. For example, Snail2 levels are highest during early transformation of melanocytes (Gupta et al. 2005a; Shirley et al. 2012). This knowledge could provide a means to more accurately identify lesions at risk for malignant transformation for further observation or removal. Additionally, in embryogenesis, these factors work in the context of various signaling pathways that keep them in check. Further exploration of how these EMT factors are regulated in embryonic development could inform potential means of controlling them in melanoma. For example, it has been shown that treatment which upregulates MITF, the master regulator of melanocyte differentiation, can drive differentiation of melanocytes expressing EMT markers, increasing susceptibility to chemotherapy and decreasing migratory capacity (Caramel et al. 2013). In addition to melanoma, EMT is present in the progression of other tumor types, and any discovery that informs the prognosis or treatment of melanoma based on these factors has the potential to be applied more broadly to other malignancies.

13.4 WNT Signaling

Wnt signaling plays a role in many aspects of embryonic development (Sadler and Langman 2010). Wnt secreted glycoproteins canonically signal through a series of intracellular steps to stabilize β-catenin so that it can translocate to the nucleus, form a complex with TCF/LEF transcription factors, and activate expression of target genes (Moon 2005). Wnt signaling regulates the melanocyte lineage at various stages of development (Lewis et al. 2004). Wnt signaling is important in neural crest specification, working in conjunction with BMP and FGF signals to prime pluripotent ectodermal cells to receive appropriate signaling to induce neural crest formation (Garnett et al. 2012; Jin et al. 2001; Sato et al. 2005). After neural crest formation, Wnt signaling plays a role in the expression of other neural crest markers and EMT factors (Garnett et al. 2012). Importantly, Wnt cooperates with Zic and Pax transcription factors to promote the expression of Snail family proteins in the neural crest, allowing appropriate neural crest migration (Sato et al. 2005). Additionally, Wnt signaling is involved in activation of Sox10, which is required for development of some nonmesenchymal neural crest derivatives, including melanocytes (Lewis et al. 2004). After neural crest migration, Wnt signaling is involved in the final specification, through multiple mechanisms, of melanocytes from precursors. Importantly, activated β-catenin itself promotes expression of MITF (Dorsky et al. 2000; Raible and Ragland 2005). Additionally, Wnt-activated expression of Sox10 increases Sox10 binding to the MITF promoter and reinforces expression of MITF. Through these mechanisms, canonical Wnt signaling promotes both neural crest and melanocyte identity.

13.4.1 Canonical Wnt Signaling in Melanoma

Canonical Wnt signaling has been implicated in the proliferation, invasion, and metastatic potential of melanoma. Multiple studies have shown Wnt ligands, ones that specifically activate the canonical pathway, are commonly overexpressed in both melanocytic nevi as well as in melanoma (Pham et al. 2003; You et al. 2004). Examination of primary human melanoma samples has shown increased nuclear localization of β-catenin (Rimm et al. 1999). Melanoma cell lines with high levels of Wnt activity also show increases in transcription of known Wnt targets, such as MITF (Widlund et al. 2002). Despite high levels of nuclear β-catenin, mutations in β-catenin, adenomatous polyposis coli (APC), and other Wnt pathway components are infrequent in melanoma, indicating alternative means of Wnt activation (Reifenberger et al. 2002; Rimm et al. 1999). Taken together, these results show that the Wnt pathway is indeed active at various stages of melanoma progression.

Canonical Wnt signaling has complex and context-dependent roles through various stages of melanoma development. Experiments examining the role of Wnt on proliferation have shown that increased Wnt signaling decreases the proliferation of both human and mouse melanoma cell lines (Chien et al. 2009). Furthermore, cells overexpressing Wnt showed a decrease in tumor size in a xenotransplantation model. Similarly, overexpression of Wntless Wnt Ligand Secretion Mediator (WLS), a protein that supports Wnt secretion, causes a decrease in the proliferation of cells in vitro, while knockdown of WLS causes an increase in proliferation (Yang et al. 2012). These results suggest that signaling by canonical Wnt ligands acts to suppress proliferation of melanoma cells. In support of this idea, studies have shown that increased Wnt activity, as measured by nuclear staining for β-catenin, is associated with improved patient survival (Chien et al. 2009). These studies provide evidence for Wnt signaling acting as an inhibitor of proliferation. However, other studies support a role for the Wnt/β-catenin pathway in promoting proliferation, suggesting that Wnt actions are dependent on biological context. Damsky et al. expressed a stabilized version of β-catenin in a $BRAF^{V600E}/PTEN^{KO}$ mouse model and showed that it increased the proliferative index and overall growth of melanomas (Damsky et al. 2011). Similarly, Delmas et al. showed expression of stabilized β-catenin, in the context of activated NRAS, was able to immortalize primary skin melanocytes and induce melanoma formation in mice (Delmas et al. 2007). These results suggest that the role of Wnt signaling is highly dependent on the context in which it is active and potentially on how the Wnt pathway itself is activated.

Similar to its effect on proliferation, regulation of invasion and metastasis by Wnt signaling is likely dependent on biological context. Experiments involving Wnt overexpressing cell lines show a decrease in metastasis in a mouse xenograft model (Chien et al. 2009). In addition, WLS knockdown cells show an increase in metastasis when applied to a mouse xenograft model, suggesting that loss of Wnt signaling increases metastasis (Yang et al. 2012). In other contexts, Wnt signaling adopts alternative roles. In $BRAF^{V600E}/PTEN^{KO}$ mice expressing stabilized β-catenin, increased metastasis was observed when compared with controls (Damsky et al. 2011). Likewise, Gallagher et al. showed that, when combined with an activated NRAS oncogene, stabilized β-catenin was able to induce more metastases in mice (Gallagher et al. 2013). As with proliferation, the effects of Wnt signaling on invasion and metastasis of melanoma depend on how Wnt activation is achieved and in which genetic background experiments are performed. These studies, as well as those on proliferation described above, suggest the mode of Wnt activation is important in its effect on tumorigenesis. Specifically, a difference exists between stabilized β-catenin and Wnt ligand-mediated activation: Wnt ligand overexpression shows a generally tumor suppressive role, while ligand-independent activation and stabilization of β-catenin promotes tumor progression.

Differential effects of Wnt signaling are also manifest in melanoma therapy. Suggesting that Wnt signaling facilitates therapeutic targeting, a Wnt3a-dependent increase in apoptosis was observed when $BRAF^{V600E}$-positive cell lines were subjected to BRAF inhibition (Biechele et al. 2012). In a later study, patients were retrospectively evaluated for response to BRAF inhibitors based on β-catenin staining prior to initiating therapy (Chien et al. 2014). Here, increased β-catenin staining prior to treatment correlated with a poorer response to BRAF inhibitors, arguing that Wnt signaling dampened the response to BRAF inhibitors. These results again suggest that the complexity of canonical Wnt signaling extends to melanoma therapy.

13.4.2 Noncanonical Wnt Signaling

Noncanonical Wnt signaling has two main sub-pathways: the planar cell polarity (PCP) pathway and the Wnt/calcium pathway (Liu et al. 2014; Veeman et al. 2003). Both pathways signal independently of β-catenin. The PCP pathway, activated by a subset of Wnt ligands binding to Wnt receptors, involves the activation of downstream factors that help rearrange cytoskeletal elements. The calcium pathway involves Wnt ligand and Frizzled receptor-induced activation of phospholipase C, leading to differential regulation of calcium within the cell. By regulating cell migration, cell polarity, and other fundamental processes, noncanonical Wnt signaling plays a role in several phases of embryonic development (Prasad et al. 2015).

The role of noncanonical Wnt signaling in promoting melanoma was first hypothesized after a screen of melanoma cell lines revealed overexpression of Wnt5a, a Wnt ligand that predominantly activates noncanonical pathways (Bittner et al. 2000). Further examination of tumor samples showed Wnt5a expression increased with melanoma progression (Bittner et al. 2000), and its expression correlated with poor patient outcomes (Forno et al. 2008). Mechanistic studies in vitro showed that exogenous Wnt5a added to melanoma cells augmented changes in polarity and migration, suggesting a role in promoting invasion and metastasis (Dissanayake et al. 2007). Supporting this result, targeting endogenous Wnt5a with an inhibitor decreased migration of melanoma cells (Jenei et al. 2009). Additional in vitro studies showed overexpression of Wnt5a caused redistribution and decreased expression of adhesion molecules (Witze et al. 2008), whereas knockdown increased adhesion molecule expression, leading to a decrease in invasion (Jenei et al. 2009). Extending these studies in vivo, Dissanayake et al. showed administration of Wnt5a in a xenograft model promoted metastasis (Dissanayake et al. 2008). Interaction of noncanonical Wnt signaling has also been implicated in resistance mechanisms to therapy. Anastas et al. have shown that elevated Wnt5a expression is correlated with a decrease in patient response to BRAF inhibitors (Anastas et al. 2014). This resistance is proposed to be mediated by an increase in AKT/PI3K signaling activation. In this study, knockdown of Wnt5a was able to rescue sensitivity to BRAF inhibition. Additionally, Webster et al. have shown Wnt5a induces a senescent, yet still invasive, phenotype in melanoma cells, allowing continued progression of tumors while avoiding conventional chemotherapy or targeted therapies (Webster et al. 2015). While Wnt5a has been shown to affect signaling independent of β-catenin, it has also been shown that there may be interactions between canonical and noncanonical Wnt signaling, especially in later-stage melanomas. In vitro experiments showed Wnt5a signaling disrupted interaction between β-catenin and N-cadherin, allowing a larger pool of available β-catenin to translocate to the nucleus and induce transcription (Grossmann et al. 2013). This interaction between canonical and noncanonical signaling pathway creates another layer of complexity in interpreting the effects of Wnt signaling.

13.5 MITF

Microphthalmia-associated transcription factor (MITF) is the master regulator of the melanocyte lineage. It activates the transcription of melanin biosynthesis genes such as the receptor MC1R, the melanosome transport protein RAB27A, the melanin biosynthetic rate limiting enzyme Tyrosinase, and other genes such as PMEL17 and MLANA (Vachtenheim and Borovanský 2010). MITF is regulated by a combination of PAX3, SOX10, and LEF1, the latter of which directly links Wnt signaling to MITF regulation (Liu et al. 2014; Vachtenheim and Borovanský 2010). Several studies in mice, zebrafish, and other systems have shown that MITF is required for melanocyte development and function (Dorsky et al. 2000; Opdecamp et al. 1997; Patton and Nairn 2010).

The role of MITF in regulating melanocyte and melanoma cell proliferation and differentiation has been extensively studied. Early studies showed a complex relationship between MITF signaling and melanoma progression. In 2005, Carreira et al. found that MITF, when expressed at low levels, acts as an anti-proliferative factor, inducing G1 cell cycle arrest via $p21^{Cip1}$ and $p16^{INK4a}$ (Carreira et al. 2005). In a follow-up study, Carreira found short-term depletion of MITF leads to $p27^{Kip1}$-dependent cell cycle arrest while simultaneously increasing the invasiveness of melanoma cells (Carreira et al. 2006). By contrast, Garraway et al. found copy number amplification of the *MITF* gene in melanomas and showed that its elevated expression promoted melanocyte transformation, suggesting MITF can act as an oncogene (Garraway et al. 2005). The results of these studies indicate that the effects of MITF in melanoma depend largely on its expression level and corresponding transcriptional activity.

To account for the differential effects of MITF, Goding and colleagues proposed the "rheostat" model to describe the observed changes in cellular phenotype based on low, moderate, or high levels of MITF signaling (Carreira et al. 2006; Hoek and Goding 2010). Under this model, cells with low levels of MITF are expected to exhibit a stem-like state where they proliferate slowly and are more invasive. Cells expressing moderate levels MITF are expected to proliferate by expressing

MITF-target genes such as *CDK2* and *BCL2*, regulating cell cycle progression and survival. Melanocytes expressing MITF at high levels are nonproliferative and non-invasive, expressing genes such as *MART1* and *Tyrosinase* that promote terminal differentiation. In sum, MITF is proposed to modulate cell activity through variable expression just as a rheostat alters resistance in a circuit.

In concordance with this new model, Cheli et al. showed that low MITF levels are associated with a greater degree of "stemness" and tumor initiation (Cheli et al. 2011). Ablation of low MITF cells from a heterogeneous tumor cell population greatly reduced tumor initiation. Additionally, the subpopulation of cells with high MITF levels were poor at initiating tumors. However, inhibition of MITF in this subpopulation upregulated the stem cell markers Oct4 and Nanog and increased tumorigenic potential. MITF inhibition led to p27 upregulation, consistent with a model in which slow growing, MITF-low cells are more stem cell-like and have the greatest potential to initiate tumors.

As an extension of the rheostat model, manipulation of MITF levels or activity has been proposed as a means of melanoma therapy. The goal of altering MITF is to change cellular phenotype, causing a switch from a stem-like phenotype to a more proliferative or differentiated phenotype. To accomplish such "phenotype-switching," methotrexate was used to increase MITF expression in melanoma cells, driving them toward a more proliferative and differentiated state (Sáez-Ayala et al. 2013). This higher rate of proliferation increased the susceptibility of the cells to treatment with the antimetabolite 3-O-(3,4,5-trimethoxybenzoyl)-(−)-epicatechin (TMECG), an inhibitor of folate metabolism. This result highlights the potential utility of using MITF-specific treatment as an adjuvant to standard of care in highly invasive and aggressive melanomas. MITF expression has also been investigated as a prognostic factor in melanoma. In 2014, Peeper and colleagues showed that a low MITF/AXL ratio was predictive of resistance to BRAF inhibitors (Müller et al. 2014). These are recent examples of how understanding MITF function in embryonic melanocyte development can further the development of clinically relevant tools and effective therapeutics.

Conclusion

Embryonic development requires many temporally and spatially regulated steps to develop mature melanocytes. From early embryonic patterning to final fate specification, multiple signaling pathways and intrinsic factors are required to complete these steps, perfectly coordinated to correctly direct development. Because embryogenesis is a unique biological scenario, many of these pathways and factors that drive proliferation and migration are only active during development, and not active in adult tissues. However, because these properties are crucial in tumor initiation and progression, the embryonic programs are often reawakened during melanoma initiation and progression. In particular, the melanocyte development program provides nascent melanomas with a toolset to promote proliferation, invasion, and metastasis. Many of the embryonic properties co-opted by melanomas are broadly shared across many forms of cancer. This common thread that connects different malignancies suggests that discoveries relating melanocyte development to melanoma could inform our understanding of biological processes underlying other cancers.

Bibliography

Anastas JN, Kulikauskas RM, Tamir T, Rizos H, Long GV, von Euw EM, Yang P-T, Chen H-W, Haydu L, Toroni RA, Lucero OM, Chien AJ, Moon RT (2014) WNT5A enhances resistance of melanoma cells to targeted BRAF inhibitors. J Clin Invest 124:2877–2890. doi:10.1172/JCI70156

Bedogni B (2014) Notch signaling in melanoma: interacting pathways and stromal influences that enhance Notch targeting. Pigment Cell Melanoma Res 27:162–168. doi:10.1111/pcmr.12194

Biechele TL, Kulikauskas RM, Toroni RA, Lucero OM, Swift RD, James RG, Robin NC, Dawson DW, Moon RT, Chien AJ (2012) Wnt/β-catenin signaling and AXIN1 regulate apoptosis triggered by inhibition of the mutant kinase BRAFV600E in human melanoma. Sci Signal 5:ra3. doi:10.1126/scisignal.2002274

Bittner M, Meltzer P, Chen Y, Jiang Y, Seftor E, Hendrix M, Radmacher M, Simon R, Yakhini Z, Ben-Dor A, Sampas N, Dougherty E, Wang E, Marincola F, Gooden C, Lueders J, Glatfelter A, Pollock P, Carpten J, Gillanders E, Leja D, Dietrich K, Beaudry C, Berens M, Alberts D, Sondak V (2000) Molecular classification of cutaneous malignant melanoma by gene expression profiling. Nature 406:536–540. doi:10.1038/35020115

Brou C, Logeat F, Gupta N, Bessia C, LeBail O, Doedens JR, Cumano A, Roux P, Black RA, Israël A (2000) A novel proteolytic cleavage involved in Notch signaling: the role of the disintegrin-metalloprotease TACE. Mol Cell 5:207–216

Cano A, Pérez-Moreno MA, Rodrigo I, Locascio A, Blanco MJ, del Barrio MG, Portillo F, Nieto MA (2000) The transcription factor Snail controls epithelial–mesenchymal transitions by repressing E-cadherin expression. Nat Cell Biol 2:76–83. doi:10.1038/35000025

Caramel J, Papadogeorgakis E, Hill L, Browne GJ, Richard G, Wierinckx A, Saldanha G, Osborne J, Hutchinson P, Tse G, Lachuer J, Puisieux A, Pringle JH, Ansieau S, Tulchinsky E (2013) A switch in the expression of embryonic EMT-inducers drives the development of malignant melanoma. Cancer Cell 24:466–480. doi:10.1016/j.ccr.2013.08.018

Carreira S, Goodall J, Aksan I, La Rocca SA, Galibert M-D, Denat L, Larue L, Goding CR (2005) Mitf cooperates with Rb1 and activates p21Cip1 expression to regulate cell cycle progression. Nature 433:764–769. doi:10.1038/nature03269

Carreira S, Goodall J, Denat L, Rodriguez M, Nuciforo P, Hoek KS, Testori A, Larue L, Goding CR (2006) Mitf regulation of Dia1 controls melanoma proliferation and invasiveness. Genes Dev 20:3426–3439. doi:10.1101/gad.406406

Cheli Y, Giuliano S, Guiliano S, Botton T, Rocchi S, Hofman V, Hofman P, Bahadoran P, Bertolotto C, Ballotti R (2011) Mitf is the key molecular switch between mouse or human melanoma initiating cells and their differentiated progeny. Oncogene 30:2307–2318. doi:10.1038/onc.2010.598

Chien AJ, Moore EC, Lonsdorf AS, Kulikauskas RM, Rothberg BG, Berger AJ, Major MB, Hwang ST, Rimm DL, Moon RT (2009) Activated Wnt/ß-catenin signaling in melanoma is associated with decreased proliferation in patient tumors and a murine melanoma model. Proc Natl Acad Sci 106:1193–1198. doi:10.1073/pnas.0811902106

Chien AJ, Haydu LE, Biechele TL, Kulikauskas RM, Rizos H, Kefford RF, Scolyer RA, Moon RT, Long GV (2014) Targeted BRAF inhibition impacts survival in melanoma patients with high levels of Wnt/β-catenin signaling. PLoS One 9:e94748. doi:10.1371/journal.pone.0094748

Comijn J, Berx G, Vermassen P, Verschueren K, van Grunsven L, Bruyneel E, Mareel M, Huylebroeck D, van Roy F (2001) The two-handed E box binding zinc finger protein SIP1 downregulates E-cadherin and induces invasion. Mol Cell 7:1267–1278. doi:10.1016/S1097-2765(01)00260-X

Conlon FL, Lyons KM, Takaesu N, Barth KS, Kispert A, Herrmann B, Robertson EJ (1994) A primary requirement for nodal in the formation and maintenance of the primitive streak in the mouse. Development 120:1919–1928

Cornell RA, Eisen JS (2002) Delta/Notch signaling promotes formation of zebrafish neural crest by repressing Neurogenin 1 function. Development (Cambridge England) 129:2639–2648

Damsky WE, Curley DP, Santhanakrishnan M, Rosenbaum LE, Platt JT, Gould Rothberg BE, Taketo MM, Dankort D, Rimm DL, McMahon M, Bosenberg M (2011) β-catenin signaling controls metastasis in braf-activated pten-deficient melanomas. Cancer Cell 20:741–754. doi:10.1016/j.ccr.2011.10.030

Delmas V, Beermann F, Martinozzi S, Carreira S, Ackermann J, Kumasaka M, Denat L, Goodall J, Luciani F, Viros A, Demirkan N, Bastian BC, Goding CR, Larue L (2007) β-catenin induces immortalization of melanocytes by suppressing p16INK4a expression and cooperates with N-Ras in melanoma development. Genes Dev 21:2923–2935. doi:10.1101/gad.450107

Dissanayake SK, Wade M, Johnson CE, O'Connell MP, Leotlela PD, French AD, Shah KV, Hewitt KJ, Rosenthal DT, Indig FE, Jiang Y, Nickoloff BJ, Taub DD, Trent JM, Moon RT, Bittner M, Weeraratna AT (2007) The Wnt5A/protein kinase C pathway mediates motility in melanoma cells via the inhibition of metastasis suppressors and initiation of an epithelial to mesenchymal transition. J Biol Chem 282:17259–17271. doi:10.1074/jbc.M700075200

Dissanayake SK, Olkhanud PB, O'Connell MP, Carter A, French AD, Camilli TC, Emeche CD, Hewitt KJ, Rosenthal DT, Leotlela PD, Wade MS, Yang SW, Brant L, Nickoloff BJ, Messina JL, Biragyn A, Hoek KS, Taub DD, Longo DL, Sondak VK, Hewitt SM, Weeraratna AT (2008) Wnt5A regulates expression of tumor-associated antigens in melanoma via changes in signal transducers and activators of transcription 3 phosphorylation. Cancer Res 68:10205–10214. doi:10.1158/0008-5472.CAN-08-2149

Dorsky RI, Raible DW, Moon RT (2000) Direct regulation of nacre, a zebrafish MITF homolog required for pigment cell formation, by the Wnt pathway. Genes Dev 14:158–162. doi:10.1101/gad.14.2.158

Edbauer D, Winkler E, Regula JT, Pesold B, Steiner H, Haass C (2003) Reconstitution of gamma-secretase activity. Nat Cell Biol 5:486–488. doi:10.1038/ncb960

Endo Y, Osumi N, Wakamatsu Y (2002) Bimodal functions of Notch-mediated signaling are involved in neural crest formation during avian ectoderm development. Development (Cambridge England) 129:863–873

Fang R, Zhang G, Guo Q, Ning F, Wang H, Cai S, Du J (2013) Nodal promotes aggressive phenotype via snail-mediated epithelial–mesenchymal transition in murine melanoma. Cancer Lett 333:66–75. doi:10.1016/j.canlet.2013.01.014

Feller J, Schneider A, Schuster-Gossler K, Gossler A (2008) Noncyclic Notch activity in the presomitic mesoderm demonstrates uncoupling of somite compartmentalization and boundary formation. Genes Dev 22:2166–2171. doi:10.1101/gad.480408

Forloni M, Dogra SK, Dong Y, Conte D, Ou J, Zhu LJ, Deng A, Mahalingam M, Green MR, Wajapeyee N (2014) miR-146a promotes the initiation and progression of melanoma by activating Notch signaling. Elife 3:e01460. doi:10.7554/eLife.01460

Forno PDD, Pringle JH, Hutchinson P, Osborn J, Huang Q, Potter L, Hancox RA, Fletcher A, Saldanha GS (2008) WNT5A expression increases during melanoma progression and correlates with outcome. Clin Cancer Res 14:5825–5832. doi:10.1158/1078-0432.CCR-07-5104

Fryer CJ, Lamar E, Turbachova I, Kintner C, Jones KA (2002) Mastermind mediates chromatin-specific transcription and turnover of the Notch enhancer complex. Genes Dev 16:1397–1411. doi:10.1101/gad.991602

Fukunaga-Kalabis M, Hristova DM, Wang JX, Li L, Heppt MV, Wei Z, Gyurdieva A, Webster MR, Oka M, Weeraratna AT, Herlyn M (2015) UV-induced Wnt7a in the human skin microenvironment specifies the fate of neural crest-like cells via suppression of Notch. J Invest Dermatol 135:1521–1532. doi:10.1038/jid.2015.59

Gallagher SJ, Rambow F, Kumasaka M, Champeval D, Bellacosa A, Delmas V, Larue L (2013) Beta-catenin inhibits melanocyte migration but induces melanoma metastasis. Oncogene 32:2230–2238. doi:10.1038/onc.2012.229

Garnett AT, Square TA, Medeiros DM (2012) BMP, Wnt and FGF signals are integrated through evolutionarily conserved enhancers to achieve robust expression of Pax3 and Zic genes at the zebrafish neural plate border. Development 139:4220–4231. doi:10.1242/dev.081497

Garraway LA, Weir BA, Zhao X, Widlund H, Beroukhim R, Berger A, Rimm D, Rubin MA, Fisher DE, Meyerson ML, Sellers WR (2005) "Lineage addiction" in human cancer: lessons from integrated genomics. Cold Spring Harb Symp Quant Biol 70:25–34. doi:10.1101/sqb.2005.70.016

Glavic A, Silva F, Aybar MJ, Bastidas F, Mayor R (2004) Interplay between Notch signaling and the homeoprotein Xiro1 is required for neural crest induction in Xenopus embryos. Development (Cambridge England) 131:347–359. doi:10.1242/dev.00945

Golan T, Messer AR, Amitai-Lange A, Melamed Z, Ohana R, Bell RE, Kapitansky O, Lerman G, Greenberger S, Khaled M, Amar N, Albrengues J, Gaggioli C, Gonen P, Tabach Y, Sprinzak D, Shalom-Feuerstein R, Levy C (2015) Interactions of melanoma cells with distal keratinocytes trigger metastasis via Notch signaling inhibition of MITF. Mol Cell 59:664–676. doi:10.1016/j.molcel.2015.06.028

Goldstein J, Horsley V (2012) Home sweet home: skin stem cell niches. Cell Mol Life Sci 69:2573–2582. doi:10.1007/s00018-012-0943-3

Grooteclaes ML, Frisch SM (2000) Evidence for a function of CtBP in epithelial gene regulation and anoikis. Oncogene 19:3823–3828. doi:10.1038/sj.onc.1203721

Grossmann AH, Yoo JH, Clancy J, Sorensen LK, Sedgwick A, Tong Z, Ostanin K, Rogers A, Grossmann KF, Tripp SR, Thomas KR, D'Souza-Schorey C, Odelberg SJ, Li DY (2013) The small GTPase ARF6 stimulates β-catenin transcriptional activity during WNT5A-mediated melanoma invasion and metastasis. Sci Signal 6:ra14. doi:10.1126/scisignal.2003398

Gupta PB, Kuperwasser C, Brunet J-P, Ramaswamy S, Kuo W-L, Gray JW, Naber SP, Weinberg RA (2005a) The melanocyte differentiation program predisposes to metastasis after neoplastic transformation. Nat Genet 37:1047–1054. doi:10.1038/ng1634

Gupta PB, Mani S, Yang J, Hartwell K, Weinberg RA (2005b) The evolving portrait of cancer metastasis. Cold Spring Harb Symp Quant Biol 70:291–297. doi:10.1101/sqb.2005.70.033

Hardy KM, Kirschmann DA, Seftor EA, Margaryan NV, Postovit L-M, Strizzi L, Hendrix MJC (2010) Regulation of the embryonic morphogen nodal by Notch4 facilitates manifestation of the aggressive melanoma phenotype. Cancer Res 70:10340–10350. doi:10.1158/0008-5472.CAN-10-0705

Hardy KM, Strizzi L, Margaryan NV, Gupta K, Murphy GF, Scolyer RA, Hendrix MJC (2015) Targeting nodal in conjunction with dacarbazine induces synergistic anticancer effects in metastatic melanoma. Mol Cancer Res 13:670–680. doi:10.1158/1541-7786.MCR-14-0077

Hartmann D, de Strooper B, Serneels L, Craessaerts K, Herreman A, Annaert W, Umans L, Lübke T, Lena Illert A, von Figura K, Saftig P (2002) The disintegrin/metalloprotease ADAM 10 is essential for Notch signalling but not for alphasecretase activity in fibroblasts. Hum Mol Genet 11:2615–2624

Hendrix MJC, Seftor REB, Seftor EA, Gruman LM, Lee LML, Nickoloff BJ, Miele L, Sheriff DD, Schatteman GC (2002) Transendothelial function of human metastatic melanoma cells: role of the microenvironment in cell-fate determination. Cancer Res 62:665–668

Hendrix MJC, Seftor EA, Seftor REB, Kasemeier-Kulesa J, Kulesa PM, Postovit L-M (2007) Reprogramming metastatic tumour cells with embryonic microenvironments. Nat Rev Cancer 7:246–255. doi:10.1038/nrc2108

Hoek KS, Goding CR (2010) Cancer stem cells versus phenotype-switching in melanoma. Pigment Cell Melanoma Res 23:746–759. doi:10.1111/j.1755-148X.2010.00757.x

James D, Levine AJ, Besser D, Hemmati-Brivanlou A (2005) TGFβ/activin/nodal signaling is necessary for the maintenance of pluripotency in human embryonic stem cells. Development 132:1273–1282. doi:10.1242/dev.01706

Jenei V, Sherwood V, Howlin J, Linnskog R, Säfholm A, Axelsson L, Andersson T (2009) A t-butyloxycarbonyl-modified Wnt5a-derived hexapeptide functions as a potent antagonist of Wnt5a-dependent melanoma cell invasion. Proc Natl Acad Sci 106:19473–19478. doi:10.1073/pnas.0909409106

Jin E-J, Erickson CA, Takada S, Burrus LW (2001) Wnt and BMP signaling govern lineage segregation of melanocytes in the avian embryo. Dev Biol 233:22–37. doi:10.1006/dbio.2001.0222

Kaufman CK, Mosimann C, Fan ZP, Yang S, Thomas AJ, Ablain J, Tan JL, Fogley RD, van Rooijen E, Hagedorn EJ, Ciarlo C, White RM, Matos DA, Puller A-C, Santoriello C, Liao EC, Young RA, Zon LI (2016) A zebrafish melanoma model reveals emergence of neural crest identity during melanoma initiation. Science 351:aad2197. doi:10.1126/science.aad2197

Kerosuo L, Bronner-Fraser M (2012) What is bad in cancer is good in the embryo: Importance of EMT in neural crest development. Semin Cell Dev Biol RNA Editing Dev Cell Behav 23:320–332. doi:10.1016/j.semcdb.2012.03.010

Kuriyama S, Mayor R (2008) Molecular analysis of neural crest migration. Philos Trans R Soc Lond B Biol Sci 363:1349–1362. doi:10.1098/rstb.2007.2252

Levin M, Johnson RL, Sterna CD, Kuehn M, Tabin C (1995) A molecular pathway determining left-right asymmetry in chick embryogenesis. Cell 82:803–814. doi:10.1016/0092-8674(95)90477-8

Lewis JL, Bonner J, Modrell M, Ragland JW, Moon RT, Dorsky RI, Raible DW (2004) Reiterated Wnt signaling during zebrafish neural crest development. Development 131:1299–1308. doi:10.1242/dev.01007

Liu J, Fukunaga-Kalabis M, Li L, Herlyn M (2014) Developmental pathways activated in melanocytes and melanoma. Arch Biochem Biophys 563:13–21. doi:10.1016/j.abb.2014.07.023

Matsuzaki F (2000) Asymmetric division of Drosophila neural stem cells: a basis for neural diversity. Curr Opin Neurobiol 10:38–44. doi:10.1016/S0959-4388(99)00052-5

Montagne C, Gonzalez-Gaitan M (2014) Sara endosomes and the asymmetric division of intestinal stem cells. Development (Cambridge England) 141:2014–2023. doi:10.1242/dev.104240

Moon RT (2005) Wnt/β-catenin pathway. Sci STKE 2005:cm1. doi:10.1126/stke.2712005cm1

Moriyama M, Osawa M, Mak S-S, Ohtsuka T, Yamamoto N, Han H, Delmas V, Kageyama R, Beermann F, Larue L, Nishikawa S-I (2006) Notch signaling via Hes1 transcription factor maintains survival of melanoblasts and melanocyte stem cells. J Cell Biol 173:333–339. doi:10.1083/jcb.200509084

Müller J, Krijgsman O, Tsoi J, Robert L, Hugo W, Song C, Kong X, Possik PA, Cornelissen-Steijger PDM, Foppen MHG, Kemper K, Goding CR, McDermott U, Blank C, Haanen J, Graeber TG, Ribas A, Lo RS, Peeper DS (2014) Low MITF/AXL ratio predicts early resistance to multiple targeted drugs in melanoma. Nat Commun 5:5712. doi:10.1038/ncomms6712

Nam Y, Weng AP, Aster JC, Blacklow SC (2003) Structural requirements for assembly of the CSL. intracellular Notch1.Mastermind-like 1 transcriptional activation complex. J Biol Chem 278:21232–21239. doi:10.1074/jbc.M301567200

Opdecamp K, Nakayama A, Nguyen MT, Hodgkinson CA, Pavan WJ, Arnheiter H (1997) Melanocyte development in vivo and in neural crest cell cultures: crucial dependence on the Mitf basic-helix-loop-helix-zipper transcription factor. Development (Cambridge England) 124:2377–2386

Patton EE, Nairn RS (2010) Xmrk in medaka: a new genetic melanoma model. J Invest Dermatol 130:14–17. doi:10.1038/jid.2009.293

Pham K, Milovanovic T, Barr RJ, Truong T, Holcombe RF (2003) Wnt ligand expression in malignant melanoma: pilot study indicating correlation with histopathological features. Mol Pathol 56:280–285. doi:10.1136/mp.56.5.280

Pinnix CC, Herlyn M (2007) The many faces of Notch signaling in skin-derived cells. Pigment Cell Res Spons Eur Soc Pigment Cell Res Int Pigment Cell Soc 20:458–465. doi:10.1111/j.1600-0749.2007.00410.x

Postovit L-M, Margaryan NV, Seftor EA, Hendrix MJC (2008) Role of nodal signaling and the microenvironment underlying melanoma plasticity. Pigment Cell Melanoma Res 21:348–357. doi:10.1111/j.1755-148X.2008.00463.x

Prasad CP, Mohapatra P, Andersson T (2015) Therapy for BRAFi-resistant melanomas: is WNT5A the answer? Cancer 7:1900–1924. doi:10.3390/cancers7030868

Quail DF, Siegers GM, Jewer M, Postovit L-M (2013) Nodal signalling in embryogenesis and tumourigenesis. Int J Biochem Cell Biol 45:885–898. doi:10.1016/j.biocel.2012.12.021

Raible DW, Ragland JW (2005) Reiterated Wnt and BMP signals in neural crest development. Semin Cell Dev Biol 16:673–682. doi:10.1016/j.semcdb.2005.06.008

Reifenberger J, Knobbe CB, Wolter M, Blaschke B, Schulte KW, Pietsch T, Ruzicka T, Reifenberger G (2002) Molecular genetic analysis of malignant melanomas for aberrations of the WNT signaling pathway genes CTNNB1, APC. ICAT BTRC Int J Cancer 100:549–556. doi:10.1002/ijc.10512

Rimm DL, Caca K, Hu G, Harrison FB, Fearon ER (1999) Frequent nuclear/cytoplasmic localization of β-catenin without Exon 3 mutations in malignant melanoma. Am J Pathol 154:325–329. doi:10.1016/S0002-9440(10)65278-9

Sadler TW, Langman J (2010) Langman's medical embryology. Lippincott William & Wilkins, Philadelphia

Sáez-Ayala M, Montenegro MF, Sánchez-del-Campo L, Fernández-Pérez MP, Chazarra S, Freter R, Middleton M, Piñero-Madrona A, Cabezas-Herrera J, Goding CR, Rodríguez-López JN (2013) Directed phenotype switching as an effective antimelanoma strategy. Cancer Cell 24:105–119. doi:10.1016/j.ccr.2013.05.009

Sato T, Sasai N, Sasai Y (2005) Neural crest determination by co-activation of Pax3 and Zic1 genes in Xenopus ectoderm. Development 132:2355–2363. doi:10.1242/dev.01823

Schouwey K, Delmas V, Larue L, Zimber-Strobl U, Strobl LJ, Radtke F, Beermann F (2007) Notch1 and Notch2 receptors influence progressive hair graying in a dosedependent manner. Dev Dyn Off Publ Am Assoc Anat 236:282–289. doi:10.1002/dvdy.21000

Shirley SH, Greene VR, Duncan LM, Torres Cabala CA, Grimm EA, Kusewitt DF (2012) Slug expression during melanoma progression. Am J Pathol 180:2479–2489. doi:10.1016/j.ajpath.2012.02.014

Strizzi L, Sandomenico A, Margaryan NV, Focà A, Sanguigno L, Bodenstine TM, Chandler GS, Reed DW, Gilgur A, Seftor EA, Seftor REB, Khalkhali-Ellis Z, Leonardi A, Ruvo M, Hendrix MJC (2015) Effects of a novel Nodal-targeting monoclonal antibody in melanoma. Oncotarget 6:34071–34086. doi:10.18632/oncotarget.6049

Topczewska JM, Postovit L-M, Margaryan NV, Sam A, Hess AR, Wheaton WW, Nickoloff BJ, Topczewski J, Hendrix MJC (2006) Embryonic and tumorigenic pathways converge via Nodal signaling: role in melanoma aggressiveness. Nat Med 12:925–932. doi:10.1038/nm1448

Vachtenheim J, Borovanský J (2010) "Transcription physiology" of pigment formation in melanocytes: central role of MITF. Exp Dermatol 19:617–627. doi:10.1111/j.1600-0625.2009.01053.x

Vallier L, Mendjan S, Brown S, Chng Z, Teo A, Smithers LE, Trotter MWB, Cho CH-H, Martinez A, Rugg-Gunn P, Brons G, Pedersen RA (2009) Activin/nodal signalling maintains pluripotency by controlling nanog expression. Development 136:1339–1349. doi:10.1242/dev.033951

Veeman MT, Axelrod JD, Moon RT (2003) A second canon: functions and mechanisms of β-catenin-independent Wnt signaling. Dev Cell 5:367–377. doi:10.1016/S1534-5807(03)00266-1

Vega S, Morales AV, Ocaña OH, Valdés F, Fabregat I, Nieto MA (2004) Snail blocks the cell cycle and confers resistance to cell death. Genes Dev 18:1131–1143. doi:10.1101/gad.294104

Webster MR, Xu M, Kinzler KA, Kaur A, Appleton J, O'Connell MP, Marchbank K, Valiga A, Dang VM, Perego M, Zhang G, Slipicevic A, Keeney F, Lehrmann E, Wood W, Becker KG, Kossenkov AV, Frederick DT, Flaherty KT, Xu X, Herlyn M, Murphy ME, Weeraratna AT (2015) Wnt5A promotes an adaptive, senescent-like stress response, while continuing to drive invasion in melanoma cells. Pigment Cell Melanoma Res 28:184–195. doi:10.1111/pcmr.12330

Widlund HR, Horstmann MA, Price ER, Cui J, Lessnick SL, Wu M, He X, Fisher DE (2002) β-catenin–induced melanoma growth requires the downstream target Microphthalmia-associated transcription factor. J Cell Biol 158:1079–1087. doi:10.1083/jcb.200202049

Witze ES, Litman ES, Argast GM, Moon RT, Ahn NG (2008) Wnt5a control of cell polarity and directional movement by polarized redistribution of adhesion receptors. Science 320:365–369. doi:10.1126/science.1151250

Wu L, Aster JC, Blacklow SC, Lake R, Artavanis-Tsakonas S, Griffin JD (2000) MAML1, a human homologue of Drosophila mastermind, is a transcriptional co-activator for NOTCH receptors. Nat Genet 26:484–489. doi:10.1038/82644

Yang J, Mani SA, Donaher JL, Ramaswamy S, Itzykson RA, Come C, Savagner P, Gitelman I, Richardson A, Weinberg RA (2004) Twist, a master regulator of morphogenesis, plays an essential role in tumor metastasis. Cell 117:927–939. doi:10.1016/j.cell.2004.06.006

Yang P-T, Anastas JN, Toroni RA, Shinohara MM, Goodson JM, Bosserhoff AK, Chien AJ, Moon RT (2012) WLS inhibits melanoma cell proliferation through the β-catenin signalling pathway and induces spontaneous metastasis. EMBO Mol Med 4:1294–1307. doi:10.1002/emmm.201201486

You L, He B, Xu Z, Uematsu K, Mazieres J, Fujii N, Mikami I, Reguart N, McIntosh JK, Kashani-Sabet M, McCormick F, Jablons DM (2004) An anti-Wnt-2 monoclonal antibody induces apoptosis in malignant melanoma cells and inhibits tumor growth. Cancer Res 64:5385–5389. doi:10.1158/0008-5472.CAN-04-1227

Zabierowski SE, Baubet V, Himes B, Li L, Fukunaga-Kalabis M, Patel S, McDaid R, Guerra M, Gimotty P, Dahmane N, Dahamne N, Herlyn M (2011) Direct reprogramming of melanocytes to neural crest stem-like cells by one defined factor. Stem Cells Dayt Ohio 29:1752–1762. doi:10.1002/stem.740

Zhu L, Marvin MJ, Gardiner A, Lassar AB, Mercola M, Stern CD, Levin M (1999) Cerberus regulates left–right asymmetry of the embryonic head and heart. Curr Biol 9:931–938. doi:10.1016/S0960-9822(99)80419-9

Tumor Microenvironment for Melanoma Cells

14

Lawrence W. Wu, Meenhard Herlyn, and Gao Zhang

14.1 Introduction

Melanoma is the most deadly cancer in the skin with a 5-year survival rate of advanced, metastatic disease at 15 %. Fortunately, recent years have witnessed breakthroughs in melanoma therapies such as targeted therapy, vemurafenib, to block the MAPK signaling pathway by specifically targeting mutated oncogenic BRAF (Bollag et al. 2010; Flaherty et al. 2010). Additionally, combining a BRAF inhibitor (Dabrafenib) with an MEK inhibitor (Trametinib) increased efficacy of treatment by overcoming certain resistance mechanisms with BRAF inhibition alone (Johnson et al. 2014; Shi et al. 2014). This increased efficacy is also seen in the combination of vemurafenib and cobimetinib, another MEK inhibitor (Larkin et al. 2014). Immune checkpoint blockade therapies targeting immune inhibitory molecules have yielded tremendous clinical responses as well. Targeting cytotoxic T-lymphocyte-associated antigen 4 (CTLA-4) using Ipilimumab (anti-CTLA-4) paved the way for other immune checkpoint blockade therapies, such as nivolumab and pembrolizumab (anti-PD1), which target programmed cell death protein 1 (PD-1) (Hodi et al. 2010). Nivolumab was found to have greater response and efficacy than Ipilimumab as a single agent therapy (Robert et al. 2015). Additionally, the combination of nivolumab and Ipilimumab is more effective than single agent ipilumumab (Postow et al. 2015). Lastly, talimogene laherparepvec (T-VEC),

L.W. Wu
Medical Scientist Training Program, University of Texas Southwestern Medical Center, 5323 Harry Hines Blvd, Dallas, TX 75390, USA

M. Herlyn (✉) • G. Zhang
Molecular and Cellular Oncogenesis Program, The Wistar Institute Melanoma Research Center, The Wistar Institute, 3601 Spruce Street, Philadelphia, PA 19104, USA
e-mail: herlynm@wistar.org

A. Bosserhoff (ed.), *Melanoma Development*,
DOI 10.1007/978-3-319-41319-8_14

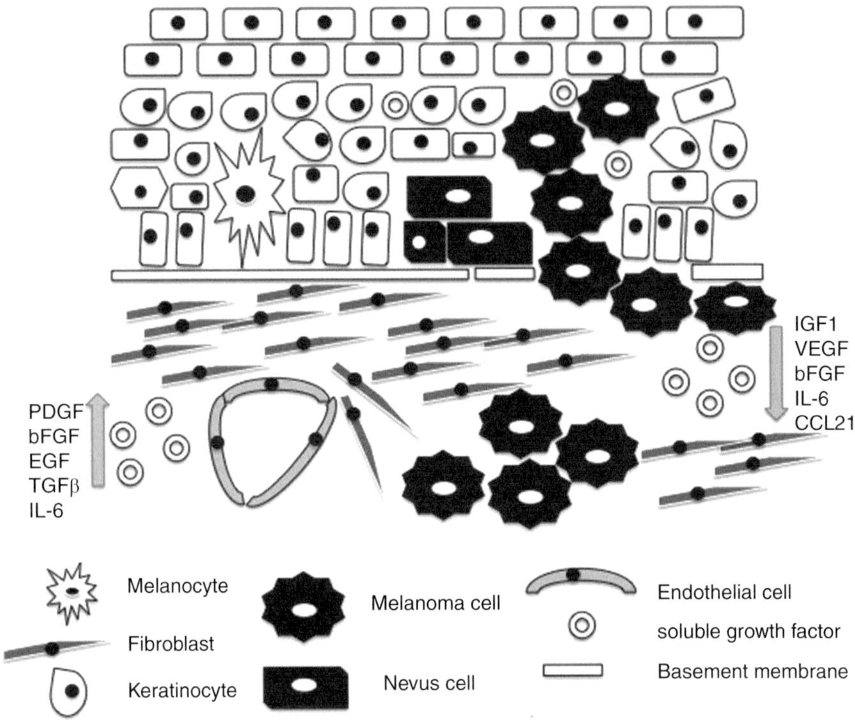

Fig. 14.1 Schematic representation of cross-talk between melanoma cells and tumor microenvironment. Normal melanocytes are localized at the basement membrane that separates epidermis from dermis and they are tightly regulated by surrounding keratinocytes through direct cell–cell contact. Upon transformation, the tight regulation mediated by E-cadherin is lost and replaced by N-cadherin between melanoma cells and adjacent cells. During melanoma development and progression, melanoma cells secrete soluble factors to recruit distant fibroblasts or immune cells in tumor microenvironment to its peritumoral zone. Stromal cells, including fibroblasts, endothelial cells, and immune cells, are activated and participate through paracrine signaling pathways to facilitate degradation of the basement membrane, invasion into the dermis, and metastatic dissemination. The dynamic communication between melanoma cells and the tumor microenvironment is mediated by direct cell–cell contact or soluble growth factors including bFGF, PDGF, VEGF, TGFβ, cytokines, and inflammatory factors

an oncolytic immunotherapy, was the first of its kind to demonstrate therapeutic benefit in a clinical trial (Andtbacka et al. 2015). The area of the immune microenvironment and mechanisms of immune-response to these checkpoint inhibitors is a very urgent topic among clinicians and scientists (see also Chaps. 16 and 17).

Melanoma cells activate, recruit, and continuously interact with other cells in the tumor microenvironment to facilitate their own growth, survival, migration, and invasion. As illustrated in Fig. 14.1, the tumor microenvironment of melanoma consists of neoplastic cells, normal cells, soluble growth factors, and extracellular matrix components that together cooperate to drive tumorigenesis. Perhaps the most striking evidence to support this notion came from our observation that metastatic melanoma cells lose their tumorigenic properties if forced to attach to keratinocytes (Hsu et al. 2000). Similarly, melanoma cells can be reprogrammed by an embryonic microenvironment to a benign phenotype (Díez-Torre et al. 2009; Gerschenson et al. 1986; Topczewska et al. 2006), further underscoring the plasticity of malignant cells and the existence of inhibitory cues in the microenvironment.

14.2 Melanocyte, Melanoma, and the Microenvironment

Human melanocytes are specialized melanin-producing cells of neural crest cell origin. They are embedded at the conjunction of epidermis and dermis. All pigmented melanocytes are derived from embryonic neural crest cells that are highly migratory (White and Zon 2008). Multipotent neural crest stem cells (NCSC) can give rise to at least six differentiated cell lineages including melanocytes, glia, sensory neurons, adrenal cells, craniofacial cartilage and bone, and smooth muscle (Bronner-Fraser and Fraser 1988; Yu et al. 2006; Li et al. 2010; Cichorek et al. 2013). Several factors play a role in establishing multipotent neural crest stem cell, restricting neural crest stem cells toward a melanoblast fate, and driving differentiation of pigmented melanocytes (White and Zon 2008) (see also Chap. 13). Melanocytes make close contacts with keratinocytes, primarily through E-cadherin. On the basement membrane, the ratio between melanocytes and keratinocytes ranges from 1:5 to 1:8. Isolated melanocytes grow relatively rapidly in culture, and display bi- or tri-polar dendrites. By contrast, melanocytes rarely grow in the physiological setting of skin and display multiple (~35) dendrites to communicate with surrounding keratinocytes. It is the cell–cell contact through E-cadherins that closely regulates growth and proliferation of melanocytes and prevents early transformation of melanocytes to nevi (see also Chap. 2). With few exceptions, melanoma cells lose contact with keratinocytes and communicate with themselves and fibroblasts, which is due to the switch from E-cadherin to N-cadherin (Hsu et al. 2000; Li et al. 2001). The restoration of E-cadherin in melanoma cells of low levels of E-cadherin led to adhesion to keratinocytes and inhibited the invasion of melanoma cells into the dermis by downregulation of invasion-related molecules (Hsu et al. 2000). Oncogenic BRAFV600E can induce repression of E-cadherin to promote melanoma cell invasion through T-Box3 transcriptional repression (Boyd et al. 2013).

There are several mechanisms for malignant transformation. Hypoxia is one of the significant characteristics of the skin and tumor microenvironment and can accelerate transformation (Bedogni et al. 2005; Monsel et al. 2010). In particular, hypoxia contributes to heterogeneity in melanoma in a HIF1α-dependent manner (Widmer et al. 2013). These experiments have provided an important hint that the surrounding tissue contributes to transformation. The combination of bFGF and ultraviolet (UV) B could readily lead to pigmented lesions, some of which resemble low-grade melanoma (Berking et al. 2001). Interestingly, melanocytes display melanoma-like aggressive phenotypes when grown on melanoma cell-derived matrix (Seftor et al. 2005), suggesting that in addition to genetic approaches, the microenvironment can also reprogram normal melanocytes into melanoma-like

Table 14.1 Growth factors or inhibitors for melanocytes derived from human epidermal keratinocytes and dermal fibroblats

Melanocyte growth regulator	Keratinocytes	Fibroblasts
α-MSH	+++	NA
bFGF	+++	++
ET-1	+++	NA
ET-3	NA	+++
HGF	NA	+++
GM-CSF	+++	++
SCF	+++	+
DKK1	NA	+++

phenotypes. Conversely, malignant cells can be reprogrammed by human or chick embryonic stem cell matrix to a benign melanocyte-like phenotype (Kulesa et al. 2006; Postovit et al. 2006) (see also Chap. 13). Sustained stress in the microenvironment may lead to epigenetic reprogramming to a malignant transformation (Molognoni et al. 2011). Together, these examples demonstrate how the surrounding microenvironment can play a major role in modulating of both normal and malignant melanocytes.

14.3 Growth Regulation of Human Melanocytes by Epidermal Keratinocytes and Dermal Fibroblasts

Human epidermal melanocytes isolated from fetal or adult skin do not propagate *in vitro* unless cultured in a defined growth medium, including phorbol ester and cholera toxin (Eisinger and Marko 1982) or growth factors that replace their activities. Conditioned medium derived from melanoma or astrocytoma cells (those selected for low TGF-ß production) support the growth of melanocytes in the absence of growth factors suggesting that malignant cells produce their own growth factors for autocrine stimulation (Table 14.1 and Eisinger et al. 1985).

Melanocytes are closely surrounded in skin by keratinocytes and survive and proliferate when co-cultured with keratinocytes or in the presence of keratinocyte-conditioned medium, suggesting that most melanocyte growth-stimulating factors are derived from keratinocytes (see also Chap. 2). Basic fibroblast growth factor (bFGF) is produced by keratinocytes to enhance melanocyte proliferation (Halaban et al. 1988). Not only does bFGF have an impact on melanocyte survival, growth, and proliferation, bFGF can also promote melanocyte migration via phosphorylation of focal adhesion kinase ($p125^{FAK}$) (Wu et al. 2006). bFGF can also be produced by dermal fibroblasts. α-MSH stimulates melanocyte growth by binding to its high affinity receptor and its activity requires bFGF and/or activation of protein kinase C (De Luca et al. 1993). Upon exposure of human keratinocytes to UVB, secreted interleukin 1-α and interleukin 1-β (IL1-α and IL1-β) from keratinocytes stimulate the secretion of endothelin (ET-1), which plays an important role in melanocyte proliferation (Imokawa et al. 1992; Jamal and Schneider 2002). Similarly, UVA/B--irradiated keratinocytes secrete granulocyte/macrophage colony-stimulating factor (GM-CSF), which also stimulates DNA synthesis and differentiation of melanocytes in a dose-dependent manner (Hirobe et al. 2004; Imokawa et al. 1996). Interestingly, direct reprogramming of mouse and human fibroblasts into melanocytes can be achieved through expression of MITF, SOX10, and PAX3 (Yang et al. 2014).

There is no apparent direct contact between epidermal melanocytes and fibroblasts in the dermis of the skin. However, fibroblasts can produce growth factors that are important for melanocytes including bFGF and hepatocyte growth factor (HGF). IL1-α from UVB-irradiated keratinocytes can stimulate the production of HGF in fibroblasts (Mildner et al. 2007). Interestingly, HGF also plays a role in promoting melanocyte motility depending on CD44v6 expression (Damm et al. 2010), protecting melanocytes from apoptosis in an MITF-dependent manner (Beuret et al. 2007), and conferring resistance to RAF inhibitors (Straussman et al. 2012). Another paracrine factor, neuregulin-1, is derived from dermal fibroblasts. It can effectively increase pigmentation of melanocytes in monolayer and the reconstructed skin model (Choi et al. 2010) and also promotes melanocyte proliferation while inhibiting differentiation (Buac et al. 2009). On the other hand, dermal fibroblasts can have an inhibitory effect on density, proliferation, and differentiation of melanocytes via secreted DKK1 (Yamaguchi et al. 2007). DKK1 is highly expressed by fibroblasts and can suppress β-catenin and MITF in melanocytes, which are essential for melanocyte growth and proliferation. Interestingly, DKK1 expression can inhibit invasiveness of melanoma cells (Chen et al. 2012). Treatment of keratinocytes with DKK1 can increase their proliferation and decrease their uptake of melanin (Yamaguchi et al. 2008).

14.4 Inflammatory Mediators on Human Melanocyte Function

The epidermal and dermal microenvironment harbors inflammatory mediators, cytokines, hormones, and growth factors that can alter human melanocyte function in a profound way. Many of these factors are released into the microenvironment after UV exposure and subsequently affect melanocyte pigmentation, proliferation, differentiation, cytokine production, and motility.

Tumor necrosis factor-α (TNF-α) is among many cytokines responsible for an inflammatory response in skin. Upon UVB irradiation, keratinocytes release TNF-α, which is likely stimulated by IL-1α. IL-1α is the primary mediator that responds to inflammation and injury in skin. Secretion of IL-1α increases as keratinocytes and fibroblasts age (Okazaki et al. 2005). It has been reported that increased secretion of IL-1α can stimulate the production of HGF by dermal fibroblasts in a paracrine manner and the production of ET-1 by keratinocytes for autocrine stimulation, which together stimulate proliferation of melanocytes and induce their tyrosinase activity. Nuclear receptor retinoid X receptor-α (RXR-α) expressed in keratinocytes is one of the upstream regulators of these cytokines and can protect keratinocytes and melanocytes from UV-induced DNA damage and enhance proliferation via modulation of secretion of heparin-binding EGF-like growth factor, GM-CSF, IL-1α, and cyclooxygenase-2 and activation of mitogen-activated protein kinase pathways (Wang et al. 2011). The depletion of RXR-α in epidermal keratinocytes leads to alterations in expression of keratinocyte-derived secreted factors such as ET-1, SCF, HGF, FGF2, and α-MSH, which modulate proliferation and activation of melanocytes after UV irradiation (Wang et al. 2011). Matrix metalloproteinases (MMP-2 and MMP-9) can also be co-up-regulated with inflammatory cytokines, serving as another important regulator in the epidermis (Decean et al. 2013).

Melanocytes express IL-8 mRNA when stimulated with TNF-α or IL-1α, and the supernatants from stimulated melanocyte cultures become positive for neutrophil and monocyte chemotactic activity, suggesting a possible role of melanocytes in participating in the initiation of an inflammatory response (Zachariae et al. 1991). The treatment of melanocytes with TNF-α, IL-1α, or IL-6 leads to the inhibition of tyrosinase activity and DNA synthesis (Swope et al. 1991), which suggests that they function as paracrine factors. Since melanocytes synthesize and transfer melanin to keratinocytes upon UV irradiation, it may implicate a negative feedback loop consisting of these factors to modulate melanocyte function. α-MSH can serve as a primary anti-inflammatory factor by opposing TNF-α-induced NF-kB activity in human melanocytes (Haycock et al. 1999). It is mainly produced by epidermal keratinocytes suggesting intricate interactions between keratinocytes, melanocytes, and inflammatory mediators.

14.5 Interplay Between Inflammation and Tumor Initiation, Promotion, and Progression

Ample evidence has pointed to a role of chronic inflammation in underlying tumor initiation and development (Grivennikov et al. 2010; Luo et al. 2004). IL-6/STAT3 and IKKβ-dependent NF-kB signaling pathways are key players linking inflammation and cancer by regulating an array of cytokines (He and Karin 2010; Yu et al. 2009). Inflammation contributes to the onset of malignancies by several potential mechanisms, including (1) stimulated cell proliferation, which can increase the likelihood of acquiring the transforming mutation, (2) production of metabolites such as reactive oxygen species (ROS) or endothelial nitric oxide synthase (eNOS), which can cause DNA damage, (3) suppression of cell-mediated immune response, which can create an environment that enhances tumor growth, and (4) inhibition of apoptosis (Kitasato et al. 2007; Rubin et al. 2004). An immunohistochemistry study demonstrated that chronic inflammation could contribute to malignant transformation in the human upper airways by the production of eNOS (Pacova et al. 2009).

UVB is regarded as an environmental carcinogen that is critical for melanoma development. UVB but not UVA can initiate melanoma using the HGF mouse genetic model (De Fabo et al. 2004). Exposure of keratinocytes to UV increases ROS production (Yoshihisa et al. 2010). In murine fibroblasts, UV irradiation enhanced ROS production via PKCdelta signaling (Bossi et al. 2008). Human epidermal keratinocytes have higher basal hydrogen peroxide (H_2O_2) levels than melanocytes and can transfer hydrogen peroxide to melanocytes (Pelle et al. 2005). UVB and UVC can differentially activate STAT3 in human keratinocytes and fibroblasts via ROS and DNA damage (Bito et al. 2010). Interestingly, IFN-γ promotes melanocytic cell survival and immune-evasion in UVB-induced melanocyte activation (Zaidi et al. 2011). Fibronectin-containing extracellular vesicles also protect against UVB radiation and associated cytotoxicity (Bin et al. 2016).

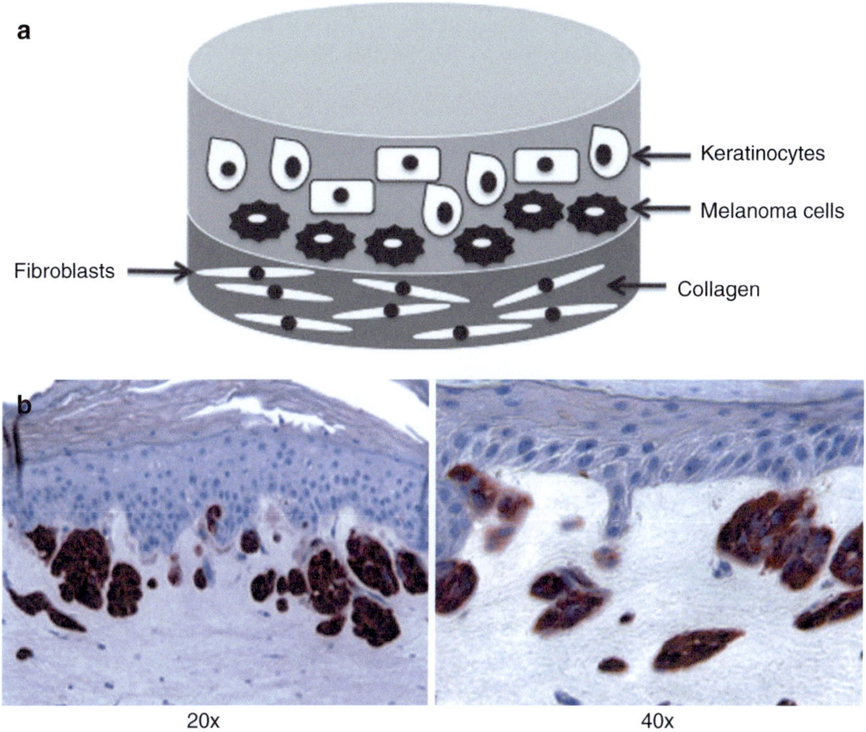

Fig. 14.2 Human skin reconstruct using the 3-D organotypic culture system. (**a**) A schematic representation of human skin reconstruct at which human melanocytes or melanoma cells are grown as 3-D with keratinocytes, fibroblasts, and collagen that mimic the microenvironment. (**b**) VGP human melanoma cells WM3248 are grown in 3-D skin reconstruct comprising of keratinocytes, fibroblasts, and collagen. Typical invasion into dermis of WM3248 cells is a characteristic of RGP melanoma line (Images are captured at 20× and 40× (Courtesy of Dr. Ling Li, the Wistar Institute))

Together, these results suggest that human epidermal keratinocytes and/or dermal fibroblasts represent major sources of ROS for epidermal melanocytes following UV irradiation and initiate inflammatory response via the STAT3 signaling pathway. The UVB radiation of primary cutaneous melanoma can promote metastatic progression (Bald et al. 2014). The release of high mobility group box 1 (HMGB1) from epidermal keratinocytes damaged by UVB and Toll-like receptor 4 (TLR4) recruit and activate neutrophils (Bald et al. 2014). This inflammatory response stimulates angiogenesis and melanoma migration toward endothelial cells. UVR targets TP53 to cooperate with oncogenic BRAFV600E to induce melanomagenesis (Viros et al. 2014). It has been noted that UVB, along with growth factor such as bFGF, can transform normal melanocytes (Berking et al. 2001, 2004). However, the underlying molecular basis of malignant transformation remains unclear. Given the evidence that ROS and DNA damage are implicated in UV irradiation-induced inflammatory response in skin keratinocytes and fibroblasts, an intriguing possibility is that UV-mediated inflammatory responses in the skin environment, including generation of ROS and release of secreted cytokines, could further cause DNA damage in epidermal melanocytes, and contribute to genetic alterations (Fig. 14.2).

Conclusion

Transformation of normal melanocytes can be partially attributed to dysregulated tissue homeostasis executed by keratinocytes. Furthermore, transformed melanocytic cells send signals throughout the microenvironment to recruit other cells types. Those cells become activated, communicate with the neoplastic cells, and elicit soluble pro-survival and anti-apoptosis signals through autocrine or paracrine signaling patterns or direct cell–cell contacts in order to create a suitable tissue microenvironment that supports melanoma progression. Over the decades, experimental studies have identified key intrinsic signaling pathways that mediate transformation of melanocytes into melanoma cells. In the skin, melanocytes are mainly surrounded by epidermal keratinocytes and they also communicate with dermal fibroblasts. How the microenvironment of melanocytes plays a role in transformation remains to be clarified. We propose to use human melanocytes as a paradigm to study and understand cell–cell communication and growth regulation between melanoma and the microenvironment. An understudied area is the role of inflammation in melanoma development and progression. The immune microenvironment is another area where we plan to explore in melanoma. We are isolating skin fibroblasts (or peripheral blood mononuclear cells) from melanoma patients or healthy individuals who are predisposed or susceptible to melanoma, reprogram them into iPS cells and then differentiate them into melanocytes. These melanocytes are being used to model how the tumor microenvironment and UV radiation trigger oncogenic transformation. These results can provide the foundation for future studies in prevention and development of new targets for therapy.

References

Andtbacka RH, Kaufman HL, Collichio F, Amatruda T, Senzer N, Chesney J, Delman KA, Spitler LE, Puzanov I, Agarwala SS, Milhem M, Cranmer L, Curti B, Lewis K, Ross M, Guthrie T, Linette GP, Daniels GA, Harrington K, Middleton MR, Miller WH Jr, Zager JS, Ye Y, Yao B, Li A, Doleman S, VanderWalde A, Gansert J, Coffin RS (2015) Talimogene laherparepvec improves durable response rate in patients with advanced melanoma. J Clin Oncol 33(25):2780–2788

Bald T, Quast T, Landsberg J, Rogava M, Glodde N, Lopez-Ramos D, Kohlmeyer J, Riesenberg S, van den Boorn-Konijnenberg D, Hömig-Hölzel C, Reuten R, Schadow B, Weighardt H, Wenzel D, Helfrich I, Schadendorf D, Bloch W, Bianchi ME, Lugassy C, Barnhill RL, Koch M, Fleischmann BK, Förster I, Kastenmüller W, Kolanus W, Hölzel M, Gaffel E, Tüting T (2014) Ultraviolet-radiation-induced inflammation promotes angiotropism and metastasis in melanoma. Nature 507(7490):109–113

Bedogni B, Welford SM, Cassarino DS, Nickoloff BJ, Giaccia AJ, Powell MB (2005) The hypoxic microenvironment of the skin contributes to Akt-mediated melanocyte transformation. Cancer Cell 8(6):443–454

Berking C, Takemoto R, Satyamoorthy K, Elenitsas R, Herlyn M (2001) Basic fibroblast growth factor and ultraviolet B transform melanocytes in human skin. Am J Pathol 158(3):943–953

Berking C, Takemoto R, Satyamoorthy K, Shirakawa T, Eskandarpour M, Hansson J, VanBelle PA, Elder DE, Herlyn M (2004) Induction of melanoma phenotypes in human skin by growth factors and ultraviolet B. Cancer Res 64(3):807–811

Beuret L, Flori E, Denoyelle C, Bille K, Busca R, Picardo M, Bertolotto C, Ballotti R (2007) Up-regulation of MET expression by alpha-melanocyte-stimulating hormone and MITF allows hepatocyte growth factor to protect melanocytes and melanoma cells from apoptosis. J Biol Chem 282(19):14140–14147

Bin BH, Kim DK, Kim NH, Choi EJ, Bhin J, Kim ST, Gho YS, Lee AY, Lee TR, Cho EG (2016) Fibronectin-Containing Extracellular Vesicles Protect Melanocytes against Ultraviolet Radiation-Induced Cytotoxicity. J Invest Dermatol 136(5):957–966

Bito T, Sumita N, Masaki T, Shirakawa T, Ueda M, Yoshiki R, Tokura Y, Nishigori C (2010) Ultraviolet light induces Stat3 activation in human keratinocytes and fibroblasts through reactive oxygen species and DNA damage. Exp Dermatol 19(7):654–660

Bollag G, Hirth P, Tsai J, Zhang J, Ibrahim PN, Cho H, Spevak W, Zhang C, Zhang Y, Habets G, Burton EA, Wong B, Tsang G, West BL, Powell B, Shellooe R, Marimuthu A, Nguyen H, Zhang KY, Artis DR, Schlessinger J, Su F, Higgins B, Iyer R, D'Andrea K, Koehler A, Stumm M, Lin PS, Lee RJ, Grippo J, Puzanov I, Kim KB, Ribas A, McArthur GA, Sosman JA, Chapman PB, Flaherty KT, Xu X, Nathanson KL, Nolop K (2010) Clinical efficacy of a RAF inhibitor needs broad target blockade in BRAF-mutant melanoma. Nature 467(7315):596–599

Bossi O, Gartsbein M, Leitges M, Kuroki T, Grossman S, Tennenbaum T (2008) UV irradiation increases ROS production via PKCdelta signaling in primary murine fibroblasts. J Cell Biochem 105(1):194–207

Boyd SC, Mijatov B, Pupo GM, Tran SL, Gowrishankar K, Shaw HM, Goding CR, Scolyer RA, Mann GJ, Kefford RF, Rizos H, Becker TM (2013) Oncogenic B-RAF V600E signaling induces the T-box3 transcriptional repressor to repress E-cadherin and enhance melanoma cell invasion. J Invest Dermatol 133(5):1269–1277

Bronner-Fraser M, Fraser SE (1988) Cell lineage analysis reveals multipotency of some avian neural crest cells. Nature 335(6186):161–164

Buac K, Xu M, Cronin J, Weeraratna AT, Hewitt SM, Pavan WJ (2009) NRG1/ERBB3 signaling in melanocyte development and melanoma: inhibition of differentiation and promotion of proliferation. Pigment Cell Melanoma Res 22(6):773–784

Choi W, Wolber R, Gerwat W, Mann T, Batzer J, Smuda C, Liu H, Kolbe L, Hearing VJ (2010) The fibroblast-derived paracrine factor neuregulin-1 has a novel role in regulating the constitutive color and melanocyte function in human skin. J Cell Sci 123(Pt 18):3102–3111

Chen J, Li H, Chen H, Hu D, Xing Q, Ren G, Luo X (2012) Dickkopf-1 inhibits the invasive activity of melanoma cells. Clin Exp Dermatol 37(4):404–410

Cichorek M, Wachulska M, Stasiewicz A, Tyminska A (2013) Skin melanocytes: biology and development. Postepy Dermatol Alergol 30(1):30–41

Damm S, Koefinger P, Stefan M, Wels C, Mehes G, Richtig E, Kerl H, Otte M, Schaider H (2010) HGF-promoted motility in primary human melanocytes depends on CD44v6 regulated via NF-kappa B, Egr-1, and C/EBP-beta. J Invest Dermatol 130(7):1893–1903

Decean H, Perde-Schrepler M, Tatomir C, Fischer-Fodor E, Brie I, Virag P (2013) Modulation of the pro-inflammatory cytokines and matrix metalloproteinases production in co-cultivated human keratinocytes and melanocytes. Arch Dermatol Res 305(8):705–714

De Fabo EC, Noonan FP, Fears T, Merlino G (2004) Ultraviolet B but not ultraviolet A radiation initiates melanoma. Cancer Res 64(18):6372–6376

De Luca M, Siegrist W, Bondanza S, Mathor M, Cancedda R, Eberle AN (1993) Alpha melanocyte stimulating hormone (alpha MSH) stimulates normal human melanocyte growth by binding to high-affinity receptors. J Cell Sci 105(Pt 4):1079–1084

Díez-Torre A, Andrade R, Eguizábal C, López E, Arluzea J, Silió M, Aréchaga J (2009) Reprogramming of melanoma cells by embryonic microenvironments. Int J Dev Biol 53(8–10):1563–1568

Eisinger M, Marko O (1982) Selective proliferation of normal human melanocytes in vitro in the presence of phorbol ester and cholera toxin. Proc Natl Acad Sci U S A 79(6):2018–2022
Eisinger M, Marko O, Ogata S, Old LJ (1985) Growth regulation of human melanocytes: mitogenic factors in extracts of melanoma, astrocytoma, and fibroblast cell lines. Science 229(4717):984–986
Flaherty KT, Puzanov I, Kim KB, Ribas A, McArthur GA, Sosman JA, O'Dwyer PJ, Lee RJ, Grippo JF, Nolop K, Chapman PB (2010) Inhibition of mutated, activated BRAF in metastatic melanoma. N Engl J Med 363(9):809–819
Gerschenson M, Graves K, Carson SD, Wells RS, Pierce GB (1986) Regulation of melanoma by the embryonic skin. Proc Natl Acad Sci U S A 83(19):7307–7310
Grivennikov SI, Greten FR, Karin M (2010) Immunity, inflammation, and cancer. Cell 140(6): 883–899
Halaban R, Langdon R, Birchall N, Cuono C, Baird A, Scott G, Moellmann G, McGuire J (1988) Basic fibroblast growth factor from human keratinocytes is a natural mitogen for melanocytes. J Cell Biol 107(4):1611–1619
Haycock JW, Wagner M, Morandini R, Ghanem G, Rennie IG, Mac Neil S (1999) Alpha-melanocyte-stimulating hormone inhibits NF-kappaB activation in human melanocytes and melanoma cells. J Invest Dermatol 113(4):560–566
He G, Karin M (2010) NF-kB and STAT3 - key players in liver inflammation and cancer. Cell Res 21(1):159–168
Hirobe T, Furuya R, Hara E, Horii I, Tsunenaga M, Ifuku O (2004) Granulocyte-macrophage colony-stimulating factor (GM-CSF) controls the proliferation and differentiation of mouse epidermal melanocytes from pigmented spots induced by ultraviolet radiation B. Pigment Cell Res 17(3):230–240
Hodi FS, O'Day SJ, McDermott DF, Weber RW, Sosman JA, Haanen JB, Gonzalez R, Robert C, Schadendorf D, Hassel JC, Akerley W, van den Eertwegh AJ, Lutzky J, Lorigan P, Vaubel JM, Linette GP, Hogg D, Ottensmeier CH, Lebbé C, Peschel C, Quirt I, Clark JI, Wolchok JD, Weber JS, Tian J, Yellin MJ, Nichol GM, Hoos A, Urba WJ (2010) Improved survival with ipilimumab in patients with metastatic melanoma. N Engl J Med 363(8):711–723
Hsu MY, Meier FE, Nesbit M, Hsu JY, Van Belle P, Elder DE, Herlyn M (2000) E-cadherin expression in melanoma cells restores keratinocyte-mediated growth control and down-regulates expression of invasion-related adhesion receptors. Am J Pathol 156(5):1515–1525
Imokawa G, Yada Y, Miyagishi M (1992) Endothelins secreted from human keratinocytes are intrinsic mitogens for human melanocytes. J Biol Chem 267(34):24675–24680
Imokawa G, Yada Y, Kimura M, Morisaki N (1996) Granulocyte/macrophage colony-stimulating factor is an intrinsic keratinocyte-derived growth factor for human melanocytes in UVA-induced melanosis. Biochem J 313(Pt 2):625–631
Jamal S, Schneider RJ (2002) UV-induction of keratinocyte endothelin-1 downregulates E-cadherin in melanocytes and melanoma cells. J Clin Invest 110(4):443–452
Johnson DB, Flaherty KT, Weber JS, Infante JR, Kim KB, Kefford RF, Hamid O, Schuchter L, Cebon J, Sharfman WH, McWilliams RR, Sznol M, Lawrence DP, Gibney GT, Burris HA 3rd, Falchook GS, Algazi A, Lewis K, Long GV, Patel K, Ibrahim N, Sun P, Little S, Cunningham E, Sosman JA, Daud A, Gonzalez R (2014) Combined BRAF (Dabrafenib) and MEK inhibition (Trametinib) in patients with BRAFV600-mutant melanoma experiencing progression with single-agent BRAF inhibitor. J Clin Oncol 32(33):3697–3704
Kitasato A, Tajima Y, Kuroki T, Tsutsumi R, Adachi T, Mishima T, Kanematsu T (2007) Inflammatory cytokines promote inducible nitric oxide synthase-mediated DNA damage in hamster gallbladder epithelial cells. World J Gastroenterol 13(47):6379–6384
Kulesa PM, Kasemeier-Kulesa JC, Teddy JM, Margaryan NV, Seftor EA, Seftor RE, Hendrix MJ (2006) Reprogramming metastatic melanoma cells to assume a neural crest cell-like phenotype in an embryonic microenvironment. Proc Natl Acad Sci U S A 103(10):3752–3757
Larkin J, Ascierto PA, Dréno B, Atkinson V, Liszkay G, Maio M, Mandalà M, Demidov L, Stroyakovskiy D, Thomas L, de la Cruz-Merino L, Dutriaux C, Garbe C, Sovak MA, Chang I, Choong N, Hack SP, McArthur GA, Ribas A (2014) Combined vemurafenib and cobimetinib in BRAF-mutated melanoma. N Engl J Med 371(20):1867–1876

Li G, Schaider H, Satyamoorthy K, Hanakawa Y, Hashimoto K, Herlyn M (2001) Downregulation of E-cadherin and Desmoglein 1 by autocrine hepatocyte growth factor during melanoma development. Oncogene 20(56):8125–8135

Li L, Fukunaga-Kalabis M, Yu H, Xu X, Kong J, Lee JT, Herlyn M (2010) Human dermal stem cells differentiate into functional epidermal melanocytes. J Cell Sci 123(Pt 6):853–860

Luo JL, Maeda S, Hsu LC, Yagita H, Karin M (2004) Inhibition of NF-kappaB in cancer cells converts inflammation-induced tumor growth mediated by TNFalpha to TRAIL-mediated tumor regression. Cancer Cell 6(3):297–305

Mildner M, Mlitz V, Gruber F, Wojta J, Tschachler E (2007) Hepatocyte growth factor establishes autocrine and paracrine feedback loops for the protection of skin cells after UV irradiation. J Invest Dermatol 127(11):2637–2644

Molognoni F, Cruz AT, Meliso FM, Morais AS, Souza CF, Xander P, Bischof JM, Costa FF, Soares MB, Liang G, Jones PA, Jasiulionis MG (2011) Epigenetic reprogramming as a key contributor to melanocyte malignant transformation. Epigenetics 6(4):450–464

Monsel G, Ortonne N, Bagot M, Bensussan A, Dumaz N (2010) c-Kit mutants require hypoxia-inducible factor 1alpha to transform melanocytes. Oncogene 29(2):227–236

Okazaki M, Yoshimura K, Uchida G, Harii K (2005) Correlation between age and the secretions of melanocyte-stimulating cytokines in cultured keratinocytes and fibroblasts. Br J Dermatol 153(Suppl 2):23–29

Pacova H, Astl J, Martinek J (2009) The pathogenesis of chronic inflammation and malignant transformation in the human upper airways: the role of beta-defensins, eNOS, cell proliferation and apoptosis. Histol Histopathol 24(7):815–820

Pelle E, Mammone T, Maes D, Frenkel K (2005) Keratinocytes act as a source of reactive oxygen species by transferring hydrogen peroxide to melanocytes. J Invest Dermatol 124(4): 793–797

Postovit LM, Seftor EA, Seftor RE, Hendrix MJ (2006) Influence of the microenvironment on melanoma cell fate determination and phenotype. Cancer Res 66(16):7833–7836

Postow MA, Chesney J, Pavlick AC, Robert C, Grossmann K, McDermott D, Linette GP, Meyer N, Giguere JK, Agarwala SS, Shaheen M, Ernstoff MS, Minor D, Salama AK, Taylor M, Ott PA, Rollin LM, Horak C, Gagnier P, Wolchok JD, Hodi FS (2015) Nivolumab and ipilimumab versus ipilimumab in untreated melanoma. N Engl J Med 372(21):2006–2017

Robert C, Schachter J, Long GV, Arance A, Grob JJ, Mortier L, Daud A, Carlino MS, McNeil C, Lotem M, Larkin J, Lorigan P, Neyns B, Blank CU, Hamid O, Mateus C, Shapira-Frommer R, Kosh M, Zhou H, Ibrahim N, Ebbinghaus S, Ribas A (2015) Pembrolizumab versus ipilimumab in advanced melanoma. N Engl J Med 372(26):2521–2532

Rubin E, Gorstein F, Schwarting R, Strayer DS (2004) Rubin's pathology: clinicopathologic foundations of medicine, 4th edn. Lippincott Williams & Wilkins, Philadelphia, p 69

Seftor EA, Brown KM, Chin L, Kirschmann DA, Wheaton WW, Protopopov A, Feng B, Balagurunathan Y, Trent JM, Nickoloff BJ, Seftor RE, Hendrix MJ (2005) Epigenetic transdifferentiation of normal melanocytes by a metastatic melanoma microenvironment. Cancer Res 65(22):10164–10169

Shi H, Hugo W, Kong X, Hong A, Koya RC, Moriceau G, Chodon T, Guo R, Johnson DB, Dahlman KB, Kelley MC, Kefford RF, Chmielowski B, Glaspy JA, Sosman JA, van Baren N, Long GV, Ribas A, Lo RS (2014) Acquired resistance and clonal evolution in melanoma during BRAF inhibitor therapy. Cancer Discov 4(1):80–93

Straussman R, Morikawa T, Shee K, Barzily-Rokni M, Qian ZR, Du J, Davis A, Mongare MM, Gould J, Frederick DT, Cooper ZA, Chapman PB, Solit DB, Ribas A, Lo RS, Flaherty KT, Ogino S, Wargo JA, Golub TR (2012) Tumour micro-environment elicits innate resistance to RAF inhibitors through HGF secretion. Nature 487(7408):500–504

Swope VB, Abdel-Malek Z, Kassem LM, Nordlund JJ (1991) Interleukins 1 alpha and 6 and tumor necrosis factor-alpha are paracrine inhibitors of human melanocyte proliferation and melanogenesis. J Invest Dermatol 96(2):180–185

Topczewska JM, Postovit LM, Margaryan NV, Sam A, Hess AR, Wheaton WW, Nickoloff BJ, Topczewski J, Hendrix MJ (2006) Embryonic and tumorigenic pathways converge via Nodal signaling: role in melanoma aggressiveness. Nat Med 12(8):925–932

Viros A, Sanchez-Laorden B, Pedersen M, Furney SJ, Rae J, Hogan K, Ejiama S, Girotti MR, Cook M, Dhomen N, Marais R (2014) Ultraviolet radiation accelerates BRAF-driven melanomagenesis by targeting TP53. Nature 511(7510):478

Wang Z, Coleman DJ, Bajaj G, Liang X, Ganguli-Indra G, Indra AK (2011) RXRα ablation in epidermal keratinocytes enhances UVR-induced DNA damage, apoptosis, and proliferation of keratinocytes and melanocytes. J Invest Dermatol 131(1):177–187

White RM, Zon LI (2008) Melanocytes in development, regeneration, and cancer. Cell Stem Cell 3(3):242–252

Widmer DS, Hoek KS, Cheng PF, Eichhoff OM, Biedermann T, Raaijmakers MI, Hemmi S, Dummer R, Levesque MP (2013) Hypoxia contributes to melanoma heterogeneity by triggering HIF1α-dependent phenotype switching. J Invest Dermatol 133(10):2436–2443

Wu CS, Lan CC, Chiou MH, Yu HS (2006) Basic fibroblast growth factor promotes melanocyte migration via increased expression of p125 (FAK) on melanocytes. Acta Derm Venereol 86(6):498–502

Yamaguchi Y, Passeron T, Watabe H, Yasumoto K, Rouzaud F, Hoashi T, Hearing VJ (2007) The effects of dickkopf 1 on gene expression and Wnt signaling by melanocytes: mechanisms underlying its suppression of melanocyte function and proliferation. J Invest Dermatol 127(5):1217–1225

Yamaguchi Y, Passeron T, Hoashi T, Watabe H, Rouzaud F, Yasumoto K, Hara T, Tohyama C, Katayama I, Miki T, Hearing VJ (2008) Dickkopf 1 (DKK1) regulates skin pigmentation and thickness by affecting Wnt/beta-catenin signaling in keratinocytes. FASEB J 22(4):1009–1020

Yang R, Zheng Y, Li L, Liu S, Burrows M, Wei Z, Nace A, Herlyn M, Cui R, Guo W, Cotsarelis G, Xu X (2014) Direct conversion of mouse and human fibroblasts to functional melanocytes by defined factors. Nat Comm 5:5807

Yoshihisa Y, Honda A, Zhao QL, Makino T, Abe R, Matsui K, Shimizu H, Miyamoto Y, Kondo T, Shimizu T (2010) Protective effects of platinum nanoparticles against UV-light-induced epidermal inflammation. Exp Dermatol 19(11):1000–1006

Yu H, Fang D, Kumar SM, Li L, Nguyen TK, Acs G, Herlyn M, Xu X (2006) Isolation of a novel population of multipotent adult stem cells from human hair follicles. Am J Pathol 168(6):1879–1888

Yu H, Pardoll D, Jove R (2009) STATs in cancer inflammation and immunity: a leading role for STAT3. Nat Rev Cancer 9(11):798–809

Zachariae CO, Thestrup-Pedersen K, Matsushima K (1991) Expression and secretion of leukocyte chemotactic cytokines by normal human melanocytes and melanoma cells. J Invest Dermatol 97(3):593–599

Zaidi MR, Davis S, Noonan FP, Graff-Cherry C, Hawley TS, Walker RL, Feigenbaum L, Fuchs E, Lyakh L, Young HA, Hornyak TJ, Arnheiter H, Trinchieri G, Meltzer PS, De Fabo EC, Merlino G (2011) Interferon-[ggr] links ultraviolet radiation to melanomagenesis in mice. Nature 469(7331):548–553

Melanoma Model Systems

15

Birgit Schittek, Miriam de Jel, and Thomas Tüting

15.1 Complex In Vitro Cell Culture Model Systems

15.1.1 Introduction

Although there is experimental evidence that human tumor cell lines grown in culture can be representative of the original tumor lesion (Masters 2000; Smalley et al. 2006b; Meier et al. 2000), it is obvious that tumor cells in vivo grow in an environment consisting of extracellular matrix components, stromal cells, inflammatory cells, and endothelial cells (Bissell and Radisky 2001). The contribution of the tumor microenvironment to tumor progression has already been recognized in 1889 by the "seed and soil" theory of Paget (Paget 1889) and later extended and confirmed by Meenhard Herlyns group (Li et al. 2003). This theory claims that not only genetic changes in the tumor cells determine an aggressive phenotype, but that microenvironmental factors have an impact on tumor cell behavior. Factors secreted by stromal cells as fibroblasts or direct cell–cell contacts between the tumor cells and the surrounding stromal cells may either inhibit malignant transformation or promote tumor progression (Li et al. 2003). Cells grown in monolayer can differ considerably in their morphology, cell–cell and cell–matrix interactions, and differentiation from those growing in more physiological three-dimensional (3-D) environments (Yamada and Cukierman 2007). Furthermore, 3-D culture gene expression profiles have been

B. Schittek (✉)
Department of Dermatology, Division of Dermatooncology, University of Tübingen, Liebermeisterstr. 25, Tübingen 72076, Germany
e-mail: birgit.schittek@med.uni-tuebingen.de

M. de Jel • T. Tüting
Friedrich-Alexander-University Erlangen-Nürnberg, Institute of Biochemistry, Biochemistry and Molecular Medicine, Erlangen, Germany
e-mail: Miriam.dejel@fau.de

A. Bosserhoff (ed.), *Melanoma Development*,
DOI 10.1007/978-3-319-41319-8_15

shown to more accurately reflect clinical expression profiles than those observed in 2-D cultures. Finally, preclinical drug screening in 3-D culture models more reliably predict clinical efficacies, and monolayer culture of tumor cells has remained a poor predictor of a patient's response toward therapeutic agents (Johnson et al. 2001; Voskoglou-Nomikos et al. 2003; Burdett et al. 2010) (Table 15.1).

Animal models are not suitable for high throughput screening but often provide definitive tests of the importance of specific molecules or drug targets. However, one has to keep in mind that animal models may not adequately reproduce features of human tumors or therapeutic responses (Kung 2007; Teicher 2006; Burdett et al. 2010). On the other hand, most 3-D in vitro models lack the complex vascular systems that perfuse tissues in vivo. Since "Life isn't flat" (Smalley et al. 2006b), in vitro 3-D tissue models provide an approach to bridge the gap between traditional cell culture and animal models (Griffith and Swartz 2006; Rangarajan et al. 2004; Yamada and Cukierman 2007).

15.1.2 Culture of Melanoma Cells in Extracellular Matrix Scaffolds

The specific extracellular matrix microenvironment provided to cells can substantially influence experimental outcome. Both the composition and stiffness of the extracellular matrix surrounding the cells have major effects on signaling and behavior (Yamada and Cukierman 2007). Therefore, a widely used strategy is to propagate cells in tissue culture and then implant them in a 3-D extracellular matrix scaffold as either single cells or as tissue-like aggregates. Three-dimensional scaffolds have been generated from purified molecules such as collagen I, Matrigel, or from native extracellular matrices secreted and isolated from fibroblasts or keratinocytes.

Because of its ubiquitous nature and relative ease of isolation, collagen was one of the earliest biomaterials to be widely used for 3-D cell culture. Collagen gel embedding involved the encapsulation of small tumor explants (1–2 mm) or of dissociated tumor cells within a collagen matrix that allowed the explants to maintain their viability and cellular architecture ex vivo (Burdett et al. 2010). Cells suspended in extracellular matrix components are easily visualized by phase contrast or immunofluorescence microscopy. In addition, the biological response of cells suspended in this 3-D system can be compared to that of cells grown in monolayer. Viable cells may also be removed from the 3-D cell culture system for further experimentation, including biological analysis and flow cytometry. Collagen gels can mimic loose or dense connective tissue depending on the concentration of collagen; such gels have been used widely in studies of fibroblast and tumor cell migration and signaling (Grinnell 2003). Since each tissue in vivo has a characteristic matrix microenvironment, for a given study, it is crucial to select an appropriately matched 3-D in vitro matrix (Yamada and Cukierman 2007). Besides collagen, the basal membrane components fibronectin, laminin, and collagen IV as well as Matrigel (BD Bioscience, San Jose, CA) have been used for melanoma cell culture. Matrigel is a basement membrane extract derived from the Engelbreth–Holm–Swarm mouse sarcoma that contains a diverse array of components, including collagen type IV, laminin, and

Table 15.1 Complex in vitro cell culture model systems

Melanoma model system	Application	Advantages	Disadvantages
Culture in extracellular matrix scaffolds	Influence of extracellular matrix components on melanoma cell growth, invasion, and drug sensitivity	Easy to perform; different matrix components can be tested	Extracellular matrix components absorb drugs or growth factors; mostly higher drug concentrations have to be used
Microcarrier bead culture	High cell density culturing in matrix components possible	Several carrier materials can be used; ideal for large-scale culturing in matrix components	Expensive and more complicated
Transwell chambers	Analysis of chemotaxis, migration, and invasion	Easy to perform when precoated transwells are used, fast assay	Expensive, high variations possible if individual coating of the inserts is performed
Organotypic explant culture	Invasion, migration, and drug response	Culturing of melanoma cells in a physiological environment	Limited culture time; patient material necessary
De-epidermized dermis (DED)	Influence of extracellular matrix components and basal membrane on melanoma cell invasion	Native extracellular matrix and basal membrane present	Limited culture time; patient material necessary
2-D coculture systems	Influence of growth factors or cell–cell contact on melanoma cell growth, survival, invasion, gene expression	Easy to perform, secreted factors as well as cell contact can be analyzed separately	Patient material necessary for primary cells; sometimes separation of the cells necessary before analysis
Mono- or multi-cellular spheroids	Influence of melanoma cells grown in aggregates on drug sensitivity, secreted factors or cell–cell contact with melanoma cells itself or other cell types	Easy to perform, fast assay, high throughput screening possible, variable platforms and conditions possible	Suboptimal physiological conditions; limited informative value about melanoma invasiveness, not all melanoma cells can be used
Organotypic skin equivalent culture	Growth, survival, migration, and invasion of melanoma cells in a physiological environment	Most sophisticated melanoma model system, physiological environment, dermal and epidermal culture systems available	Laborious, expertise needed, not all melanoma cells can be used

other ECM molecules, as well as various soluble factors, such as cytokines and growth factors (Burdett et al. 2010). However, because Matrigel is a largely undefined and variable mixture of proteins, Matrigel culture has not been widely used for drug screening purposes.

More sophisticated models use other biomaterial scaffolds for culturing melanoma cells on other natural substrates (Fischbach et al. 2007; Zhang et al. 2010). Prototypical scaffolds were developed, in which freeze-dried and then cross-linked solutions of collagen and glycosaminoglycans create biodegradable, sponge-like structures (Griffith and Swartz 2006). Hyaluronic acid can also be used as a scaffold for bioengineered skin (Scuderi et al. 2008). Furthermore, native extracellular matrix components secreted by fibroblasts can be isolated by a protocol described by Beacham et al. (2007). The advantage of using native extracellular matrix components is that the natural composition and 3-D structure of the matrix molecules remain intact. Extracellular matrix components can serve as a reservoir for growth factors secreted by neighboring cells or melanoma cells and by this can influence morphology and growth of neighboring cells. Together with fibroblasts, immune cells, and blood vessels, the extracellular matrix builds the tumor stroma and influences tumor progression, invasion, and metastasis (Mueller and Fusenig 2004).

15.1.3 Microcarrier Bead Culture

Microcarrier beads are also widely used (Smit et al. 1995). A microcarrier is a support matrix allowing for the growth of adherent cells in bioreactors. Carrier materials for cells may be composed by gelatin, porous glass, collagen, or cellulose, with dimensions of 170–6,000 μm. In microcarrier culture, cells grow as monolayers on the surface of small spheres or as multilayers in the pores of macroporous structures that are usually suspended in culture medium by gentle stirring. By using microcarriers in simple suspension culture, fluidized or packed bed systems, yields of up to 200 million cells per milliliter are possible. Therefore, microcarriers provide convenient surfaces for growing animal cells or increasing the yield of cells from standard monolayer culture vessels and perfusion chambers. The high cell density confers more stability and improves the longevity of the culture, making macroporous microcarriers suitable for long-term culture. It has been described that normal human melanocytes or melanoma cells can be coated on microcarrier beads and polymerized within fibrin or fibrin–collagen hydrogels. A layer of dermal fibroblasts was added to more accurately simulate the microenvironment. Invasion can be monitored over a time period of 7 days. This model shows that the melanoma cell lines recapitulate their in situ growth patterns in this environment (Ghajar et al. 2007).

Microcarrier beads can also be rolled on a lymph node endothelial surface, which was created by growing endothelial cells on a differentiating extract of lymph node biomatrix, and testing the ability of tumor cells to invade across Matrigel-coated filters. Interestingly, compared to the contact with plastic, Lewis lung carcinoma and B16 melanoma cell invasiveness were increased after exposure to "lung endothelial surface." This indicates that a lymph node environment may modulate the metastatic potential of tumor cells (Whalen et al. 1994).

15.1.4 Transwell Chambers

Transwell chambers are often used to study migration or invasion of tumor cells. This system is also called Boyden chamber assay, originally introduced by Boyden for the analysis of leukocyte chemotaxis (Boyden 1962). It is based on a cylindrical cell culture insert nested inside the well of a cell culture plate. It consists of chambers of two medium-filled compartments separated by a microporous membrane. The insert contains a polycarbonate membrane at the bottom with a defined pore size. Depending on the composition of the porous membrane, either migration or invasion of tumor cells can be studied. Usually, cells are seeded in the upper compartment in serum-free media, while serum or similar chemoattractants are placed in the well below. Migratory cells move through the pores toward the chemoattractant below. The number of cells that have migrated to the lower side of the membrane is determined after staining the membrane and quantified in a plate reader. Therefore, the Boyden chamber-based cell migration assay has also been called filter membrane migration assay, transwell migration assay, or chemotaxis assay. A number of different Boyden chamber devices are commercially available (Chen 2005). Such a system can be used to obtain an objective numerical readout to assess the effects of drugs or the modulation of target gene expression on cell migration. Furthermore, by the addition of a Matrigel layer on top of the membrane, this assay can be modified to measure invasion, such that cells have to invade through the matrix to reach the underside of the filter.

15.1.5 Organotypic Explant Culture: Ex Vivo Cultures

Organ explant slices can be cultured on a semiporous membrane or are embedded in a 3-D collagen gel (Pampaloni et al. 2007). Tumor tissue slices can be cultivated for up to 7 days and have been mainly used to determine drug responses and to predict tumor responses (Hickman et al. 2014; Gerlach et al. 2014). Organotypic slice cultures preserve the cytoarchitecture and cellular differentiation of the original tissue. Although this approach benefits, in that epithelial/endothelial cells are cultured in a relatively physiologically normal microenvironment, the culture period during which the organ remains viable is limited. A problem is also how to obtain the starting material, especially if it is of human origin (Hegerfeldt et al. 2002; Berry et al. 1975; Friedl et al. 2004). With this method one can also perform 3-D invasion assays, which support the invasion of tumor cell clusters from cancer explants.

15.1.6 De-epidermized Dermis (DED)

The skin model based on de-epidermized human dermis populated with keratinocytes and fibroblasts was originally developed for resurfacing burned patients (Ghosh et al. 1997; Chakrabarty et al. 1999; Sahota et al. 2003; Harrison et al. 2006). On de-epidermized dermis (DED) stromal cells, keratinocytes, or melanoma cells can be seeded and cultured for several days and the invasive capacity of melanoma cells in this environment can be analyzed (Dekker et al. 2000). Using this model one can evaluate the contribution of the extracellular matrix, the basal membrane or normal skin cells on melanoma cell invasion. The advantage of this system is that the de-epidermized dermis retains a native extracellular matrix and basal membrane and the contribution of the basal membrane in the invasive properties of melanoma cells can be analyzed easily. This in vitro system showed reliable invasion of highly invasive cells and was used to investigate the proteolytic mechanisms involved in melanoma cell invasion into dermal connective tissue (Dennhofer et al. 2003). By culturing melanoma cells either on the dermal side of the DED or on the basal membrane side, one can study the influence of the basement membrane on the invasive behavior of melanoma cells (Van Kilsdonk et al. 2010). It is also possible to study the role of matrix metalloproteases in this model on melanoma cell invasion (Dennhofer et al. 2003). The basement membrane components can also be removed by treatment of the DED by incubation with dispase (Harrison et al. 2006). Using this model, it has been shown that the dermoepidermal basement membrane can prevent invasion of metastatic melanoma cell lines in the absence of a stratified epidermis (Van Kilsdonk et al. 2010).

15.1.7 2-D Coculture Systems

The 2-D coculture system is ideally suited to analyze the effect of defined factors or genes especially on melanocyte transformation in an environment in which at least a quasi in vivo like cellular communication can take place. It is known that melanocytes cultured in vitro display different phenotypic characteristics than melanocytes in vivo. This suggests a role of microenvironmental signals in controlling the melanocytic phenotype. Indeed, it was shown that upon coculture with undifferentiated keratinocytes, melanocytes regain their normal phenotype resembling those in situ, indicating that keratinocytes regulate cell growth, dendricity, and antigen expression of melanocytes in vitro (Hsu et al. 2002; Shih et al. 1994). Following malignant transformation, the dominance of keratinocytes over the melanocytic phenotype is lost and melanoma cells become more and more autonomous (Valyi-Nagy et al. 1993; Shih et al. 1994; Hsu et al. 2000, 2002). To analyze independently the effects of soluble factors, the coculture can be performed in Transwell systems where melanocytes and keratinocytes are seeded in two compartments of a tissue culture well, which is separated by a semiporous membrane. By this, it was shown that E-cadherin-mediated cell adhesion is required for keratinocyte-mediated control of melanocytic cells (Li et al. 2004).

The cultivation of melanoma cells with normal dermal fibroblasts indicates that melanoma cells can direct gene expression in fibroblasts (Gallagher et al. 2005; Loffek et al. 2005; Ntayi et al. 2003). Interestingly, highly aggressive melanoma cells cannot only direct the activation and functional differentiation of stromal fibroblasts and endothelial cells but also can transdifferentiate by masquerading as endothelial cells to take over all or part of stromal functions, a phenomenon termed as vasculogenic mimicry (Maniotis et al. 1999; Hendrix et al. 2003, 2007).

15.1.8 Mono- or Multicellular Spheroids

Spheroids, or tumor cell aggregates, have been used since the 1970s, mostly for investigations into the mechanisms of action of radiotherapy and chemotherapeutic drugs as well as drug resistance (Hirschhaeuser et al. 2010; Mueller-Klieser 1997; Smalley et al. 2006b). The principle is that melanoma cells are grown under non-adherent conditions, which permits the formation of 3-D aggregations or spheroids. Once formed, the spheroids are implanted into a matrix of collagen I, which mimics the microenvironment of human skin.

Cellular spheroids take advantage of many cell types to aggregate. The cellular aggregates can range in size from 20 to 1 μm in diameter, depending on the cell type and growth conditions. However, fewer than 100 human tumor cell lines have been shown to have the capacity to grow in spheroid cultures (Friedrich et al. 2007, 2009). Melanoma cells are more suitable for spheroid formation since it was shown that 18 of the 26 analyzed melanoma cell lines can form spheroids (Smalley et al. 2006a, b). Spheroids more closely resemble the in vivo situation than monolayer conditions due to the architecture and the extensive cell–cell contacts provided by the spheroids. Spheroids exhibit many of the biological properties of solid tumors, including cell morphology, growth kinetics, gene expression, and drug response (Friedrich et al. 2007, 2009; Hirschhaeuser et al. 2010; Kunz-Schughart et al. 2004; Mueller-Klieser 1997). Human tumor spheroids are widely used for drug screening since cancer cells grown in these spheroids show greater resistance toward several anticancer drugs compared to cells grown in monolayer (Smalley et al. 2006b). This may be explained in part by increased cell–cell contact, 3-D cellular architecture, enhanced deposition of tumor-derived ECM within the spheroid, a lower overall cell proliferation rate, or a combination of these factors (Bates et al. 2000; Hamilton 1998; Burdett et al. 2010). Interestingly, similar to the situation in a tumor, a diffusion gradient exists within spheroids for oxygen and nutrients limiting the availability of these compounds to the innermost cells (Lin and Chang 2008).

In spheroids, melanoma cells form concentric, spherical structures that contain large proliferating cells in the periphery and smaller quiescent cells on the interior of the sphere (Fig. 15.1a, b). These spheroids can be implanted into a collagen-based matrix where they exhibit an invasive phenotype that is indicative of the progression stage of melanoma (Smalley et al. 2006b). This system can be further explored by interspersing fibroblasts into the collagen before imbedding into a spheroid. These fibroblasts infiltrate the spheroid and produce ECM proteins (Smalley et al. 2005) (Fig. 15.1a, b). Spheroids can be established from a single cell type or can be multicellular mixtures of tumor, stromal, and immune cells (Hirschhaeuser et al. 2010). Several cell types such as fibroblasts and immune cells have been described, which can be successfully mixed with tumor spheroids under

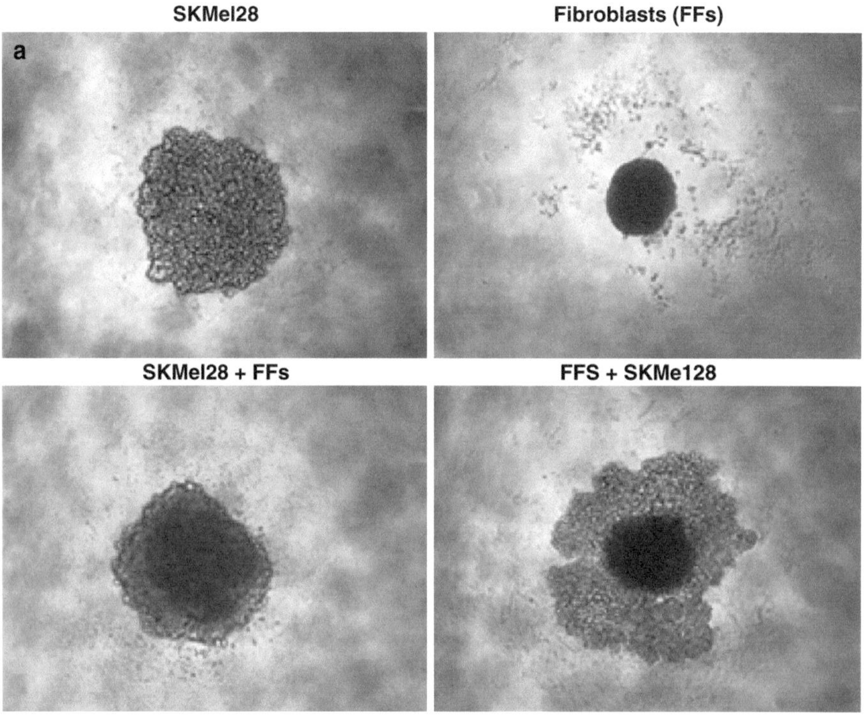

Fig. 15.1 Spheroid and organotypic skin equivalent models. (**a**) Phase contrast pictures of spheroids of SKMel28 melanoma cells or primary dermal fibroblasts (FFs) 48 h after aggregation. *Lower left* picture: Spheroids of SKMel28 melanoma cells were formed for 24 h and afterward cocultivated for 24 h with dissociated fibroblasts for further 24 h. *Lower right* picture: Spheroids of primary fibroblasts were formed for 24 h and afterward cocultivated for 24 h with SKMel28 melanoma cells for further 24 h. (**b**) Melanoma spheroids either untreated (control) or treated with a beta-catenin inhibitor (Sinnberg et al. 2010). Spheroids were stained with the vitality stains calcein-AM and ethidium bromide to visualize live and dead cells, respectively. As a measure of cell death induction ethidium bromide fluorescence indicates dead cells. (**c**) Organotypic epidermal skin equivalents (SE). Shown are hematoxylin/eosin stainings of organotypic epidermal skin reconstructs with either integrated primary melanocytes (marked with an *arrow*), a radial growth phase (RGP), vertical growth phase (VGP), or metastatic melanoma cell line. We have observed that skin reconstructs consisting of human fibroblasts and keratinocytes simulate human skin in vivo and that human melanocytes or melanoma cells from different stages of melanoma development and progression recapitulate in skin reconstructs the biological behavior in vivo. In the skin reconstructs, only an irregular basement membrane is formed as seen by the collagen IV staining (pictures taken with permission from (Meier et al. 2000)

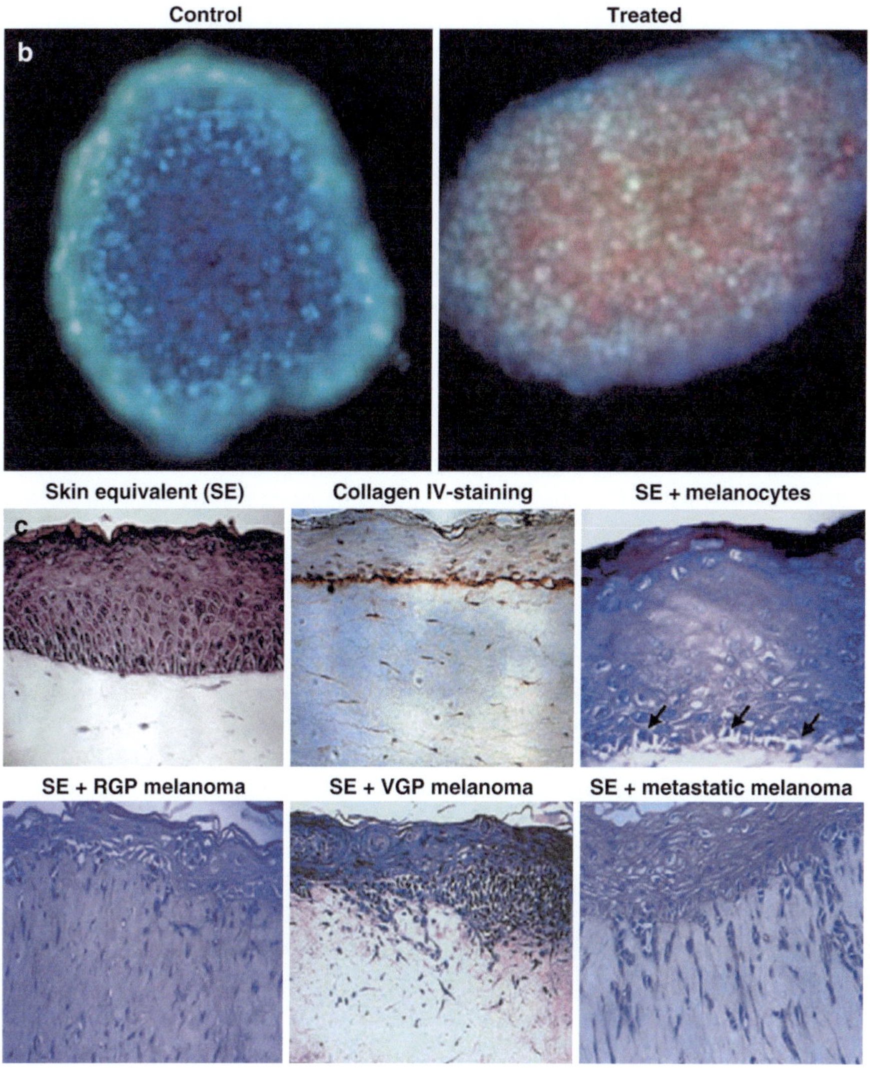

Fig. 15.1 (continued)

coculture conditions (Smalley et al. 2006b). Using this model system it was also shown that zebrafish embryo extracts promote sphere-forming ability of human melanoma cell lines (Na et al. 2009). Preformed multicellular tumor spheroids can be incubated with immune cells that migrate into the spheroid. As a result, tumor-associated migration and differentiation processes as well as cytotoxic and cytostatic activity of migrated immune cell populations can be examined (Konur et al. 1996; Gottfried et al. 2006; Pampaloni et al. 2007).

Spheroid formation can be induced by a variety of different techniques. In the spinner flask culture, fluid turbulence prevents attachment and promotes cellular aggregation (Sutherland et al. 1971). In the rotary wall vessel, reactor cells are placed between rotating cylindrical walls to mimic microgravity (Lin and Chang 2008; Friedrich et al. 2007). A simpler method, which does not need specialized equipment or additional processing, is the liquid overlay method. This involves the liquid overlay of a cell suspension over a non-adherent surface, such as agar-coated plates (Yuhas et al. 1977; Burdett et al. 2010). The absence of fluid flow using this method results in a more pronounced diffusional gradient within the spheroids. Additionally, the spheroids formed through liquid overlay are more varied in size and number. To optimize this and to get more consistent spheroid size and composition, recent adaptations involve spheroid formation within hanging drops (Kelm et al. 2003; Timmins and Nielsen 2007) and microfluidic chips (Wu et al. 2008; Burdett et al. 2010). However, these methods need again specialized equipment and additional handling steps.

By contrast, the collagen-implanted spheroid model is easier and faster to perform and is suited to high throughput drug screening studies. This assay takes account of both cell–cell contact between adjacent tumor cells and the need for 3-D supporting matrix. It is based on the liquid overlay method in which a uniform cell suspension is plated on top of hard (1.5 %) agar, which prevents the tumor cells from adhering to the underlying tissue culture plastic. After 48–72 h, the tumor cells form small aggregates, or spheroids. These spheroids can be used directly for drug toxicity studies. The protocol developed by Smalley et al. (2006a) differs in that the spheroids are harvested and mixed with a suspension of bovine collagen type I. These are then plated on a 24-well plate, which is already layered with collagen to prevent the spheroids from settling onto the underlying plastic. These collagen-implanted spheroids can be used for the analysis of the invasive capability of melanoma cells. It was shown that the extent of collagen invasion correlated with the tumor stage and the cells from the early stages were poorly invasive, whereas the cells from the metastasis colonized the entire collagen gel (Smalley et al. 2006a, b). The spheroids are scored for cell survival by removing the cell culture media, washing in PBS, and then staining using calcein-AM and ethidium bromide (Fig. 15.1b).

15.1.9 Organotypic Skin Equivalent Culture Model

The organotypic skin equivalent culture model is the most advanced and complex model currently available. The Fusenig lab was the first to use the organotypic skin model to study invasion of squamous cell carcinoma cells (Borchers et al. 1997). In simplest term, an organotypic culture of skin can be engineered using its four major components, collagen, dermal fibroblasts, melanocytes, and epidermal keratinocytes (Parenteau et al. 1992). This model is ideally suited to study the effect of inhibitors or gene expression or UV on toxic effects or on invasive capability of tumor cells or melanocytes. These organotypic cultures have been extended to different tumor types, including breast, prostate, and ovarian cancer (Chioni and Grose 2008).

The experimental protocols for creating human skin reconstructs have been described elsewhere (Meier et al. 2000, 2003; Berking et al. 2001). In brief, for the creation of an epidermal skin reconstruct, a mixture of collagen and human skin fibroblasts are seeded out into 6- or 24-well plates. After the fibroblasts have constricted the collagen, a mixture of keratinocytes and melanocytes are overlaid on top of the stromal layer. After the culture is established, the tray is lifted and the top exposed to the air, which induces keratinocyte differentiation. At maturity, the human skin reconstruct has near identical histology to normal human skin and a basal membrane like structure is built (Meier et al. 2000, 2003) (Fig. 15.1c). For the generation of a dermal skin reconstruct, one processes only until the fibroblasts have been seeded on the collagen layer (Sinnberg et al. 2010). When melanoma cells from the different defined tumor stages are introduced into the epidermal reconstruct, they exhibit progression-specific behavior. Cells derived from the radial growth phase melanoma stay within the epidermal keratinocyte layer and do not breach the basement membrane (Meier et al. 2000, 2003). Cells from the vertical growth phase of melanoma invade through the basement membrane into the dermal fibroblast layer, and cells from metastatic lesions invade rapidly throughout the dermis (Fig. 15.1c). It is possible to include melanocytes or melanoma cells in which gene expression was modulated, and it was shown that this can have dramatic effects on aggressiveness or invasive capability (Meier et al. 2003; Berking et al. 2001). The human reconstruct is a very useful model for modeling not only the growth of melanoma cells in a 3-D microenvironment but also the interaction of melanoma cells with the surrounding keratinocytes and fibroblasts. This approach can also be applied to other tissues as human breast, colon, and esophagus (Smalley et al. 2006b). Thus, the composite culture model enables functional studies of individual genes and interactions between specific gene products in various skin cell types in a biologically relevant milieu (Hsu et al. 2002; Meier et al. 2000; Sinnberg et al. 2010).

Skin reconstructs have a maximal life span of approximately 1 month in vitro, which can be extended to several months once grafted to living hosts (Javaherian et al. 1998; Satyamoorthy et al. 1999; Berking et al. 2001; Hsu et al. 2002). In these models, melanocytes regain their physiological localization at the level of the basal layer in the epidermis (Fig. 15.1c). They preserve all their functionality since in response to UV rays they proliferate, synthesize, and secrete melanin (Auxenfans et al. 2009). Further advancements are the endothelialized skin equivalents in which human endothelial cells from umbilical vessels are seeded together with fibroblasts, which organize themselves into tubular structures with a well-defined lumen resulting in an endothelialized skin equivalent (Hudon et al. 2003; Auxenfans et al. 2009). Seeding of keratinocytes on this endothelialized dermis results in the formation of capillary structures (Velazquez et al. 2002; Smalley et al. 2006b). Finally, the immunocompetent skin equivalent model is available. The reconstruct is a novel 3-D culture system in which the migration of leukocytes toward tumor cells and the factors that influence leukocyte migration can be studied under in vivo-like conditions (Berencsi et al. 2007; Zhang et al. 2006).

15.2 Experimental Animal Models

15.2.1 Introduction

In melanoma research, a great variety of experimental animal models is available. Each model has distinct advantages for the investigation of particular scientific questions regarding melanoma formation, genetics, and therapy as reviewed recently (van der Weyden et al. 2016). Melanomas naturally occur in horses, dogs, minipigs, and fish. Already at the end of the 1920s melanoma development was documented in interspecies hybrids of the fish genus *Xiphophorus* (Gordon 1927; Häussler 1928; Kosswig 1928). Since then the genetics of melanoma susceptibility was intensively studied in this model with successful identification of relevant oncogenes like *Xmrk*. Zebrafish and medaka are other well-studied melanoma fish models which have helped to unravel the underlying mechanisms of spontaneous as well as carcinogen and ultraviolet (UV) induced melanoma formation. Mouse models are also widely used in melanoma research, as mice exhibit short breeding cycles with a relatively large number of offspring, are easily manipulated genetically, and can be treated with UV and chemical carcinogens. A major benefit of modeling melanoma in mice is its ability to investigate the role of different genetic abnormalities observed in patients on disease progression due to the high degree of homology with the human genome. Mice have been generated that develop melanoma in the skin which metastasize early and are highly resistant to chemo- and radiotherapy, a fundamental characteristic of malignant melanoma. Experimental models in the laboratory mouse have been of critical importance to understand the biologic mechanisms how melanoma cells migrate in and out of blood and lymph vessels, evade immune defense, and colonize distant organs. In addition to the study of gene function on an organismal level, mouse models have also been widely used to evaluate the efficacy of novel treatment strategies in controlling metastatic disease progression. Experimental mouse models for cancer research can principally be subdivided into three different categories:

- Transplantation of human tumor cells into immunodeficient mice
- Transplantation of mouse tumor cells into syngeneic immunocompetent mice
- Primary autochthonous ("genetically engineered") mouse models of cancer

We will briefly sketch the historical development of each category and provide a few selected examples how technical advances have enabled new insights in different areas of melanoma research over the years. We do not intend to provide a comprehensive catalog of all possible model systems but hope to give the reader a broad and stimulating overview (Table 15.2).

Table 15.2 Experimental mouse models

Melanoma model systems	Application	Advantages	Disadvantages
Transplantation of human melanoma cells into immunodeficient mice	Analysis of gene functions in human melanoma cells for invasive and metastatic tumor growth in vivo; preclinical evaluation of new drug candidates	Fast, reliable assay that portrays important aspects of human melanoma biology	Excludes the role of immune cells in the tumor microenvironment, does not portray the early steps of malignant transformation
Transplantation of mouse melanoma cells into syngeneic immunocompetent mice	Analysis of gene functions in mouse melanoma cells for invasive and metastatic tumor growth in vivo; preclinical evaluation of drug efficacy	Fast, reliable assay that includes the role of immune cells in the tumor microenvironment	Does not portray the early steps of malignant transformation, may not adequately portray all aspects of human melanoma biology
Primary autochthonous (genetically engineered) mouse melanoma models	Analysis of gene functions in the pathogenesis of melanoma on an organismal level; preclinical confirmation of drug efficacy	Allows for the investigation of early steps in malignant transformation in a fully immunocompetent tumor microenvironment	Time consuming and costly experimental setting, may not adequately portray all aspects of human melanoma biology

15.2.2 Transplantation of Human Melanoma Cells into Immunodeficient Mice

The successful engraftment of human tumors onto immunodeficient mice was first reported in 1969 using the athymic nude mouse (Rygaard and Povlsen 1969). This approach was widely used in subsequent years to study the morphological and biochemical characteristics of different tumor cells in vivo and the response of such xenografts to antineoplastic agents (Giovanella et al. 1973; Seaman et al. 1975). Several groups investigated the ability of human melanoma cells to grow metastastically in nude mice either following intravenous injection ("experimental pulmonary metastasis assay" or "lung colonization assay") or following subcutaneous injection ("spontaneous metastasis assay"). In each case, the development of lung metastases was assessed over time. It was noted that melanomas, like most malignant neoplasms, were composed of heterogeneous tumor cell populations with different capacities for invasion and metastasis. Intrinsic features of a given tumor line appeared to be major determinants in regulating metastatic spread (Kozlowski et al. 1984). These features could be selected for by serial in vivo passaging. In addition, it was noted that growth of melanoma metastases was limited by residual immune reactivity of nude mice against xenogeneic human tumor cells, which was mediated particularly by NK cells.

Over the years, a number of melanoma cell lines were established (e.g., A375, MeWo, SKMel28, 1205Lu, and many others), which could be transplanted in nude mice as well as in mice with severe combined immunodeficiency (SCID), which were described a few years later. With the emerging ability to genetically modify tumor cells in vitro, these model systems have been successfully used to functionally assess the role of individual gene products on invasive growth and metastatic spread of melanoma cells in vivo until today. As an example, Clark et al. serially transplanted A375-M cells in nude mice and used cDNA microarray analyses to identify RhoC as a protein associated with melanoma metastases. Retroviral overexpression confirmed that RhoC indeed promotes the ability of melanoma cells to metastasize in mice in vivo (Clark et al. 2000). The ability to stably knock down the expression of a target gene using RNA interference has provided an additional valuable tool to study gene function not only on the cellular but also on the organismal level in mice. This technology was used to show that the CYLD protein regulates the ability of a human melanoma cell line to grow invasively and metastasize in vivo (Massoumi et al. 2009).

Several technical advances have expanded the range of experimental possibilities for the study of human tumor cells in immunodeficient mice. To more adequately model the tumor microenvironment, the group of Meenhard Herlyn transplanted human skin onto SCID mice and injected melanoma cells into the xenografts. This "orthotopic" tumor transplantation model circumvented the significant anatomic and physiologic differences between mouse and human skin and recapitulated the close interaction between melanocytes and keratinocytes (Juhasz Albelda et al. 1993). Crossing SCID mice onto the nonobese diabetic (NOD) genetic background improved tumor engraftment rates because NOD/SCID mice show reduced macrophage and NK function, as well as an absence of complement-dependent hemolytic activity. These mice were used by the group of Weinberg to study the in vivo growth properties of human melanocytes, which were transformed by defined genetic modifications in vitro (Gupta et al. 2005). Using this experimental approach, they provided evidence that the developmental origins of melanocytes in the neural crest might be relevant to their metastatic propensity. By combining both approaches it has today become possible to transplant complex skin reconstructs generated in vitro onto immunodeficient mice to study their behavior in vivo as mentioned in Sect. 15.1 above.

Another technical improvement for studying human tumor cells in immunodeficient mice has been developed by hematologists investigating the development and function of hematopoietic stem cells in immunodeficient mice. To further facilitate the permanent engraftment of bone marrow precursors, they tested various mice with additional genetic changes affecting the immune system. It was found that NOD/SCID mice, which lack the IL2 receptor common γ chain (NOD/SCID/γc mice), show extremely high engraftment rates using human hematopoietic cells (Ito et al. 2002). The reason for the high engraftment rates was attributed to multiple immunological functional defects that affect dendritic cells in addition to the absence of T, B, and NK cells. Using these highly immunocompromised NOD/SCID/γc mice, Carreno et al. demonstrated that the residual immunity in NOD as well as NOD/SCID mice affected the metastatic growth of A375 melanoma cells (Carreno et al. 2009). They used tumor cells stably expressing a luciferase gene and monitored tumor growth in the lungs in real time by measuring in vivo bioluminescence with a highly sensitive CCD camera. In addition, they demonstrated human melanoma recognition by residual NOD/SCID NK cells, which correlates with MICA/B expression and could be blocked by anti-mouse NKG2D antibodies.

The importance of using different immunodeficient mouse strains became prominently evident when analyzing the ability of different subpopulations of malignant cells derived from primary melanomas to generate tumor xenografts. The group of Markus Frank showed that only very few human melanoma cells can form tumors when transplanted into NOD/SCID mice, and that melanoma cells expressing the chemoresistance mediator ABCB5 were highly enriched for such "melanoma-initiating cells." Importantly, they demonstrated that this minor tumorigenic cell population could be therapeutically targeted and destroyed in vivo with a specific monoclonal antibody (Schatton et al. 2008). Sean Morrison's group showed that a slight modification of the xenotransplantation assay conditions and the use of more highly immunocompromised NOD/SCID/γc mice greatly increased the detection of tumorigenic melanoma cells (Quintana et al. 2008). The mechanisms underlying melanoma cell heterogeneity (which had already been observed in the early days of melanoma xenografting) can now be studied using genetically modified transplantable melanoma cell lines in NOD/SCID/γc mice. The group of Meenhard Herlyn reported that a dynamically regulated JARID1B-expressing subpopulation of melanoma cells is essential for continuous tumor growth (Roesch et al. 2010). These results suggest a new understanding of melanoma heterogeneity with tumor maintenance as a dynamic process mediated by spatially and temporarily distinct subpopulations. Highly sophisticated imaging techniques are currently being employed to monitor in vivo in real time the proliferation and migration of transplanted melanoma cells expressing various fluorescent and bioluminescent reporter genes placed under the control of constitutive or dynamically regulated promoters.

Recent trials aim at facilitating a personalized cancer therapy generating individualized tumor models by means of melanoma patient-derived xenografts (PDX). These PDXs serve as preclinical models to test drug response, unravel resistance mechanisms, and offer the possibility for new drug and biomarker discovery. Especially therapeutic strategies for patients with mutations of the BRAF and NRAS oncogene and accompanying resistance to targeted therapies by inhibitors like vemurafenib are frequently investigated (Das Thakur et al. 2013;

Guerreschi et al. 2013). In addition, as some melanomas are not easily accessible or difficult to biopsy an alternative method was established by using circulating tumor cell-derived xenografts (CDX), which is suitable for studying late-stage melanoma (Girotti et al. 2016). The high similarity between PDXs and the corresponding biopsies of the patient with regard to mutation and expression patterns as well as histopathologic and immunohistochemical properties was proven in many studies. Moreover, PDXs show similar resistance mechanisms as the donor tumor (Kemper et al. 2015) allowing for detailed analysis of the underlying processes. However, one has to keep in mind that PDXs may not display the whole genetic heterogeneity of the patient's tumor (Kemper et al. 2015) and therefore provide only a partial prediction of the patient's disease progression and treatment response. Although the clinical feasibility and translatability of PDXs could be demonstrated (Einarsdottir et al. 2014; Gao et al. 2015), their use is technically challenging with some cases of engraftment failure and a quite time-consuming and costly procedure.

Taken together, the transplantation of human melanoma cells into immunodeficient mice can be generally considered as a rather rapid, reliable, and reproducible experimental approach to functionally study the role of genes in the process of malignant progression to metastatic disease. Importantly, this experimental system most closely reflects the intrinsic biology of human melanomas and partly recapitulates the tumor microenvironment in vivo. Furthermore, it is of critical importance for preclinical testing of novel therapeutics to develop personalized treatment strategies and understand drug resistance. However, work with human tumors in immunodeficient mice has two major inherent drawbacks. Firstly, it excludes the interaction of tumor cells with the immune system, which is of critical importance in shaping the tumor microenvironment and the process of tumor progression. Secondly, transplanted tumors grow rapidly and do not portray the early events during tumor initiation.

15.2.3 Transplantation of Mouse Melanoma Cells into Syngeneic Immunocompetent Mice

To experimentally include the role of the immune system in tumor progression requires the use of immunocompetent animals. However, in mice, melanoma develops only very rarely. One of these rare events occurred at the base of the ear in a C57BL/6 mouse at the Jackson Laboratories in 1954. This tumor was serially transplanted and subsequently established in vitro as the B16 melanoma cell line by Isaiah Fidler in the early 1970s. B16 melanoma cells readily form solid tumors when injected s.c. or i.v. into syngeneic C57BL/6 mice and were widely used from the early 1970s on as a model for metastases research to investigate the steps involved in tumor dissemination. Following the concept of "seed and soil," originally proposed by Stephen Paget in the late nineteenth century (Paget 1889), Fidler and colleagues showed that both host factors and properties of the tumor cells contribute to the success or failure of the metastatic process. Already in 1977, it was reported that different B16 melanoma cell subclones derived in vitro varied greatly in their ability to form lung metastases upon intravenous inoculation into syngeneic mice. This observation suggested that B16 melanoma cells were heterogeneous and that highly metastatic tumor cell variants preexisted in the parental population (Fidler and Kripke 1977). The origins of tumor cell heterogeneity were also analyzed using K1735 melanoma cells, which were established from a UV-irradiated C3H mouse (Fidler and Hart 1982). These transplantable mouse melanoma cell lines are still used today to understand the cellular and molecular mechanisms underlying the process of metastatic progression utilizing modern tools of molecular genetics to overexpress or silence individual genes and of in vivo imaging to follow fluorescent and bioluminescent reporter genes as described in the previous section.

The most important application of tumor transplantation models in immunocompetent mice, however, was to understand the role of innate and adaptive immune responses in tumor progression. Because B16 melanoma cells are poorly immunogenic and do not efficiently stimulate antigen-specific tumor immunity, they were widely used as a model to study tumor vaccine adjuvants, including various microbial extracts. Molecular insights into the mechanisms how immune responses against tumor cells develop was gained from studies with B16 melanoma cells genetically modified to secrete immunostimulatory cytokines. Unexpected at the time, the expression of GM-CSF effectively promoted the induction of tumor immunity (Dranoff et al. 1993). It later became clear that this cytokine acted as a potent growth factor for antigen-presenting dendritic cells, which are critically required to initiate adaptive immunity. The experimental strategy to overexpress (or knock down) immune-related genes in B16 melanoma cells continues to reveal important insights into the interaction between tumor and immune cells until today. This is best illustrated by a recent report showing that the expression of the chemokine CCL21 by B16 melanoma cells induces a lymphoid-like reticular stromal network and recruits regulatory leukocyte populations to promote an immunotolerant microenvironment in mice (Shields et al. 2010).

The transplantable B16 melanoma model has also been used to study antigen-specific vaccination strategies, including the use of synthetic peptides as well as recombinant proteins and genes. Initially, investigators targeted model foreign antigens such as chicken ovalbumin, which were stably transfected into B16 cells (Mayordomo et al. 1995). In our own work, we found that efficient induction of cellular immune responses against clinically relevant melanocytic self-antigens such as TRP2 or gp100, which are naturally expressed by B16 melanoma cells, required strong activation of dendritic antigen-presenting cells either by culture from bone marrow precursors in vitro or by recombinant viral vaccines in vivo (Tüting et al. 1999; Steitz et al. 2000). Importantly, by combining antigen-specific vaccination with genetic modification of B16 melanoma cells, we could show that the expression of type I IFNs promoted T cell effector functions in the tumor microenvironment (Steitz et al. 2001). Type I IFNs could also be efficiently stimulated in tumor tissue by adjuvant peritumoral injections of immunostimulatory nucleic acids such as polyI:C and CpG-rich DNA, which imitate viral RNA and DNA and activate the innate immune system through the Toll-like receptors (TLR) 3 and 9 (Tormo et al. 2006a; Bald et al. 2014a).

The B16 model is also very suitable to study biological processes and therapeutic agents, which simultaneously affect both tumor and host cells, particularly immune cells. In addition to using genetically modified tumor cells, researchers have also employed genetically engineered hosts and injected specific monoclonal antibodies to dissect the underlying molecular and cellular mechanisms. Our own work with therapeutic oligonucleotides exemplifies this strategy. We explored the use of small immunostimulatory siRNA molecules, which simultaneously can silence a target gene in tumor cells, in our case the antiapoptotic gene Bcl2, and activate retinoic acid-inducible gene-I (RIG-I), a cytosolic sensor of viral RNA, in immune cells (Poeck et al. 2008). Silencing Bcl2 promoted tumor cell apoptosis and activation of RIG-I stimulated cytotoxic immune cells to destroy tumor cells. Surprisingly, we found that activation of RIG-I also contributed to apoptosis induction directly in tumor cells. Experiments in mice, genetically lacking the interferon alpha receptor 1 chain, demonstrated that this response was critically dependent on a functional type I IFN system. The injection of cytotoxic antibodies against NK cells showed that this cell type largely mediated the antitumor response.

The interaction between melanoma cells and T cells in the tumor microenvironment in vivo can be studied in greater detail using adoptive lymphocyte transfer approaches. This experimental strategy has been facilitated by the development of T cell receptor transgenic mice, which carry large numbers of genetically marked T cells that specifically recognize melanocytic antigens (Overwijk et al. 2003; Xie et al. 2010). The adoptive transfer and in vivo activation of T cells in mice bearing macroscopically detectable B16 melanomas enables investigations of the mechanisms that determine the balance between tumor regression and progressive disease, including the various possibilities of tumor immune escape. To more closely imitate the clinical situation, mice have been genetically engineered to express the human HLA-A2 molecule and T cells have been genetically engineered to express human T cell receptors (Frankel et al. 2010). These highly sophisticated experimental models have been of considerable help to translate this therapeutic approach into clinical reality for melanoma patients.

In summary, the transplantation of mouse melanoma cells into syngeneic immunocompetent mice also represents a rapid, reliable, and reproducible experimental approach to functionally study the role of genes in the process of malignant progression to metastatic disease. This experimental system may not fully reflect the biology of human melanomas, but it much more adequately portrays the role of the immune system in shaping the tumor microenvironment in vivo. It has been of critical importance for preclinical development and testing of novel therapeutics, including melanoma vaccines with dendritic cells and immunomodulatory agents such as the anti-CTLA4 mAb, which is currently evaluated in clinical phase III studies. However, transplanted mouse melanomas also progress very rapidly following tumor inoculation and do not recapitulate the gradual series of cellular changes from premalignant to malignant pathologies.

15.2.4 Primary Autochthonous (Genetically Engineered) Mouse Melanoma Models

Advances in molecular genetics and stem cell biology have made it possible to study the functional role of oncogenes and tumor suppressor genes in the pathogenesis of melanoma on an organismal level. Work over the last decade has shown that genetic alterations observed in human melanomas also promote the malignant transformation of melanocytes in mice. This most likely reflects the fact that the genetic control of melanocyte proliferation, migration, and differentiation in embryonic development is highly conserved during the evolution of vertebrates. Genetically engineered mouse tumor models initially involved the transgenic expression of viral or cellular oncogenes under the control of tissue-specific promoters. The transgenic expression of certain growth factors or growth factor receptors also promoted tumor development. Subsequently, it became possible to delete tumor suppressor genes by gene targeting. More recently, the conditional deletion of tumor suppressor genes or activation of oncogenes has been achieved via Cre-lox technology. Because genetically engineered mouse models for melanoma have been extensively reviewed (Chin et al. 2006; Larue and Beerman 2008; Zaidi et al. 2008), we will only briefly sketch their historical development and highlight some of the more important recent advances in the field.

The transformation of melanocytes in mice was first achieved by Beatrice Mintz's group who placed the oncogenic SV40 large T antigen under the control of a tyrosinase promoter construct specifically in melanocytes. Founder lines expressing high transgene levels developed eye melanomas very early while lines expressing low transgene levels developed eye melanomas much later. Grafting experiments of skin derived from mice with high melanoma susceptibility onto mice with low melanoma susceptibility revealed proliferating pigment cells close to areas of greatest wound healing, which subsequently evolved into invasively growing melanomas (Mintz and Silvers 1993). These observations strongly suggested that pro-inflammatory growth factors and cytokines known to be produced in wound repair can promote growth and malignant conversion of genetically susceptible melanocytes in vivo.

Lynda Chin and colleagues generated mice that expressed the activated $Hras^{G12V}$ oncogene under a tyrosinase promoter in mice, which carried a deletion of the $p16^{INK4a}/p19^{ARF}$ tumor suppressor gene locus (Chin et al. 1997). These mice spontaneously developed cutaneous melanomas after a short latency and with high penetrance. Her results indicated that activation of Ras and loss of $p16^{INK4a}/p19^{ARF}$ can cooperate to accelerate the development of melanoma and provided the first in vivo experimental evidence for a role of $p16^{INK4a}/p19^{ARF}$ deficiency in the pathogenesis of melanoma. In our own work, we could demonstrate the critical role of the $p16^{Ink4a}$–Cdk4 interaction in suppressing the transformation of melanocytes following oncogene activation (Tormo et al. 2006b). The transgenic overexpression of the hepatocyte growth factor (Hgf), which drives Ras signaling via its receptor tyrosine kinase c-Met, cooperates with a mutated oncogenic cyclin-dependant kinase 4 ($Cdk4^{R24C}$) knocked into the germline, which abrogates p16 binding. Hgf-$Cdk4^{R24C}$

mice spontaneously develop multiple small (benign) nevi and subsequently single progressively growing (malignant) melanomas, indicating that impairment of the p16^{Ink4a}-Cdk4 axis affects the complete spectrum of stepwise malignant transformation of melanocytes (Landsberg et al. 2010).

With the recent development of techniques allowing for tamoxifen-inducible conditional activation of oncogenes specifically in melanocytes, it became possible to show that the mutated oncogenic Braf^{V600E}, which is frequently found in human melanomas, also strongly drives melanocyte proliferation in the skin of mice leading to the development of multiple melanocytic nevi (Dhomen et al. 2009; Dankort et al. 2009). The simultaneous deletion of the tumor suppressor genes PTEN or p16^{INK4a} led to a decreased latency and increased penetrance of melanoma. These novel models will undoubtedly help to dissect the molecular mechanisms regulating melanocyte proliferation, oncogene-induced senescence and tumor progression in the microenvironment of nevi and melanoma in vivo. The introduction of fluorescent or bioluminescent marker genes that are specifically expressed by melanocytes will enable the in vivo imaging of early proliferative events during melanocyte transformation, particularly following neonatal UV irradiation which has been shown to significantly promote melanomagenesis in several models, including Hgf-transgenic mice (Noonan et al. 2001).

Another transgenic mouse model showing spontaneous melanoma development was generated by the insertion of a *Dct* promoter-Grm1 construct leading to an aberrant expression of the metabotropic glutamate receptor 1 (Grm1) in melanocytes (Pollock et al. 2003). With complete penetrance Tg(*Grm1*) mice develop pigmented lesions at hairless skin regions, including ear, tail, and anus within 4–6 months. Furthermore, not only local metastasis but also metastatic spread in distant organs like lung, liver, lymph node, and spleen occurs (Schiffner et al. 2012). Interestingly, the majority of these disseminated cells display phenotypic changes during metastasis in form of de-pigmentation as is also found frequently in human melanoma. During the last years, a variety of human melanoma cell lines and tissue samples were screened with respect to their Grm1 expression showing overall high levels in contrast to normal melanocytes or benign nevi emphasizing the importance of ectopic Grm1 expression in melanoma development. Indeed, the malignant transformation of murine melanocytes could be induced by solely stable Grm1 expression (Shin et al. 2008). The activation of the Grm1 receptor results in a constitutive activation of the MAPK and PI3K/AKT signaling pathway. Both can be suppressed by treatment with the glutamate release inhibitor riluzole with the effect of a reduced colony formation, migration and invasion ability of human melanoma cell lines (Le et al. 2010). Hence, GRM1 seems to be a promising therapeutic target for future clinical trials. In addition, GRM1 expression was detected recently in human uveal melanoma samples and in accordance Tg(*Grm1*) mice were shown to develop melanocytic hyperproliferation within the uveal tract resulting in some cases of choroideal melanoma (Schiffner et al. 2014). Therefore, Tg(*Grm1*) mice open up the new opportunity to analyze spontaneous uveal melanoma development and metastasis in a murine model system.

Genetically engineered mouse melanoma models also provide novel opportunities to experimentally investigate the regulation of immune cell functions in the tumor microenvironment and understand the role of "cancer immunosurveillance" and "cancer-associated inflammation" in the pathogenesis of primary and metastatic melanoma. This is nicely illustrated by a recent report that primary melanomas developing in mice expressing the Ret oncogene as a transgene disseminate early but remain dormant for varying periods of time (Eyles et al. 2010). The control of tumor growth is mediated at least in part by cytotoxic T cells, since antibody-mediated depletion of these cells resulted in faster outgrowth of visceral metastases. These findings suggest that immune responses can be essential for prolonging the survival of early stage melanomas and that therapeutic strategies designed to reinforce such immune responses may produce marked survival benefits.

However, the immune system can be a double-edged sword because an inflammatory response can also promote tumor growth as has been first observed by Beatrice Mintz almost 20 years ago. Pro-inflammatory mediators capable of activating NF-kB signaling may not only support tumor cell survival, regenerative proliferation, and migration but can also enhance neoangiogenesis. An important role for NF-kB signaling in melanomagenesis has indeed been obtained by the group of Ann Richmond (Yang et al. 2010a). They generated mice, which allowed the inducible genetic ablation of Ikkβ (a kinase which phosphorylates IkB leading to NF-kB nuclear translocation and activation), specifically in melanocytes expressing the oncogenic $HRas^{G12V}$ mutation on the $p16^{INK4a}/p19^{ARF}$-deficient background. The deletion of Ikkβ significantly inhibited the development of melanomas in these mice in vivo and promoted p53-dependent apoptosis and cell cycle arrest in cultured melanocytes in vitro. These results support a role for tumor cell-intrinsic activation of NF-kB signaling in the pathogenesis of melanoma in agreement with reports in genetically engineered mouse models for other tumor types (Grivennikov et al. 2010). NF-kB-driven inflammatory responses may also participate in the development of melanoma following burning doses of UV irradiation. This interesting question can now be experimentally addressed using UV-sensitive mouse models.

The impact of tumor-associated inflammatory responses on T cell-mediated immunosurveillance has been addressed by Anne-Marie Schmitt-Verhulst's group in mice where activation of oncogenic $HRas^{G12V}$ and deletion of $p16^{INK4a}/p19^{ARF}$ can be induced simultaneously by tamoxifen treatment (Soudja et al. 2010). These "TiRP" mice develop two different types of melanoma: slowly growing, pigmented melanomas and more rapidly growing, nonpigmented melanomas that are infiltrated by $Gr1^+/CD11b^+$ inflammatory immune cells. TiRP mouse melanomas also express the T cell-defined tumor antigen P1A in melanocytes, which allows investigations with adoptively transferred T cells specifically recognizing the P1A antigen on melanoma cells. Using this experimental system, it could be shown that an initially protective adaptive immune response is subsequently suppressed by chronic tumor-associated inflammation associated with infiltrating bone marrow-derived immature myeloid cells and a systemic Th2/Th17-oriented cytokine production profile.

In our own work, we found that primary $Hgf\text{-}Cdk4^{R24C}$ melanomas can effectively escape recognition and destruction by cytotoxic effector T cells. To experimentally introduce T cell-mediated immunosurveillance, we adoptively transferred melanoma-specific TCR-transgenic cytotoxic T lymphocytes in the context of a combination treatment protocol consisting of host preconditioning, viral vaccination, and adjuvant peritumoral injections with immunostimulatory nucleic acids, which trigger innate immune responses in the tumor microenvironment (Kohlmeyer et al. 2009). This frequently resulted in complete and long-term regression of primary cutaneous melanomas. However, primary tumors eventually recurred indicating that some melanoma cells survived. Importantly, we observed large areas of poorly melanotic, proliferating melanoma cells in recurring melanomas suggesting that cytotoxic inflammation caused a phenotypic switch in subpopulations of tumor cells reminiscent of inflammatory melanomas in the TiRP mice (Landsberg et al. 2010). This phenomenon might represent a conversion of tumor cells toward a mesenchymal, invasive phenotype, which has been shown to result in the suppression of adaptive immune responses (Kudo-Saito et al. 2009). Similar phenomena were observed in response to adoptive T cell therapy, which allowed tumor cells to escape immune destruction through reversible inflammation-induced dedifferentiation (Landsberg et al. 2012). Moreover, an inflammatory environment following UV irradiation of the skin promoted melanoma cell invasion and metastasis (Bald et al. 2014b).

Taken together, genetically engineered mouse melanoma models imitate the multistep pathogenesis of melanoma in man where primary tumor cells establish in a unique microenvironment, and naturally progress toward metastatic disease. These models are ideally suited to adequately address many of the key issues in melanoma biology, including the regulation of proliferation, differentiation, and senescence of melanocytes following oncogene activation; the origin of tumor cell heterogeneity and the mechanisms of phenotype switching; the relationship of melanoma cells with neural crest-derived precursor cells; the initiation of innate and adaptive immunity leading to immunosurveillance and inflammation; the role of pro-inflammatory mediators for tumor cell survival, proliferation, and migration as well as neoangiogenesis; and the dynamics of tumor cell migration, dormancy, and metastatic colonization.

15.2.5 Experimental Mouse Models: Conclusions

A number of observations in the clinic suggest a close relationship between the activation of oncogenic signaling pathways driving the malignant transformation of melanocytes and the activation of immune responses in the tumor microenvironment. Future work in different experimental mouse models will help to dissect the role of innate immune signaling pathways in tumor and immune cells, which determine the balance between tumor regression and tumor progression. Even more importantly, work in these model systems will inform us how targeted inhibition of signaling pathways will affect the survival of tumor cells in vivo in the tumor microenvironment, including the response of immune cells. While genetically engineered mouse models adequately recapitulate many aspects of the early genetic events of melanocyte transformation, including the important role of the immune system in melanomagenesis, it must be kept in mind that they only partly reflect the features of human melanoma. Some of the more obvious shortcomings such as the low number of melanocytes in the interfollicular melanocytes may be overcome experimentally. Nevertheless, considerable differences will always remain in the molecular hardwiring of mouse tumor and immune cells that will have to be appreciated in each experimental setting. Furthermore, work with these model systems requires a long-term commitment since they are extremely time consuming, labor intensive, and costly. This may be alleviated in part by the generation of transplantable cell lines from primary melanomas with defined genetic alterations.

Conclusion

In this chapter, we have presented many of the commonly used complex in vitro cell culture model systems and the in vivo experimental mouse models that are employed by research groups today to study the various aspects of melanoma biology and to evaluate novel therapeutic strategies. The relative importance of each experimental approach depends largely on two important aspects: Firstly, how well does the model recapitulate the process it attempts to emulate? Secondly, how well does the model itself offer the flexibility to expand our knowledge relating to the pathologic process being evaluated? Today, researchers are more and more combining the strengths of new in vitro cell culture models, new "humanized" mouse strains for the transplantation of human melanomas, and new "genetically engineered" mouse models for primary melanoma to comprehensively analyze their particular aspect of melanoma biology.

References

Auxenfans C, Fradette J, Lequeux C, Germain L, Kinikoglu B, Bechetoille N, Braye F, Auger FA, Damour O (2009) Evolution of three dimensional skin equivalent models reconstructed in vitro by tissue engineering. Eur J Dermatol 19:107–113

Bald T, Landsberg J, Lopez-Ramos D, Renn M, Glodde N, Jansen P, Gaffal E, Steitz J, Tolba R, Kalinke U, Limmer A, Jönsson G, Hölzel M, Tüting T (2014a) Immune-cell poor melanomas benefit from PD-1 blockade after targeted type I IFN activation. Cancer Discov 4:674–687

Bald T, Quast T, Landsberg J, Rogava M, Glodde N, Lopez-Ramos D, Kohlmeyer J, Riesenberg S, van den Boorn-Konijnenberg D, Hömig-Hölzel C, Reuten R, Schadow B, Weighardt I, Wenzel D, Helfrich I, Schadendorf D, Bloch W, Bianchi ME, Koch M, Fleischmann BK, Förster I, Kastenmüller W, Kolanus W, Hölzel M, Gaffal E, Tüting T (2014b) Ultraviolet radiation-induced inflammation promotes angiotropism and metastasis in melanoma. Nature 507:109–113

Bates RC, Edwards NS, Yates JD (2000) Spheroids and cell survival. Crit Rev Oncol Hematol 36:61–74

Beacham DA, Amatangelo MD, Cukierman E (2007) Preparation of extracellular matrices produced by cultured and primary fibroblasts. Curr Protoc Cell Biol Chapter 10:Unit 10.9

Berencsi K, Meropol NJ, Hoffman JP, Sigurdson E, Giles L, Rani P, Somasundaram R, Zhang T, Kalabis J, Caputo L, Furth E, Swoboda R, Marincola F, Herlyn D (2007) Colon carcinoma cells induce CXCL11-dependent migration of CXCR3-expressing cytotoxic T lymphocytes in organotypic culture. Cancer Immunol Immunother 56:359–370

Berking C, Takemoto R, Schaider H, Showe L, Satyamoorthy K, Robbins P, Herlyn M (2001) Transforming growth factor-beta1 increases survival of human melanoma through stroma remodeling. Cancer Res 61:8306–8316

Berry RJ, Laing AH, Wells J (1975) Fresh explant culture of human tumours in vitro and the assessment of sensitivity to cytotoxic chemotherapy. Br J Cancer 31:218–227

Bissell MJ, Radisky D (2001) Putting tumours in context. Nat Rev Cancer 1:46–54

Borchers AH, Steinbauer H, Schafer BS, Kramer M, Bowden GT, Fusenig NE (1997) Fibroblast-directed expression and localization of 92-kDa type IV collagenase along the tumor-stroma interface in an in vitro three-dimensional model of human squamous cell carcinoma. Mol Carcinog 19:258–266

Boyden S (1962) The chemotactic effect of mixtures of antibody and antigen on polymorphonuclear leucocytes. J Exp Med 115:453–466

Burdett E, Kasper FK, Mikos AG, Ludwig JA (2010) Engineering tumors: a tissue engineering perspective in cancer biology. Tissue Eng Part B Rev 16:351–359

Carreno BM et al (2009) Immunodeficient mouse strains display marked variability in growth of human melanoma lung metastases. Clin Cancer Res 15:3277–3286

Chakrabarty KH, Dawson RA, Harris P, Layton C, Babu M, Gould L, Phillips J, Leigh I, Green C, Freedlander E, Mac NS (1999) Development of autologous human dermal-epidermal composites based on sterilized human allodermis for clinical use. Br J Dermatol 141:811–823

Chen HC (2005) Boyden chamber assay. Methods Mol Biol 294:15–22

Chin L, Pomerantz J, Polsky D, Jacobson M, Cohen C, Cordon-Cardo C, Horner JW 2nd, DePinho RA (1997) Cooperative effects of INK4a and ras in melanoma susceptibility in vivo. Genes Dev 11:2822–2834

Chin L, Garraway LA, Fisher DE (2006) Malignant melanoma: genetics and therapeutics in the genomic era. Genes Dev 20:2149–2182

Chioni AM, Grose R (2008) Organotypic modelling as a means of investigating epithelial-stromal interactions during tumourigenesis. Fibrogenesis Tissue Repair 1:8

Clark EA, Golub TR, Lander ES, Hynes RR (2000) Genomic analysis of metastasis reveals an essential role for RhoC. Nature 406:532–535

Dankort D, Curley DP, Cartlidge RA, Nelson B, Karnezis AN, Damsky WE Jr, You MJ, DePinho RA, McMahon M, Bosenberg M (2009) Braf(V600E) cooperates with Pten loss to induce metastatic melanoma. Nat Genet 41:544–552

Das Thakur M, Salangsang F, Landman AS, Sellers WR, Pryer NK, Levesque MP, Dummer R, McMahon M, Stuart DD (2013) Modelling vemurafenib resistance in melanoma reveals a strategy to forestall drug resistance. Nature 494:251–255

Dekker SK, van Doorn R, Kempenaar J, Gruis NA, Vermeer BJ, Ponec M (2000) Skin equivalent: an attractive model to evaluate early melanoma metastasis. Melanoma Res 10:127–140

Dennhofer R, Kurschat P, Zigrino P, Klose A, Bosserhoff A, Krieg T, van Muijen G, Mauch C, Hunzelmann N (2003) Invasion of melanoma cells into dermal connective tissue in vitro: evidence for an important role of cysteine proteases. Int J Cancer 106:316–323

Dhomen N, Reis-Filho JS, Da Rocha DS, Hayward R, Savage K, Delmas V, Larue L, Pritchard C, Marais R (2009) Oncogenic Braf induces melanocyte senescence and melanoma in mice. Cancer Cell 15:294–303

Dranoff G, Jaffee E, Lazenby A, Golumbek P, Levitsky H, Brose K, Jackson V, Hamada H, Pardoll D, Mulligan RC (1993) Vaccination with irradiated tumor cells engineered to secrete murine GM-CSF stimulates potent, specific, and long-lasting tumor immunity. Proc Natl Acad Sci U S A 90:3539–3543

Einarsdottir BO, Bagge RO, Bhadury J, Jespersen H, Mattsson J, Nilsson LM, Truve K, Lopez MD, Naredi P, Nilsson O et al (2014) Melanoma patient-derived xenografts accurately model the disease and develop fast enough to guide treatment decisions. Oncotarget 5:9609–9618

Eyles J, Puaux AL, Wang X, Toh B, Prakash C, Hong M, Tan TG, Zheng L, Ong LC, Jin Y, Kato M, Prévost-Blondel A, Chow P, Yang H, Abastado JP (2010) Tumor cells disseminate early, but immunosurveillance limits metastatic outgrowth, in a mouse model of melanoma. J Clin Invest 120:2030–2039

Fidler IJ, Hart IR (1982) Biological diversity in metastatic neoplasms: origins and implications. Science 217:998–1003

Fidler IJ, Kripke ML (1977) Metastasis results from preexisting variant cells within a malignant tumor. Science 197:893–895

Fischbach C, Chen R, Matsumoto T, Schmelzle T, Brugge JS, Polverini PJ, Mooney DJ (2007) Engineering tumors with 3D scaffolds. Nat Methods 4:855–860

Frankel TL, Burns WR, Peng PD, Yu Z, Chinnasamy D, Wargo JA, Zheng Z, Restifo NP, Rosenberg SA, Morgan RA (2010) Both CD4 and CD8 T cells mediate equally effective in vivo tumor treatment when engineered with a highly avid TCR targeting tyrosinase. J Immunol 184: 5988–5998

Friedl P, Hegerfeldt Y, Tusch M (2004) Collective cell migration in morphogenesis and cancer. Int J Dev Biol 48:441–449

Friedrich J, Ebner R, Kunz-Schughart LA (2007) Experimental anti-tumor therapy in 3-D: spheroids – old hat or new challenge? Int J Radiat Biol 83:849–871

Friedrich J, Seidel C, Ebner R, Kunz-Schughart LA (2009) Spheroid-based drug screen: considerations and practical approach. Nat Protoc 4:309–324

Gallagher PG, Bao Y, Prorock A, Zigrino P, Nischt R, Politi V, Mauch C, Dragulev B, Fox JW (2005) Gene expression profiling reveals cross-talk between melanoma and fibroblasts: implications for host-tumor interactions in metastasis. Cancer Res 65:4134–4146

Gao H, Korn JM, Ferretti S, Monahan JE, Wang Y, Singh M, Zhang C, Schnell C, Yang G, Zhang Y et al (2015) High-throughput screening using patient-derived tumor xenografts to predict clinical trial drug response. Nat Med 21:1318–1325

Gerlach MM, Merz F, Wichmann G, Kubick C, Wittekind C, Lordick F, Dietz A, Bechmann I (2014) Slice cultures from head and neck squamous cell carcinoma: a novel test system for drug susceptibility and mechanisms of resistance. Br J Cancer 110:479–488

Ghajar CM, Suresh V, Peyton SR, Raub CB, Meyskens FL Jr, George SC, Putnam AJ (2007) A novel three-dimensional model to quantify metastatic melanoma invasion. Mol Cancer Ther 6:552–561

Ghosh MM, Boyce S, Layton C, Freedlander E, Mac NS (1997) A comparison of methodologies for the preparation of human epidermal-dermal composites. Ann Plast Surg 39:390–404

Giovanella BC, Yim SO, Morgan AC, Stehlin JS, Williams LJ (1973) Metastasis of human melanomas transplanted in "nude" mice. J Natl Cancer Inst 50:1051–1053

Girotti MR, Gremel G, Lee R, Galvani E, Rothwell D, Viros A, Mandal AK, Lim KH, Saturno G, Furney SJ et al (2016) Application of sequencing, liquid biopsies, and patient-derived xenografts for personalized medicine in melanoma. Cancer Discov 6:286–299

Gordon M (1927) The genetics of a viviparous top-minnow platypoecilus; the inheritance of two kinds of melanophores. Genetics 12:253–283

Gottfried E, Kunz-Schughart LA, Andreesen R, Kreutz M (2006) Brave little world: spheroids as an in vitro model to study tumor-immune-cell interactions. Cell Cycle 5:691–695

Griffith LG, Swartz MA (2006) Capturing complex 3D tissue physiology in vitro. Nat Rev Mol Cell Biol 7:211–224

Grinnell F (2003) Fibroblast biology in three-dimensional collagen matrices. Trends Cell Biol 13:264–269

Grivennikov SI, Greten FR, Karin M (2010) Immunity, inflammation, and cancer. Cell 140:883–899

Guerreschi P, Scalbert C, Qassemyar A, Kluza J, Ravasi L, Huglo D, Martinot-Duquennoy V, Formstecher P, Marchetti P, Mortier L (2013) Patient-derived tumor xenograft model to guide the use of BRAF inhibitors in metastatic melanoma. Melanoma Res 23:373–380

Gupta PB, Kuperwasser C, Brunet JP, Ramaswamy S, Kuo WL, Gray JW, Naber SP, Weinberg RA (2005) The melanocyte differentiation program predisposes to metastasis after neoplastic transformation. Nat Med 37:1047–1054

Hamilton G (1998) Multicellular spheroids as an in vitro tumor model. Cancer Lett 131:29–34

Harrison CA, Heaton MJ, Layton CM, Mac NS (2006) Use of an in vitro model of tissue-engineered human skin to study keratinocyte attachment and migration in the process of reepithelialization. Wound Repair Regen 14:203–209

Häussler G (1928) Über Melanombildungen bei Bastarden von Xiphophorus maculatus var. rubra. Klin Wochenschr 7:1561–1562

Hegerfeldt Y, Tusch M, Brocker EB, Friedl P (2002) Collective cell movement in primary melanoma explants: plasticity of cell-cell interaction, beta1-integrin function, and migration strategies. Cancer Res 62:2125–2130

Hendrix MJ, Seftor EA, Hess AR, Seftor RE (2003) Vasculogenic mimicry and tumour-cell plasticity: lessons from melanoma. Nat Rev Cancer 3:411–421

Hendrix MJ, Seftor EA, Seftor RE, Kasemeier-Kulesa J, Kulesa PM, Postovit LM (2007) Reprogramming metastatic tumour cells with embryonic microenvironments. Nat Rev Cancer 7:246–255

Hickman JA, Graeser R, de Hoogt R, Vidic S, Brito C, Gutekunst M, van der Kuip H, IMI PREDECT Consortium (2014) Three-dimensional models of cancer for pharmacology and cancer cell biology: capturing tumor complexity in vitro/ex vivo. Biotechnol J 9:1115–1128

Hirschhaeuser F, Menne H, Dittfeld C, West J, Mueller-Klieser W, Kunz-Schughart LA (2010) Multicellular tumor spheroids: an underestimated tool is catching up again. J Biotechnol 148:3–15

Hsu MY, Meier FE, Nesbit M, Hsu JY, Van BP, Elder DE, Herlyn M (2000) E-cadherin expression in melanoma cells restores keratinocyte-mediated growth control and down-regulates expression of invasion-related adhesion receptors. Am J Pathol 156:1515–1525

Hsu MY, Meier F, Herlyn M (2002) Melanoma development and progression: a conspiracy between tumor and host. Differentiation 70:522–536

Hudon V, Berthod F, Black AF, Damour O, Germain L, Auger FA (2003) A tissue-engineered endothelialized dermis to study the modulation of angiogenic and angiostatic molecules on capillary-like tube formation in vitro. Br J Dermatol 148:1094–1104

Ito M, Hiramatsu H, Kobayashi K, Suzue K, Kawahata M, Hioki K, Ueyama Y, Koyanagi Y, Sugamura K, Tsuji K, Heike T, Nakahata T (2002) NOD/SCID/γc null mouse: an excellent recipient mouse model for engraftment of human cells. Blood 100:3175–3182

Javaherian A, Vaccariello M, Fusenig NE, Garlick JA (1998) Normal keratinocytes suppress early stages of neoplastic progression in stratified epithelium. Cancer Res 58:2200–2208

Johnson JI, Decker S, Zaharevitz D, Rubinstein LV, Venditti JM, Schepartz S, Kalyandrug S, Christian M, Arbuck S, Hollingshead M, Sausville EA (2001) Relationships between drug activity in NCI preclinical in vitro and in vivo models and early clinical trials. Br J Cancer 84:1424–1431

Juhasz Albelda SM, Elder DE, Murphy GF, Adachi K, Herlyn D, Valyi-Nagy IT, Herlyn M (1993) Growth and invasion of human melanomas in human skin grafted to immunodeficient mice. Am J Pathol 142:528–537

Kelm JM, Timmins NE, Brown CJ, Fussenegger M, Nielsen LK (2003) Method for generation of homogeneous multicellular tumor spheroids applicable to a wide variety of cell types. Biotechnol Bioeng 83:173–180

Kemper K, Krijgsman O, Cornelissen-Steijger P, Shahrabi A, Weeber F, Song JY, Kuilman T, Vis DJ, Wessels LF, Voest EE et al (2015) Intra- and inter-tumor heterogeneity in a vemurafenib-resistant melanoma patient and derived xenografts. EMBO Mol Med 7:1104–1118

Kohlmeyer J, Cron M, Landsberg J, Bald T, Renn M, Mikus S, Bondong S, Wikasari D, Gaffal E, Hartmann G, Tüting T (2009) Complete regression of advanced primary and metastatic mouse melanomas following combination chemoimmunotherapy. Cancer Res 69:6265–6274

Konur A, Kreutz M, Knuchel R, Krause SW, Andreesen R (1996) Three-dimensional co-culture of human monocytes and macrophages with tumor cells: analysis of macrophage differentiation and activation. Int J Cancer 66:645–652

Kosswig C (1928) Über Kreuzungen zwischen den Teleostiern Xiphophorus helleri und Platypoecilus maculatus. Z Indukt Abstammungs-Vererbungsl 47:150–158

Kozlowski JM, Fidler IJ, Campbell D, Xu Z, Kaighn M-E, Hart IJ (1984) Metastatic behavior of human tumor cell lines grown in the nude mouse. Cancer Res 44:3522–3529

Kudo-Saito C, Shirako H, Takeuchi T, Kawakami Y (2009) Cancer metastasis is accelerated through immunosuppression during snail-induced EMT of cancer cells. Cancer Cell 15: 195–206

Kung AL (2007) Practices and pitfalls of mouse cancer models in drug discovery. Adv Cancer Res 96:191–212

Kunz-Schughart LA, Freyer JP, Hofstaedter F, Ebner R (2004) The use of 3-D cultures for high-throughput screening: the multicellular spheroid model. J Biomol Screen 9:273–285

Landsberg J, Gaffal E, Cron M, Kohlmeyer J, Renn M, Tüting T (2010) Autochthonous primary and metastatic melanomas in Hgf-Cdk4^{R24C} mice evade T cell-mediated immune surveillance. Pigment Cell Melanoma Res 23:649–660

Landsberg J, Kohlmeyer J, Renn M, Bald T, Rogava M, Cron M, Fatho M, Lennerz V, Wölfel T, Hölzel H, Tüting T (2012) Melanomas resist T-cell therapy through inflammation-induced reversible dedifferentiation. Nature 490:412–416

Larue L, Beerman F (2008) Cutaneous melanoma in genetically modified animals. Pigment Cell Melanoma Res 20:485–497

Le MN, Chan JL, Rosenberg SA, Nabatian AS, Merrigan KT, Cohen-Solal KA, Goydos JS (2010) The glutamate release inhibitor Riluzole decreases migration, invasion, and proliferation of melanoma cells. J Invest Dermatol 130:2240–2249

Li G, Satyamoorthy K, Meier F, Berking C, Bogenrieder T, Herlyn M (2003) Function and regulation of melanoma-stromal fibroblast interactions: when seeds meet soil. Oncogene 22:3162–3171

Li G, Fukunaga M, Herlyn M (2004) Reversal of melanocytic malignancy by keratinocytes is an E-cadherin-mediated process overriding beta-catenin signaling. Exp Cell Res 297:142–151

Lin RZ, Chang HY (2008) Recent advances in three-dimensional multicellular spheroid culture for biomedical research. Biotechnol J 3:1172–1184

Loffek S, Zigrino P, Angel P, Anwald B, Krieg T, Mauch C (2005) High invasive melanoma cells induce matrix metalloproteinase-1 synthesis in fibroblasts by interleukin-1alpha and basic fibroblast growth factor-mediated mechanisms. J Invest Dermatol 124:638–643

Maniotis AJ, Folberg R, Hess A, Seftor EA, Gardner LM, Pe'er J, Trent JM, Meltzer PS, Hendrix MJ (1999) Vascular channel formation by human melanoma cells in vivo and in vitro: vasculogenic mimicry. Am J Pathol 155:739–752

Massoumi R, Kuphal S, Hellerbrand C, Haas B, Wild P, Spruss T, Pfeifer A, Fässler R, Bosserhoff AK (2009) Down-regulation of CYLD expression by Snail promotes tumor progression in malignant melanoma. J Exp Med 206:221–232

Masters JR (2000) Human cancer cell lines: fact and fantasy. Nat Rev Mol Cell Biol 1:233–236

Mayordomo JI, Zorina T, Storkus WJ, Zitvogel L, Celluzzi C, Falo LD, Melief CJ, Ildstad ST, Kast WM, Deleo AB et al (1995) Bone marrow-derived dendritic cells pulsed with synthetic tumour peptides elicit protective and therapeutic antitumour immunity. Nat Med 1:1297–1302

Meier F, Nesbit M, Hsu MY, Martin B, Van BP, Elder DE, Schaumburg-Lever G, Garbe C, Walz TM, Donatien P, Crombleholme TM, Herlyn M (2000) Human melanoma progression in skin reconstructs: biological significance of bFGF. Am J Pathol 156:193–200

Meier F, Caroli U, Satyamoorthy K, Schittek B, Bauer J, Berking C, Moller H, Maczey E, Rassner G, Herlyn M, Garbe C (2003) Fibroblast growth factor-2 but not Mel-CAM and/or beta3 integrin promotes progression of melanocytes to melanoma. Exp Dermatol 12:296–306

Mintz B, Silvers WK (1993) Transgenic mouse model of malignant skin melanoma. Proc Natl Acad Sci U S A 90:8817–8821

Mueller MM, Fusenig NE (2004) Friends or foes – bipolar effects of the tumour stroma in cancer. Nat Rev Cancer 4:839–849

Mueller-Klieser W (1997) Three-dimensional cell cultures: from molecular mechanisms to clinical applications. Am J Physiol 273:C1109–C1123

Na YR, Seok SH, Kim DJ, Han JH, Kim TH, Jung H, Park JH (2009) Zebrafish embryo extracts promote sphere-forming abilities of human melanoma cell line. Cancer Sci 100:1429–1433

Noonan FP, Recio JA, Takayama H, Duray P, Anver MR, Rush WL, De Fabo EC, Merlino G (2001) Neonatal sunburn and melanoma in mice. Nature 413:271–272
Ntayi C, Hornebeck W, Bernard P (2003) Influence of cultured dermal fibroblasts on human melanoma cell proliferation, matrix metalloproteinase-2 (MMP-2) expression and invasion in vitro. Arch Dermatol Res 295:236–241
Overwijk WW, Theoret MR, Finkelstein SE, Surman DR, de Jong LA, Vyth-Dreese FA, Dellemijn TA, Antony PA, Spiess PJ, Palmer DC, Heimann DM, Klebanoff CA et al (2003) Tumor regression and autoimmunity after reversal of a functionally tolerant state of self-reactive CD8+ T cells. J Exp Med 198:569–580
Paget G (1889) Remarks on a case of alternate partial anaesthesia. Br Med J 1:1–3
Pampaloni F, Reynaud EG, Stelzer EH (2007) The third dimension bridges the gap between cell culture and live tissue. Nat Rev Mol Cell Biol 8:839–845
Parenteau NL, Bilbo P, Nolte CJ, Mason VS, Rosenberg M (1992) The organotypic culture of human skin keratinocytes and fibroblasts to achieve form and function. Cytotechnology 9:163–171
Poeck H, Besch R, Maihoefer C, Renn M, Tormo D, Morskaya SS, Kirschnek S, Gaffal E, Landsberg J, Hellmuth J, Schmidt A, Anz D et al (2008) 5′-Triphosphate-siRNA: turning gene silencing and Rig-I activation against melanoma. Nat Med 14:1256–1263
Pollock PM, Cohen-Solal K, Sood R, Namkoong J, Martino JJ, Koganti A, Zhu H, Robbins C, Makalowska I, Shin SS et al (2003) Melanoma mouse model implicates metabotropic glutamate signaling in melanocytic neoplasia. Nat Genet 34:108–112
Quintana E et al (2008) Efficient tumour formation by single human melanoma cells. Nature 456:593–598
Rangarajan A, Hong SJ, Gifford A, Weinberg RA (2004) Species- and cell type-specific requirements for cellular transformation. Cancer Cell 6:171–183
Roesch A, Fukunaga-Kalabis M, Schmidt EC, Zabierowski SE, Brafford PA, Vultur A, Basu D, Gimotty P, Vogt T, Herlyn M (2010) A temporarily distinct subpopulation of slow-cycling melanoma cells is required for continuous tumor growth. Cell 141:583–594
Rygaard J, Povlsen CO (1969) Heterotransplantation of a human malignant tumor to nude mice. Acta Pathol Microbiol Scand 77:758–760
Sahota PS, Burn JL, Heaton M, Freedlander E, Suvarna SK, Brown NJ, Mac NS (2003) Development of a reconstructed human skin model for angiogenesis. Wound Repair Regen 11:275–284
Satyamoorthy K, Meier F, Hsu MY, Berking C, Herlyn M (1999) Human xenografts, human skin and skin reconstructs for studies in melanoma development and progression. Cancer Metastasis Rev 18:401–405
Schatton T, Murphy GF, Frank NY, Yamaura K, Waaga-Gasser AM, Gasser M, Zhan Q, Jordan S, Duncan LM, Weishaupt C, Fuhlbrigge RC, Kupper TS, Sayegh MH, Frank MH (2008) Identification of cells initiating human melanomas. Nature 451:345–349
Schiffner S, Chen S, Becker JC, Bosserhoff AK (2012) Highly pigmented Tg(Grm1) mouse melanoma develops non-pigmented melanoma cells in distant metastases. Exp Dermatol 21: 786–788
Schiffner S, Braunger BM, de Jel MM, Coupland SE, Tamm ER, Bosserhoff AK (2014) Tg(Grm1) transgenic mice: a murine model that mimics spontaneous uveal melanoma in humans? Exp Eye Res 127:59–68
Scuderi N, Onesti MG, Bistoni G, Ceccarelli S, Rotolo S, Angeloni A, Marchese C (2008) The clinical application of autologous bioengineered skin based on a hyaluronic acid scaffold. Biomaterials 29:1620–1629
Seaman WE, Blackman MA, Gindhart TD, Roubinia JR, Loeb JM, Povlsen CO, Jacobsen GK (1975) Chemotherapy of a human malignant melanoma transplanted in the nude mouse. Cancer Res 35:2790–2796
Shields JD, Kourtis IC, Tomei AA, Roberts JM, Swartz MA (2010) Induction of lymphoidlike stroma and immune escape by tumors that express the chemokine CCL21. Science 328:749–752

Shih IM, Elder DE, Hsu MY, Herlyn M (1994) Regulation of Mel-CAM/MUC18 expression on melanocytes of different stages of tumor progression by normal keratinocytes. Am J Pathol 145:837–845

Shin SS, Namkoong J, Wall BA, Gleason R, Lee HJ, Chen S (2008) Oncogenic activities of metabotropic glutamate receptor 1 (Grm1) in melanocyte transformation. Pigment Cell Melanoma Res 21:368–378

Sinnberg T, Menzel M, Kaesler S, Biedermann T, Sauer B, Nahnsen S, Schwarz M, Garbe C, Schittek B (2010) Suppression of casein kinase 1alpha in melanoma cells induces a switch in beta-catenin signaling to promote metastasis. Cancer Res 70:6999–7009

Smalley KS, Lioni M, Herlyn M (2005) Targeting the stromal fibroblasts: a novel approach to melanoma therapy. Expert Rev Anticancer Ther 5:1069–1078

Smalley KS, Haass NK, Brafford PA, Lioni M, Flaherty KT, Herlyn M (2006a) Multiple signaling pathways must be targeted to overcome drug resistance in cell lines derived from melanoma metastases. Mol Cancer Ther 5:1136–1144

Smalley KS, Lioni M, Herlyn M (2006b) Life isn't flat: taking cancer biology to the next dimension. In Vitro Cell Dev Biol Anim 42:242–247

Smit NP, Westerhof W, Smit W, Nanninga B, Pavel S (1995) Some aspects of melanin formation of melanocytes cultured on collagen-coated microcarrier beads. Pigment Cell Res 8:89–96

Soudja SM, Wehbe M, Mas A, Chasson L, de Tenbossche CP, Huijbers I, Van den EB, Schmitt-Verhulst AM (2010) Tumor-initiated inflammation overrides protective adaptive immunity in an induced melanoma model in mice. Cancer Res 70:3515–3525

Steitz J, Bruck J, Steinbrink K, Enk A, Knop J, Tüting T (2000) Genetic immunization of mice with human tyrosinase-related protein 2: implications for the immunotherapy of melanoma. Int J Cancer 86:89–94

Steitz J, Bruck J, Lenz J, Knop J, Tüting T (2001) Depletion of CD25(+) CD4(+) T cells and treatment with tyrosinase-related protein 2-transduced dendritic cells enhance the interferon alpha-induced, CD8(+) T-cell-dependent immune defense of B16 melanoma. Cancer Res 61:8643–8646

Sutherland RM, McCredie JA, Inch WR (1971) Growth of multicell spheroids in tissue culture as a model of nodular carcinomas. J Natl Cancer Inst 46:113–120

Teicher BA (2006) Tumor models for efficacy determination. Mol Cancer Ther 5:2435–2443

Timmins NE, Nielsen LK (2007) Generation of multicellular tumor spheroids by the hanging-drop method. Methods Mol Med 140:141–151

Tormo D, Ferrer A, Bosch P, Gaffal E, Basner-Tschakarjan E, Wenzel J, Tüting T (2006a) Therapeutic efficacy of antigen-specific vaccination and toll-like receptor stimulation against established transplanted and autochthonous melanoma in mice. Cancer Res 66:5427–5435

Tormo D, Ferrer A, Gaffal E, Wenzel J, Basner-Tschakarjan E, Steitz J, Heukamp LC, Gutgemann I, Buettner R, Malumbres M, Barbacid M, Merlino G et al (2006b) Rapid growth of invasive metastatic melanoma in carcinogen-treated hepatocyte growth factor/scatter factor-transgenic mice carrying an oncogenic CDK4 mutation. Am J Pathol 169:665–672

Tüting T, Steitz J, Bruck J, Gambotto A, Steinbrink K, Deleo AB, Robbins P, Knop J, Enk AH (1999) Dendritic cell-based genetic immunization in mice with a recombinant adenovirus encoding murine TRP2 induces effective anti-melanoma immunity. J Gene Med 1:400–406

Valyi-Nagy IT, Hirka G, Jensen PJ, Shih IM, Juhasz I, Herlyn M (1993) Undifferentiated keratinocytes control growth, morphology, and antigen expression of normal melanocytes through cell-cell contact. Lab Invest 69:152–159

Van der Weyden L, Patton EE, Wood GA, Foote AK, Brenn T, Arends MJ, Adams DJ (2016) Cross-species models of human melanoma. J Pathol 238:152–165

Van Kilsdonk JW, Bergers M, Van Kempen LC, Schalkwijk J, Swart GW (2010) Keratinocytes drive melanoma invasion in a reconstructed skin model. Melanoma Res 20:372–380

Velazquez OC, Snyder R, Liu ZJ, Fairman RM, Herlyn M (2002) Fibroblast-dependent differentiation of human microvascular endothelial cells into capillary-like 3-dimensional networks. FASEB J 16:1316–1318

Voskoglou-Nomikos T, Pater JL, Seymour L (2003) Clinical predictive value of the in vitro cell line, human xenograft, and mouse allograft preclinical cancer models. Clin Cancer Res 9:4227–4239
Whalen GF, Gordon C, Yeshion C, Juers D, Yurt R (1994) Influence of a lymph node environment on invasiveness of metastatic tumor cells. J Am Coll Surg 179:145–150
Wu LY, Di CD, Lee LP (2008) Microfluidic self-assembly of tumor spheroids for anticancer drug discovery. Biomed Microdevices 10:197–202
Xie Y, Akpinarli A, Maris C, Hipkiss EL, Lane M, Kwon EK, Muranski P, Restifo NP, Antony PA (2010) Naive tumor-specific CD4(+) T cells differentiated in vivo eradicate established melanoma. J Exp Med 207:651–667
Yamada KM, Cukierman E (2007) Modeling tissue morphogenesis and cancer in 3D. Cell 130:601–610
Yang J, Splittgerber R, Yull FE, Kantrow S, Ayers GD, Karin M, Richmond A (2010a) Conditional ablation of Ikkb inhibits melanoma tumor development in mice. J Clin Invest 120:2563–2574
Yang H, Higgins B, Kolinsky K, Packman K, Go Z, Iyer R, Kolis S, Zhao S, Lee R, Grippo JF, Schostack K, Simcox ME, Heimbrook D, Bollag G, Su F (2010b) RG7204 (PLX4032), a selective BRAFV600E inhibitor, displays potent antitumor activity in preclinical melanoma models. Cancer Res 70:5518–5527
Yuhas JM, Li AP, Martinez AO, Ladman AJ (1977) A simplified method for production and growth of multicellular tumor spheroids. Cancer Res 37:3639–3643
Zaidi MR, Chi-Ping D, Merlino G (2008) From UVs to metastases: modeling melanoma initiation and progression in the mouse. J Invest Dermatol 128:2381–2391
Zhang T, Somasundaram R, Berencsi K, Caputo L, Gimotty P, Rani P, Guerry D, Swoboda R, Herlyn D (2006) Migration of cytotoxic T lymphocytes toward melanoma cells in three-dimensional organotypic culture is dependent on CCL2 and CCR4. Eur J Immunol 36: 457–467
Zhang Y, Cai X, Choi SW, Kim C, Wang LV, Xia Y (2010) Chronic label-free volumetric photoacoustic microscopy of melanoma cells in three-dimensional porous scaffolds. Biomaterials 31:8651–8658

New Approaches to Signaling

16

Ryan J. Sullivan and Keith T. Flaherty

16.1 New Therapeutic Approaches in Signaling

16.1.1 Introduction

The emergence of selective BRAF inhibitors for the treatment of metastatic melanoma changed the therapeutic landscape of this disease. For decades, the melanoma field lagged others in achieving significant alteration in the natural history of metastatic disease with conventional cytotoxic chemotherapy. However, with the emergence of immune checkpoint inhibitor therapy, in particular anti-programmed death 1 (PD1) and anti-PD ligand 1 (PD-L1), monoclonal antibodies alone or in combination with the anti-cytotoxic T-lymphocyte antigen 4 (CTLA4), and the development of combined BRAF/MEK inhibitor therapy, the treatment landscape has dramatically changed. Still, the majority of patients will still die from this disease, and optimizing treatment of metastatic melanoma remains a critical need. It is hoped that the discovery of somatic genetic alterations in signal transduction pathways that regulate proliferation, cell cycle, differentiation, and survival will provide further opportunities for expanding the reach of targeted therapy (Table 16.1).

R.J. Sullivan, MD • K.T. Flaherty, MD (✉)
Harvard Medical School, Massachusetts General Hospital Cancer Center,
55 Fruit Street, Boston, MA 02114, USA
e-mail: kflaherty@partners.org

A. Bosserhoff (ed.), *Melanoma Development*,
DOI 10.1007/978-3-319-41319-8_16

Table 16.1 Oncogenes and tumor suppressor genes in melanoma and therapeutic strategies

Oncogene	Pathway	Drug targeting strategy
BRAF	MAP kinase	Direct, ATP competitive kinase inhibitors Downstream, allosteric MEK inhibitors
NRAS	RAS	Combinations targeting RAS effecter pathways
C-KIT	RAS	Direct, ATP competitive kinase inhibitors
AKT3	PI3 kinase	Direct, allosteric AKT inhibitors
Cyclin D	P16/Rb	Indirect, ATP competitive CDK4 inhibitors
CDK4	P16/Rb	Direct, ATP competitive kinase inhibitors
GNAQ/GNA11	G-protein coupled receptors	Indirect, PKC, MAP kinase, PI3 kinase pathway inhibitors

Tumor suppressor gene	Pathway	Drug targeting strategy
NF1	RAS	Combinations targeting RAS effecter pathways
PTEN	PI3 kinase	PI3K, AKT, mTOR inhibitors
P16	P16/Rb	Indirect, ATP competitive CDK4 inhibitors
BAP1	Polycomb repressive complex 1	Indirect, histone deacetylase inhibitors

16.2 Oncogenes Amenable to Direct Targeting

16.2.1 TCGA and the MAP Kinase Pathway

The Cancer Genome Atlas (TCGA) in melanoma recently reported its first comprehensive profiling using whole exome sequencing (WES), RNA sequencing (RNA Seq), and proteomics from 331 patients with cutaneous melanoma (Cancer Genome Atlas 2015). The most important conclusions from this work were that four subsets of melanoma patients were defined based on the driving mutation (BRAF, NRAS, NF1, and triple wild-type) and that the great majority of tumors activate the mitogen-activated protein kinase (MAPK) pathway through oncogene (BRAF, NRAS, MEK1/2) or tumor suppressor gene mutation (NF1) mutations and/or at the gene expression level. These findings confirm that the most important targets of small molecule inhibitor therapy in melanoma are the mediators of the MAPK pathway. However, a deeper look at the data suggests that other key regulators of cancer biology are also potential targets, including the phosphoinositol-3-kinase (PI3K) pathway, the cell cycle regulation mediators cyclin D (CCND1) and cyclin-dependent kinase 4 (CDK4), regulators of apoptosis such as mouse double minute 2 homolog (MDM2) and B-cell lymphoma 2 (BCL2) family members, and even epigenetic regulators.

16.2.2 The Development of BRAF Inhibitors in Melanoma

The identification of activating mutations in the searing threonine kinase, BRAF, in 50–60 % of melanomas in 2002 was the watershed event that opened the door for investigations of molecularly targeted therapy in melanoma (Davies et al. 2002). BRAF is a constituent of the long-studied MAP kinase pathway, a known mediator of growth factor signals in cancer (also refer to Chap. 7 (Fisher)). However, prior to the identification of BRAF mutations, only RAS mutations were known to constrictively activate the pathway in a subset of cancers, including melanoma (Albino et al. 1984). Therefore, when BRAF mutations were screened for in a large series of diverse tumor types, and found, it was immediately apparent that these mutations might underlie the biologic importance of this pathway in 7–8 % of all cancers (Davies et al. 2002). The fundamental challenges that confronted the field were (1) understanding the potential vulnerability of BRAF inhibition despite the presence of numerous additional genetic alterations in the same tumors and (2) the development of potent and selective inhibitors.

In the immediate years following the identification of BRAF mutations, sorafenib was the only targeted therapy in clinical development known to have some capacity for inhibiting RAF kinases including BRAF (Wilhelm et al. 2006). Laboratory evidence suggested that sorafenib was able to have a cytotoxic effect on melanoma cell lines; however, this effect did not seem to depend on the presence or absence of BRAF mutations (Whittaker et al. 2010). This lack of cellular selectivity suggested the possibility that BRAF might be the important point of intervention even in tumors that lacked a RAF mutation. However, it was also known that non-pharmacologic methods for limiting the production of BRAF protein only impacted the growth and survival of melanoma cell lines with a BRAF mutation (Hingorani et al. 2003; Wellbrock et al. 2004). Clinical trials were rapidly designed and executed even before significant preclinical testing had occurred. Early in clinical testing, it was revealed that sorafenib was not associated with tumor regression when administered as a single-agent and only modestly inhibited the MAP kinase pathway in tumors analyzed during the first few weeks of therapy (Flaherty et al. 2005). Still, two large Phase III trials were opened evaluating the combination of chemotherapy (carboplatin and paclitaxel) with or without sorafenib, both in the front-line and second-line setting. These trials both showed no benefit of adding sorafenib to chemotherapy and successfully ended the era of non-specific inhibitors of RAF in patients with metastatic melanoma (Hauschild et al. 2009; Flaherty et al. 2013). This did, however, leave open the possibility that more potent and selective BRAF inhibitors might yield superior molecular effects as well as evidence of clinical efficacy.

Several BRAF inhibitors subsequently entered clinical trials that were developed and optimized in preclinical tumor models that harbor BRAF mutations. The most successful of these were agents are highly selective for BRAF. In fact, three selective BRAF inhibitors (vemurafenib, dabrafenib, and encorafenib) have emerged from

Phase I clinical trials and demonstrated clear antitumor activity (Flaherty et al. 2010; Kefford et al. 2010; Dummer et al. 2013). Further, both vemurafenib and dabrafenib have been shown, in randomized Phase III trials, to be superior to chemotherapy in patients with advanced (unresectable Stage III or Stage IV) melanoma harboring $BRAF^{V600E}$ or $BRAF^{V600K}$ mutations. Specifically, in the BRIM3 study, 675 patients with $BRAF^{V600E/K}$ mutations were randomized 1:1 to receive vemurafenib or dacarbazine (DTIC) (Chapman et al. 2011). The initial primary endpoint was overall survival; however, at the first interim analysis, the trial design was changed to use a composite endpoint of OS and progression-free survival (PFS) and allow for crossover from DTIC to vemurafenib at the time of progression. The initial analysis demonstrated the superiority of vemurafenib versus DTIC with respect to response rate (48 % vs 5 %), PFS (hazard ratio [HR] 0.26; 95 % confidence interval [CI] 0.20–0.33, p value < 0.001), and OS (HR 0.37, 95 % CI 0.26–0.55, $p < 0.001$). Similarly, in the BREAK3 study, 250 patients with advanced BRAFV600E/K mutant melanoma were randomized to receive either dabrafenib or DTIC; though as opposed to the BRIM3 study, patients were randomized at 3:1 to receive dabrafenib, patients were allowed to cross over from DTIC to dabrafenib from the beginning, and the primary endpoint was PFS (Hauschild et al. 2012). Not surprisingly, patients randomized to dabrafenib had superior outcomes to those randomized to DTIC and specifically had improved PFS (HR 0.30, 95 % CI 0.18–0.51, $p < 0.0001$) and RR (50 % vs 4 %). Based on the data from BRIM3 and BREAK3, the United States Food and Drug Administration (FDA) approved vemurafenib in 2011 and dabrafenib in 2013.

The efficacy of the BRAF inhibitors vemurafenib and dabrafenib were unprecedented and balanced by a favorable toxicity profile (Chapman et al. 2011; Flaherty et al. 2010; Hauschild et al. 2012; Sosman et al. 2012; Falchook et al. 2012). With that said, a number of toxicities are seen with therapy including those commonly seen with small molecule inhibitors such as nausea, diarrhea, and fatigue to those quite specific for BRAF inhibitors including hyperkeratosis, palmar–plantar erythema, arthralgia, and squamous cell carcinomas of the skin (cuSCC). These latter adverse effects have since been determined to be related to paradoxical upregulation of the pathway in tissues that are dependent on MAPK pathway signaling (Oberholzer et al. 2012; Su et al. 2012; Heidorn et al. 2010; Poulikakos et al. 2010). This occurs through the interaction of the BRAF inhibitor with wild-type BRAF in these cells that triggers a conformational change in BRAF that leads to robust homo- and hetero-dimerization with RAF isoforms and subsequent pathway activation (Poulikakos et al. 2010; Heidorn et al. 2010). This is best understood in the setting of cuSCC, where an upstream mutation in HRAS has been seen in the majority of these cases (Oberholzer et al. 2012; Su et al. 2012).

16.2.3 Building upon BRAF Inhibition and the Development of MEK Inhibitor Therapy in BRAF Mutant Melanoma

In tumor biopsy samples initially collected from patients treated with vemurafenib and dabrafenib, some degree of residual MAP kinase pathway activity persists even when patients are administered maximum tolerated doses. Similarly, residual ERK activity can be detected in vitro when BRAF mutant cell lines are treated with high concentrations of the tool compound, PLX4720 (Paraiso et al. 2010). So, even before turning to combination regimens, it was felt that that there may be value in finding agents that inhibit the MAPK pathway at distinct points. MEK inhibitors were developed in BRAF mutant melanoma for this express purpose. The first such inhibitor to be evaluated was trametinib, which quickly was developed from Phase I trials to a randomized Phase III trial in patients with advanced $BRAF^{V600E/K}$ mutant melanoma. In the METRIC study, 322 patients were randomized on a 2:1 ratio to receive either trametinib or chemotherapy (single agent DTIC or paclitaxel) (Flaherty et al. 2012b). The trial met its primary endpoint of improved overall survival (HR 0.54, 95 % CI 0.32–0.92, $p=0.01$), as well as secondary endpoints of improved PFS (HR 0.45, 95 % CI 0.33–0.63, $p<0.001$) and RR (22 % compared to 9 %). Additionally, trametinib was well tolerated with most common toxicities, which were related to inhibition of the MAPK pathway in normal tissues, such as acneiform rash, diarrhea, fatigue, peripheral edema, nausea, and hypertension with rare toxicities including reduced ejection fraction and ophthalmologic effects such as central serous retinopathy and, less commonly, retinal vein thrombosis. Based on these data, the FDA approved trametinib for the treatment of advanced $BRAF^{V600E/K}$ melanoma in 2013.

With the FDA approval of BRAF inhibitors (vemurafenib and dabrafenib) and a MEK inhibitor (trametinib), an important issue that arose was how to use these types of drugs in relation to the other. For example, would sequencing or combination of BRAF and MEK inhibitors be more effective and if combination were effective, would it be tolerable. To address this issue, it is important to understand the status of the MAPK pathway at the time of resistance to BRAF inhibitors. For example, if the MAPK pathway were active at the time of BRAF inhibitor resistance, than perhaps targeting the pathway downstream might be a useful endeavor, whereas if the pathway were not reactivated, targeting alternative pathways rather than the MAPK pathway would likely be more fruitful. Over the years, following the availability of BRAF inhibitors on clinical trials and commercially, a number of mechanisms of resistance have been identified including adaptive changes in receptor tyrosine kinase activity (AXL, IGFR1, PDGFR, etc.) and genetic aberrations that lead to MAPK pathway reactivation and/or upregulation of other pro-survival signaling pathways including the phosphoinositide-3-kinase (PI3K) pathway (Montagut et al. 2008; Smalley et al. 2008; Emery et al. 2009; Johannessen et al. 2010; Nazarian et al. 2010; Paraiso et al. 2010, 2011; Villanueva et al. 2010; Poulikakos et al. 2011; Shi et al. 2012; Wilson et al. 2012). Importantly, reactivation of the MAPK pathway, through a multitude of mechanisms (including upstream RAS mutation, BRAF amplification, alternative splicing of BRAF, and downstream MEK1/2 mutations), occurs in up to 70 % of cases, though nearly 20 % of the time both MAPK and PI3K activation is seen (Shi et al. 2014; Van Allen et al. 2014). These data predict that effective, downstream inhibition of the MAPK pathway after BRAF inhibitor therapy would be an effective therapy in most patients with BRAF inhibitor-resistant, BRAF mutant melanoma.

To test the hypothesis that downstream MAPK pathway inhibition would be effective in the setting of BRAF inhibitor resistance, a Phase II trial of trametinib following BRAF inhibitor therapy was performed in patients with BRAF mutant melanoma who had either received prior BRAF inhibitor therapy (Cohort A) or had not received prior BRAF inhibitor therapy but had been treated with chemotherapy or immune therapy (Cohort B) (Kim et al. 2013). In Cohort A, no responses were seen in any of the 40 patients treated, and the median PFS was 1.8 months. In Cohort B, responses were seen in 25 % of the 57 patients enrolled and the median PFS was 4 months, which was similar to the data for patients treated in the METRIC study. The conclusion from this trial is that MEK inhibitor therapy, in this case trametinib, is not effective in patients with BRAF mutant melanoma who have previously received BRAF inhibitor therapy.

The next issue to be addressed was whether combined BRAF and MEK inhibitor therapy would be tolerable and effective. It was hoped that such a combination would suppress MAPK signaling to even greater degrees than are achievable with either agent alone. Additionally, it was hypothesized that the co-administration of a MEK inhibitor with a selective BRAF inhibitor would counter the paradoxical upregulation of the MAPK pathway that occurs in normal tissues following selective BRAF inhibitor therapy. Thus, it was thought that the consequence of dual BRAF and MEK blockade may be less toxicity, whereas the prediction is for most combination regimens to engender greater toxicity. The first such trial was the combination of dabrafenib and trametinib, which in a Phase I/II trial, was shown to be tolerable at the maximum tolerable dose (MTD) levels of each individual drug and was associated with high response rates (~70 %) and median PFS in excess of 9 months (Flaherty et al. 2012a). Two additional BRAF/MEK combinations have shown to be tolerable and effective, vemurafenib and combimetinib (MEK inhibitor), and encorafenib and binimetinib (MEK inhibitor) (Ribas et al. 2014; Sullivan et al. 2015b). In all three combinations, the rate of symptoms thought to be related to paradoxical activation of MAPK pathway in non-BRAF mutant cells by the BRAF inhibitors were abrogated by the MEK inhibitor. Specifically, the rate of hyperkeratosis, palmar–plantar erythema, and cuSCC are greatly reduced in the combination compared to single-agent BRAF inhibitors.

More recently, three Phase III trials have been completed showing the superiority of the combination of BRAF/MEK inhibitor therapy to single-agent BRAF inhibitors. In COMBI-d, 423 patients with previously untreated and advanced $BRAF^{V600E/K}$ mutant melanoma were randomized to the combination of dabrafenib and trametinib versus dabrafenib and placebo (Long et al. 2015). Patients treated with the combination had improved RR (69 % vs 53 %), PFS (median 11 months vs. 8.8 months; HR 0.67, 95 % CI 0.53–0.84, $p=0.0004$), and OS (median 25.1 months vs. 18.7 months; HR 0.71, 95 % CI 0.55–0.92, $p=0.0107$). In COMBI-v, 704 patients were randomized to either dabrafenib plus trametinib versus vemurafenib and placebo (Robert et al. 2015). Similar to COMBI-d, patients treated with the combination had superior RR (64 % vs. 51 %), PFS (median 11.4 months vs. 7.3 months; HR 0.56, 95 % CI 0.46–0.69, $p<0.001$), and OS (1 year rate 72 % vs. 65 %; HR 0.69, 95 % CI 0.53–0.89, $p=0.005$) compared to those treated with vemurafenib and placebo. The third such trial, coBRIM, compared the combination of vemurafenib plus cobimetinib versus vemurafenib plus placebo and, like the COMBI-d and COMBI-v trials, demonstrated superiority compared to vemurafenib plus placebo in RR (65 % vs. 59 %), PFS (median 12.5 months vs. 6.2 months; HR 0.58, 95 % CI 0.46–0.72), and OS (median 22.3 months vs. 17.4 months; HR 0.70, 95 % CI 0.55–0.90) (Larkin et al. 2014). A fourth trial, COLUMBUS, is ongoing and randomizing patients to encorafenib plus binimetinib, encorafenib plus placebo, and vemurafenib plus placebo (NCT01909453).

16.2.4 Adding to the BRAF/MEK Inhibitor Backbone in BRAF Mutant Melanoma

Given the myriad mechanisms of resistance to BRAF-targeted therapy in melanoma, which are often seen in the same tumor or in multiple tumors in a patient, it is hard to imagine that targeting one specific signaling pathway mediator (ERK, PI3K, AKT, etc.) will be associated with dramatic clinical benefit. Notwithstanding, targeting ERK with the ERK1/2 inhibitor BVD523 has been associated with transient responses in some patients with BRAF mutant melanoma who were previously treated with BRAF/MEK inhibitor therapy (Infante et al. 2005). While this is predictable given that the majority of patients will have reactivation of the MAPK pathway, it is also not surprising that the benefit was transient, given that multiple mechanisms are often involved. It is this pervasive heterogeneity in the mechanism of resistance to BRAF-targeted therapy that forces researchers and clinical investigators to think about alternative targets (immune system, apoptosis, oncogene chaperones, early adaptive changes to therapy) as opposed to the traditional targets, namely mediators of signal transduction pathways (e.g., PI3K pathway or MAPK pathway).

16.2.4.1 Dual BRAF and Immune Targeting

Combination of BRAF-targeted therapy with immunotherapies is an attractive approach for several reasons. First, BRAF does not appear to be an important constituent of the MAP kinase pathway in mature immune cells, including T cells (Tsukamoto et al. 2008). Second, emerging evidence suggests that inhibition of the MAPK pathway in patients with melanoma, through inhibition of BRAF and/or MEK, leads to increased melanoma antigen expression, decreased immunosuppressive cytokines, increased trafficking of CD8+ T-lymphocytes, and increased expression of programmed death 1 (PD1) and its ligand (PDL1) (Donia et al. 2012; Cooper et al. 2013; Frederick et al. 2013; Wilmott et al. 2012). Also, it has recently been shown that patients with a higher proportion of preexisting tumor-infiltrating lymphocyte clones, determined by T-cell receptor (TCR) rearrangement sequencing (so-called ImmunoSeq), have better outcomes with BRAF/MEKi therapy, although nearly all patients have an increase in TCR clonality in the setting of BRAF/MEKi therapy (Cooper et al. 2013). The major conclusion from these data is that MAPK pathway targeting enhances antitumor immunity within the tumor microenvironment, providing a strong rationale for combination of MAPK-targeted therapy with immunotherapy.

The first wave of combined BRAF-targeted therapy plus ipilimumab studies have been performed and limited by tolerability. Specifically, the vemurafenib plus ipilimumab study was closed in dose escalation when it was observed that six of the ten evaluable patients had developed grade 3 or 4 elevation of transaminases (Ribas et al. 2013). Interestingly, when dabrafenib was combined with ipilimumab, there was less hepatic toxicity, though when the triple combination of dabrafenib, trametinib, and ipilimumab was tested, two of nine patients developed bowel perforation (Puzanov et al. 2014). Based on the results of these trials, the development of ipilimumab-based targeted therapy–immunotherapy trials has been halted.

The next wave of combined targeted-immunotherapy trials has been evaluating various combinations of BRAF plus or minus MEK inhibitors with anti-PDL1 antibodies. The first such trial explored the safety and efficacy of vemurafenib plus the anti-PDL1 antibody atezolizumab. In the initial cohort, concomitant initiation of therapy was associated with excess toxicity (elevated liver enzymes, fatigue, rash); however, with employing a lead-in of 28 days to perform the combination phase of the trial, the combination has been shown to be well tolerated and associated with responses in the majority (76 %) of the 17 patients evaluable for response, including three complete responders (Hamid et al. 2015). This trial is now evaluating the triple combination of vemurafenib, cobimetinib, and atezolizumab (NCT01656642). The second trial to explore the utility of anti-PDL1 antibodies with targeted therapy is the Phase I/II trial of durvalumab with either trametinib (in BRAF wild-type patients) or dabrafenib/trametinib (in BRAF mutant patients). In the cohort of BRAF mutant patients, the response rate was 69 % (18/26 patients), with all patients having control of disease (response or stable disease) at first imaging (Ribas et al. 2015). Whether these combinations are associated with a more durable benefit rate than BRAF/MEK inhibitor therapy is unknown, but the initial results are promising that combined BRAF/MEK plus anti-PDL1 therapy is tolerable and associated with response in the great majority of patients. As durability of response will be the next clinical endpoint by which these combinations will be judged, substantially greater sample sizes and follow-up will be needed to glean the impact of these regimens.

16.2.4.2 Targeting Apoptosis

Constitutive activation of the MAPK pathway in the context of a BRAFV600 mutation is associated with a number of pro-survival consequences including inhibition of proapoptotic BCL-2 family members, inactivation of BAD, and downregulation of BIM to enhance cell survival (Boisvert-Adamo and Aplin 2008; Cartlidge et al. 2008). Preclinically, inhibition of BRAF or MEK leads to apoptosis, at least in part, through the upregulation of BIM and its inhibition of the antiapoptotic proteins BCL-2 and MCL-1 (VanBrocklin et al. 2009; Haq et al. 2013; Wroblewski et al. 2013; Frederick et al. 2014). Further, gene expression analyses of patient tumor biopsies demonstrate that treatment with either vemurafenib or dabrafenib and trametinib reduces MCL-1 mRNA levels and increases BIM mRNA and protein levels in most patients (Frederick et al. 2014). Nonetheless, the degree of apoptosis in the setting of BRAF inhibitor therapy is variable and likely attenuated by the antiapoptotic BCL-2 family members, BCL-x_L and BCL-w, both of which also increase with BRAF-directed therapy (Trunzer et al. 2013; Long et al. 2013; Frederick et al. 2014). These findings support the addition of an agent that can augment BRAF and MEK inhibitor-induced apoptosis and serves as the preliminary evidence for a Phase I/II trial of dabrafenib, trametinib, and navitoclax, a small molecule inhibitor of BCL-2, BCL-x_L, and BCL-w (NCT01989585).

Another important mechanism of promoting cell survival in melanoma is the inactivation of the tumor suppressor gene/protein, p53. While p53 is mutated in a minority of patients (~15 %), it is functionally inactivated by MDM2 or MDM4 in approximately half of patients with melanoma (Cancer Genome Atlas 2015; Gembarska et al. 2012; Ji et al. 2012; Muthusamy et al. 2006; Polsky et al. 2001). Thus, small molecule targeting of MDM2 in combination with BRAF and/or MEK inhibitors is rational and supported by preclinical evidence showing synergy of the combination in both in vitro and in vivo studies (Ji et al. 2012; Saiki et al. 2014). Based on the rationale and preclinical data, clinical trials are being developed to evaluate this combination, and one such trial is actively enrolling patients with either trametinib plus or minus dabrafenib in combination with tMDM2 inhibitor AMG232 (NCT02110355).

16.2.4.3 Targeting an Oncogenic Chaperone (Heat Shock Protein 90)

Heat shock proteins act as cellular chaperones for client proteins and facilitate cellular signaling. Heat shock protein 90 (HSP90) serves as a molecular chaperone to a number of mediators of growth factor pathways and is a potential therapeutic target in the setting of BRAF inhibitor resistance. Included among its client proteins are insulin-like growth factor 1 receptor (IGF1R), BRAF, CRAF, AKT, cyclin D, and cyclin-dependent kinase 4 (CDK4), all of which have been implicated in BRAF inhibitor resistance. Supporting this is data showing that the HSP inhibitor XL888 blocks growth and survival, in vitro and in vivo, in BRAF-mutant melanoma cell lines that harbor acquired resistance mechanisms to BRAF inhibitor including COT overexpression, platelet-derived growth factor receptor beta (PDGFR-b) overexpression, concomitant BRAF and NRAS mutations, and cyclin D amplifications. Additionally, a reduction in levels of a number of both client proteins and growth pathway mediators was seen, as was a favorable change in the pro- and antiapoptotic molecules, respectively, BIM and MCL1. Similar data also have been generated with the HSP90 inhibitor AT13387, showing activity in cell lines with BRAF inhibitor acquired-resistance mechanisms and suppression of acquired resistance in BRAF mutant melanoma cell lines in xenograft models when mice are treated with both a BRAF inhibitor and AT13387 (Smyth et al. 2014). Based on these data, clinical trials have been launched evaluating single-agent BRAF inhibition (vemurafenib) with XL888 (NCT01657591), as well as the combination of dabrafenib, trametinib, and AT13387 (NCT02097225).

16.2.5 PI3 Kinase Pathway

The PI3 kinase pathway is another RAS effecter pathway that has been implicated in the pathophysiology of numerous cancers, including melanoma. Melanomas commonly feature loss of PTEN function, a negative regulator of AKT activation by

PI3 kinase (Guldberg et al. 1997). Hemizygous and homozygous deletion appear to be the most common type of genetic alteration in PTEN in melanoma. Additionally, numerous point mutations, thought to inactivate PTEN, and thereby permitting higher PI3 kinase pathway activity, have also been described in some melanomas (Celebi et al. 2000). A point of continued controversy is whether silencing of PTEN expression by promoter hypermethylation might also be a mechanism of gene silencing in melanoma (Mirmohammadsadegh et al. 2006; Furuta et al. 2004). In any case, it is clear that a substantial subset of melanomas have genetic alterations in PTEN, and the preponderance of evidence suggests that it is the consequence of overactivity in the PI3 kinase pathway that is of pathophysiologic significance. It should be noted that numerous other cytoplasmic and nuclear sites of PTEN activity have been described, but it is unclear if any of those are important to melanoma biology (Zhang and Yu 2010). Some evidence has been produced from array comparative genome hybridization experiments to support the presence of AKT3 amplification in a distinct subset of melanomas from those that have PTEN loss, and rare activating mutations in AKT3 have been reported (Stahl et al. 2004; Davies et al. 2008). This is further genetic evidence that the PI3 kinase pathway plays a critical role in a subset of melanomas. Notably, it appears that PTEN loss is frequently seen concomitant with BRAF mutation (Tsao et al. 2004). This suggests that both of these RAS effecter pathways are needed to contribute to melanoma formation.

Experimental evidence supports a role for the PI3 kinase pathway in melanoma invasion into the dermis, and potentially in metastatic spread. In particular, the introduction of activated AKT results in the conversion from a radial growth to vertical growth phase phenotype in primary melanoma in animal models (Govindarajan et al. 2007). Conversely, restoration of PTEN expression or blockade of PI3K/AKT signaling in melanoma cells blocks invasion and induces apoptosis (Stewart et al. 2002; Ruth et al. 2006). Introduction of AKT3 into melanoma cell lines promotes proliferation and survival, whereas knockdown of AKT3 mRNA, but not AKT1 or AKT2, inhibits both phenotypes (Stahl et al. 2004). Introduction of myristylated AKT prevented the expression of proapoptotic mediators such as Bim and Bmf and knockdown of AKT3 with siRNA greatly enhances the degree of apoptosis seen in BRAF mutant cell lines treated with a selective BRAF inhibitor (Shao and Aplin 2010).

The development of therapeutic agents targeting the PI3 kinase pathway, and particularly the components within it that are critical to melanoma pathophysiology, is at a very early stage. Due to the overall prevalence of PTEN loss, activating mutations in PI3 kinase itself, and activating mutations or amplification in AKT, significant efforts have been made in the pharmaceutical industry to develop antagonists of this pathway. Three classes of PI3 kinase inhibitors have emerged in clinical development: (1) inhibitors of specific PI3 kinase isoforms, (2) agents that inhibit with near equal potency all PI3 kinase isoforms, and (3) dual inhibitors of PI3 kinase and mTOR. When considering which of these agents might be most relevant in melanoma, the deficiency in our knowledge regarding which isoform or isoforms of PI3 kinase to target becomes apparent. In lymphocytes, it appears that the catalytic subunit p110delta (the delta isoform) is the one whose activity is most markedly upregulated in the setting of PTEN deletion (Janas et al. 2008). However, in breast cancer models, it appears that PI3 beta is the most relevant isoform in mediating cell invasion in response to RAS activation (De Laurentiis et al. 2011). These observations remain to be confirmed, specifically in melanomas.

The therapeutic strategy at the level of AKT may be somewhat more straightforward based on available genetic and experimental evidence. Given that the most common activating mutations in AKT across cancers are in AKT1, the focus of pharmaceutical development has been on agents with preferential inhibitory effects on this isoform (Carpten et al. 2007). AKT2 appears to be the most critical isoform in glucose homeostasis, and therefore would be the one isoform to avoid targeting (Altomare et al. 1998). The first generation of AKT inhibitors in clinical development have fairly uniform potency against the three AKT isoforms. This may be problematic, as dose-limiting toxicity may be rendered by AKT2 inhibition, or possibly co-inhibition of all isoforms. The ideal AKT inhibitor for melanoma might be one that is relatively AKT3-specific, and such an agent has not yet been developed. In fact, the AKT inhibitor that is furthest into clinical development, MK-2206, is equally potent against AKT1 and AKT2, but fivefold less potent against AKT3 (Yap 2009). Thus, the melanoma field awaits the development of additional AKT inhibitors with more optimal properties relevant to the biology of AKT signaling in this disease.

16.2.6 Beyond BRAF: Targeting Other Molecular Subsets

16.2.6.1 NRAS Mutant Melanoma

Activating mutations in NRAS continue to be an elusive target in melanoma, more than 30 years after their initial identification (Albino et al. 1984). Approximately 25 % of all advanced melanoma cases harbor an activating mutation in and RAS, with Q61R mutation being the most common and mutations at position 12 in the amino acid sequence being the next most commonly affected (Curtin et al. 2006; Cancer Genome Atlas 2015). NRAS is not amenable to targeting with drugs of the sort that can compete with ATP binding as RAS does not consume ATP as an energy source. Rather, RAS is a GTPase, and the common mutation found in cancer impairs GTPase activity. Thus, an effective pharmacologic inhibitor of mutated ras would need to restore the lost GTPase activity, and such compounds have not been readily discovered to date. Experimental evidence demonstrating the biologic significance of RAS in melanoma stems from at siRNA knockdown experiments as well as genetically engineered models demonstrating its contribution to melanoma pathophysiology (Eskandarpour et al. 2009; Nogueira et al. 2010). More indirect evidence supporting the therapeutic potential of antagonizing RAS comes from experiments using farnesyltransferase inhibitors, which block one of the key post-translational modifications required for RAS to localize to the plasma membrane (Smalley and Eisen 2003). The introduction of mutated NRAS into melanocytes induces senescence, or transformation in the appropriate genetic background (Whitwam et al. 2007). In transgenic models, introduction of activating NRAS mutations combined with either p53 or p16 loss of function through genetic inactivation results in proliferative and invasive melanocytic lesions (Nogueira et al. 2010). In cell lines, knockdown of NRAS mRNA results in growth arrest and apoptosis selectively in melanoma cell lines that harbor activating NRAS mutations (Eskandarpour et al. 2009). At exposures that inhibit the farnesylation of many signaling molecules, farnesyltransferase inhibitors will arrest the cell cycle and induce cell death in melanoma cells that harbor NRAS mutations. Additionally, this intervention sensitizes such cells to the cytotoxic effects of chemotherapy. Unfortunately, chemical trials with farnesyltransferase inhibitors have been largely disappointing, owing to the lack of evidence of single-agent efficacy in patients with RAS-mutated cancers when these agents are administered at maximum tolerated doses (Gajewski et al. 2006). While there is some evidence that partial inhibition of RAS signaling can be achieved with these agents, it appears that the degree of innovation is insufficient to significantly perturb these tumors (Sebti and Hamilton 2000). Thus, agents with more selectivity for RAS are anxiously awaited but for the reasons noted above continue to be a major technical challenge.

An alternative strategy would be to block the downstream signal transduction pathways that are activated in the setting of RAS mutation. There are numerous RAS effecter pathways, the MAP kinase and PI3K pathways being the best described, but the relative importance of each has not been elucidated. As drug targeting of RAS effecter pathways has been a major priority in pharmaceutical development, there are numerous agents emerging targeting the MAP kinase and PI3K pathways, which might be useful for NRAS mutant melanoma. In particular, potent and selective MEK inhibitors have demonstrated single agent activity in NRAS mutant melanoma. Specifically, binimetinib was associated with responses in over 20 % of patients with metastatic, NRAS mutant melanoma, and with a median PFS of 3.7 months (Ascierto et al. 2013). While these data are not dramatic, this was a notable benefit in a previously hard-to-treat subgroup of patients and provided the justification for a randomized, Phase III trial of binimetinib versus DTIC (so-called NEMO trial). The initial findings of this trial were recently publicized as part of a press release stating that treatment with binimetinib was associated with improved PFS (median 2.8 months vs. 1.5 months; HR 0.62, 95 % CI 0.47–0.80, $p<0.0001$) compared to DTIC treatment.

The data with single-agent binimetinib is an encouraging first step, but better regimens are still needed for this patient population. One such regimen is the combination of MEK inhibitors with CDK4 inhibitors. There is ample preclinical data suggesting that cell cycle progression is a key mechanism of resistance to single-agent MEK inhibition in NRAS mutant melanoma. In patients, two trials of MEK and CDK4 inhibitors have been performed to date. The first is the combination of binimetinib with the CDK4/6 inhibitor ribociclib. In this Phase I/II trial exclusively enrolling patients with advanced NRAS mutant melanoma, the majority of patients across all dose cohorts experienced tumor regression, and responses were seen in 7 of the 22 patients enrolled, with another 11 experiencing stable disease (Van Herpen et al. 2015). The second trial evaluated the combination of trametinib plus the CDK4/6 inhibitor palbociclib. The difference with this study was that it allowed the enrollment of patients with any advanced solid tumor. In this dose escalation study, only two responses were seen (one in an NRAS mutant colon cancer patient and the other in a NRAS/BRAF/NF1 wild-type melanoma patient) among the 26 patients treated (Sullivan et al. 2015a). In eight NRAS mutant patients, one responded (the aforementioned colon cancer patient), four had stable disease, and three had progression of disease as a best response.

16.2.6.2 CDK/Cyclin/p16

Germline mutation in CDKN2A, the gene that encodes both p16 and p14, have long been known to confer susceptibility to melanoma and is the highest penetrance allele yet discovered in familial melanoma (Hussussian et al. 1994). Mutations in CDKN2A, as well as hemizygous and homozygous deletions, are also observed in sporadic cases of melanoma (Wagner et al. 1998; Fujimoto et al. 1999). The best characterized point mutations identified in familial melanoma result in a disruption of the p16/CDK4 inhibitory interaction, suggesting that this may be the critical interaction related to melanoma formation (Haferkamp et al. 2008). The net consequence of p16 loss or mutation is that CDK4 is dysinhibited and pushes cells through the cell cycle without the usual checkpoint regulation. In cases where CDKN2A is wild-type, a distinct subset of melanomas harbor cyclin D amplification (Curtin et al. 2005). Cyclin D is another binding partner for CDK4 and is a critical co-activator of CDK4 activity. Thus, cyclin D application results in overactivity of CDK4, analogous to loss of p16 function. Lastly, CDK4 itself has been found to be amplified in some cases of sporadic melanoma and to contain activating mutations in the kinase domain in another subset (Muthusamy et al. 2006). This genetic evidence would support that the CDK4 cell cycle checkpoint is a critical suppressor of melanoma formation and, conversely, its overactivity appears to contribute to melanoma pathophysiology. In vitro as well as mouse transgenic models support cooperative the between activating BRAF mutations and genetic aberrations in p16/cyclin D/CDK4 (Dhomen et al. 2009; Robinson et al. 2010). What remains to be determined is whether dual targeting of this axis combined with an inhibitor of the MAP kinase pathway, such as BRAF, will have greater therapeutic value then inhibiting either target alone.

Restoring p16 function in the setting of mutation or deletion is beyond the scope of what current pharmacologic development can achieve. Additionally, cyclin D lacks an enzymatic function against which drugs could be readily generated. That leaves CDK4, with its kinase activity, as a potentially relevant point of intervention in tumors with p16/cyclin D/CDK4 aberrations. Potent and selective CDK4 inhibitors have been developed and completed or are in the process of completing Phase I clinical trials. An example of this class of drugs is PD032991, which is an orally available CDK4/6 inhibitor (Fry et al. 2004). As one might project for a cell cycle targeted therapy, this agent produced mild to moderate–mild suppression that was reversible during planned treatment interruptions in Phase I (Schwartz et al. 2007). This agent and other CDK4 inhibitors are actively being tested clinically in patients with melanoma. It is of particular interest to evaluate the efficacy of single-agent CDK4 inhibitor therapy in patients with p16/cyclin D/CDK4 alterations, though there are no such data that have been presented or published to date. As noted above for NRAS mutant melanoma, the genetic evidence supporting CDK4 dysregulation as being critical to melanoma formation supports further clinical investigation in combination with other approaches. Now that BRAF and MEK inhibitors have established their own evidence of efficacy as single agents and in combination in BRAF mutant and NRAS mutant subtypes, the most feasible approach would be to test a combination of a selective CDK4 inhibitor with a BRAF with or without a MEK inhibitor in BRAF mutant patients (or with MEK inhibitor in NRAS mutant patients as described above). This is occurring as part of an additional dose escalation and expansion cohort in the Phase I/II trial of encorafenib plus binimetinib that was described above as well as in other trials as well (Sullivan et al. 2015b).

16.2.6.3 KIT

By the time CKIT mutations were reported in melanoma in 2006, KIT had already been validated as a therapeutic target in gastrointestinal stromal tumor (GIST) (Demetri et al. 2002). And subsequently, several second-generation KIT inhibitors established therapeutic benefit in this population as well (Fig. 16.1) (Demetri et al. 2006). However, it was not known whether the somatic genetic changes that might accompany KIT mutation in melanoma, perhaps differently than GIST, might render melanoma more or less susceptible to single-agent KIT-targeted therapy.

Imatinib was the first KIT inhibitor to demonstrate single-agent activity in GIST, and was the first agent to be evaluated clinically in melanoma (Hodi et al. 2008). In the years prior to the discovery of KIT and mutations in melanoma, three Phase II clinical trials were conducted with imatinib as a single agent in metastatic

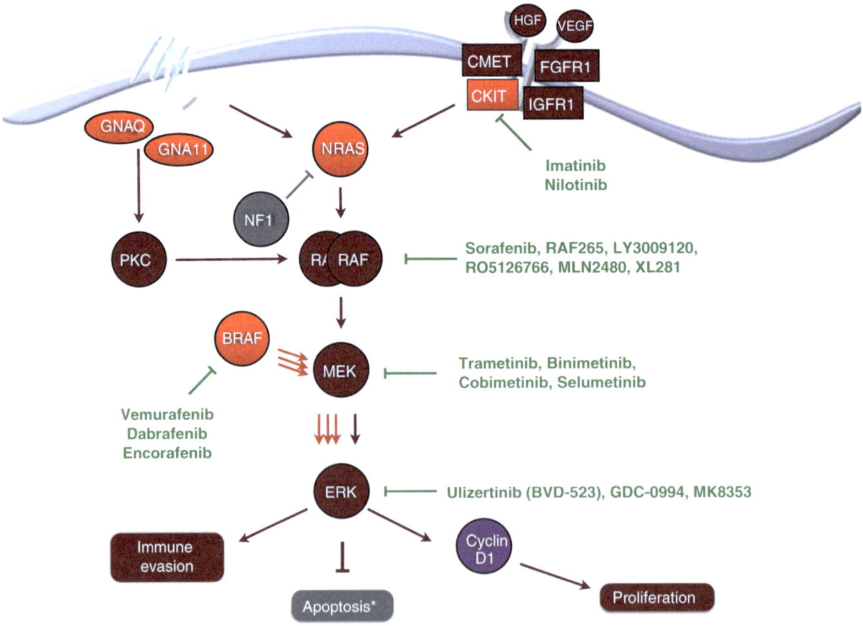

Fig. 16.1 c-KIT, RAF, and MEK inhibitors in clinical development for melanoma

melanoma (Ugurel et al. 2005; Wyman et al. 2006; Kim et al. 2008). However, nearly all of the patients enrolled on trials did not have melanoma that arose from the clinical subtypes in which KIT mutations can be found, mucosal, acral/lentiginous, and those associated with chronic sun damage. So, although KIT mutation analysis was not performed in the context of these trials, one would estimate that very few, if any, of these patients had KIT mutations. Only one patient experienced an objective response in those trials and this patient had a prior history of a mucosal melanoma primary. In addition to activating mutations in KIT, amplification has also been described, and can occur in the presence or absence of mutation. So, the hypotheses addressed in clinical trials with KIT inhibitors in melanoma are whether mutation and/or amplification might serve as predictive markers for response to these therapies. It should be noted that many of the mutations in KIT described in melanoma overlap with those previously seen in GIST. Some of these mutations have been described as imatinib-sensitive in the context of GIST, while others have not. And novel mutations in KIT have been described in some cases of melanoma as well. Thus, new questions remain to be answered in the context of KIT inhibitor trials in melanoma to understand not only whether mutations previously described as sensitive to existing drugs would be so in melanoma but also to determine if amplification or novel mutations are similarly predictive of response to therapy.

A single patient with mucosal melanoma whose tumor was found to harbor an internal tandem duplication in the juxtamembrane domain of KIT was treated with imatinib and an objective response lasting for at least several months was observed (Hodi et al. 2008). This first report established that KIT targeted therapy could be effective in melanoma.

There are now three Phase II trials with imatinib in KIT mutant or amplified melanoma that have been completed. In one of those trials, Carvajal and colleagues screened 295 patients with metastatic melanoma whose primary tumors were mucosal, acral/lentiginous, or arose from chronic sun-damaged skin (Carvajal et al. 2011). Archival tumor specimens were screened for the presence of amplification in KIT or mutations in exons 9, 11, 13, 17, and 18. A total of 51 of 295 (17 %) of these patients were found to have aberrations in KIT and 28 were treated with imatinib. Two patients experienced complete responses and two had partial responses (16 % response rate) among the 25 evaluable patients. The median time to progression was 12 weeks and median overall survival was 46.3 weeks. All of the responders had either an exon 11 or 13 mutation. In another Phase II trial, Guo and colleagues enrolled 43 patients with KIT mutation in exons 9, 11, 13, 17, and 18 or amplification only (Guo et al. 2011). The starting dose of imatinib was 400 mg daily, with escalation of the dose to 600–800 mg daily upon disease progression. Forty-three patients were enrolled, all of whom had a response evaluation by the time of publication. Ten patients (23 %) had an objective response, and nine had either an exon 11 or 13 mutation. In patients with exon 11 or 13 mutations, the response rate was 35 % (6 of 17) and 33 % (3 of 9), respectively. A third Phase II trial of imatinib in patients with CKIT aberrations treated patients with 400 mg daily to be escalated to 400 mg twice daily in the setting of no initial response (Hodi et al. 2013). Twenty-five patients were enrolled, and all but one was evaluable for response. Seven patients had disease response; all but one had either an exon 11 or 13 mutation (there was one responder with an exon 17 point mutation).

Based on these two trials, several preliminary conclusions can be made: (1) the previously described imatinib-sensitive mutations in GIST also predict responsiveness to imatinib in melanoma, (2) several patients with predicted imatinib sensitivity did not respond, and (3) on the basis of response rates in the 20–25 % range, patients with CKIT exon 11 and 13 mutations are a subgroup worthy of further investigation.

Additionally, Phase II trials of nilotinib in patients with CKIT mutant melanoma who have progressed or who are intolerant of first-line KIT inhibitor therapy has been completed (Carvajal et al. 2015). In this trial, 20 patients were enrolled to one of two cohorts, Cohort A prior KIT inhibitor therapy or Cohort B patient with brain metastases. The primary endpoint was 4 months of disease control, and three of eleven patients treated in cohort A and one of eight in Cohort B met this endpoint. The conclusion of this trial was that nilotinib may be associated with clinical benefit in patients with CKIT mutant melanoma but is associated with limited benefit in patients with brain metastases.

Clearly, the proof of concept has been established that KIT mutant melanoma can be responsive to imatinib. However, much work remains to be done to understand the response rate for particular mutations or in particular exons. KIT amplification alone remains of uncertain significance with regard to connoting responsiveness to therapy. And the durability of response or disease stabilization and its impact on overall survival remains to be determined. The pace with which these questions can be answered is limited by the rarity of genetic alterations in KIT in the overall melanoma population, and their presence in a minority of patients with the relevant clinical subtypes in which they can be found.

16.2.7 Oncogenes Not Readily Amenable to Direct Targeting

16.2.7.1 MITF

The microopthalmia transcription factor, MITF, is the master regulator of melanocyte differentiation and expression of melanocyte-specific antigens (see also Chap. 9 (Abdel-Malek)). Its potential role as an oncogene in melanoma has recently been suggested based on the discovery of high-level amplification of the MITF locus in approximately 15 % of melanomas (Garraway et al. 2005). In such tumors, and some others without amplification, knockdown of MITF with siRNA impairs proliferation. Being a member of the transcription factor superfamily that includes MYC, a contribution to cancer pathophysiology would not be unprecedented. However, targeting MITF with pharmacologic inhibitors is not currently possible. This molecule lacks an enzymatic domain against which small molecules could readily be developed. Rather, agents that block the association of MITF with cofactors, or key promoter regions in MITF target genes, would be needed. In order to avoid pleiotropic effects on the expression of a vast array of genes, likely resulting in unacceptable toxicity, a deeper understanding of which MITF target genes contribute most significantly to melanoma biology is required. Such a detailed understanding would potentially generate alternative targets that are amenable to pharmacologic therapy. In the meantime, there is evidence that epigenetic regulation of MITF may be apparent in the cancer setting and could be ameliorated to some degree with the use of the histone deacetylase inhibitor (Yokoyama et al. 2008). A clinical trial is currently ongoing in metastatic melanoma patients using a class to specific histone deacetylase inhibitor (LBH589).

16.2.7.2 GNAQ/GNA11

In 2008, activating mutations in the G protein-coupled receptor signaling molecule, GNAQ, were first described in a large subset of uveal melanomas (Van Raamsdonk et al. 2009). The same mutations are not found in other melanoma subtypes. The following year, analogous mutations in the highly homologous GNA11 were described in initial in an additional portion of uveal melanoma cases. In total, either of these mutations appears to be present in approximately 80 % of uveal melanomas. It had previously been shown that BRAF and NRAS mutations are not found in uveal melanoma, so the discovery of these activating mutations filled a significant void in the understanding of oncogenic drivers in this clinical subtype of melanoma. Like RAS, these proteins are GTPases, in which the GTPase activity is disabled by the mutation that had been described. Therefore, pharmacologic agents would need to restore the GTPase activity in order to antagonize the signaling capacity of these molecules. As has been noted, such an approach appears to be extremely technically challenging, and such candidate therapies do not currently exist.

Outside of the context of cancer, these G protein alpha subunits (GNAQ and GNA11) are known to activate several downstream signal transduction pathways, including the MAP kinase and PI3 kinase pathways (Van Raamsdonk et al. 2004). Early experimental evidence in melanoma cell lines harboring a GNAQ mutation suggested that the MAP kinase pathway may be a point of vulnerability for therapeutic purposes (Van Raamsdonk et al. 2009). Given the availability of potent and selective MEK inhibitors, clinical trials employing single agent MEK inhibitor therapy were performed. The first of these studies randomized 101 patients with metastatic uveal melanoma to either the MEK1/2/inhibitor selumetinib or chemotherapy (both temozolomide and DTIC were allowable) (Carvajal et al. 2014). The primary endpoint, PFS was superior in the selumetinib arm (HR 0.46, 95 % CI 0.30–0.91; $p<0.001$) compared to the chemotherapy arm, though the OS was not statistically significantly different (HR 0.66; 95 % CI 0.41–1.06; $p=0.09$). The follow-up trial randomized patients to chemotherapy or chemotherapy plus selumetinib and failed to meet its primary endpoint of improved PFS. Obviously, further preclinical work is needed to understand more about the hierarchy of signal transduction pathways downstream of these G proteins so that rational combination drug strategies can be formulated.

16.2.7.3 BAP1

The most recent genetic discovery in melanoma also comes in the uveal melanoma subpopulation. It has long been known that the short arm of chromosome 3 is frequently deleted in uveal melanomas, and particularly those that metastasize and result in fatality (van Gils et al. 2008). However, a potential candidate tumor suppressor gene on this chromosome had not been described. Recently, massively parallel exome sequencing has uncovered mutations in BRCA1-associated protein 1 (BAP1) in more than 80 % of metastatic uveal melanomas (Harbour et al. 2010). The distribution of these mutations in regions of the gene/protein that interacts with two distinct deubiquitinases, UCH and ULD, suggests that that BAP1 is indeed a tumor suppressor gene. As with any other tumor suppressor gene in cancer, we currently lack the ability to restore the function that is lost through inactivating mutations or deletion. However, a greater mechanistic understanding of the activities of BAP1 binding partners may provide opportunities for therapeutic intervention. The two deubiquitinases that the genetic evidence suggests to be important in BAP1 function are likely not ideal therapeutic targets as ubiquination and deubiquination are fundamental levels of regulating protein stability that pharmacologic inhibitors of such molecules may have far-reaching and toxic effects. One observation made in previous mechanistic studies regarding BAP1 function suggests that BAP1 regulates the activity of the polycomb repressive complex 1 (PRC1), which regulates histone acetylation and acetylation (Scheuermann et al. 2010). Experimental evidence suggests that in BAP1-mutated uveal melanoma cell lines, histone deacetylase inhibitors have a growth-inhibitory effect (Harbour et al. 2010). This approach is certainly possible to investigate in clinical trials, as numerous histone deacetylase inhibitors have been developed.

Conclusion

The discovery of somatic genetic changes in oncogenes and tumor suppressor genes, and the subsequent biological validation of their significance, has opened the door for the development of molecularly targeted therapies aiming to antagonize the very genetic underpinnings of melanoma. The proof of principle has been established with BRAF-targeted therapy, that melanoma can be vulnerable to such an approach, despite the vast array of genetic alterations present within any one tumor. However, it is equally clear that no single point of intervention will eradicate metastatic melanoma, and that understanding the hierarchy of oncogenes and signal transduction pathways becomes critical to develop rational combination therapies, which might make an even more significant impact. Numerous challenges and hurdles remain, and the development of more effective molecularly targeted therapies for each of the recently described molecular subsets of melanoma remains a major focus of investigation. Clearly, combination targeted therapy strategies will require that each component within the combination be highly selective for its intended target, or that the target is uniquely relevant to melanoma biology and not normal physiology. Given our increasingly detailed understanding of the network of genetic changes and aberrant signal transduction and the downstream phenotypic consequences on various cellular processes, there is no shortage of essential points of intervention or types of combinations. It will be critical for the melanoma field to remain mindful of the ultimate goal, which is to tailor the therapeutic approach to the individual patient based on the unique constellation of alterations within their tumor.

References

Albino AP, Le Strange R, Oliff AI, Furth ME, Old LJ (1984) Transforming ras genes from human melanoma: a manifestation of tumour heterogeneity? Nature 308:69–72

Altomare DA, Lyons GE, Mitsuuchi Y, Cheng JQ, Testa JR (1998) Akt2 mRNA is highly expressed in embryonic brown fat and the AKT2 kinase is activated by insulin. Oncogene 16:2407–2411

Ascierto PA, Schadendorf D, Berking C, Agarwala SS, van Herpen CM, Queirolo P, Blank CU, Hauschild A, Beck JT, St-Pierre A, Niazi F, Wandel S, Peters M, Zubel A, Dummer R (2013) MEK162 for patients with advanced melanoma harbouring NRAS or Val600 BRAF mutations: a non-randomised, open-label phase 2 study. Lancet Oncol 14:249–256

Boisvert-Adamo K, Aplin AE (2008) Mutant B-RAF mediates resistance to anoikis via Bad and Bim. Oncogene 27:3301–3312

Cancer Genome Atlas Network (2015) Genomic classification of cutaneous melanoma. Cell 161:1681–1696

Carpten JD, Faber AL, Horn C, Donoho GP, Briggs SL, Robbins CM, Hostetter G, Boguslawski S, Moses TY, Savage S, Uhlik M, Lin A, Du J, Qian YW, Zeckner DJ, Tucker-Kellogg G, Touchman J, Patel K, Mousses S, Bittner M, Schevitz R, Lai MH, Blanchard KL, Thomas JE (2007) A transforming mutation in the pleckstrin homology domain of AKT1 in cancer. Nature 448:439–444

Cartlidge RA, Thomas GR, Cagnol S, Jong KA, Molton SA, Finch AJ, Mcmahon M (2008) Oncogenic BRAF(V600E) inhibits BIM expression to promote melanoma cell survival. Pigment Cell Melanoma Res 21:534–544

Carvajal RD, Antonescu CR, Wolchok JD, Chapman PB, Roman RA, Teitcher J, Panageas KS, Busam KJ, Chmielowski B, Lutzky J, Pavlick AC, Fusco A, Cane L, Takebe N, Vemula S, Bouvier N, Bastian BC, Schwartz GK (2011) KIT as a therapeutic target in metastatic melanoma. JAMA 305:2327–2334

Carvajal RD, Sosman JA, Quevedo JF, Milhem MM, Joshua AM, Kudchadkar RR, Linette GP, Gajewski TF, Lutzky J, Lawson DH, Lao CD, Flynn PJ, Albertini MR, Sato T, Lewis K, Doyle A, Ancell K, Panageas KS, Bluth M, Hedvat C, Erinjeri J, Ambrosini G, Marr B, Abramson DH, Dickson MA, Wolchok JD, Chapman PB, Schwartz GK (2014) Effect of selumetinib vs chemotherapy on progression-free survival in uveal melanoma: a randomized clinical trial. JAMA 311:2397–2405

Carvajal RD, Lawrence DP, Weber JS, Gajewski TF, Gonzalez R, Lutzky J, O'day SJ, Hamid O, Wolchok JD, Chapman PB, Sullivan RJ, Teitcher JB, Ramaiya N, Giobbie-Hurder A, Antonescu CR, Heinrich MC, Bastian BC, Corless CL, Fletcher JA, Hodi FS (2015) Phase II study of nilotinib in melanoma harboring KIT alterations following progression to prior KIT inhibition. Clin Cancer Res 21:2289–2296

Celebi JT, Shendrik I, Silvers DN, Peacocke M (2000) Identification of PTEN mutations in metastatic melanoma specimens. J Med Genet 37:653–657

Chapman PB, Hauschild A, Robert C, Haanen JB, Ascierto P, Larkin J, Dummer R, Garbe C, Testori A, Maio M, Hogg D, Lorigan P, Lebbe C, Jouary T, Schadendorf D, Ribas A, O'day SJ, Sosman JA, Kirkwood JM, Eggermont AM, Dreno B, Nolop K, Li J, Nelson B, Hou J, Lee RJ, Flaherty KT, Mcarthur GA (2011) Improved survival with vemurafenib in melanoma with BRAF V600E mutation. N Engl J Med 364:2507–2516

Cooper ZA, Frederick DT, Juneja VR, Sullivan RJ, Lawrence DP, Piris A, Sharpe AH, Fisher DE, Flaherty KT, Wargo JA (2013) BRAF inhibition is associated with increased clonality in tumor-infiltrating lymphocytes. Oncoimmunology 2:e26615

Curtin JA, Fridlyand J, Kageshita T, Patel HN, Busam KJ, Kutzner H, Cho KH, Aiba S, Brocker EB, Leboit PE, Pinkel D, Bastian BC (2005) Distinct sets of genetic alterations in melanoma. N Engl J Med 353:2135–2147

Curtin JA, Busam K, Pinkel D, Bastian BC (2006) Somatic activation of KIT in distinct subtypes of melanoma. J Clin Oncol 24:4340–4346

Davies H, Bignell GR, Cox C, Stephens P, Edkins S, Clegg S, Teague J, Woffendin H, Garnett MJ, Bottomley W, Davis N, Dicks E, Ewing R, Floyd Y, Gray K, Hall S, Hawes R, Hughes J,

Kosmidou V, Menzies A, Mould C, Parker A, Stevens C, Watt S, Hooper S, Wilson R, Jayatilake H, Gusterson BA, Cooper C, Shipley J, Hargrave D, Pritchard-Jones K, Maitland N, Chenevix-Trench G, Riggins GJ, Bigner DD, Palmieri G, Cossu A, Flanagan A, Nicholson A, Ho JW, Leung SY, Yuen ST, Weber BL, Seigler HF, Darrow TL, Paterson H, Marais R, Marshall CJ, Wooster R, Stratton MR, Futreal PA (2002) Mutations of the BRAF gene in human cancer. Nature 417:949–954

Davies MA, Stemke-Hale K, Tellez C, Calderone TL, Deng W, Prieto VG, Lazar AJ, Gershenwald JE, Mills GB (2008) A novel AKT3 mutation in melanoma tumours and cell lines. Br J Cancer 99:1265–1268

De Laurentiis A, Pardo OE, Palamidessi A, Jackson SP, Schoenwaelder SM, Reichmann E, Scita G, Arcaro A (2011) The catalytic class I(A) PI3K Isoforms play divergent roles in breast cancer cell migration. Cell Signal 23(3):529–541

Demetri GD, von Mehren M, Blanke CD, Van den Abbeele AD, Eisenberg B, Roberts PJ, Heinrich MC, Tuveson DA, Singer S, Janicek M, Fletcher JA, Silverman SG, Silberman SL, Capdeville R, Kiese B, Peng B, Dimitrijevic S, Druker BJ, Corless C, Fletcher CD, Joensuu H (2002) Efficacy and safety of imatinib mesylate in advanced gastrointestinal stromal tumors. N Engl J Med 347:472–480

Demetri GD, van Oosterom AT, Garrett CR, Blackstein ME, Shah MH, Verweij J, Mcarthur G, Judson IR, Heinrich MC, Morgan JA, Desai J, Fletcher CD, George S, Bello CL, Huang X, Baum CM, Casali PG (2006) Efficacy and safety of sunitinib in patients with advanced gastrointestinal stromal tumour after failure of imatinib: a randomised controlled trial. Lancet 368: 1329–1338

Dhomen N, Reis-Filho JS, da Rocha Dias S, Hayward R, Savage K, Delmas V, Larue L, Pritchard C, Marais R (2009) Oncogenic Braf induces melanocyte senescence and melanoma in mice. Cancer Cell 15:294–303

Donia M, Fagone P, Nicoletti F, Andersen RS, Hogdall E, Straten PT, Andersen MH, Svane IM (2012) BRAF inhibition improves tumor recognition by the immune system: potential implications for combinatorial therapies against melanoma involving adoptive T-cell transfer. Oncoimmunology 1: 1476–1483

Dummer R, Robert C, Nyakas M, Mcarthur GA, Kudchadkar RR, Gomez-Roca C, Sullivan RJ, Flaherty KT, Murer C, Michel D, Tang Z, de Parseval LA, Delord JP (2013) Initial results from a phase I, open-label, dose escalation study of the oral BRAF inhibitor LGX818 in patients with BRAF V600 mutant advanced or metastatic melanoma. ASCO, 2013 Chicago. J Clin Oncol

Emery CM, Vijayendran KG, Zipser MC, Sawyer AM, Niu L, Kim JJ, Hatton C, Chopra R, Oberholzer PA, Karpova MB, Macconaill LE, Zhang J, Gray NS, Sellers WR, Dummer R, Garraway LA (2009) MEK1 mutations confer resistance to MEK and B-RAF inhibition. Proc Natl Acad Sci U S A 106:20411–20416

Eskandarpour M, Huang F, Reeves KA, Clark E, Hansson J (2009) Oncogenic NRAS has multiple effects on the malignant phenotype of human melanoma cells cultured in vitro. Int J Cancer 124:16–26

Falchook GS, Long GV, Kurzrock R, Kim KB, Arkenau TH, Brown MP, Hamid O, Infante JR, Millward M, Pavlick AC, O'day SJ, Blackman SC, Curtis CM, Lebowitz P, Ma B, Ouellet D, Kefford RF (2012) Dabrafenib in patients with melanoma, untreated brain metastases, and other solid tumours: a phase 1 dose-escalation trial. Lancet 379:1893–1901

Flaherty KT, Redlinger M, S LM, Lathia CD, Weber BL, O'Dwyer PJ (2005) Phase I/II, pharmacokinetic and pharmacodynamic trial of BAY 43–9006 alone in patients with metastatic melanoma. J Clin Oncol 23:3037

Flaherty KT, Puzanov I, Kim KB, Ribas A, Mcarthur GA, Sosman JA, O'dwyer PJ, Lee RJ, Grippo JF, Nolop K, Chapman PB (2010) Inhibition of mutated, activated BRAF in metastatic melanoma. N Engl J Med 363:809–819

Flaherty KT, Infante JR, Daud A, Gonzalez R, Kefford RF, Sosman J, Hamid O, Schuchter L, Cebon J, Ibrahim N, Kudchadkar R, Burris HA 3rd, Falchook G, Algazi A, Lewis K, Long GV, Puzanov I, Lebowitz P, Singh A, Little S, Sun P, Allred A, Ouellet D, Kim KB, Patel K,

Weber J (2012a) Combined BRAF and MEK inhibition in melanoma with BRAF V600 mutations. N Engl J Med 367:1694–1703

Flaherty KT, Robert C, Hersey P, Nathan P, Garbe C, Milhem M, Demidov LV, Hassel JC, Rutkowski P, Mohr P, Dummer R, Trefzer U, Larkin JM, Utikal J, Dreno B, Nyakas M, Middleton MR, Becker JC, Casey M, Sherman LJ, Wu FS, Ouellet D, Martin AM, Patel K, Schadendorf D (2012b) Improved survival with MEK inhibition in BRAF-mutated melanoma. N Engl J Med 367(2):107–114

Flaherty KT, Lee SJ, Zhao F, Schuchter LM, Flaherty L, Kefford R, Atkins MB, Leming P, Kirkwood JM (2013) Phase III trial of carboplatin and paclitaxel with or without sorafenib in metastatic melanoma. J Clin Oncol Off J Am Soc Clin Oncol 31:373–379

Frederick DT, Piris A, Cogdill AP, Cooper ZA, Lezcano C, Ferrone CR, Mitra D, Boni A, Newton LP, Liu C, Peng W, Sullivan RJ, Lawrence DP, Hodi FS, Overwijk WW, Lizee G, Murphy GF, Hwu P, Flaherty KT, Fisher DE, Wargo JA (2013) BRAF inhibition is associated with enhanced melanoma antigen expression and a more favorable tumor microenvironment in patients with metastatic melanoma. Clin Cancer Res Off J Am Assoc Cancer Res 19:1225–1231

Frederick DT, Salas Fragomeni RA, Schalck A, Ferreiro-Neira I, Hoff T, Cooper ZA, Haq R, Panka DJ, Kwong LN, Davies MA, Cusack JC, Flaherty KT, Fisher DE, Mier JW, Wargo JA, Sullivan RJ (2014) Clinical profiling of BCL-2 family members in the setting of BRAF inhibition offers a rationale for targeting de novo resistance using BH3 mimetics. PLoS One 9:e101286

Fry DW, Harvey PJ, Keller PR, Elliott WL, Meade M, Trachet E, Albassam M, Zheng X, Leopold WR, Pryer NK, Toogood PL (2004) Specific inhibition of cyclin-dependent kinase 4/6 by PD 0332991 and associated antitumor activity in human tumor xenografts. Mol Cancer Ther 3:1427–1438

Fujimoto A, Morita R, Hatta N, Takehara K, Takata M (1999) p16INK4a inactivation is not frequent in uncultured sporadic primary cutaneous melanoma. Oncogene 18:2527–2532

Furuta J, Umebayashi Y, Miyamoto K, Kikuchi K, Otsuka F, Sugimura T, Ushijima T (2004) Promoter methylation profiling of 30 genes in human malignant melanoma. Cancer Sci 95:962–968

Gajewski TF, Salama AK, Niedzwiecki D, Johnson J, Linette G, Bucher C, Blaskovich MA, Sebti SM, Haluska F; Cancer and Leukemia Group B. Phase II study of the farnesyltransferase inhibitor R115777 in advanced melanoma (CALGB 500104). J Transl Med. 2012 Dec 10;10:246. doi:10.1186/1479-5876-10-246.

Garraway LA, Widlund HR, Rubin MA, Getz G, Berger AJ, Ramaswamy S, Beroukhim R, Milner DA, Granter SR, Du J, Lee C, Wagner SN, Li C, Golub TR, Rimm DL, Meyerson ML, Fisher DE, Sellers WR (2005) Integrative genomic analyses identify MITF as a lineage survival oncogene amplified in malignant melanoma. Nature 436:117–122

Gembarska A, Luciani F, Fedele C, Russell EA, Dewaele M, Villar S, Zwolinska A, Haupt S, de Lange J, Yip D, Goydos J, Haigh JJ, Haupt Y, Larue L, Jochemsen A, Shi H, Moriceau G, Lo RS, Ghanem G, Shackleton M, Bernal F, Marine JC (2012) MDM4 is a key therapeutic target in cutaneous melanoma. Nat Med 18:1239–1247

Govindarajan B, Sligh JE, Vincent BJ, Li M, Canter JA, Nickoloff BJ, Rodenburg RJ, Smeitink JA, Oberley L, Zhang Y, Slingerland J, Arnold RS, Lambeth JD, Cohen C, Hilenski L, Griendling K, Martinez-Diez M, Cuezva JM, Arbiser JL (2007) Overexpression of Akt converts radial growth melanoma to vertical growth melanoma. J Clin Invest 117:719–729

Guldberg P, thor Straten P, Birck A, Ahrenkiel V, Kirkin AF, Zeuthen J (1997) Disruption of the MMAC1/PTEN gene by deletion or mutation is a frequent event in malignant melanoma. Cancer Res 57:3660–3663

Guo J, Si L, Kong Y, Flaherty KT, Xu X, Zhu Y, Corless CL, Li L, Li H, Sheng X, Cui C, Chi Z, Li S, Han M, Mao L, Lin X, Du N, Zhang X, Li J, Wang B, Qin S (2011) Phase II, open-label, single-arm trial of imatinib mesylate in patients with metastatic melanoma harboring c-Kit mutation or amplification. J Clin Oncol Off J Am Soc Clin Oncol 29:2904–2909

Haferkamp S, Becker TM, Scurr LL, Kefford RF, Rizos H (2008) p16INK4a-induced senescence is disabled by melanoma-associated mutations. Aging Cell 7:733–745

Hamid O, Patel M, Hodi FS, Amaria R, Sullivan R, Boasberg P, Wallin J, He X, Cha E, Richie N, Ballinger M, Hwu P (2015) Preliminary clinical safety, tolerability and activity results from a

Phase Ib study of atezolizumab (anti-PDL1) combined with vemurafenib in BRAFV600 mutant metastatic melanoma. Society for Melanoma Research Congress, San Francisco

Haq R, Yokoyama S, Hawryluk EB, Jonsson GB, Frederick DT, Mchenry K, Porter D, Tran TN, Love KT, Langer R, Anderson DG, Garraway LA, Duncan LM, Morton DL, Hoon DS, Wargo JA, Song JS, Fisher DE (2013) BCL2A1 is a lineage-specific antiapoptotic melanoma oncogene that confers resistance to BRAF inhibition. Proc Natl Acad Sci U S A 110:4321–4326

Harbour JW, Onken MD, Roberson ED, Duan S, Cao L, Worley LA, Council ML, Matatall KA, Helms C, Bowcock AM (2010) Frequent mutation of BAP1 in metastasizing uveal melanomas. Science 330(6009):1410–1413

Hauschild A, Agarwala SS, Trefzer U, Hogg D, Robert C, Hersey P, Eggermont A, Grabbe S, Gonzalez R, Gille J, Peschel C, Schadendorf D, Garbe C, O'day S, Daud A, White JM, Xia C, Patel K, Kirkwood JM, Keilholz U (2009) Results of a phase III, randomized, placebo-controlled study of sorafenib in combination with carboplatin and paclitaxel as second-line treatment in patients with unresectable stage III or stage IV melanoma. J Clin Oncol Off J Am Soc Clin Oncol 27:2823–2830

Hauschild A, Grob JJ, Demidov LV, Jouary T, Gutzmer R, Millward M, Rutkowski P, Blank CU, Miller WH Jr, Kaempgen E, Martin-Algarra S, Karaszewska B, Mauch C, Chiarion-Sileni V, Martin AM, Swann S, Haney P, Mirakhur B, Guckert ME, Goodman V, Chapman PB (2012) Dabrafenib in BRAF-mutated metastatic melanoma: a multicentre, open-label, phase 3 randomised controlled trial. Lancet 380:358–365

Heidorn SJ, Milagre C, Whittaker S, Nourry A, Niculescu-Duvas I, Dhomen N, Hussain J, Reis-Filho JS, Springer CJ, Pritchard C, Marais R (2010) Kinase-dead BRAF and oncogenic RAS cooperate to drive tumor progression through CRAF. Cell 140:209–221

Hingorani SR, Jacobetz MA, Robertson GP, Herlyn M, Tuveson DA (2003) Suppression of BRAF(V599E) in human melanoma abrogates transformation. Cancer Res 63:5198–5202

Hodi FS, Friedlander P, Corless CL, Heinrich MC, Mac Rae S, Kruse A, Jagannathan J, Van den Abbeele AD, Velazquez EF, Demetri GD, Fisher DE (2008) Major response to imatinib mesylate in KIT-mutated melanoma. J Clin Oncol 26:2046–2051

Hodi FS, Corless CL, Giobbie-Hurder A, Fletcher JA, Zhu M, Marino-Enriquez A, Friedlander P, Gonzalez R, Weber JS, Gajewski TF, O'Day SJ, Kim KB, Lawrence D, Flaherty KT, Luke JJ, Collichio FA, Ernstoff MS, Heinrich MC, Beadling C, Zukotynski KA, Yap JT, Van den Abbeele AD, Demetri GD, Fisher DE (2013) Imatinib for melanomas harboring mutationally activated or amplified KIT arising on mucosal, acral, and chronically sun-damaged skin. J Clin Oncol 31:3182–3190

Hussussian CJ, Struewing JP, Goldstein AM, Higgins PA, Ally DS, Sheahan MD, Clark WH Jr, Tucker MA, Dracopoli NC (1994) Germline p16 mutations in familial melanoma. Nat Genet 8:15–21

Infante JR, Janku F, Tolcher AW, Patel MR, Sullivan RJ, Flaherty K, Carvajal RD, Varghese AK, Wong DJ, Sznol M, Sosman JA, Wang-Gillam A, Burris HA, Ribas A, Patel SP, Welsch DJ, Saha S (2005) Dose escalation stage of a first-in-class phase I study of the novel oral ERK 1/2 kinase inhibitor BVD-523 (ulixertinib) in patients with advanced solid tumors. ASCO annual meeting, 2005 Chicago. J Clin Oncol, abstr 2506

Janas ML, Hodson D, Stamataki Z, Hill S, Welch K, Gambardella L, Trotman LC, Pandolfi PP, Vigorito E, Turner M (2008) The effect of deleting p110delta on the phenotype and function of PTEN-deficient B cells. J Immunol 180:739–746

Ji Z, Njauw CN, Taylor M, Neel V, Flaherty KT, Tsao H (2012) p53 rescue through HDM2 antagonism suppresses melanoma growth and potentiates MEK inhibition. J Invest Dermatol 132:356–364

Johannessen CM, Boehm JS, Kim SY, Thomas SR, Wardwell L, Johnson LA, Emery CM, Stransky N, Cogdill AP, Barretina J, Caponigro G, Hieronymus H, Murray RR, Salehi-Ashtiani K, Hill DE, Vidal M, Zhao JJ, Yang X, Alkan O, Kim S, Harris JL, Wilson CJ, Myer VE, Finan PM, Root DE, Roberts TM, Golub T, Flaherty KT, Dummer R, Weber BL, Sellers WR, Schlegel R, Wargo JA, Hahn WC, Garraway LA (2010) COT drives resistance to RAF inhibition through MAP kinase pathway reactivation. Nature 468:968–972

Kefford R, Arkenau H, Brown MP, Millward M, Infante JR, Long GV, Ouellet D, Curtis M, Lebowitz PF, Falchook GS (2010) Phase I/II study of GSK2118436, a selective inhibitor of oncogenic mutant BRAF kinase, in patients with metastatic melanoma and other solid tumors. J Clin Oncol 28 Suppl:611s

Kim KB, Eton O, Davis DW, Frazier ML, Mcconkey DJ, Diwan AH, Papadopoulos NE, Bedikian AY, Camacho LH, Ross MI, Cormier JN, Gershenwald JE, Lee JE, Mansfield PF, Billings LA, Ng CS, Charnsangavej C, Bar-Eli M, Johnson MM, Murgo AJ, Prieto VG (2008) Phase II trial of imatinib mesylate in patients with metastatic melanoma. Br J Cancer 99:734–740

Kim KB, Kefford R, Pavlick AC, Infante JR, Ribas A, Sosman JA, Fecher LA, Millward M, Mcarthur GA, Hwu P, Gonzalez R, Ott PA, Long GV, Gardner OS, Ouellet D, Xu Y, Demarini DJ, Le NT, Patel K, Lewis KD (2013) Phase II study of the MEK1/MEK2 inhibitor Trametinib in patients with metastatic BRAF-mutant cutaneous melanoma previously treated with or without a BRAF inhibitor. J Clin Oncol Off J Am Soc Clin Oncol 31:482–489

Larkin J, Ascierto PA, Dreno B, Atkinson V, Liszkay G, Maio M, Mandala M, Demidov L, Stroyakovskiy D, Thomas L, de la Cruz-Merino L, Dutriaux C, Garbe C, Sovak MA, Chang I, Choong N, Hack SP, Mcarthur GA, Ribas A (2014) Combined vemurafenib and cobimetinib in BRAF-mutated melanoma. N Engl J Med 371:1867–1876

Long GV, Wilmott JS, Haydu LE, Tembe V, Sharma R, Rizos H, Thompson JF, Howle J, Scolyer RA, Kefford RF (2013) Effects of BRAF inhibitors on human melanoma tissue before treatment, early during treatment, and on progression. Pigment Cell Melanoma Res 26:499–508

Long GV, Stroyakovskiy D, Gogas H, Levchenko E, de Braud F, Larkin J, Garbe C, Jouary T, Hauschild A, Grob JJ, Chiarion-Sileni V, Lebbe C, Mandala M, Millward M, Arance A, Bondarenko I, Haanen JB, Hansson J, Utikal J, Ferraresi V, Kovalenko N, Mohr P, Probachai V, Schadendorf D, Nathan P, Robert C, Ribas A, Demarini DJ, Irani JG, Swann S, Legos JJ, Jin F, Mookerjee B, Flaherty K (2015) Dabrafenib and trametinib versus dabrafenib and placebo for Val600 BRAF-mutant melanoma: a multicentre, double-blind, phase 3 randomised controlled trial. Lancet 386:444–451

Mirmohammadsadegh A, Marini A, Nambiar S, Hassan M, Tannapfel A, Ruzicka T, Hengge UR (2006) Epigenetic silencing of the PTEN gene in melanoma. Cancer Res 66:6546–6552

Montagut C, Sharma SV, Shioda T, Mcdermott U, Ulman M, Ulkus LE, Dias-Santagata D, Stubbs H, Lee DY, Singh A, Drew L, Haber DA, Settleman J (2008) Elevated CRAF as a potential mechanism of acquired resistance to BRAF inhibition in melanoma. Cancer Res 68: 4853–4861

Muthusamy V, Hobbs C, Nogueira C, Cordon-Cardo C, Mckee PH, Chin L, Bosenberg MW (2006) Amplification of CDK4 and MDM2 in malignant melanoma. Genes Chromosomes Cancer 45:447–454

Nazarian R, Shi H, Wang Q, Kong X, Koya RC, Lee H, Chen Z, Lee MK, Attar N, Sazegar H, Chodon T, Nelson SF, Mcarthur G, Sosman JA, Ribas A, Lo RS (2010) Melanomas acquire resistance to B-RAF(V600E) inhibition by RTK or N-RAS upregulation. Nature 468:973–977

Nogueira C, Kim KH, Sung H, Paraiso KH, Dannenberg JH, Bosenberg M, Chin L, Kim M (2010) Cooperative interactions of PTEN deficiency and RAS activation in melanoma metastasis. Oncogene 29(47):6222–6232

Oberholzer PA, Kee D, Dziunycz P, Sucker A, Kamsukom N, Jones R, Roden C, Chalk CJ, Ardlie K, Palescandolo E, Piris A, Macconaill LE, Robert C, Hofbauer GF, Mcarthur GA, Schadendorf D, Garraway LA (2012) RAS mutations are associated with the development of cutaneous squamous cell tumors in patients treated with RAF inhibitors. J Clin Oncol 30:316–321

Paraiso KH, Fedorenko IV, Cantini LP, Munko AC, Hall M, Sondak VK, Messina JL, Flaherty KT, Smalley KS (2010) Recovery of phospho-ERK activity allows melanoma cells to escape from BRAF inhibitor therapy. Br J Cancer 102:1724–1730

Paraiso KH, Xiang Y, Rebecca VW, Abel EV, Chen YA, Munko AC, Wood E, Fedorenko IV, Sondak VK, Anderson AR, Ribas A, Palma MD, Nathanson KL, Koomen JM, Messina JL, Smalley KS (2011) PTEN loss confers BRAF inhibitor resistance to melanoma cells through the suppression of BIM expression. Cancer Res 71:2750–2760

Polsky D, Bastian BC, Hazan C, Melzer K, Pack J, Houghton A, Busam K, Cordon-Cardo C, Osman I (2001) HDM2 protein overexpression, but not gene amplification, is related to tumorigenesis of cutaneous melanoma. Cancer Res 61:7642–7646
Poulikakos PI, Zhang C, Bollag G, Shokat KM, Rosen N (2010) RAF inhibitors transactivate RAF dimers and ERK signalling in cells with wild-type BRAF. Nature 464:427–430
Poulikakos PI, Persaud Y, Janakiraman M, Kong X, Ng C, Moriceau G, Shi H, Atefi M, Titz B, Gabay MT, Salton M, Dahlman KB, Tadi M, Wargo JA, Flaherty KT, Kelley MC, Misteli T, Chapman PB, Sosman JA, Graeber TG, Ribas A, Lo RS, Rosen N, Solit DB (2011) RAF inhibitor resistance is mediated by dimerization of aberrantly spliced BRAF(V600E). Nature 480:387–390
Puzanov I, Callahan MK, Linette GP, Patel SP, Luke JJ, Sosman JA, Wolchok JD, Hamid O, Minor DR, Orford KW, Hug BA, Ma B, Matthys GM, Hoos A (2014) Phase 1 study of the BRAF inhibitor dabrafenib (D) with or without the MEK inhibitor trametinib (T) in combination with ipilimumab (Ipi) for V600E/K mutation–positive unresectable or metastatic melanoma (MM). ASCO annual meeting, 2014 Chicago. J Clin Oncol
Ribas A, Hodi FS, Callahan M, Konto C, Wolchok J (2013) Hepatotoxicity with combination of vemurafenib and ipilimumab. N Engl J Med 368:1365–1366
Ribas A, Gonzalez R, Pavlick A, Hamid O, Gajewski TF, Daud A, Flaherty L, Logan T, Chmielowski B, Lewis K, Kee D, Boasberg P, Yin M, Chan I, Musib L, Choong N, Puzanov I, Mcarthur GA (2014) Combination of vemurafenib and cobimetinib in patients with advanced BRAF(V600)-mutated melanoma: a phase 1b study. Lancet Oncol 15:954–965
Ribas A, Butler M, Lutzky J, Lawrence DP, Robert C, Miller W, Linette GP, Ascierto PA, Kuzel T, Algazi AP, Postow MA, Nathan PD, Curti BD, Robbins PB, Li X, Blake-Haskins JA, Gordon MS (2015) Phase I study combining anti-PD-L1 (MEDI4736) with BRAF (dabrafenib) and/or MEK (trametinib) inhibitors in advanced melanoma. ASCO annual meeting, 2015 Chicago. 3003
Robert C, Karaszewska B, Schachter J, Rutkowski P, Mackiewicz A, Stroiakovski D, Lichinitser M, Dummer R, Grange F, Mortier L, Chiarion-Sileni V, Drucis K, Krajsova I, Hauschild A, Lorigan P, Wolter P, Long GV, Flaherty K, Nathan P, Ribas A, Martin AM, Sun P, Crist W, Legos J, Rubin SD, Little SM, Schadendorf D (2015) Improved overall survival in melanoma with combined dabrafenib and trametinib. N Engl J Med 372:30–39
Robinson JP, Vanbrocklin MW, Guilbeault AR, Signorelli DL, Brandner S, Holmen SL (2010) Activated BRAF induces gliomas in mice when combined with Ink4a/Arf loss or Akt activation. Oncogene 29:335–344
Ruth MC, Xu Y, Maxwell IH, Ahn NG, Norris DA, Shellman YG (2006) RhoC promotes human melanoma invasion in a PI3K/Akt-dependent pathway. J Invest Dermatol 126:862–868
Saiki AY, Caenepeel S, Yu D, Lofgren JA, Osgood T, Robertson R, Canon J, Su C, Jones A, Zhao X, Deshpande C, Payton M, Ledell J, Hughes PE, Oliner JD (2014) MDM2 antagonists synergize broadly and robustly with compounds targeting fundamental oncogenic signaling pathways. Oncotarget 5:2030–2043
Scheuermann JC, de Ayala Alonso AG, Oktaba K, Ly-Hartig N, Mcginty RK, Fraterman S, Wilm M, Muir TW, Muller J (2010) Histone H2A deubiquitinase activity of the Polycomb repressive complex PR-DUB. Nature 465:243–247
Schwartz GK, LoRusso PM, Dickson MA, Randolph SS, Shaik MN, Wilner KD, Courtney R, O'Dwyer PJ. Phase I study of PD 0332991, a cyclin-dependent kinase inhibitor, administered in 3-week cycles (Schedule 2/1). Br J Cancer. 2011 Jun 7;104(12):1862–8.
Sebti SM, Hamilton AD (2000) Farnesyltransferase and geranylgeranyltransferase I inhibitors and cancer therapy: lessons from mechanism and bench-to-bedside translational studies. Oncogene 19:6584–6593
Shao Y, Aplin AE (2010) Akt3-mediated resistance to apoptosis in B-RAF-targeted melanoma cells. Cancer Res 70:6670–6681
Shi H, Moriceau G, Kong X, Lee MK, Lee H, Koya RC, Ng C, Chodon T, Scolyer RA, Dahlman KB, Sosman JA, Kefford RF, Long GV, Nelson SF, Ribas A, Lo RS (2012) Melanoma whole-exome sequencing identifies (V600E)B-RAF amplification-mediated acquired B-RAF inhibitor resistance. Nat Commun 3:724

Shi H, Hugo W, Kong X, Hong A, Koya RC, Moriceau G, Chodon T, Guo R, Johnson DB, Dahlman KB, Kelley MC, Kefford RF, Chmielowski B, Glaspy JA, Sosman JA, van Baren N, Long GV, Ribas A, Lo RS (2014) Acquired resistance and clonal evolution in melanoma during BRAF inhibitor therapy. Cancer Discov 4:80–93

Smalley KS, Eisen TG (2003) Farnesyl transferase inhibitor SCH66336 is cytostatic, pro-apoptotic and enhances chemosensitivity to cisplatin in melanoma cells. Int J Cancer 105:165–175

Smalley KS, Lioni M, Dalla Palma M, Xiao M, Desai B, Egyhazi S, Hansson J, Wu H, King AJ, van Belle P, Elder DE, Flaherty KT, Herlyn M, Nathanson KL (2008) Increased cyclin D1 expression can mediate BRAF inhibitor resistance in BRAF V600E-mutated melanomas. Mol Cancer Ther 7:2876–2883

Smyth T, Paraiso KH, Hearn K, Rodriguez-Lopez AM, Munck JM, Haarberg HE, Sondak VK, Thompson NT, Azab M, Lyons JF, Smalley KS, Wallis NG (2014) Inhibition of HSP90 by AT13387 delays the emergence of resistance to BRAF inhibitors and overcomes resistance to dual BRAF and MEK inhibition in melanoma models. Mol Cancer Ther 13:2793–2804

Sosman JA, Kim KB, Schuchter L, Gonzalez R, Pavlick AC, Weber JS, Mcarthur GA, Hutson TE, Moschos SJ, Flaherty KT, Hersey P, Kefford R, Lawrence D, Puzanov I, Lewis KD, Amaravadi RK, Chmielowski B, Lawrence HJ, Shyr Y, Ye F, Li J, Nolop KB, Lee RJ, Joe AK, Ribas A (2012) Survival in BRAF V600-mutant advanced melanoma treated with vemurafenib. N Engl J Med 366:707–714

Stahl JM, Sharma A, Cheung M, Zimmerman M, Cheng JQ, Bosenberg MW, Kester M, Sandirasegarane L, Robertson GP (2004) Deregulated Akt3 activity promotes development of malignant melanoma. Cancer Res 64:7002–7010

Stewart AL, Mhashilkar AM, Yang XH, Ekmekcioglu S, Saito Y, Sieger K, Schrock R, Onishi E, Swanson X, Mumm JB, Zumstein L, Watson GJ, Snary D, Roth JA, Grimm EA, Ramesh R, Chada S (2002) PI3 kinase blockade by Ad-PTEN inhibits invasion and induces apoptosis in RGP and metastatic melanoma cells. Mol Med 8:451–461

Su F, Viros A, Milagre C, Trunzer K, Bollag G, Spleiss O, Reis-Filho JS, Kong X, Koya RC, Flaherty KT, Chapman PB, Kim MJ, Hayward R, Martin M, Yang H, Wang Q, Hilton H, Hang JS, Noe J, Lambros M, Geyer F, Dhomen N, Niculescu-Duvaz I, Zambon A, Niculescu-Duvaz D, Preece N, Robert L, Otte NJ, Mok S, Kee D, Ma Y, Zhang C, Habets G, Burton EA, Wong B, Nguyen H, Kockx M, Andries L, Lestini B, Nolop KB, Lee RJ, Joe AK, Troy JL, Gonzalez R, Hutson TE, Puzanov I, Chmielowski B, Springer CJ, Mcarthur GA, Sosman JA, Lo RS, Ribas A, Marais R (2012) RAS mutations in cutaneous squamous-cell carcinomas in patients treated with BRAF inhibitors. N Engl J Med 366:207–215

Sullivan RJ, Amaria RN, Lawrence DP, Brennan J, Leister C, Singh R, Legos J, Thurm HC, Yan L, Flaherty KT, Davies MA, Sosman J (2015a) Phase 1b dose-escalation study of trametinib (MEKi) plus palbociclib (CDK4/6i) in patients with advanced solid tumors. Molecular targets and cancer therapeutics, Boston

Sullivan RJ, Weber J, Patel SP, Dummer R, Miller WH, Cosgrove D, Carlino MS, Tan D, Lebbe C, Cipani T, Elez E, Maacke H, Nikolopoulos P, Aout M, Moutouh-De Parseval L, Ascierto P (2015b) A Phase 1b/2 Study of BRAF Inhibitor (BRAFi) Encorafenib (ENCO) Plus MEK Inhibitor (MEKi) Binimetinib (BINI) in cutaneous melanoma patients naive to BRAFi treatment. ASCO, Chicago

Trunzer K, Pavlick AC, Schuchter L, Gonzalez R, Mcarthur GA, Hutson TE, Moschos SJ, Flaherty KT, Kim KB, Weber JS, Hersey P, Long GV, Lawrence D, Ott PA, Amaravadi RK, Lewis KD, Puzanov I, Lo RS, Koehler A, Kockx M, Spleiss O, Schell-Steven A, Gilbert HN, Cockey L, Bollag G, Lee RJ, Joe AK, Sosman JA, Ribas A (2013) Pharmacodynamic effects and mechanisms of resistance to vemurafenib in patients with metastatic melanoma. J Clin Oncol 31:1767–1774

Tsao H, Goel V, Wu H, Yang G, Haluska FG (2004) Genetic interaction between NRAS and BRAF mutations and PTEN/MMAC1 inactivation in melanoma. J Invest Dermatol 122:337–341

Tsukamoto H, Irie A, Senju S, Hatzopoulos AK, Wojnowski L, Nishimura Y (2008) B-Raf-mediated signaling pathway regulates T cell development. Eur J Immunol 38:518–527

Ugurel S, Hildenbrand R, Zimpfer A, La Rosee P, Paschka P, Sucker A, Keikavoussi P, Becker JC, Rittgen W, Hochhaus A, Schadendorf D (2005) Lack of clinical efficacy of imatinib in metastatic melanoma. Br J Cancer 92:1398–1405

van Allen EM, Wagle N, Sucker A, Treacy DJ, Johannessen CM, Goetz EM, Place CS, Taylor-Weiner A, Whittaker S, Kryukov GV, Hodis E, Rosenberg M, Mckenna A, Cibulskis K, Farlow D, Zimmer L, Hillen U, Gutzmer R, Goldinger SM, Ugurel S, Gogas HJ, Egberts F, Berking C, Trefzer U, Loquai C, Weide B, Hassel JC, Gabriel SB, Carter SL, Getz G, Garraway LA, Schadendorf D, Dermatologic Cooperative Oncology Group of Germany (DeCOG) (2014) The genetic landscape of clinical resistance to RAF inhibition in metastatic melanoma. Cancer Discov 4:94–109

van Gils W, Lodder EM, Mensink HW, Kilic E, Naus NC, Bruggenwirth HT, van Ijcken W, Paridaens D, Luyten GP, de Klein A (2008) Gene expression profiling in uveal melanoma: two regions on 3p related to prognosis. Invest Ophthalmol Vis Sci 49:4254–4262

van Herpen C, Postow MA, Carlino MS, Kalkavan H, Weise A, Amaria RN, de Vos F, Carvajal RD, Matano A, Bhansali S, Lam L, Yerramilli-Rao P, Sosman JA (2015) A phase 1b/2 study of ribociclib (LEE011; CDK4/6 inhibitor) in combination with binimetinib (MEK162; MEK inhibitor) in patients with NRAS-mutant melanoma. European Cancer Congress, 2015 Vienna

van Raamsdonk CD, Fitch KR, Fuchs H, de Angelis MH, Barsh GS (2004) Effects of G-protein mutations on skin color. Nat Genet 36:961–968

van Raamsdonk CD, Bezrookove V, Green G, Bauer J, Gaugler L, O'brien JM, Simpson EM, Barsh GS, Bastian BC (2009) Frequent somatic mutations of GNAQ in uveal melanoma and blue naevi. Nature 457:599–602

Vanbrocklin MW, Verhaegen M, Soengas MS, Holmen SL (2009) Mitogen-activated protein kinase inhibition induces translocation of Bmf to promote apoptosis in melanoma. Cancer Res 69:1985–1994

Villanueva J, Vultur A, Lee JT, Somasundaram R, Fukunaga-Kalabis M, Cipolla AK, Wubbenhorst B, Xu X, Gimotty PA, Kee D, Santiago-Walker AE, Letrero R, D'andrea K, Pushparajan A, Hayden JE, Brown KD, Laquerre S, Mcarthur GA, Sosman JA, Nathanson KL, Herlyn M (2010) Acquired resistance to BRAF inhibitors mediated by a RAF kinase switch in melanoma can be overcome by cotargeting MEK and IGF-1R/PI3K. Cancer Cell 18:683–695

Wagner SN, Wagner C, Briedigkeit L, Goos M (1998) Homozygous deletion of the p16INK4a and the p15INK4b tumour suppressor genes in a subset of human sporadic cutaneous malignant melanoma. Br J Dermatol 138:13–21

Wellbrock C, Ogilvie L, Hedley D, Karasarides M, Martin J, Niculescu-Duvaz D, Springer CJ, Marais R (2004) V599EB-RAF is an oncogene in melanocytes. Cancer Res 64:2338–2342

Whittaker S, Kirk R, Hayward R, Zambon A, Viros A, Cantarino N, Affolter A, Nourry A, Niculescu-Duvaz D, Springer C, Marais R (2010) Gatekeeper mutations mediate resistance to BRAF-targeted therapies. Sci Transl Med 2:35ra41

Whitwam T, Vanbrocklin MW, Russo ME, Haak PT, Bilgili D, Resau JH, Koo HM, Holmen SL (2007) Differential oncogenic potential of activated RAS isoforms in melanocytes. Oncogene 26:4563–4570

Wilhelm S, Carter C, Lynch M, Lowinger T, Dumas J, Smith RA, Schwartz B, Simantov R, Kelley S (2006) Discovery and development of sorafenib: a multikinase inhibitor for treating cancer. Nat Rev Drug Discov 5:835–844

Wilmott JS, Long GV, Howle JR, Haydu LE, Sharma RN, Thompson JF, Kefford RF, Hersey P, Scolyer RA (2012) Selective BRAF inhibitors induce marked T-cell infiltration into human metastatic melanoma. Clin Cancer Res Off J Am Assoc Cancer Res 18:1386–1394

Wilson TR, Fridlyand J, Yan Y, Penuel E, Burton L, Chan E, Peng J, Lin E, Wang Y, Sosman J, Ribas A, Li J, Moffat J, Sutherlin DP, Koeppen H, Merchant M, Neve R, Settleman J (2012) Widespread potential for growth-factor-driven resistance to anticancer kinase inhibitors. Nature 487:505–509

Wroblewski D, Mijatov B, Mohana-Kumaran N, Lai F, Gallagher SJ, Haass NK, Zhang XD, Hersey P (2013) The BH3-mimetic ABT-737 sensitizes human melanoma cells to apoptosis induced by selective BRAF inhibitors but does not reverse acquired resistance. Carcinogenesis 34:237–247

Wyman K, Atkins MB, Prieto V, Eton O, Mcdermott DF, Hubbard F, Byrnes C, Sanders K, Sosman JA (2006) Multicenter phase II trial of high-dose imatinib mesylate in metastatic melanoma: significant toxicity with no clinical efficacy. Cancer 106:2005–2011

Yap TA, Yan L, Patnaik A, Fearen I, Olmos D, Papadopoulos K, Baird RD, Delgado L, Taylor A, Lupinacci L, Riisnaes R, Pope LL, Heaton SP, Thomas G, Garrett MD, Sullivan DM, de Bono JS, Tolcher AW. First-in-man clinical trial of the oral pan-AKT inhibitor MK-2206 in patients with advanced solid tumors. J Clin Oncol. 2011 Dec 10;29(35):4688–95.

Yokoyama S, Feige E, Poling LL, Levy C, Widlund HR, Khaled M, Kung AL, Fisher DE (2008) Pharmacologic suppression of MITF expression via HDAC inhibitors in the melanocyte lineage. Pigment Cell Melanoma Res 21:457–463

Zhang S, Yu D (2010) PI(3)king apart PTEN's role in cancer. Clin Cancer Res 16:4325–4330

Immune Checkpoint Inhibitors in Melanoma Define a New Era in Immunotherapy Aiming for Cure

17

Alexander M.M. Eggermont, Dirk Schadendorf, and Caroline Robert

17.1 The New Paradigm: Breaking Tolerance Is the Prerequisite

Advances in melanoma therapies are at present mainly in the field of immunotherapy and mutation-driven drug development (Eggermont et al. 2014). Breaking tolerance represents a major paradigm shift and the impact of the first checkpoint inhibitors, i.e. anti-CTLA-4 (cytotoxic T lymphocyte antigen-4) and anti-PD1/anti-PDL1 (programmed death-1 receptor and its ligand PD-L1) is unprecedented (Pardoll 2012). In only 5 years, advanced melanoma has been transformed from an incurable disease into a curable disease (Eggermont et al. 2013; Robert et al. 2013). Breaking tolerance has a transversal impact throughout solid tumor oncology.

17.2 Anti-CTLA4

17.2.1 Ipilimumab in the Therapeutic Setting of Advanced Melanoma

Monoclonal antibody blocking of cytotoxic T lymphocyte antigen 4 (CTLA-4) leads to breaking immune tolerance and can induce tumor regressions. In 2011, the fully humanized monoclonal anti-CTLA4 antibody ipilimumab was approved in the USA in first- and second- line for patients with advanced melanoma and in second

A.M.M. Eggermont, MD, PhD (✉) • C. Robert
Gustave Roussy Cancer Campus Grand Paris and University Paris-Sud, 114 Rue Edouard Vaillant, 94805 Villejuif, France
e-mail: alexander.eggermont@gustaveroussy.fr

D. Schadendorf
University Medical Center Essen, Dermatology Clinic, Essen, Germany

A. Bosserhoff (ed.), *Melanoma Development*,
DOI 10.1007/978-3-319-41319-8_17

line in Europe at a dose of 3 mg/kg. The approval was based on randomized controlled trial (RCT) results that showed that ipilimumab alone or combined with a peptide vaccination provided a significant survival benefit of about 33 % compared to vaccination alone (Hodi et al. 2010). In another RCT, but in first-line, ipilimumab at 10 mg/kg combined with dacarbazine provided only a small, albeit statistically significant, benefit over treatment with dacarbazine alone, but there seems no reason to advocate the use of this combination (Robert et al. 2011). Mature data in thousands of patients indicate that about 20 % of patients treated with ipilimumab have the potential to survive for at least 3 years and up to 10 years from treatment initiation (Schadendorf et al. 2015). Also the efficacy in patients with brain metastases has been established and reported (Margolin et al. 2012). Ipilimumab responses can occur after the initial tumor progression or the appearance of new lesions. For this reason, immune-related response criteria (irRC) have been developed to avoid premature treatment cessation (Wolchok et al. 2009; Hoos et al. 2010).

Adverse events (AE) occur in about 40 % of patients and are mostly immune-related (irAE), such as skin rashes, colitis, hepatitis, and hypophysitis. Grades 3–4 adverse events occur in about 20 % of patients and can, in rare cases, be fatal. Usually, they resolve spontaneously or after steroid therapy. Endocrinopathies behave differently and pituitary–adrenal axis failure usually requires permanent hormonal substitution. High-dose steroids are indicated for severe irAEs, but other immunosuppressive agents, like anti-TNF-alpha antibodies may also be needed, especially in the context of severe colitis (Weber et al. 2012).

Good biomarkers for response to ipilimumab therapy still remain to be established. Immune-related adverse events, an increase in lymphocyte counts, an increase in eosinophil counts, the presence of NY-ESO-1 antigen, and the resistance in vitro to T-regulatory cell functions seem to be associated with higher response rates (Attia et al. 2005; Ku et al. 2010; Delyon et al. 2013; Ménard et al. 2008). Recently, the high levels of soluble CD25 in the serum, especially in combination with high levels of LDH, were demonstrated to be a very strong prognostic factor for poor outcome (Hannani et al. 2015).

Even the optimal dose and schedule for ipilimumab remain to be established. A randomized phase II trial comparing 0.3 mg/kg, 3 mg/kg, and 10 mg/kg suggested 10 mg/kg to be the more effective dose, but associated it with more toxicity (Wolchok et al. 2010). The results of the RCT comparing 3 mg/kg versus 10 mg/kg are not yet mature. The value of four thrice-weekly administrations (induction) compared to induction followed by further administrations (maintenance) has not been established.

17.2.2 Ipilimumab in the Adjuvant Setting of Resected Stage III Melanoma

The results of a double-blind placebo-controlled adjuvant trial EORTC18071 in stage III patients at high risk for relapse were recently published (Eggermont et al. 2015). In 951 patients with high-risk stage III disease (palpable nodal disease or sentinel node positive disease with metastases >1 mm in diameter according to the

Rotterdam Criteria (van Akkooi et al. 2008; van der Ploeg et al. 2011, 2014)), ipilimumab was dosed at 10 mg/kg and administered every 3 weeks over the first 12 weeks (induction) and thereafter every 12 weeks for up to 3 years or relapse. A significant impact on RFS (HR 0.75, $p=0.0013$) for the ITT population was reported. Most patients came off treatment after four to five administrations of ipilimumab. The potential value of maintenance therapy will therefore remain unanswered. irAEs were consistent with what has been observed in advanced melanoma trials, but at a higher frequency, especially regarding endocrinopathies. Post hoc analyses demonstrated a significant impact both in patients with sentinel node-positive disease and palpable node-positive disease. Similar to EORTC adjuvant trials 18952 and 18991 with IFN and pegylated-IFN, patients with sentinel-positive disease derived a greater benefit (Eggermont et al. 2005, 2008, 2012a). Patients with an ulcerated primary derived the greatest benefit like in the meta-analysis of the IFN trials 18952 and 18991, indicating that ulcerated melanoma is a separate biologic entity (Eggermont et al. 2012b, c). In contrast, however, to the experience in the adjuvant IFN trials EORTC 18952 and 18991, patients with non-ulcerated melanomas also derived a benefit in the adjuvant ipilimumab setting (van Akkooi et al. 2008). This is in contrast to the total lack of benefit in IFN trials, which has also recently been confirmed in the individual patient data (IPD) meta-analysis of all adjuvant IFN versus observation trials (Suciu et al. 2014).

17.2.3 Combination Therapies with Ipilimumab

Various combinations of ipilimumab with other immune-modulating, anti-angiogenic or chemotherapeutic, or targeted agents have been reported or are ongoing. Guiding principles for combination treatment designs could be to use drugs that lead to immunogenic cell death (Kroemer et al. 2013; Vacchelli et al. 2014a; Galluzzi et al. 2012; Zitvogel et al. 2013). Since radiotherapy can also induce immunogenic cell death, the reported observation of abscopal antitumor effects after radiotherapy and ipilimumab has led to a number of clinical studies to further investigate this phenomenon (Postow et al. 2012).

17.2.3.1 Chemotherapy

Three studies regarding the combination of chemotherapy with ipilimumab in melanoma patients have been published thus far.

1. *Dacarbazine*: A phase III trial comparing DTIC versus DTIC plus ipilimumab at 10 mg/kg in first-line in patients with advanced melanoma showed a survival benefit for patients treated with the combination (Robert et al. 2011). The median benefit of only 2.1 months was, however, disappointing and the combination is not believed to bring a benefit over ipilimumab alone.
2. *Fotemustine*: In an open-label, single-arm phase II trial, 86 patients with advanced melanoma, 20 of them with asymptomatic brain metastases, received induction treatment of 10 mg/kg intravenous ipilimumab every 3 weeks for a total of four

doses, and 100 mg/m² intravenous fotemustine weekly for 3 weeks and then every 3 weeks from week 9 to week 24 (Di Giacomo et al. 2012). Patients with a confirmed clinical response were eligible for maintenance treatment from week 24, with ipilimumab every 12 weeks and fotemustine every 3 weeks. Forty patients (46.5 %) in the study population achieved disease control, as did 10 patients with brain metastases (50 %). Toxicity was considerable with 47 patients (55 %) having grade 3 or 4 treatment-related adverse events.

3. *Carboplatin/taxol*: Very preliminary results of a randomized phase II trial comparing concurrent carboplatin plus paclitaxel and ipilimumab (four doses at 3 mg/kg) with sequential treatment of these agents were reported recently (Jamal et al. 2014). In 31 patients, response rates (RR) and disease control rates (DCR) for 14 evaluable patients at 24 weeks were 21.4 % and 42.9 % by mWHO, and 35.7 % and 64.3 % by irRC, respectively. Grades 3 to 4 AEs were observed in 63 % of patients.

17.2.3.2 Antiangiogenic Agents

Bevacizumab Four dosing cohorts of ipilimumab (3 or 10 mg/kg) with four doses at 3-week intervals and then every 12 weeks, and bevacizumab (7.5 or 15 mg/kg) every 3 weeks, were studied in 46 patients with metastatic melanoma (Hodi et al. 2014a). There were 8 PRs and 22 SDs, and a disease control rate of 67.4 %. Median survival was 25.1 months. Extensive CD8(+) and macrophage cell infiltration were observed in on-treatment tumor biopsies. From this initial experience, it appears that the combination of bevacizumab and ipilimumab can be safely administered. VEGF-A blockade influences inflammation, lymphocyte trafficking, and immune regulation that should be studied further.

17.2.3.3 Cytokines

1. *Interleukin-2 (IL-2):* The most mature data on the combination of IL-2 and ipilimumab regard 36 patients treated at the NCI Surgery Branch (Prieto et al. 2012). There were six complete responders (17 %), which was higher than the 6 % CR rate in 56 patients treated with ipilimumab alone and the 7 % CR rate among 85 patients who received ipilimumab with gp100 peptide vaccination. All CRs except one were ongoing at 54+ to 99+ months at the time of the report. The combination with IL-2 did not seem to increase toxicity. The combination with IL-2 should be explored further.
2. *Interferon-alpha (IFN):* The first phase II trial report on the combination of IFN was a study with the anti-CTLA4 drug tremelimumab (Tarhini et al. 2012). In this study, 37 stage IV melanoma patients received tremelimumab 15 mg/kg/course (three cycles [one cycle = 4 weeks]) intravenously every 12 weeks. High-dose interferon alfa-2b (HDI) was administered concurrently, at 20 MU/m²/day i.v. for 5 days/week for 4 weeks followed by 10 MU/m²/day s.c. three times a week for 8 weeks per course. In 35 evaluable patients, overall response rate was 24 % (four CRs and five PRs), 38 % SD, with a median progression-free survival of 6.4 months and a median overall survival of 21 months. These results seemed to indicate additive antitumor activity.

3. *Pegylated-IFN*: In 31 patients, ipilimumab (3 mg/kg for four doses) was administered in combination with peg-interferon alfa-2b at 3 mcg/kg weekly for up to 156 weeks (Kudchadkar et al. 2014). Among 26 evaluable patients, there were two CRs, nine PRs, three SDs, and twelve PDs. Peg-interferon alfa-2b added to ipilimumab resulted in a response rate of 42.3 % and was well tolerated except for a high grade 3 rash rate of 20 %. The combination warrants further exploration.
4. *GM-CSF:* In a randomized phase II trial, conducted by ECOG in 245 patients with unresectable stage III/IV melanoma, ipilimumab plus GM-CSF (sargramostim) treatment was compared with ipilimumab alone (Hodi et al. 2014b). Patients received ipilimumab at 10 mg/kg, intravenously on day 1 plus sargramostim, 250 μg subcutaneously, on days 1–14 of a 21-day cycle versus ipilimumab alone. Ipilimumab treatment included induction for four cycles followed by maintenance every fourth cycle. At a rather short median follow-up of 13.3 months, overall survival was superior for the combination treatment (17.5 months versus 12.7 months), the 1-year survival rates were 68.9 % versus 52.9 %. Surprisingly, no differences for PFS were observed (median PFS of 3.1 months for both treatment arms). The combination treatment was associated with less toxicity. Further studies are needed to elucidate these observations, which is true for all combinations with cytokines (Vacchelli et al. 2014b).

17.2.3.4 Vaccines

1. *gp100 vaccines*: Theoretically, a combination of a vaccine with anti-CTLA4 is very attractive. Yet the results from the RCT comparing ipilimumab versus ipilimumab plus gp100 vaccine versus gp100 vaccination alone did not show a benefit for the combination of ipilimumab plus the vaccine compared to ipilimumab alone (Hodi et al. 2010) and similar observations were made with the mature results of the NCI Surgery Branch experience (Prieto et al. 2012).
2. *Laherparepvec (T-VEC):* The first combination study of ipilimumab with the vaccine laherparepvec (T-VEC) was reported at the 2014 ASCO annual meeting (Puzanov et al. 2014a). In 17 patients, the response rate was 41 % (24 % CR, 18 % PR); and 35 % had SD. Median time to response was 2.9 months. No DLTs were reported. Grade 3/4 AEs occurred in 32 %, with only two patients having irAEs at grades 3/4. These very preliminary results seem promising, but more mature data are awaited.

17.2.4 BRAF and MEK Inhibitors

Combinations of BRAF inhibitors and MEK inhibitors with immune checkpoint inhibitors such as anti-CTLA are theoretically attractive, but have, in practice, proven to be not so simple to develop.

1. *Vemurafenib*: A phase I trial combining vemurafenib and ipilimumab was stopped early, after only 11 patients, because of several cases of grades 3–4 hepatitis (Ribas et al. 2013).

2. *Dabrafenib + Trametenib*: A phase I trial with dabrafenib + ipilimumab did not evoke a high rate of hepatitis, and an expansion cohort is ongoing (Puzanov et al. 2014b). However, the combination of dabrafenib + trametenib + ipilimumab phase I study was stopped because of life-threatening colitis in three of the first seven patients (Puzanov et al. 2014b).

17.2.5 Anti-PD1 and Anti-PDL1

PD1 protein is another immune checkpoint expressed in many tumor-infiltrating lymphocytes in response to inflammation. It has two ligands, PD-L1 (B7-H1) and PD-L2 (B7-DC). The engagement of PD1 on the lymphocyte surface by PD-L1 on melanoma cells delivers inhibitory signals down-regulating T-cell function (Topalian et al. 2012a). Remarkable results of phase I trials evaluating two anti-PD1 antibodies (nivolumab and pembrolizumab) reported response rates of 30 % (Topalian et al. 2012b; Robert et al. 2014). Anti-PD-L1 antibody also gave an encouraging long-term response rate of 17.3 % in melanoma patients in a phase I study (Brahmer et al. 2012). Importantly, the safety profile is very favorable compared to ipilimumab, with much lower rates of irAEs, in particular the troublesome colitis and hypophysitis. Both pembrolizumab and nivolumab have been reported to induce response rates around 30 % in advanced melanoma patients, even in patients that previously failed ipilimumab (Hamid et al. 2013; Topalian and Sznol 2014). Responses tend to be very durable, up to 2 years. Moreover, PDL-1 expression in the tumor is a good biomarker for response for monotherapy with either agent. Nivolumab proved to be vastly superior dacarbazine in first-line in a RCT in 418 patients with advanced non-BRAF-mutant melanoma (Robert et al. 2015a). Pembrolizumab proved to be superior to therapy of choice in ipilimumab failures (Ribas et al. 2015). Moreover, in a cohort of 655 patients treated with pemborlizumab it was demonstrated that response rates in BRAF wild-type patients and in BRAF-mutant patients are similar (45 % and 50 %, respectively) (Daud et al. 2015). Moreover, pembrolizumab has been shown to be superior to ipilimumab in a phase III trial (Robert et al. 2015b). Overall, it leads to the conclusion that anti-PD1 can be considered to be proposed to all patients with advanced melanoma in first-line, irrespective of mutational status, perhaps with the only exception of patients with bulky rapidly progressive BRAF-mutant melanoma. However, the incredible impact of anti-PD1 and anti-PDL1 monoclonal antibodies lies in its broad transversal impact in oncology, now with activity demonstrated against a wide panel of neoplasms other than melanoma, including lung cancer, renal cell cancer, bladder cancer, stomach cancer, head and neck cancer, ovarian cancer, and colorectal cancer with microsatellite instability and Hodgkin lymphoma (Lorenzo Galluzzi et al. 2014).

17.2.6 Anti-PD1 Plus Anti-CTLA4

Very impressive data have been reported on the efficacy of the combination of ipilimumab and nivolumab in the last 2 years (Wolchok et al. 2013; Sznol et al. 2014). The rationale to combine these two checkpoint inhibitors is that they have different mechanisms of action, with anti-CTLA4 mainly acting at the central level in the lymph node compartment, perpetuating and/or restoring the induction and proliferation of activated T-cells, and with anti-PD1 mainly acting at the peripheral level at the tumor site, preventing the neutralization of cytotoxic T cells by PDL1 expressing tumor cells and PDL2 expressing plasmoid dendritic cells in the tumor infiltrate. Very deep and long-lasting responses are observed, and in the update on the current experience presented by Sznol et al. at the 2014 ASCO annual meeting, with impressive survival rates of >90 % at 1 year and >80 % at 2 years in advanced melanoma patients (Sznol et al. 2014). In 2015, the RCT comparing nivolumab + ipilimumab versus nivolumab versus ipilimumab in advanced melanoma patients was published and demonstrated that the combination is superior to either monotherapy and that nivolumab alone is superior to ipilimumab regarding PFS (Larkin et al. 2015). The trial is not mature regarding OS data. Importantly, patients with PDL1-positive tumors seemed to benefit equally from nivolimumab monotherapy compared with combination therapy. PDL-1-negative patients had the best results with the combination therapy. It will be very interesting to have the mature results of this trial in 1–1.5 years' time. Clearly, all these results are unprecedented in the melanoma world and demonstrate the power of the current concepts of breaking tolerance.

Immunotherapy combinations in general are expected to be perhaps the most dynamic drug development field for years to come. Once breaking tolerance is achieved, or even further improved with candidate molecules such as anti-LAG3 and others, the door is open to combine with agonists such as OX40, CD137, and others. Deepening breaking tolerance and combining with various agonistic approaches is a complex scenario to work out, but obviously, smart immune combos are the future (Eggermont and Robert 2014).

References

Attia P, Phan GQ, Maker AV et al (2005) Autoimmunity correlates with tumor regression in patients with metastatic melanoma treated with anti-cytotoxic T-lymphocyte antigen-4. J Clin Oncol 23:6043–6053

Brahmer JR, Tykodi SS, Chow LQM et al (2012) Safety and activity of anti-PD-L1 antibody in patients with advanced cancer. N Engl J Med 366:2455–2465

Daud A, Ribas A, Robert C, et al (2015) Long-term efficacy of pembrolizumab (pembro; MK-3475) in a pooled analysis of 655 patients (pts) with advanced melanoma (MEL) enrolled in KEYNOTE-001. J Clin Oncol 33, (suppl; abstr 9005)

Delyon J, Mateus C, Lefevres D et al (2013) Experience in daily practice with ipilimumab for the treatment of patients with metastatic melanoma: an early increase in lymphocytes and eosinophils is associated with improved survival. Ann Oncol 24:1697–1703

Di Giacomo AM, Ascierto PA, Pilla L et al (2012) Ipilimumab and fotemustine in patients with advanced melanoma (NIBIT-M1): an open-label, single-arm phase 2 trial. Lancet Oncol 13(9):879–886

Eggermont AM, Robert C (2014) Melanoma: smart therapeutic strategies in immuno-oncology. Nat Rev Clin Oncol 11:181–182

Eggermont AMM, Suciu S, MacKie R et al (2005) Post-surgery adjuvant therapy with intermediate doses of interferon alfa 2b versus observation in patients with stage IIb/III melanoma (EORTC 18952): randomised controlled trial. Lancet 366:1189–1196

Eggermont AMM, Suciu S, Santinami M et al (2008) Adjuvant therapy with pegylated interferon alfa-2b versus observation alone in resected stage III melanoma: final results of EORTC 18991, a randomised phase III trial. Lancet 372:117–126

Eggermont AM, Suciu S, Testori A et al (2012a) Long term results of the randomized phase III trial EORTC 18991 of adjuvant therapy with pegylated interferon alfa-2b versus observation in resected stage III melanoma. J Clin Oncol 30:3810–3818

Eggermont AMM, Suciu S, Testori A et al (2012b) Ulceration and stage are predictive of interferon efficacy in melanoma: Results of the phase III adjuvant trials EORTC 18952 and EORTC 18991. Eur J Cancer 48:218–225

Eggermont AM, Spatz A, Lazar V, Robert C (2012c) Is ulceration in cutaneous melanoma just a prognostic and predictive factor or is ulcerated melanoma a distinct biologic entity? Curr Opin Oncol 24:137–140

Eggermont AM, Kroemer G, Zitvogel L (2013) Immunotherapy and the concept of a clinical cure. Eur J Cancer 49(14):2965–2967

Eggermont AM, Spatz A, Robert C (2014) Cutaneous melanoma. Lancet 383(9919):816–827. doi:10.1016/S0140-6736(13)60802-8

Eggermont AM, Chiarion-Sileni V, Grob JJ et al (2015) Adjuvant ipilimumab versus placebo after complete resection of high-risk stage III melanoma (EORTC 18071): a randomised, double-blind, phase 3 trial. Lancet Oncol 16(5):522–530

Galluzzi L, Senovilla L, Zitvogel L, Kroemer G (2012) The secret ally: immunostimulation by anticancer drugs. Nat Rev Drug Discov 11:215–233

Hamid O, Robert C, Daud A et al (2013) Safety and tumor responses with lambrolizumab (anti-PD-1) in melanoma. N Engl J Med 369(2):134–144

Hannani D, Vétizou M, Enot D et al (2015) Anticancer immunotherapy by CTLA-4 blockade: obligatory contribution of IL-2 receptors and negative prognostic impact of soluble CD25. Cell Res 25(2):208–224. doi:10.1038/cr.2015.3, Epub 2015 Jan 13. Erratum in: Cell Res. 2015 Mar;25(3):399–400. Zörnig, Inka [added]; Hassel, Jessica [added]

Hodi FS, O'Day SJ, McDermott DF et al (2010) Improved survival with ipilimumab in patients with metastatic melanoma. N Engl J Med 363:711–723

Hodi FS, Lawrence D, Lezcano C et al (2014a) Bevacizumab plus ipilimumab in patients with metastatic melanoma. Cancer Immunol Res 2:632–642

Hodi FS, Lee S, McDermott DF et al (2014b) Ipilimumab plus sargramostim vs ipilimumab alone for treatment of metastatic melanoma: a randomized clinical trial. JAMA 312:1744–1753

Hoos A, Eggermont AMM, Janetzki S et al (2010) Improved endpoints for cancer immunotherapy trials. J Natl Cancer Inst 102:1388–1397

Jamal R, Belanger K, Friedmann JE et al (2014) A randomized phase II study of ipilimumab (IPI) with carboplatin and paclitaxel (CP) in patients with unresectable stage III or IV metastatic melanoma (MM). J Clin Oncol 32(5s): abstract 9066

Kroemer G, Galluzzi L, Kepp O, Zitvogel L (2013) Immunogenic cell death in cancer therapy. Ann Rev Immunol 31:51–72

Ku GY, Yuan J, Page DB et al (2010) Single-institution experience with ipilimumab in advanced melanoma patients in the compassionate use setting: lymphocyte count after 2 doses correlates with survival. Cancer 116:1767–1775

Kudchadkar RR, Gibney GT, Dorman D, et al (2014) A phase IB study of ipilimumab with peginterferon alfa-2b for patients with unresectable stages IIIB/C/IV melanoma. J Clin Oncol 32(5s): abstract 9098

Larkin J, Chiarion-Sileni V, Gonzalez R et al (2015) Combined Nivolumab and Ipilimumab or Monotherapy in Untreated Melanoma. N Engl J Med 373(1):23–34

Lorenzo Galluzzi L, Kroemer G, Eggermont A (2014) Novel immune checkpoint blocker approved for the treatment of advanced melanoma. Oncoimmunology 3:e29030

Margolin K, Ernstoff MS, Hamid O et al (2012) Ipilimumab in patients with melanoma and brain metastases: an open-label, phase 2 trial. Lancet Oncol 13:459–465

Ménard C, Ghiringhelli F, Roux S et al (2008) Ctla-4 blockade confers lymphocyte resistance to regulatory T-cells in advanced melanoma: surrogate marker of efficacy of tremelimumab? Clin Cancer Res 14:5242–5249

Pardoll D (2012) The blockade of immune checkpoints in immunotherapy. Nat Rev Cancer 12(4):252–264

Postow MA, Callahan MK, Barker CA et al (2012) Immunologic correlates of the abscopal effect in a patient with melanoma. N Engl J Med 366:925–931

Prieto PA, Yang JC, Sherry RM et al (2012) CTLA-4 blockade with ipilimumab: long-term follow-up of 177 patients with metastatic melanoma. Clin Cancer Res 18:2039–2047

Puzanov I, Milhem MM, Andtbacka RH, et al (2014) Primary analysis of a phase 1b multicenter trial to evaluate safety and efficacy of talimogene laherparepvec (T-VEC) and ipilimumab (ipi) in previously untreated, unresected stage IIIB-IV melanoma. J Clin Oncol 32 suppl: Abstract 9092

Puzanov I, Callahan ML, Linette GP, et al (2014) Phase 1 study of the BRAF inhibitor dabrafenib (D) with or without the MEK inhibitor trametinib (T) in combination with ipilimumab (Ipi) for V600E/K mutation–positive unresectable or metastatic melanoma (MM). J Clin Oncol;32 suppl: abstract 2511

Ribas A, Hodi FS, Callahan M et al (2013) Hepatotoxicity with combination of vemurafenib and ipilimumab. N Engl J Med 368:1365–1366

Ribas A, Puzanov I, Dummer R et al (2015) Pembrolizumab versus investigator-choice chemotherapy for Ipilimumab-refractory melanoma (KEYNOTE-002): a randomised, controlled, phase 2 trial. Lancet Oncol 16:908–918

Robert C, Thomas L, Bondarenko I et al (2011) Ipilimumab plus dacarbazine for previously untreated metastatic melanoma. N Engl J Med 364:2517–2526

Robert C, Soria JC, Eggermont AM (2013) Drug of the year: programmed death-1 receptor/programmed death-1 ligand-1 receptor monoclonal antibodies. Eur J Cancer 49(14):2968–2971

Robert C, Ribas A, Wolchok JD et al (2014) Anti-programmed-death-receptor-1 treatment with pembrolizumab in ipilimumab-refractory advanced melanoma: a randomised dose-comparison cohort of a phase 1 trial. Lancet 384:1109–1117

Robert C, Long GV, Brady B et al (2015a) Nivolumab in previously untreated melanoma without BRAF mutation. N Engl J Med 372(4):320–330

Robert C, Schachter J, Long GV et al (2015b) KEYNOTE-006 investigators. Pembrolizumab versus Ipilimumab in Advanced Melanoma. N Engl J Med 372(26):2521–2532

Schadendorf D, Hodi FS, Robert C, Weber JS, Margolin K, Hamid O, Patt D, Chen TT, Berman DM, Wolchok JD (2015) Pooled Analysis of Long-Term Survival Data From Phase II and Phase III Trials of ipilimumab in Unresectable or Metastatic Melanoma. J Clin Oncol 33(17): 1889–1894

Suciu S, Ives N, Eggermont AM, et al (2014) Predictive importance of ulceration on the efficacy of adjuvant interferon-a (IFN): An individual patient data (IPD) meta-analysis of 15 randomized trials in more than 7,500 melanoma patients (pts). J Clin Oncol 32(5s): abstract 9067

Sznol M, Kluger HM, Callahan MK et al (2014) Survival, response duration, and activity by BRAF mutation (MT) status of nivolumab (NIVO, anti-PD-1, BMS-936558, ONO-4538) and ipilimumab (IPI) concurrent therapy in advanced melanoma (MEL). J Clin Oncol 32(18_suppl):LAB9003

Tarhini AA, Cherian J, Moschos SJ et al (2012) Safety and efficacy of combination immunotherapy with interferon alfa-2b and tremelimumab in patients with stage IV melanoma. J Clin Oncol 30(3):322–328

Topalian SL, Sznol M (2014) McDermott DF, et al Survival, durable tumor remission, and long-term safety in patients with advanced melanoma receiving nivolumab. J Clin Oncol 32:1020–1030

Topalian SL, Drake CG, Pardoll DM (2012a) Targeting the PD-1/B7-H1(PD-L1) pathway to activate anti-tumor immunity. Curr Opin Immunol 24:207–212

Topalian SL, Hodi FS, Brahmer JR et al (2012b) Safety, activity, and immune correlates of anti-PD-1 antibody in cancer. N Engl J Med 366:2443–2454

Vacchelli E, Aranda F, Eggermont A, Galon J, Sautes-Fridman C, Cremer I et al (2014a) Trial Watch: Chemotherapy with immunogenic cell death inducers. Oncoimmunology 3:e27878

Vacchelli E, Aranda F, Obrist F et al (2014b) Trial watch: Immunostimulatory cytokines in cancer therapy. Oncoimmunology 3:e29030

van Akkooi AC, Nowecki ZI, Voit C et al (2008) Sentinel node tumor burden according to the Rotterdam criteria is the most important prognostic factor for survival in melanoma patients: a multicenter study in 388 patients with positive sentinel nodes. Ann Surg 248(6):949–955

van der Ploeg AP, van Akkooi AC, Rutkowski P et al (2011) Prognosis in patients with sentinel node-positive melanoma is accurately defined by the combined Rotterdam tumor load and Dewar topography criteria. J Clin Oncol 29(16):2206–2214
van der Ploeg AP, van Akkooi AC et al (2014) The prognostic significance of sentinel node tumour burden in melanoma patients: an international, multicenter study of 1539 sentinel node-positive melanoma patients. Eur J Cancer 50(1):111–120
Weber JS, Kaehler KC, Hauschild A (2012) Management of immune-related adverse events and kinetics of response with ipilimumab. J Clin Oncol 30:2691–2697
Wolchok JD, Hoos A, O'Day S et al (2009) Guidelines for the evaluation of immune therapy activity in solid tumors: immune-related response criteria. Clin Cancer Res 15:7412–7420
Wolchok JD, Neyns B, Linette G et al (2010) Ipilimumab monotherapy in patients with pretreated advanced melanoma: a randomised, double-blind, multicentre, phase 2, dose-ranging study. Lancet Oncol 11:155–164
Wolchok JD, Kluger H, Callahan MK et al (2013) Nivolumab plus ipilimumab in advanced melanoma. N Engl J Med 369:122–133
Zitvogel L, Galluzzi L, Smyth MJ, Kroemer G (2013) Mechanism of action of conventional and targeted anticancer therapies: reinstating immunosurveillance. Immunity 39:74–88

Index

A. Bosserhoff (ed.), *Melanoma Development*,
DOI 10.1007/978-3-319-41319-8

MIX
Papier aus verantwortungsvollen Quellen
Paper from responsible sources
FSC® C105338

FSC
www.fsc.org

If you have any concerns about our products,
you can contact us on
ProductSafety@springernature.com

In case Publisher is established outside the EU,
the EU authorized representative is:
Springer Nature Customer Service Center GmbH
Europaplatz 3, 69115 Heidelberg, Germany

Printed by Libri Plureos GmbH
in Hamburg, Germany